S0-BPI-634

Supportive Care in Cancer

BASIC AND CLINICAL ONCOLOGY

Editor

Bruce D. Cheson, M.D.

National Cancer Institute
National Institutes of Health
Bethesda, Maryland

1. Chronic Lymphocytic Leukemia: Scientific Advances and Clinical Developments, *edited by Bruce D. Cheson*
2. Therapeutic Applications of Interleukin-2, *edited by Michael B. Atkins and James W. Mier*
3. Cancer of the Prostate, *edited by Sakti Das and E. David Crawford*
4. Retinoids in Oncology, *edited by Waun Ki Hong and Reuben Lotan*
5. Filgrastim (r-metHuG-CSF) in Clinical Practice, *edited by George Morstyn and T. Michael Dexter*
6. Cancer Prevention and Control, *edited by Peter Greenwald, Barnett S. Kramer, and Douglas L. Weed*
7. Handbook of Supportive Care in Cancer, *edited by Jean Klastersky, Stephen C. Schimpff, and Hans-Jörg Senn*
8. Paclitaxel in Cancer Treatment, *edited by William P. McGuire and Eric K. Rowinsky*
9. Principles of Antineoplastic Drug Development and Pharmacology, *edited by Richard L. Schilsky, Gérard A. Milano, and Mark J. Ratain*
10. Gene Therapy in Cancer, *edited by Malcolm K. Brenner and Robert C. Moen*
11. Expert Consultations in Gynecological Cancers, *edited by Maurie Markman and Jerome L. Belinson*
12. Nucleoside Analogs in Cancer Therapy, *edited by Bruce D. Cheson, Michael J. Keating, and William Plunkett*
13. Drug Resistance in Oncology, *edited by Samuel D. Bernal*
14. Medical Management of Hematological Malignant Diseases, *edited by Emil J Freireich and Hagop M. Kantarjian*
15. Monoclonal Antibody-Based Therapy of Cancer, *edited by Michael L. Grossbard*
16. Medical Management of Chronic Myelogenous Leukemia, *edited by Moshe Talpaz and Hagop M. Kantarjian*
17. Expert Consultations in Breast Cancer: Critical Pathways and Clinical Decision Making, *edited by William N. Hait, David A. August, and Bruce G. Haffty*

18. Cancer Screening: Theory and Practice, *edited by Barnett S. Kramer, John K. Gohagan, and Philip C. Prorok*
19. Supportive Care in Cancer: A Handbook for Oncologists: Second Edition, Revised and Expanded, *edited by Jean Klastersky, Stephen C. Schimpff, and Hans-Jörg Senn*
20. Integrated Cancer Management: Surgery, Medical Oncology, and Radiation Oncology, *edited by Michael H. Torosian*

ADDITIONAL VOLUMES IN PREPARATION

AIDS-Related Cancers and Their Treatment, *edited by Ellen Feigal, Alexandra Levine, and Robert Biggar*

The Graft Versus Leukemia Effect in Allogeneic Stem Cell Transplantation, *edited by John Barrett and Yin-Zheng Jiang*

Cancer in the Elderly, *edited by Carrie P. Hunter, Karen A. Johnson, and Hyman B. Muss*

Supportive Care in Cancer

A Handbook for Oncologists

Second Edition, Revised and Expanded

edited by

Jean Klastersky
Institut Jules Bordet
Université Libre de Bruxelles
Brussels, Belgium

Stephen C. Schimpff
University of Maryland Medical System
and University of Maryland School of Medicine
Baltimore, Maryland

Hans-Jörg Senn
Center for Tumor Detection and Prevention
St. Gallen
and Basel University Medical School
Basel, Switzerland

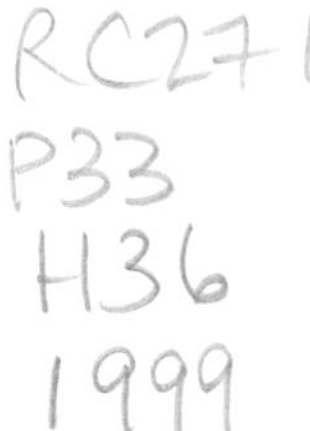

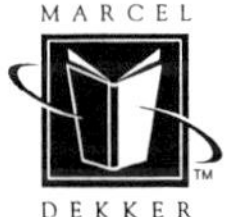

Marcel Dekker, Inc. New York • Basel

ISBN: 0-8247-1998-0

First edition published as *Handbook of Supportive Care in Cancer.*

This book is printed on acid-free paper.

Headquarters
Marcel Dekker, Inc.
270 Madison Avenue, New York, NY 10016
tel: 212-696-9000; fax: 212-685-4540

Eastern Hemisphere Distribution
Marcel Dekker AG
Hutgasse 4, Postfach 812, CH-4001 Basel, Switzerland
tel: 41-61-261-8482; fax: 41-61-261-8896

World Wide Web
http://www.dekker.com

The publisher offers discounts on this book when ordered in bulk quantities. For more information, write to Special Sales/Professional Marketing at the headquarters address above.

Current printing (last digit):
10 9 8 7 6 5 4 3 2 1

PRINTED IN THE UNITED STATES OF AMERICA

Series Introduction

The current volume, *Supportive Care in Cancer: A Handbook for Oncologists, Second Edition, Revised and Expanded,* is Volume 19 in the Basic and Clinical Oncology series. Many of the advances in oncology have resulted from close interaction between the basic scientist and the clinical researcher. The current volume follows, expands on, and illustrates the success of this relationship as demonstrated by new therapies and promising areas for scientific research.

As editor of the series, my goal has been to recruit volume editors who not only have established reputations based on their outstanding contributions to oncology, but also have an appreciation for the dynamic interface between the laboratory and the clinic. To date, the series has consisted of monographs on topics such as chronic lymphocytic leukemia, nucleoside analogs in cancer therapy, therapeutic applications of interleukin-2, retinoids in onclogy, gene therapy of cancer, and principles of antineoplastic drug development and pharmacology. *Supportive Care in Cancer: A Handbook for Oncologists, Second Edition, Revised and Expanded,* is certainly a most important addition to the series.

Volumes in progress include works on AIDS-related malignancies, secondary malignancies, chronic lymphoid leukemias, and controversies in gynecologic oncology. I anticipate that these volumes will provide a valuable contribution to the oncology literature.

Bruce D. Cheson, M.D.

Preface

It is expected that the number of people afflicted with cancer will increase substantially over the next decades. However, it is not expected that significant progress in presently available antineoplastic therapies will take place rapidly enough to substantially alter their prognostic outlook. This is especially true for the vast number of middle-aged and elderly cancer patients with epithelial neoplasias, for whom truly curative therapeutic options are not, and in all likelihood will not be, available during the years to come. Even if the present boom in molecular biology and preclinical gene-therapy projects in the laboratory lends to real progress at the clinical level, it will take many years for significant prognostic gains to ''pay off'' in community oncology practice.

In other words, more patients in the near future will be receiving present-day, mostly intensive antineoplastic therapies from surgeons, radiotherapists, and medical oncologists, and at least half of them will finally die from various life-threatening complications of their ultimately ''incurable'' disease. These patients will often pass through a more or less prolonged phase of chronic cancer characterized not only by the manifestations of the illness itself, but by repeated episodes of side effects from various therapies. The emotional burden of the potentially fatal outcome, preceded by episodes of mostly partial and transient remissions, as well as the progressive deterioration of physical and social capabilities, are additional reasons for concern. This reality, faced by too many of our adult cancer patients, is why we developed this text.

Supportive care is difficult to define. It is the totality of medical, nursing, psychosocial, and rehabilitative support that our patients need from the onset of their disease through various active therapeutic phases for long-term cure—or until death. The scope of supportive care is therefore inevitably very wide and heterogeneous, as it encompasses care of cancer manifestations, prevention and management of therapeutic side effects, and psychological and spiritual support, in the broadest sense.

Supportive care is part of the management of cancer and other presently incurable diseases, such as chronic neurological diseases, AIDS, and so on. One could argue that *basic* supportive care is part of any general practitioner's, and at least practicing oncologist's, medical armamentarium: every internist and medical oncologist treats infections and other complications or manifestations of cancer or its therapies, diagnoses hypercalcemia, and provides pain therapy and some kind of psychosocial assistance.

Given the importance of supportive care (in many instances more than specific antineoplastic therapy itself), extensive clinical research and specialized teaching are necessary for its improvement and success, and require motivated specialists involved in active investigation, professionalization, and teaching of its various areas.

These areas are extremely heterogeneous and, as such, extremely challenging! Supportive care branches out to many subspecialties of the traditional medical and nursing care system and encompasses a broad and highly interesting variety of facets, such as those discussed in this book.

Supportive care differs considerably from palliative care, although these fields may overlap, and semantics may play a role. Palliation of symptoms, by either active prevention or therapeutic intervention, is certainly a main goal of any supportive care strategy. However, the term *palliative care*, as used today by its proponents and in the literature, is normally reserved for the approach to the terminal, and especially dying, patient. Thus, palliative care addresses only the "terminal" aspect (although clearly an important one) of the broad umbrella of supportive care, which is concerned with the optimal well-being of the cancer patient in all stages of this usually long and complicated disease.

Such a definition carries many practical difficulties, as it brings under a "common hat" many different specialties that differ considerably in approach, technique, and health care personnel. The infectious disease specialist might not be interested in pain control, and the nurse providing stomach care might not necessarily be attentive to research on bisphosphonates in patients with osteolytic bone metastases. Nevertheless, all these approaches are applicable to a patient with neoplastic disease, be it limited or extensive, early or late, curable or not! A common—interdisciplinary and multiprofessional—forum is thus necessary to bridge these various aspects, all of which have one common aim: comprehensive supportive care in cancer.

Early attempts to bring together on a multiprofessional level those who are interested in oncological supportive care have been made through various international meetings. These meetings have been attended by hundreds of doctors, oncology nurses, and other health care workers interested in cancer patients' well-being.

Another constructive step was taken in 1991 by creating a new interdisciplinary society, the Multinational Association of Supportive Care in Cancer (MASCC). MASCC aims to provide the common ground on which people with different expertise and interest meet with the basic goal of improving supportive care in cancer through mutual education and common research. MASCC plans to achieve its goals by organizing annual supportive care symposia where specialized and also more general information will be exchanged at an international, multiprofessional level. MASCC has also created its own official journal, *Supportive Care in Cancer,* which is open to important contributions from any field of supportive care in oncology.

Finally, the board of the young and dynamic MASCC society and several additional international experts felt the need to publish an authoritative handbook on supportive care in cancer. This textbook should complete the educational structures already available for scientific and professional interaction and cooperation in this essential field of cancer medicine. The chapters were provided by internationally known experts, who have attempted to cover all relevant aspects of supportive care in cancer, mainly from the viewpoint of medical oncology and oncology nursing.

The second edition is justified not only by the overall excellent performance of the first edition but also by the need for continuously updated information in the broad field of supportive care in oncology. Our concept of supportive care continues to encompass all the aspects that make life more tolerable for the patients who undergo curative or palliative treatment for cancer. Terminal care—too often improperly called palliative care—is a part of supportive care, but the latter goes well beyond it. Following this conception of supportive care, we are dealing with a very broad spectrum and heterogeneous group of activities and individuals, whose interest in the various aspects of supportive care may overlap—although rarely completely. A comprehensive book such as this will be useful to many professionals engaged in the management of cancer patients provided it is didactic and easily accessible.

For the second edition, we have increased the readability by including clear summaries for each chapter and by increasing the number of tables, figures, and algorithms. The content of the handbook has also been changed by the addition of new chapters dealing with fatigue, home care, complementary approaches, hospices, and terminal care.

This second issue of the handbook will be useful for oncologists, general physicians, nurses, psychologists, social workers, pharmacists, and all who provide care to cancer patients because it tries to mirror what supportive care is: a combination of multiple approaches aimed at maintaining an adequate quality of life for the patient suffering from a neoplasia.

It is our hope, and that of all the dedicated contributors to this handbook, that our message cuts across the traditional professional boundaries of specialized care in cancer, in order to truly optimize comprehensive supportive care for all cancer patients.

Jean Klastersky
Stephen C. Schimpff
Hans-Jörg Senn

Contents

Contributors

Ahmad Awada, M.D. Medical Oncology Attending, Department of Internal Medicine, Institut Jules Bordet, Brussels, Belgium

Gerald P. Bodey, M.D., F.A.C.P., F.C.C.P. Emeritus Professor of Medicine, Department of Medical Specialties, The University of Texas M.D. Anderson Cancer Center, Houston, Texas

J. J. Body, M.D., Ph.D. Professor, Department of Medicine, Supportive Care Clinic, Institut Jules Bordet, Université Libre de Bruxelles, Brussels, Belgium

D. Bron, M.D., Ph.D. Professor, Department of Hematology, Institut Jules Bordet, Université Libre de Bruxelles, Brussels, Belgium

Nathalie Cornez, M.D. Attending, Department of Internal Medicine, Institut Jules Bordet, Université Libre de Bruxelles, Brussels, Belgium

Ben E. De Pauw, M.D., Ph.D. Professor, Hematology and Blood Transfusion Service, University Hospital St. Radboud, Nijmegen, The Netherlands

M. Dicato, M.D. Head, Department of Hematology-Oncology, Centre Hospitalier de Luxembourg, Luxembourg

James T. D'Olimpio, M.D. Director, Comprehensive Program in Palliative Medicine and Cancer Pain, Department of Medicine, Don Monti Division of Medical Oncology, North Shore University Hospital, Manhasset, New York

C. Duhem, M.D. Department of Hematology-Oncology, Centre Hospitalier de Luxembourg, Luxembourg

Kenji Eguchi, M.D., Ph.D. Vice-Director, Department of Internal Medicine and Thoracic Oncology, National Shikoku Cancer Center Hospital, Matsuyama, Japan

Michael E. Frederich, M.D. Staff Physician, San Diego Hospice, San Diego, California

Nobukazu Fujimoto, M.D. Clinician Department of Internal Medicine II, Okayama University Medical School, Okayama, Japan

James G. Gallagher, M.D., Ph.D., F.A.C.P. Professor of Clinical Medicine, Cancer Center, Penn State—Geisenger Health System, Danville, Pennsylvania

Patricia A. Ganz, M.D. Professor, UCLA Schools of Medicine and Public Health & Control Research, University of California, Los Angeles, and Associate Director, Jonsson Comprehensive Cancer Center, Los Angeles, California

Agnes Glaus, M.Sc., Ph.D., R.N. Center for Tumor Detection and Prevention, St. Gallen, Switzerland

Gertrude Grahn, Ph.D., R.N.T. Associate Professor, Lund University, Lund, Sweden

Stuart A. Grossman, M.D. Professor of Oncology, Medicine and Neurosurgery, Department of Oncology, The Johns Hopkins Oncology Center, Baltimore, Maryland

Jerzy G. Hildebrand, M.D., Ph.D. Professor and Chair, Department of Neurology, Hôpital Erasme and Universite Libre de Bruxelles, Brussels, Belgium

Debra Broadwell Jackson, Ph.D., R.N. Professor, Office for SACS Accreditation and University Assessment, Clemson University, Clemson, South Carolina

Jean Klastersky, M.D., Ph.D. Chief, Department of Medicine, and Professor of Medicine, Institut Jules Bordet, Université Libre de Bruxelles, Brussels, Belgium

Pavel Klener, M.D., Ph.D., D.Sc. Professor of Medicine and Oncology, 1st Department of Medicine, Charles University Hospital, Prague, Czech Republic

Elizabeth LeTourneau-Lee, B.A., R.N., C.R.N.H. Hospice of the Valley and Associate Professor, GateWay Community College, School of Nursing, Phoenix, Arizona

J. Norelle Lickiss, M.D., F.R.A.C.P., F.R.C.P.E. Professor (Medicine), University of Sydney and Director, Sydney Institute of Palliative Medicine, Central Sydney Area Palliative Care Services, Royal Prince Alfred Hospital, Camperdown, New South Wales, Australia

Charles L. Loprinzi, M.D. Chair, Division of Medical Oncology, Mayo Clinic, Rochester, Minnesota

Beth E. Meyerowitz, Ph.D. Assoicate Professor, Department of Psychology, University of Southern California, Los Angeles, California

Anne O'Donnell, M.B.Ch.B., B.Sc., F.R.A.C.P. Registrar, Department of Medical Oncology, Central Sydney Area Palliative Care Services, Royal Prince Alfred Hospital, Camperdown, New South Wales, Australia

C. Daniel Overholser, D.D.S., M.S.D. Professor and Chair, Department of Oral Medicine and Diagnostic Sciences, University of Maryland, Baltimore, Maryland

Prema P. Peethambaram, M.D., B.S. Senior Associate Consultant, Division of Medical Oncology, Mayo Clinic, Rochester, Minnesota

J. C. Pector, M.D., Ph.D. Department of Surgery, Institut Jules Bordet, Université Libre de Bruxelles, Brussels, Belgium

Martin A. Perez, M.A. Graduate Student, Department of Psychology, University of Southern California, Los Angeles, California

Martine J. Piccart, M.D., Ph.D. Chair of the Chemotherapy Department, Department of Internal Medicine, Institut Jules Bordet, Université Libre de Bruxelles, Brussels, Belgium

Stefan Rauh, M.D. Department of Hematology-Oncology, Centre Hospitalier de Luxembourg, Luxembourg

Darius Razavi, M.D., Ph.D. Professor and Head, Department of Psychiatry, Centre Hospitalier Universitaire Saint-Pierre, Brussels, Belgium

Pierre Reusser, M.D. Assistant Professor Medicine, Department of Medicine, University Hospital, Basel, Switzerland

F. Ries, M.D. Physician, Department of Hematology-Oncology, Centre Hospitalier de Luxembourg, Luxembourg

Fausto Roila, M.D. Vice-Director, Medical Oncology Division, Policlinico Hospital, Perugia, Italy

Edward B. Rubenstein, M.D. Chief, Section of Medical Supportive Care, Department of Anesthesiology and Critical Care, The University of Texas M.D. Anderson Cancer Center, Houston, Texas

Stephen C. Schimpff, M.D. Executive Vice President, University of Maryland Medical System, CEO, University of Maryland Medical Center, and Professor of Medicine and Oncology, University of Maryland School of Medicine, Baltimore, Maryland

Jean-Paul Sculier, M.D., Ph.D. Professor, Department of Medicine, Institut Jules Bordet, Université Libre de Bruxelles, Brussels, Belgium

Friedrich Steifel, M.D. Privat-Docent and Médicin Adjoint, Service de Psychiatrie, de Liason, University Hospital, Lausanne, Switzerland

Charlotte C. Sun, M.P.H. The University of Texas M.D. Anderson Cancer Center, Houston, Texas

Martin H. N. Tattersall, M.D., M.Sc. Professor of Cancer Medicine, University of Sydney, Sydney, New South Wales, Australia

Maurizio Tonato, M.D. Director, Medical Oncology Division, Policlinico Hospital, Perugia, Italy

Vincent Vinciguerra, M.D. Professor and Chief, Don Monti Division of Medical Oncology, North Shore University Hospital, Manhasset, New York

Stephen H. Zinner, M.D. Professor of Medicine and Director, Division Infectious Diseases, Department of Medicine, Brown University, Providence, Rhode Island

Supportive Care in Cancer

1

Therapy of Infections in Cancer Patients

Jean Klastersky
Institut Jules Bordet, Université Libre de Bruxelles, Brussels, Belgium

I. APPROACH TO FEVER IN CANCER PATIENTS

A. Patterns of Fever

Fever has long been associated with malignancy and remains a common problem in cancer patients. With the advent of cytotoxic therapy, fever in the cancer patient has been closely linked with infection, especially when the patient is granulocytopenic. Because fever can be the only sign of infection in neutropenic patients, its appearance necessitates that a series of diagnostic and therapeutic measures be taken empirically (i.e., without the precise knowledge of the nature and cause of the infection). This approach is different from that which is usually recommended for fever in nonneutropenic patients. First, it is important to decide whether fever is caused by infection or another process. Second, the site of the infection and the offending pathogen are sought through a series of microbiological techniques. Third, when a precise clinical and microbiological diagnosis is available, a rational choice of therapy can be made. Depending on the acuteness of the disease, these diagnostic steps can be accelerated and, occasionally, presumptive therapy is prescribed in nonneutropenic patients.

If the diagnostic work-up is negative and fever persists for more than 7 days, it is customary to speak about fever of unknown origin (FUO). A series of specific diagnostic possibilities, as discussed later, is then considered.

The pattern of fever is usually unimportant for making a causal diagnosis

(1). In cancer patients, just as in those without malignancies, fever is usually the consequence of an infection. Fever, however, can be caused by the cancer itself through tumor-related necrosis, hemorrhage, or pyrogens, but this is a less common cause of pyrexia than infection. These pyrexias are often considered as FUOs because the direct causal relationship between the tumor and the fever is not obvious.

Finally, fever in cancer patients can be caused by any disease other than infection or cancer, just as in noncancer patients, and by various medical interventions (Table 1).

B. Fever Caused by Infection

Fevers caused by infection must be distinguished between fever that occurs during neutropenia or in nonneutropenic cancer patients. Acute fever in nonneutropenic cancer patients, if clinical signs suggest infection, should not be managed differently than similar episodes in patients without cancer, with special attention being given to a possible cancer-caused obstruction of natural passages. There are several examples of such infections caused by obstructions, for example, pneumonia in bronchial cancer, pyelitis in bladder or prostatic cancer, and cholangitis in pancreatic carcinoma. Obstruction is also frequently responsible for relapses of infection after successful therapy. Surgery and various less invasive techniques (e.g., laser for ear-nose-throat [ENT] or bronchial tumors; tube or stent for cystic duct or ureter obstructions) can relieve such obstructions.

Obstruction often leads to the development of infection by the local mucosal flora; *Streptococcus pneumoniae* remains a major pathogen in lung cancer pa-

Table 1 Fever in Cancer Patients

Infection
Bacterial
Fungal
Viral
Protozoal
Tumor
Necrosis
Hemorrhage
Pyrogens
Obstruction → infection
Other causes
Unrelated to cancer
Related to the tumor or its therapy

tients and *Escherichia coli* and *Streptococcus faecalis* are often isolated in patients with pancreatic and hepatobiliary tumors. Colon carcinomas are associated with an increased frequency of *Streptococcus bovis* bacteremia and endocarditis. However, the patients can also be heavily colonized by the nosocomial flora, namely by the Enterobacteriaceae from the gastrointestinal tract, which accounts for the frequency of gram-negative bacillary infections in those patients, regardless of the nature of the underlying neoplastic disease.

In neutropenic patients, the pyrexial episode requires prompt intervention, on an empirical basis, as is discussed later. Neutropenia and fever should be clearly defined using criteria such as those used by the Immunocompromised Host Society (2): an oral temperature >38.5°C once or >38°C on two or more occasions during a 12-hour period. The major risk for acute bacterial infections occurs when the polymorphonuclear leukocytes (PMNL) are <500/mm^3. However, patients with >500 but <1000 PMNL/mm^3 and whose counts are anticipated to decrease below 500/mm^{3}within 24 to 48 hours are also at risk. Any analysis should evaluate separately patients with <100 PMNL/mm^3 in whom the risk of frequent and severe infection is maximal.

Neutropenia predisposes the patient to severe and rapidly progressing infection by bacterial and fungal pathogens; it also interferes with the usual clinical manifestations of sepsis. Therefore, empirical therapy has become an accepted practice and has been initially designed to cover the most likely pathogens, namely gram-negative rods, especially *Pseudomonas aeruginosa*. Besides these ''microbiologically defined infections,'' no microbiological or clinical cause for the infection is found in some patients (''unexplained fever'' or FUO); in others, only clinical clues lead to a presumptive diagnosis of infection (''clinically defined infection''). The criteria for these categories have been established and are widely accepted (2). In Table 2, the proportion of microbiologically documented and clinically defined infections and that of unexplained fevers are indicated, as

Table 2 Infection Documentation in IATCG Trials VIII and IX

Microbiologically defined		
Bacteremia	314	(24%)
Bacterial-nonbacteremic	61	(5%)
Viral	12	(1%)
Fungal	23	(2%)
Mixed	8	(0.5%)
Clinically defined	332	(26%)
Unexplained fever	493	(38%)
Fever not related to infection	47	(3.5%)
Total	1290	

observed in recent European Organization for Research on Treatment of Cancer (EORTC) trials. During the past 2 decades, there has been a progressive reduction of gram-negative bacillary infections and a gradual increase of infections caused by gram-positive microorganisms, namely *Staphylococcus epidermidis* and various strains of streptococci (Table 3).

Although gram-negative bacilli represent less than 30% of the pathogens responsible for sepsis in granulocytopenic patients, these infections can be fulminant, especially when *P. aeruginosa* is involved. Empirical therapy of febrile neutropenia thus requires a broad-spectrum coverage that includes gram-negative bacilli. If neutropenia is severe and expected to be prolonged, a combination of a beta-lactam with an aminoglycoside might be superior to single-drug therapy (3). The EORTC group has successfully used ceftazidime with amikacin under these circumstances. Because the aminoglycosides carry a risk of ototoxicity or nephrotoxicity, especially when other toxic agents are used, they should not be continued beyond 48 to 72 hours, unless microbiological data strongly support their use. Moreover, recent studies suggest that single-drug therapy with ceftazidime, cefepime, imipenem, or meropenem might be as effective as combination therapy (4,5).

The question of whether the gram-positive cocci should be covered from the start is unsettled. Most studies used vancomycin or teicoplanin because most strains of *S. epidermidis* are resistant to other drugs. However, infections caused by *S. epidermidis* are often indolent and cause a low mortality rate; thus, they do not require therapy before microbiological documentation. On the other hand, there is a high morbidity and serious mortality rate (±15%) with streptococcal infections, and most authors recommend either prophylaxis or empirical therapy when streptococcal infection is a possibility (6).

Fungal infection can be documented in 5% of the neutropenic patients as the cause of the initial febrile episode; that figure has not changed much for many years. Bacterial and fungal infection can coexist in the neutropenic host and the bacteremia might overshadow the more difficult to document fungal infection. The fungal infection manifests as a persisting or recurring fever after the eradication of bacteremia by empirically prescribed antibiotics. It has become accepted to administer empirically amphotericin B (AmB) to those granulocytopenic patients who remain febrile after a few days of broad-spectrum antimicrobial therapy and in whom no bacteremia can be documented (7). As neutropenia persists, the risk of fungal infection increases; many fevers in patients with prolonged neutropenia are caused by fungal infection.

Viral infection is uncommonly diagnosed in neutropenic patients without concomitant immunosuppression after bone marrow transplantation. Herpes simplex virus (HSV) is an exception because it causes fever early after transplantation, usually during the initial neutropenic episode; therefore, in most centers involved in bone marrow transplantation, prophylactic acyclovir is administered

Table 3 Microbiological Nature of Febrile Neutropenia: Single Organism Bacteremia in EORTC Trials

	I (1973–1978)	III (1980–1983)	V (1986–1988)	XI (1993–1994)
Bacteremias/no febrile episodes	145/453 (32%)	141/582 (24%)	213/749 (28%)	227/958 (23%)
Gram-negative bacteremias	103 (71%)	83 (59%)	78 (37%)	61 (26%)
Gram-positive bacteremias	42 (29%)	58 (41%)	135 (63%)	138 (74%)

early during the course of neutropenia to prevent HSV infection. Acyclovir also protects to a certain degree against cytomegalovirus (CMV) infection, although the most active drug is ganciclovir (8). One hesitates to use it for prophylaxis because it causes neutropenia. Cytomegalovirus causes infection, which, in cancer patients at least, most often manifests as a diffuse interstitial pneumonitis. These infections usually occur when the patient is no longer neutropenic but still severely immunosuppressed. Fever in these patients, especially if associated with pulmonary symptoms, is an indication for bronchoalveolar lavage (BAL) and subsequent therapy based on the findings. In many centers handling bone marrow transplanted patients, it has become customary to perform BAL 30 days after the transplant even in asymptomatic patients. The sensitivity of the detection of CMV infection and *Pneumocystis carinii* pneumonia (PCP) has been improved by the use of polymerase chain reaction (PCR) and search of CMV antigenemia, although BAL examination remains the most sensitive technique (9). If BAL is not available or feasible, CMV and *P. carinii* should both be covered with ganciclovir and cotrimoxazole in immunocompromised cancer patients with diffuse pulmonary involvement.

C. Fever Caused by Cancer

Neoplasms are reported as a frequent cause of fever in most reviews (10); however, the neoplasm itself is not always the source of the fever in that the tumor predisposes the patient to local or systemic infection. As mentioned, obstruction and neutropenia are among the most important cancer-related or treatment-related factors that predispose the patient to infection and are indirectly responsible for cancer-caused fever.

Fever caused directly by the tumor itself was actually rarely found in neutropenic young patients with leukemia or lymphoma. On the other hand, in the same study, the underlying malignancy could be implicated in 25% of fevers in nongranulocytopenic solid tumor patients (11).

Two older studies reported on prolonged FUO in 83 cancer patients, most of whom were not neutropenic. About 50% of the febrile episodes were eventually caused by an infection (12,13). The data are summarized in Table 4. In patients with underlying lymphomas, the tumor was responsible for prolonged fever in 69%, whereas it was the case only for 17% among the leukemic patients, who were usually neutropenic.

A variety of solid tumors were also considered to be responsible for FUO; the numbers in each category are small and no firm conclusions can be made. Nevertheless, fever caused by the tumor was found in 7 of 12 of patients with breast cancer but in only two of nine of those with pulmonary or head and neck tumors. A striking feature of the patients with neoplastic fever in the two series was the extension and the aggressive nature of the underlying neoplasm. All the

Table 4 Noninfectious Febrile Episodes Caused by the Underlying Cancer

Lymphoma	18/26 (69%)	
Hodgkin's disease		12/18
Non-Hodgkin's lymphoma		6/8
Leukemia	5/29 (17%)	
Acute lymphocytic		3/7
Acute granulocytic		2/13
Chronic lymphocytic		0/4
Chronic granulocytic		0/5
Solid tumors	13/28 (46%)	
Breast		7/12 (58%)
Head and neck[a]		2/5
Lung		0/4
Gynecological tract[b]		2/3
Rhabdomyosarcoma		1/1
Melanoma		0/1
Kidney		1/1
Prostate		0/1

[a] Larynx: 3; esophagus: 1; thyroid: 1.
[b] Cervix: 1; vulva: 1; uterus: 1.
Source: Refs. 12 and 13.

lymphomas presented visceral involvement or new nodes; all the cases of leukemia were in relapse; solid tumors were widely metastatic and were often associated with extensive liver involvement. Liver involvement as a cause of neoplastic fever has been reported in the past; however, the mechanisms remain unknown.

Why lymphomas, renal carcinoma, and some other tumors produce fever is unclear. Although it is often stated that inflammation and necrosis of tumors are responsible for the pyrexia in most patients with neoplastic fever, it appears that such an explanation is not valid in many patients. In these cases, fever is probably mediated by the same cytokines as other pyrexias. Endogenous pyrogen (interleukin-1 [IL-1]) production has been suspected in febrile patients with Hodgkin's disease; how and why these substances are produced remain to be answered.

It is difficult to be certain that a fever is due to the neoplasia itself. The diagnosis rests, in most cases, on the absence of demonstration of an infection or other pyrogenic process. Clinical characteristics may be useful to distinguish between infectious and neoplastic fevers; the infected patient is often ill, or even toxic, with chills, tachycardia, and possible hypotension. In the case of fever related to neoplasia, chills and tachycardia are lacking or minimal; the patient may feel well and be unaware of the pyrexia, which is often intermittent. However, these criteria are not sufficient, in most cases, to make a firm diagnosis.

Although the rapidity of microbiological diagnosis of infection is constantly improving, it still may take time, and many febrile patients with cancer, especially if neutropenia is present, receive empirical treatment for a hidden infection while awaiting the microbiological work-up.

Other workers have proposed the use of anti-inflammatory agents to make the differential diagnosis between infectious and neoplastic causes of FUO. Aspirin and acetaminophen have little effect on fever caused by a malignant tumor. On the other hand, it has been reported that indomethacin dramatically and completely eliminates such fevers. Naproxen has been found to be very effective for such purposes; a prompt and complete lysis of fever was obtained in 20 patients within 12 hours and was maintained with adequate doses (14). Based on these observations, the ''naproxen test'' (three doses of 375 mg naproxen at 12-hour intervals) has been proposed for the diagnosis of neoplastic fever; it should result in complete lysis of pyrexia, and the patient should experience sustained normal temperature while receiving naproxen. However, the claim that fevers caused by infections, allergic drug reactions, or collagen diseases do not respond to naproxen is not supported by prospective and comparative studies on adequate numbers of patients. It is clear that naproxen and other similar agents can control fever in patients for which no other cause than the tumor itself can be found. Whether this effect is really specific and, thus, can be used as a diagnostic tool remains to be proven.

D. Noninfectious Nonneoplastic Causes of Fever in Cancer Patients

The spectrum of FUO has not changed significantly over the past 40 years (10). Besides infections and neoplasms, which are the two most common causes of FUO, multisystem diseases (e.g., systemic lupus erythematosus [SLE], Still's disease, temporal arteritis and other vasculitides, granulomatous diseases) accounted for 10% to 20% of the cases in several studies. Drug-related fevers and factitious pyrexias are reported in 1% to 3% and 3% to 5% of cases, respectively. Miscellaneous causes are found in approximately 15% of patients (Table 5).

Fevers of uncertain etiology that persist for prolonged periods of time carry a different type of differential diagnosis (15). An FUO of more than 1 year's duration is rarely caused by infection or lymphoma, but it is associated more often with granulomatous disease such as granulomatous hepatitis, Crohn's disease, or a hidden neoplasm such as colonic carcinoma.

E. Protracted Fevers in Cancer Patients

Persistent FUO after recovery from granulocytopenia in acute leukemia was found in 15% of 168 patients; fungal infections were the most common cause

Table 5 Causes of Fever of Unidentified Origin (%)

	1961 (n = 100)	1973 (n = 80)	1982 (n = 105)	1984 (n = 133)	1992 (n = 100)
Infection	36	34	30	31	23
Neoplasm	20	19	31	18	7
Multisystem disease	17	10	10	14	21
Drug-related	1	1	0	0	3
Factitious	3	3	3	4	3
Miscellaneous[a]	15	9	8	10	17
No diagnosis	9	25	16	22	26

[a] For example, aneurysm, emboli, Crohn's disease, atrial myxoma, Mediterranean fever, thyroiditis, hypersensitivity.
Source: Ref. 10.

(9 of 26 patients) (16). A common late infection during the course of protracted granulocytopenia, as seen in the aggressively treated hematological patients, is hepatosplenic candidiasis. These patients have prolonged fevers not responding to antibiotics; they usually are in the process of recovering from prolonged and severe neutropenia. Characteristic are the multiple hepatic and splenic abscess-like lesions seen on ultrasound or computed tomography (CT) scan, from which the microorganisms are not always cultured.

As discussed, other workers have studied prolonged fevers of uncertain origin in cancer patients (12,13). Findings are summarized in Table 6. Although such a retrospective analysis implies some simplifications, it can be seen that abscesses and pneumonias were the most common clinical presentations. Abscesses were mainly intra-abdominal and associated with cancer, surgery, or disseminated infections. Gram-negative bacilli predominated but cultures often revealed mixed infections with gram-positive pathogens, *Bacteroides* sp., and occasionally HSV.

Of the pneumonia cases, 7 of 17 were due to fungi, one to CMV, and, in the others, the diagnosis was not microbiologically documented. Possibly, some of these pneumonias were not caused by infectious agents or they were due to pathogens that are difficult to isolate such as viruses, fungi, or protozoans.

Some series reviewed were reported before extensive practice of bone marrow transplantation and before the advent of modern diagnostic tools such as CT scan, magnetic resonance imaging (MRI), and various sophisticated microbiological procedures. More recent studies show that protracted fever following resolution of neutropenia is not uncommon and is caused by infection in about 40% of patients. Fungal infections occur frequently after recovery from myelosuppression despite widespread use of prophylactic antifungal therapy (17).

Table 6 Persistent Fever in Cancer Patients

	Bacteria			Fungi			Viruses				
Sites of infection	G+	G−	TB	Candida	Aspergillus	Others	HSV	CMV	Others	Presumed infections	Total
Endocarditis or catheter-related	4										4
Disseminated infection			1	3		3[a]					7
Abscesses	2	12	1[b]	2			1[c]			4	22
Pneumonia				1	5	1		1		9	17
Urinary tract infection		1		1							2
Gastrointestinal infection		1							1[d]	4	6
Meningitis						1[e]					1
Ear-nose-throat infection							1			1	2
Arthritis osteomyelitis		1					1[f]				2
Total	7	15	1	7	5	6	2	1	1	18	63

[a] Histoplasmosis (disseminated).
[b] Tuberculous pericarditis.
[c] Herpetic perirectal cellulitis.
[d] Non-A, non-B hepatitis.
[e] Cryptococcal meningitis.
[f] Sporotrichosis (arthritis).
Source: Adapted from Refs. 12, 13, and 16. *Abbreviations*: HSV, herpes simplex virus; CMV, cytomegalovirus.

The frequency of fungal infection in cancer patients with protracted fever is high enough to recommend the empirical use of antifungal agents when bacterial, viral, or protozoal infections have been reasonably ruled out. This applies mainly to cases without clinical or radiobiological documentation; if a possible focus for infection (abscess, pneumonia) is detected, it should be aggressively approached to seek a specific diagnosis. An overall algorithm for the management of fever in nonneutropenic cancer patients is proposed in Fig. 1.

F. Role of Colony-Stimulating Factors in Cancer Chemotherapy

Granulocyte colony-stimulating factor (G-CSF) and granulocyte-macrophage colony-stimulating factor (GM-CSF) are hemopoietic growth factors available

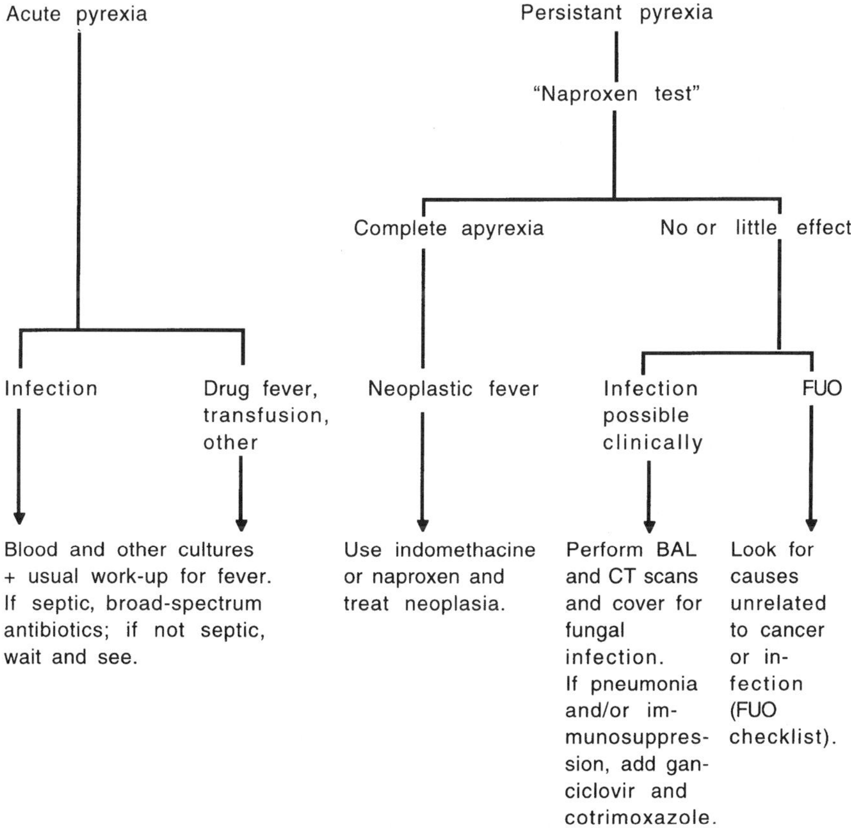

Figure 1 Fever in nonneutropenic cancer patients with no clinical documentation.

commercially for use in patients. The predominant effects of G-CSF are to stimulate the survival, proliferation, differentiation, and function of neutrophil granulocyte precursors or mature cells. A GM-CSF acts not only on cells of the neutrophil lineage but also on cells of the eosinophil and monocyte/macrophage lineages. The distinctive properties of each agent have been recently reviewed (18).

Although these effects on neutrophil levels would be expected to correlate with reduced risk of infection, it was important to demonstrate that these hematological effects of CSFs do indeed translate into clinical benefits. A large number of clinical studies are available and allow the following main recommendations.

First, these agents are probably useful in the setting of autologous bone marrow transplantation for reducing the nadir and the duration of severe granulocytopenia. They might also be appropriate for patients receiving aggressive therapy that would be likely to cause more than a week of significant granulocytopenia ($<$500 granulocytes/mm^3).

Next, these factors might also prevent recurrence of sepsis that occurred during a preceding episode of neutropenia and can allow the administration of chemotherapy at regular doses without delay, which may be caused by excessive or persisting neutropenia. The accepted indications for the use of the colony stimulating agents, as endorsed by the American Society of Clinical Oncology (ASCO), are summarized in Table 7 (19).

The value of GM-CSF or G-CSF commenced at the time of onset of a febrile neutropenic episode along with empirical antibiotics has been studied. As an adjunct therapy for septicemia in children with acute leukemia, G-CSF was not associated with a reduction of the mortality rate (20). In another earlier controlled study in adults with chemotherapy-induced febrile neutropenia, G-CSF used with antibiotics accelerated neutrophil recovery and shortened the duration of neutropenia; infectious morbidity and mortality rates were not affected (21).

Until more data become available, a sensible approach to the question of whether GM-CSF or G-CSF should be added to empirical antibiotics might be to use GM-CSF or G-CSF only in patients expected to have neutrophil levels of 100/mm^3 or less for 1 week. Few patients with febrile neutropenia would thus

Table 7 Indications for Colony-Stimulating Factors

Primary prophylaxis if expected incidence of neutropenic fever $<$40%
Secondary prophylaxis if dose reduction is not considered reasonable
After high-dose chemotherapy with bone marrow or progenitor cell transplantation
Mobilization of progenitor cells into peripheral blood
In addition to empirical antibiotics if there is a high risk of septic complications (?)

receive both empirical therapy with antibiotics and cytokines, but those who do should have the greatest opportunity for benefit (22).

Other possible applications for the control of infection by the granulopoiesis stimulating growth factors might be the use of stimulated donor granulocytes for the diagnosis of infectious sites or therapy for neutropenic sepsis. Both indications need controlled studies before being possibly recommended. Claims that the use of GM-CSF might favorably alter the course of antifungal therapy in neutropenic patients with fungal infections also need to be confirmed in large controlled trials.

G. Ambulatory and Home Care of Febrile Neutropenia

Febrile neutropenic patients have traditionally received hospital-based parenteral antibiotic therapy because of the risk of serious complications and death. Recently, a low-risk population among febrile neutropenic patients has been identified (23), and several alternatives to hospital-based therapy have been evaluated in such patients. These include early discharge to home antibiotic therapy after initial stabilization in the hospital or treatment of the entire febrile episode with intravenous and/or oral antibiotics in an ambulatory setting. A multidisciplinary approach involving the physician and other health care providers, the patients, and their families, ensures the success of this therapeutic modality. Careful patient selection, daily follow-up, close monitoring for the development of complications or adverse reactions, and informed consent, along with detailed instructions to patients, minimize the risk of the development of serious complications. Outpatient antibiotic therapy for febrile episodes in low-risk neutropenic patients should be considered an acceptable alternative to hospital-based therapy (24).

Attempts to shorten the hospital stay have been successfully made by discontinuing intravenous antibiotics in patients with negative blood cultures who remained clinically stable and afebrile for 48 hours and replacing them with orally administered drugs. In other low risk patients, especially in children, early discontinuation of antibiotics or early discharge have been used successfully, under adequate monitoring and follow-up.

The question of optimal duration of therapy of febrile neutropenia is important and includes adequate prediction of the duration of neutropenia. Early circulating mononuclear cells have been found predictive of neutrophil recovery, and other clinically predictive factors can probably be used. The use of the granulocyte-stimulating cytokines may alter the duration of neutropenia and allow a reduction of hospital-based treatment. The type of chemotherapy and early lymphopenia after cytotoxic chemotherapy are definite risk factors for febrile neutropenia (25). All these aspects should be taken into account for deciding how and where therapy of febrile neutropenia is to be conducted.

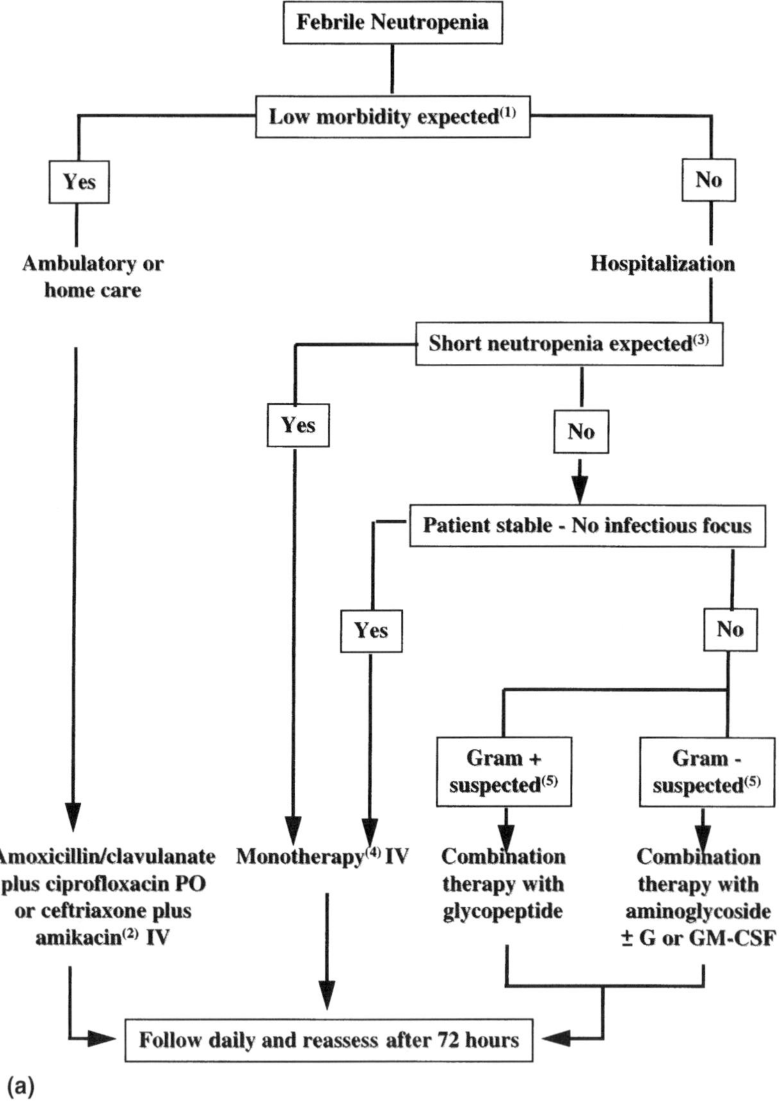

Figure 2 An algorithm for therapy of febrile neutropenia taking into account cost-effectiveness.

Notes: (1) Talcott's group IV

(2) Once daily administration possible

(3) *Source*: Ref. 25

(4) Ceftazidime, cefepime, imipenem, meropenem, piperacillin-tazobactam

(5) *Source*: Ref. 28

(6) Aminoglycoside to be discontinued after 72 hours if no evidence of bacteremia; G- or GM-CSF to be discontinued if neutrophil count $>1000/mm^3$. Glycopeptide for gram-positive bacteremia to be discontinued after 72 hours if no evidence of bacteremia

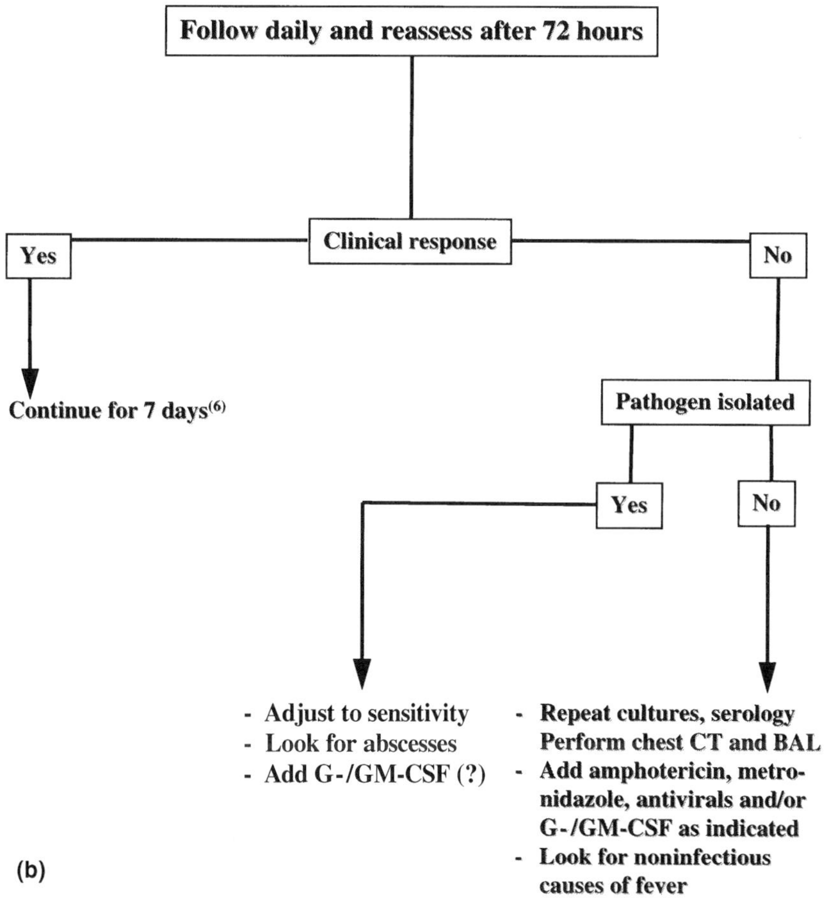

(b)

H. Cost-Effectiveness of the Management of Febrile Neutropenia

Cost-effectiveness has become an important aspect of managed care, and considerations relating to febrile neutropenia have been reviewed recently (Fig. 2). At present, the mortality rate resulting from the infection itself during an episode of febrile neutropenia is approximately 3%; in addition, further infection and progressive cancer account for the overall 10% mortality rate in patients with febrile neutropenia. Most patients, especially if neutropenia is of short duration, have an uneventful course once treated with antibiotics. About 50% become afebrile 3 to 4 days after the onset of therapy; in the others, it is common to have modifications of the initial treatment made at that time, ensuring an eventual favorable outcome. The usual duration of hospitalization is 7 to 8 days and the average cost, under these circumstances, is approximately $4600.

There is a trend toward monotherapy for the treatment of febrile neutropenia; third generation cephalosporins and penems are preferred to the classic combination therapy of beta-lactams and aminoglycosides. However, if one takes into account that combination therapy is associated with a shorter stay of bacteremic patients in the hospital, which reduces the cost and leads to a better response rate in those patients with gram-negative becillary bacteremia and prolonged severe neutropenia, it might be wise to recommend initial combination therapy for febrile episodes in patients whose neutropenia is expected to last for more than 10 days. In these patients, if gram-negative bacillary bacteremia is not documented or if the duration of neutropenia is actually shorter than expected, combination therapy is no longer needed and can be discontinued early, avoiding potential problems associated with prolonged administration of aminoglycosides.

However, gram-negative bacillary sepsis is presently found in only about 5% of the patients with febrile neutropenia. It may be asked whether it is advisable to prescribe aminoglycosides to all patients for the benefit of only few. However, using the Talcott's criteria and predictive rules for prolonged neutropenia, one should be able to limit the prescription of combination therapy to relatively small numbers of patients at high risk. As discussed, aminoglycosides can be safely discontinued after 48 to 78 hours if blood cultures do not confirm the presumptive diagnosis of gram-negative bacillary bacteremia or if granulocytopenia subsides.

Empirical prescription of a glycopeptide is not only useless (provided some coverage of streptococcal infections is given) but also expensive. The addition of a glycopeptide to the initial empirical therapy is effective only when it is dictated by the isolation of a microorganism specifically sensitive to it. The observation that patients with gram-positive bacteremia who receive a glycopeptide from the onset of therapy stay less long in the hospital and thus reduce costs cannot justify the systematic use of glycopeptides for empirical therapy. Gram-positive bacteremia occurs in only 15% of the episodes of febrile neutropenia; moreover, the emergence of vancomycin-resistant enterococci and staphylococci, which has been linked to excess prescription glycopeptides and cephalosporins, represents a major threat.

The demonstration by Talcott et al. (23) that among febrile neutropenic patients a subgroup exists with a better prognosis in terms of mortality opened the way for ambulatory therapy of febrile neutopenia. This group represents about 25% of patients with febrile neutropenia.

Outpatient treatment either in a day care facility ($285 daily) or under close supervision at home ($148) with ceftriaxone/amikacin, an active regimen that can be given once a day, reduces daily cost substantially as compared to the administration of the same regimen within the hospital. Furthermore, in patients who can take oral antibiotics (amoxicillin/clavulanate and ciprofloxacin) the costs can be reduced further to $43 per day, including daily surveillance at home by a physician and a nurse (26).

The use of G-CSF is not cost-effective for the prevention of febrile neutropenia. In a recent meta-analysis by Messori et al. (27), the average cost associated with the prevention of one episode of neutropenic fever was $14,372 using the Italian price of the drug converted to dollars and $41,088 using the U.S. price. It is possible, but not proven, that this therapy might be more cost-effective in patients with prolonged neutropenia. On the other hand, the addition of GM-CSF or G-CSF to antibiotics for the treatment of febrile neutropenia is associated with a significantly more rapid recovery of adequate neutrophil counts and a significantly reduced duration of hospitalization. In two studies (26), there was a substantial reduction of the cost in the patients receiving the CSF compared to a placebo.

Based on the aforementioned considerations, we developed an algorithm (Figs. 2a and b) for the treatment of febrile neutropenia, which takes into account the cost-effectiveness, as well as the possibility to predict the overall prognosis of febrile neutropenia (23), the severity of neutropenia (25) and the likehood of bacteremia (28).

II. BLOOD-BORNE INFECTIONS

A. Bacteremias Caused by Common Pathogens

Bacteremia is still the most common type of infection related to neutropenia in cancer patients; it is usually caused by common bacteria such as the staphylococci, streptococci, gram-negative enteric rods, and *P. aeruginosa*. The clinical signs and symptoms, with the exception of fever, may be inconspicuous and the initial site of infection is often not obvious because the granulocytopenia reduces inflammatory reactions. The usual work-up for blood-borne infections is summarized in Table 8.

The bacteremia can progress rapidly, especially if *P. aeruginosa* is involved, into vasomotor collapse and death; at least 50% of neutropenic patients infected with *P. aeruginosa* die within 48 hours after the first clinical manifestations if no effective therapy is prescribed. Other microorganisms (streptococci, Enterobacteriaceae) can also occasionally cause a rapidly fatal infection in neutropenic patients. These observations make up the rationale for empirical coverage of all these pathogens in febrile neutropenic cancer patients, as mentioned previously.

The drugs and their dosage for febrile neutropenia, as used in the EORTC studies and at the Institut Jules Bordet, are indicated in Table 9 and the costs for these various interventions are summarized in Table 10.

There are limited data on restrictive adjustments of initial therapy, once the offending pathogen is known. Most investigators would agree that, if a patient is on both anti–gram-positive (vancomycin or teicoplanin) and anti–gram-negative

Table 8 Diagnostic Microbiological Work-Up of Bacteremia, Fungemia, and Viremia in Immunocompromised Cancer Patients

Methods of proven efficacy	Remarks
Anaerobic broth blood cultures (2–3 samples at 30-min interval and 5 days of observation)	High volume and resin are better (at higher cost) Longer observation required for rare fastidious bacteria and *Histoplasma caspulatum*
Anaerobic broth blood cultures	Restrict to high-risk patients (gastrointestinal, gynecological, head and neck); aerobic bottle can detect *Bacteroides fragilis* group and clostridia but slower
Lysis-centrifugation blood culture	Best for yeasts and mycobacteria (high cost)
Quantitative blood cultures through central catheter + peripheral vein samples (catheter-related infections)	For coagulase-negative staphylococci only (controversial for other pathogens)
Buffy-coat culture for cytomegalovirus (CMV) (shell-vial), polymerase chain reaction (PCR) and antigenemia on whole blood, and direct immunofluorescence detection of CMV in polymorphonuclear leukocytes	In patients with bone marrow and organ transplantation (heavy workload)
Viral cultures in urine	
Blood culture for *Toxoplasma gondii*	

	Microbiological diagnosis by PCR or antigenemia detection	
PCR	*Chlamydia pneumoniae* (BAL)	
	Culture is possible and fastidious	
	A four-fold increase in antibody titer is diagnostic	
	HSV type 1, 2/6, and 7 (blood, CSF)	
	Culture is easy and rapid	
	Herpes zoster (CSF)	
	Hepatitis C (blood)	
	Parvovirus B19 (blood, CSF)	
	Poliomavirus JC (CSF)	
	Poliomavirus BK (urine)	
	Specificity might be questioned (reactivation)	
	Pneumocystis carinii (BAL)	
	Toxoplasma gondii (CSF)	
Antigen detection		
	Haemophilus Influenzae (CSF)	Cost-effectiveness has been challenged; useful if patient is receiving antibiotics
	Streptococcus pneumoniae (CSF)	
	Neisseria meningitis group A, B and C (CSF)	
	Cryptococcus neoformans (blood, CSF)	
	HBS (blood)	
	RSV (LBA)	
	Specificity and sensitivity still unsatisfactory with enzyme-linked immunosorbent assays	

Abbreviations: BAL, bronchoalveolar lavage; CSF, cerebrospinal fluid.

Table 9 Drugs Used at the Institut Jules Bordet or in the EORTC Protocols for the Empirical Therapy of Infections in Neutropenic Patients

Drug	Dosage
Ceftazidime	2 g IV tid
Cefepime	2 g IV tid
Imipenem	500 mg IV qid (or 12.5 mg/kg IV qid)
Meropenem	1 g IV tid
Amikacin	20 mg/kg IV once daily (maximum 1.5 g/d)
Ceftriaxone	2 g IV once daily
Piperacillin-Tazobactam	4 g IV qid
Vancomycin	1 g IV bid
Teicoplanin	400 mg IV q $8^h \times 3$ doses (loading dose) followed by 400 mg IV once daily
Ciprofloxacin	750 mg PO bid
Amoxicillin clavulanate	625 mg PO tid
Amphotericin B	1.2 mg/kg once daily
Fluconazole	200 to 400 mg IV or PO once daily
Itraconazole	200 mg PO bid
Acyclovir	5 to 10 mg/kg IV tid
Ganciclovir	5 mg/kg IV bid
G-CCF	5 gamma/kg SC once daily

Table 10 Daily Cost of Various Interventions for the Management of Febrile Neutropenia

Intervention/treatment	Cost ($US)
Hospital stay	350
Day care clinic	177
At home nurse's visit	14
At home doctor's visit	16
Ceftazidime (6 g)	101
Meropenem (3 g)	92
Ceftriaxone (4 g)	70
Amikacin (1.5 g)	38
Vancomycin (2 g)	80
Amoxicillin/clavulanate (1875 mg)	7
Ciprofloxacine (1500 mg)	6
Filgrastim (300 μg)	113
Amphotericin B (75 mg)	11

coverage, the former can be discontinued if a gram-negative pathogen is isolated. On the other hand, under the same conditions, if a gram-positive organism is isolated, one would hesitate to discontinue anti–gram-negative coverage. Older studies showed that early discontinuation of such therapy in patients who remain febrile and granulocytopenic can occasionally lead to fulminant gram-negative infection, even if initially obtained blood cultures were negative. Anti–gram-negative therapy can be simplified at that point and, in most cases, a single beta-lactam or penem drug appears sufficient as a companion antibiotic to the anti–gram-positive coverage; the latter has to be adapted to the nature and sensitivity of the isolated microorganism, as previously stated.

The algorithm shown in Fig. 3 is helpful in most cases of documented bacteremias occurring in neutropenic patients. It does not take into account the case of bacteremia caused by unusual microorganisms with unexpected sensitivities; in addition, the physician must be aware of the possible changes in susceptibility of more usual pathogens that often occur as the result of antibiotic pressure.

B. Bacteremias Caused by Opportunistic Pathogens

Isolated humoral-immunity dysfunction has been associated with infections caused by encapsulated bacteria. Patients with multiple myeloma and hypogammaglobulinemia are more vulnerable to *Pneumococcus* and *Haemophilus influenzae* infections. *Salmonella* infections are more severe in patients with impaired cellular immunity. This includes patients at extreme of age, malnutrition, malignancy, and acquired immunodeficiency syndrome (AIDS), and those receiving corticosteroids or other immunosuppressive therapy. Despite in vitro susceptibility, cephalosporins result in a high rate of failure and fluoroquinolones constitute the first choice for salmonellosis.

Corynebacterium jekeium is a lipophylic saprophyte of the skin with a preferential colonization of the rectal, inguinal, and axillary areas. Colonization is associated with underlying malignancy, mainly hematological, long duration of hospitalization, and broad-spectrum antibiotic treatment. Septicemia can also develop in granulocytopenic patients with indwelling catheters. Infected perianal fissure, as well as cellulitis of bone marrow biopsy or insertion of catheter sites, has been reported as primary sources of septicemia. Secondary cutaneous lesions, rashes, necrotic lesions, and abscesses of soft tissue have also been described. *C. jekeium* is characterized by its high degree of resistance to antibiotics such as penicillins and cephalosporins; it is susceptible to glycopeptides. Removal of infected catheter and treatment with vancomycin constitute the optimal management of these infections.

Rothia dentocariosa, Capnocytophaga sp., and *Eikenella corrodens* are part of the mouth flora. Bacteremia in granulocytopenic patients with oral mucositis or ulcerations has been reported with these organisms.

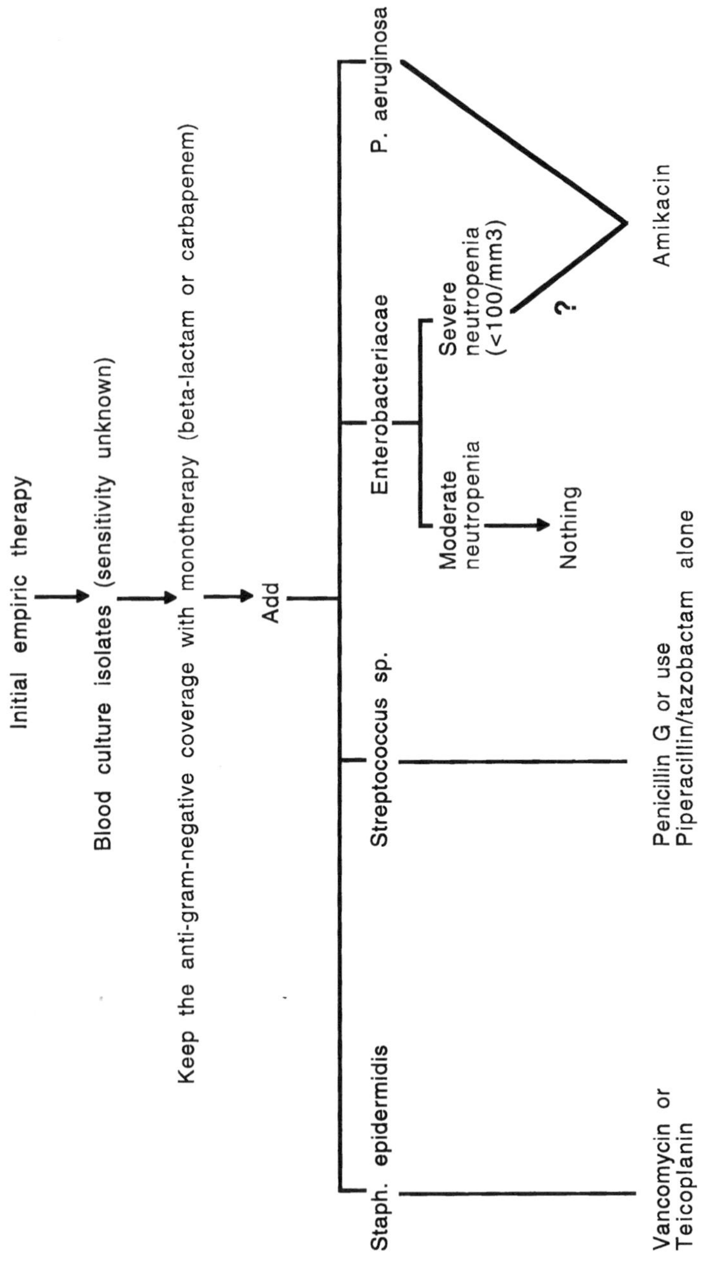

Figure 3 Modification of Empiric therapy according to microbiological results.

Several other bacteria have emerged as new causes of infection in neutropenic and nonneutropenic patients with cancer. *Xanthomonas maltophilia* is increasing as a cause of nosocomial infections in these patients and may be resistant to multiple antibiotics; trimethoprim-sulfamethoxazole and some of the new fluoroquinolones may be effective. *Pseudomonas putrefaciens (Alteromonas putrefaciens)* is a non–glucose-fermenting gram-negative rod that is known to cause otitis media and infect leg ulcers; this organism was recently described as a cause of fulminant sepsis in a neutropenic patient with metastatic carcinoma.

Leuconostoc sp., which are gram-positive cocci with high-level vancomycin resistance, have recently been described as a cause of bacteremia in patients with underlying diseases, including leukemia and human immunodeficiency virus (HIV) infection.

Leptotrichia buccalis, an anaerobic gram-negative rod, has been reported as a cause of bacteremia in patients with advanced malignancies and who have oral mucosal ulceration or inflammation; this organism is usually susceptible to penicillins, cephalosporins, tetracyclines, clindamycin, and metronidazole.

C. Bacteremias Associated with Catheters

Since the 1980s, indwelling intravenous Silastic catheters have become used increasingly in the management of cancer patients. As foreign bodies, however, they are a source of both infectious and noninfectious complications. Although the incidence of catheter-associated infections varies among studies, the risk for development of a bacteremia whenever a patient has a catheter appears to be increased several-fold among both neutropenic and nonneutropenic patients. The coagulase-negative staphylococci are the most common cause of catheter-associated bacteremia, but *S. aureus, Bacillus* sp., corynebacteria, and gram-negative organisms (especially *Acinetobacter* sp. and *Pseudomonas* sp.) can also cause these infections. *Candida* sp. and *Mycobacterium fortuitum* are two additional opportunistic causative agents of catheter-related bacteremia in cancer patients.

For the neutropenic cancer patient with an indwelling catheter in whom bacteremia, develops it is often possible to treat the infection without removing the catheter. This is particularly true when the infection is caused by coagulase-negative staphylococci but even some cases of gram-negative infections can be successfully treated without removing the catheter. The antibiotics should be rotated to include all of the ports and lumens, because the infection can be restricted to only one of these and treatment failure can otherwise occur (29). However, several caveats must be noted. Certain bacterial organisms (e.g., *Bacillus* sp.) may not be eradicated, even when they are sensitive to the antibiotics being delivered, and thus, when isolated, it is generally necessary to remove the device. The presence of candidemia is an indication for catheter removal because failure to do so is associated with a higher incidence of systemic sequelae. Patients with tunnel infections, whether caused by bacteria, mycobacteria, or fungi, virtually always requires the removal of the device and administration of systemic antibiotics to treat the infection.

Clinical studies have suggested that using subcutaneously implanted devices may lower the risk for infection as compared to the externalized (i.e., Hickman-Broviac) type catheters (30).

D. Fungemias and Disseminated Fungal Infection

The incidence of candidiasis is high in cancer patients. Studies from Memorial Sloan-Kettering Cancer Center and MD Anderson reported 12 candidiasis cases per 100 leukemia admissions, and candidemia represented 5% to 7% of all positive blood cultures in several cancer centers. One of the more recent autopsy series reported that 25% of leukemia and bone marrow transplant recipients had fungal infections, 58% being attributed to *Candida* sp.

Acute hematogenous candidiasis is the most common presentation of fungal diseases in neutropenic patients, and most cases are due to *Candida albicans*, although at some institutions it is being supplanted by *Candida tropicalis. C. krusei* has emerged recently, and the role of fluconazole has been suspected in its emergence because *C. krusei* is resistant to it; however, colonization by that species has been reported before the use of fluconazole and *C. krusei* infections can occur in patients who did not receive fluconazole. *Candida parapsilosis* is associated with total parenteral nutrition. *Candida guillermondii, Torulopsis glabrata*, and *Candida lusitaniae* may infrequently cause fungemia; candidal fungemia with multiple organisms is uncommon. Blood cultures are positive in only one third of autopsy-proven candidiasis; therefore, even one single blood positive culture should be taken into consideration in neutropenic patients; indeed, mortality rate is not lower than in patients with three or more positive blood cultures. Serological tests have low sensitivity, although the recent detection of D-arabinitol seems to be promising as demonstrated in an animal model of disseminated candidiasis. Surveillance cultures have a positive predictive value for *C. tropicalis*, but not for other *Candida* species.

For all these reasons, it is important to recognize the clinical manifestations: persistence or relapse of fever despite broad-spectrum antibiotic therapy in neutropenic patients, hypotension, myalgia, and development of small red maculopapular cutaneous lesions are suggestive of acute hematogenous candidiasis. Endophthalmitis causes orbital pain, blurred vision, scotomas, photophobia, and loss of vision. Fundic lesions similar to Roth spots, with extension to the vitreous, are characteristic. Candidal endophthalmitis requires vitrectomy and local instillation of 5 to 10 μg of amphotericin B.

Chronic disseminated candidiasis is another important complication of fungemia, which usually goes undetected until recovery from neutropenia. Early manifestations are relapse of fever and increase of alkaline phosphatase. Hepatic and splenic abscesses and occasionally renal and pulmonary abscesses can be demonstrated by CT scan. Diagnosis is confirmed by histological demonstration of fungi on liver biopsy, but cultures of biopsy tissue often remain negative.

Amphotericin B is the therapy of choice for fungemia caused by *Candida* other than *C. lusitaniae*; the daily dose ranges from 0.5 to 1 mg/kg. Fluconazole, 6 to 12 mg/kg, is indicated for *C. lusitaniae* infections but might probably be used for the infections caused by the other sensitive *Candida* sp. as well.

For chronic disseminated candidiasis, liposomal AmB and fluconazole appear to be better tolerated and less toxic than amphotericin B; therapy needs often to be prolonged for weeks or months (Table 11).

Other fungi than *Candida* sp., namely *Aspergillus* sp. and *Cryptococcus neoformans* may cause disseminated infection and extensive invasion of various tissues and organs in cancer patients; these pathogens are rarely detected in blood cultures.

Aspergillus infection is extremely common in patients with prolonged neutropenia, especially if they are immunosuppressed by corticoids. As is discussed later, it usually starts in the lung or in the sinuses; metastatic extension to the brain is common. So far, microbiological and serological tests have been disappointing and, as is discussed later, a high level of clinical suspicion is needed to allow early diagnosis (31).

C. neoformans is a yeast that causes principally meningitis in severely immunocompromised patients such as those with AIDS or lymphomas. It is extremely rare in neutropenic patients or after allogeneic bone marrow transplantation. A disseminated presentation of cryptococcal infection exists as well. It causes usually disseminated cutaneous nodules; lung and liver involvement has been described as well. The diagnosis of cryptococcosis can be made by the demonstration or culture of the yeast in the spinal fluid or in a biopsy. Serological testing for the cryptococcal antigen in blood or spinal fluid is both sensitive and specific.

Malassezia furfur is a lipophylic cutaneous saprophytic that has caused fungemia in debilitated patients taking total parenteral nutrition. Supplementation of conventional media with olive oil is necessary for growth of this fungus, although blood culture withdrawn through the catheter used for parenteral nutrition contains sufficient fatty acids. Removal of infected catheter, discontinuation of parenteral nutrition, and treatment with amphotericin B are important measures. In neutropenic cancer patients, fatal cases with pulmonary involvement have been reported.

Trichosporonosis, mainly caused by *Trichosporon beigelii*, is very similar to candidiasis. Clinically, undistinguishable cutaneous lesions may occur, but here they evolve into necrotic ulcers. Renal involvement seems to be more frequent, with possible early renal failure. Cryptococcal antigen test is positive in trichosporonosis at a low titer level (<1 in 32) and may be a clue for the diagno-

Table 11 Therapy for Disseminated Fungi that Do Not Usually Present as Pneumonia

	First-choice therapy	Alternative therapy
Candidiasis		
Acute hematogenous	Amphotericin B (0.5–1 mg/kg/d)	Ampholiposomes or fluconazole
Chronic hepatosplenic	Fluconazole (6–12 mg/kg)	Ampholiposomes
Cryptococcosis	Amphotericin B + 5 fluorocytosine (0.5 mg/kg/d + 100 mg/kg/d)	Fluconazole or itraconazole
Mucormycosis	Surgical debridement or excision + Amphotericin B (1 mg/kg/d)	
Trichosporonosis	Fluconazole (400 mg/d)	Ampholiposomes or combination therapy with Amphotericin B + fluconazole
Sporotrichosis	Iodides	Amphotericin B (1 mg/kg/d) or itraconazole (400 mg/d)

sis. Most of the cases reported in neutropenic patients have been fatal because *T. beigelii* is resistant in vitro to amphotericin B. Experience with triazoles alone, or combined with amphotericin B or 5-fluorocytosine, is still limited.

Other unusual opportunistic yeasts responsible for fungemia in neutropenic patients have been reported increasingly during the past decade. These include *Geotrichum, Hansenula*, and *Rhodotorula*. A handful of cases are reported and the epidemiological, clinical, and prognostic factors are not well defined. In most cases, involved catheters were removed and patients received amphotericin B therapy.

Protothecosis, an algal infection, has been reported recently in a child with Hodgkin's disease; *Pr. wickerhamii*, mixed with *T. glabrata*, was isolated in blood obtained through a Hickman catheter.

Amphotericin B deoxycholate has remained the drug of choice for severe invasive fungal infections for nearly 40 years (Table 12). However, its infusion-related side effects, as well as its chronic toxicity, may lead to dose reduction or early discontinuation of the treatment. The introduction of the new triazoles—fluconazole and itraconazole—has improved the therapeutic chances against several fungal infections; however, the need for a broad-spectrum drug for empirical antifungal therapy, the emergence of fluconazole-resistant *Candida* sp., and the limitations of itraconazole in terms of speed of action and erratic oral absorption still make AmB important for broad-spectrum coverage of suspected fungal infection.

Despite the increasing use of fluconazole and itraconazole as therapy for systemic mycoses, direct comparison of the efficacy of these drugs with that of AmB in the treatment of life-threatening infections is still lacking. In recent years, however, AmB and fluconazole have been compared in various large studies for the treatment of candidemia. In a multicenter randomized trial of 206 nonneutropenic patients with various underlying diseases, fluconazole and AmB were not significantly different in their effectiveness in treating candidemia (32). However, an invasive infection was documented in only a minority of cases. Therefore, the question of whether treatment with fluconazole and treatment with AmB in patients with candidemia and deep-seated infection are comparable remains unanswered. Both in a large, multicenter, prospective observational study and in a matched cohort study of cancer patients, fluconazole was shown to be better tolerated than AmB.

Fluconazole is a selective antifungal drug with no activity against molds at the standard dosages. A trial of high dosages (800–2000 mg/d) of fluconazole was conducted in 28 cancer patients with mold infections (33). Fluconazole was well tolerated at total daily doses up to 1600 mg, but its activity seemed to be limited. Itraconazole is active in vitro against *Aspergillus* sp. Its clinical efficacy, which is hampered by the lack of an injectable preparation, seems equivalent to that of AmB, although no large studies are available.

Table 12 Clinical Characteristics and Specific Therapy of Fungal Opportunistic Pneumonia

	Clinical patterns	Recommended therapy
Aspergillus sp.	Acute onset, chest pain, cutaneous ulcerations (rare), CNS abscesses. Nodular X-ray inflitrates unique or multiple, with halo-sign or cavitation.	Amphotericin B: 1 mg/kg/d IV up to 2 g of total dose and/or itraconazole: 400 mg/d PO
Mucorales	Acute onset and fulminant course; palate necrotic ulcer. Ecthyma gangrenosum-like or nodular cutaneous lesions (disseminated). X-ray findings similar to aspergillosis.	Amphotericin B: 1 mg/kg/d IV up to 2 g of total dose
Coccidioides sp.	Travel to endemic area is important. Acute progressive pneumonia and miliary dissemination.	Amphotericin B: 1 mg/kg/d IV up to 2 g of total dose
Histoplasma capsulatum	Hepatospenomegaly, patchy infiltrates or miliary dissemination, chest radiograph may be normal.	Amphotericin B (as for *Coccidioides*), ketoconazole or itraconazole 400 mg 400 mg/d orally, can be given for moderate disease.
Fusarium and *Pseudoallescheria*	Similar to aspergillosis, with more frequent cutaneous ulcerations; both can be isolated from blood.	Both are invariably resistant to amphotericin B. No standard therapy for *Fusarium*.
		Miconazole 60–90 mg/kg/d IV for 6 weeks is the therapy of choice of pseudoallerscheriosis.

The combination of AmB and flucytosine has been used in the treatment of cryptococcal meningitis and has frequently also been extended to other yeast and mold infections. Its efficacy under these circumstances has not been studied in controlled fashion and favorable reports remain anectodal.

Despite some evidence of in vitro antagonism between AmB and azoles in animal models, in a study of murine invasive candidiasis, combination therapy with AmB and fluconazole was superior to therapy with fluconazole alone and at least as efficacious as therapy with AmB alone, thus suggesting the absence of in vitro antagonism (34). The possible role of that combination in the treatment of invasive *Candida* infections in humans should be evaluated.

For the past 10 years, evidence has existed that encapsulating AmB into liposomes or binding AmB to other lipid carriers is associated with a significant reduction of AmB toxicity. Consequently, the new formulation of AmB promises to have a higher therapeutic index than conventional AmB. Three lipid formulations of AmB are under clinical investigation: liposomal AmB, AmB lipid complex (ABLC), and AmB colloidal dispersion (ABCD; Amphocil).

The clinical efficacy of liposomal AmB in the treatment of fungal infections in cancer patients was evaluated in several noncomparative, retrospective studies. In a single-center experience, AmBisome was used for the treatment of 133 suspected or confirmed fungal infections in neutropenic patients (35). The drug was well tolerated, even at the dosage of 5 mg/kg/d, and no significant renal impairment was observed. The fungal infection was resolved with AmBisome treatment in 81 (61%) of the cases. In particular, a complete or excellent partial resolution of the signs of infection was obtained in 32 of 57 (56%) patients with proven or suspected aspergillosis, including 6 of 11 patients who failed to respond to a previous treatment with AmB.

In an open-label trial, 168 patients with invasive mycoses underwent treatment with ABCD at dosages up to 6 mg/kg/d (36). The patients had failed to respond to a previous AmB treatment, had experienced treatment-limiting toxic effects of AmB, or had preexisting renal impairment. Complete clinical response or improvement was observed in 49% of the patients (48 of 97 evaluable cases), and ABCD was associated with little renal toxicity. Clinical efficacy appeared to correlate significantly with the degree and persistence of neutropenia; therefore, it is difficult to assess from this experience the contribution of recovery from neutropenia to the response to ABCD.

Several experiences with the use of AmB plus lipid emulsions (Intralipid) have been reported from both Europe and United States (37). The use of that preparation is criticized by some authors who showed that AmB does not mix well with the fat emulsion Intralipid. The formation of particles in the solution requires filtration to avoid fat embolism; such filtration could also remove AmB bound to these aggregates, thus resulting in the administration of an unpredictably lower dose than intended.

New azoles and new classes of antifungal agents are under investigation in in vitro and in vivo experimental studies, and phase I and II clinical studies are in progress for some of them. The broad spectrum of action, the favorable pharmacokinetics, and the low toxicity are the primary expected characteristics of these drugs. Voriconazole was found to be 10 to 100 times more potent than fluconazole in an in vivo study against *Candida* sp. Because of its favorable pharmacokinetics and its broad spectrum of antifungal activity, including activity against *Candida* sp., *Aspergillus* sp., and *C. neoformans*, voriconazole seems to be a promising antifungal drug, particularly in the setting of infections resulting from resistant fungal species (38).

Profound, persistent neutropenia is a major risk factor for invasive fungal infections, and recovery of neutropenia is a determinant in the prognosis. As discussed in a recent review, in experimental animal models, and in a preliminary study, the administration of colony-stimulating factors combined with antifungal drugs might possibly improve the treatment of invasive fungal infections in neutropenic cancer patients (39,40).

G-CSF and GM-CSF have been successfully used as adjuvant therapy in some cases of invasive zygomycosis or fusariosis, which are opportunistic fungal infections associated with a particularly high mortality rate in patients with persistent neutropenia. The improvement of clinical manifestations was closely related to neutrophil recovery, probably favored by G-CSF administration.

These factors have also been administered to donors to markedly increase the leukocyte yields. Some patients with fungal infections that do not respond to adequate antifungal therapy, do respond after being transfused with polymorphonuclear neutrophil concentrates collected from G-CSF–primed donors. However, it was difficult to prove that the clinical response was directly due to G-CSF–stimulated white blood cell transfusion.

Although encouraging, the published experiences on the use of growth factors as adjuvant therapy of invasive mycoses are only anecdotal reports. Randomized clinical trials are needed to clarify the role of these expensive drugs in the strategies of antifungal therapy.

III. OPPORTUNISTIC PNEUMONIAS

A. Bacterial Pneumonias

Pulmonary infections are frequent among immunocompromised patients. Granulocytopenic patients may lack symptoms of infection, such as cough and sputum production, and more than one third do not have rales or consolidation signs. About 50% of the neutropenic patients with bacterial pneumonia have a bacteremia; this is the most reliable way to establish the microbiological diagnosis and to orient therapy. The combination of gram-negative bacteremia and pneumonia makes the prognosis worse as compared to having bacteremia alone. Recently, bronchoalveolar lavage (BAL) has been shown to be a reliable tool for the diagnosis of opportunistic pneumonias in cancer patients (Table 13) (41).

Most patients with bacterial pneumonia complicating severe neutropenia require empirical therapy similar to that described for blood-borne infections because bacterial pneumonia in neutropenic patients is caused by the same spectrum of pathogens that is involved in bacteremias except *S. epidermidis*. The symptoms and signs of systemic sepsis often overshadow the specific pulmonary manifestations. Therapy should be instituted empirically, as in the case of suspected bacteremia, taking into account that bacterial pneumonia during severe neutropenia carries a poor prognosis.

The incidence of tuberculosis has increased during the past decade in relation with the AIDS epidemic. Because the diagnosis is often delayed, transmission of the disease to the immunocompromised patient is possible, although, in cancer patients, reactivation of a long-dormant disease is more frequent. Patients with Hodgkin's disease, lung cancer, leukemia, head and neck cancer, and stomach cancer appear to have an increased risk of tuberculosis. Most of the cases are suspected on routine chest radiograph with apical pulmonary infiltrates and cavitation. Rarely, tuberculosis may present with disseminated granulomas and be confused with metastasis. Miliary tuberculosis is rare and tends to occur among leukemic patients.

A 6-month course of double-drug (isoniazid and rifampicin) therapy is probably adequate in immunocompromised patients, with pyrazinamide also being given in the first 2 months of therapy. Pulmonary infection caused by mycobact-

Table 13 Etiology of Pulmonary Infiltrates as Demonstrated by Bronchoalveolar Lavage in Patients with Leukemia

	%
Gram-positive and/or gram-negative bacteria	61
Fungi[a]	32
Mycobacteria (*Mycobacterium tuberculosis*)	3
Legionella pneumophila	1
Viruses[b]	8
Pneumocystis carinii	19

[a] 24 patients: *Candida albicans*, 11; *Rhizopus* sp., 1; *Aspergillus fumigatus*, 1; *Cephalosporium* sp., 1; *Candida pseudotropicalis*, 1; *Candida krusei*, 1.

[b] 6 patients: herpes simplex, 3; cytomegalovirus, 3.

Source: Adapted from Ref. 41.

eria other than tuberculosis or by resistant strains is rare and occurs in association with chronic pulmonary disease and lung cancer.

Nocardiosis, mainly caused by *Nocardia asteroides*, is an uncommon pulmonary infection in cancer patients. Traditionally, it has been associated with lymphoma and leukemia, but it has also been reported in patients with solid tumors. The radiographic appearance of pulmonary nocardiosis is variable and includes solitary or multiple cavitary lesions, diffuse bronchopneumonia, reticulonodular infiltrates, and empyema. Upper lobes are commonly involved. Nodular subcutaneous lesions and cerebral abscesses may be associated with nocardial pneumonia and should alert the clinician to the possibility of the diagnosis. Sulfonamides at a dosage of 6 to 8 g/d intravenously (IV) or trimethoprim-sulfamethoxazole (TMP-SMX) at a dosage of 480 mg (TMP) and 2,400 mg (SMX) daily, either IV or orally, is the therapy of choice. Diagnosed early and treated adequately, nocardiosis usually has a favorable outcome.

Legionellosis accounts for about 6% of nosocomial pneumonias and 3% of community-acquired pneumonias. A frequency of 13% was reported among bone marrow transplant recipients, and, overall, a greater frequency of legionellosis has been documented in immunocompromised patients. In some institutions, it has been associated with contaminated cooling-tower reservoirs and hospital potable water. High fever with relative bradycardia and extrapulmonary manifestations, such as nausea, diarrhea, headache, and changes in mental status, constitute the principal characteristics of the disease. Radiological findings are variable and include unilobar or multilobar consolidation, lung abscess, and empyema. Laboratory studies may reveal hyponatremia, hypophosphatemia, abnormal liver tests, proteinuria, and microscopic hematuria. Legionella is diagnosed by culture of sputum or BAL on semiselective charcoal-yeast medium or by direct fluorescent antibody test and by serum antibody and urinary antigen detection. If legionellosis is untreated, mortality rate is high in immunosuppressed patients. Erythromycin combined with rifampicin or fluoroquinolones combined with rifampicin constitute the therapy of choice.

B. Fungal Pneumonias

Invasive aspergillosis, mainly caused by *Aspergillus fumigatus* and *Aspergillus flavus*, is one of the most common fatal infections in neutropenic cancer patients. The risk of infection increases proportionally to the duration of neutropenia. The two major sites of infection are the lungs and the paranasal sinuses. The clinical manifestations include persistent or recurrent fever, despite broad-spectrum antibiotics therapy, pleuritic chest pain, and dry cough. Dyspnea and hypoxemia appear late and are indicative of extensive invasion and poor prognosis. Nasal discharge, epistaxis, facial swelling, and tenderness indicate sinus involvement. Chest CT scans are superior to standard radiographs and should be performed early. Radiological patterns include solitary nodular lesion, multiple nodular lesions, triangular peripheral infiltrates with tendency to cavitation, and diffuse pulmonary infiltrates. Dissemination to the major organs has been reported, the most common and often fatal being to the central nervous system, which occurs in 10% to 15% of cases. Many epidemics of invasive aspergillosis have been described in relation with building construction around hospitals (42). Prevention of aspergillosis consists of isolation of the patient in a protected environment. The value of aerosolized AmB is disputed. The diagnosis of pulmonary aspergillosis and other similar fungal infections is very difficult; one should have a high degree of diagnostic suspicion in patients who are predisposed to these complications. High-resolution chest computed tomographic scanning combined with microbiological examination of the product of BAL probably represents the best chance for precise diagnosis (30). AmB at 1 mg/kg/d IV, for a total dose of 2 g, is the therapy of choice. Mortality rate is highest among bone marrow recipients: more than 80%.

Mucormycosis produces similar clinical manifestations to aspergillosis but often produces pansinusitis. It is less frequent, with a more fulminant course, and survival rate is very rare, despite AmB therapy. Coccidioidomycosis, histoplasmosis, and blastomycosis are restricted to geographically well-defined areas in northwest America and in Africa. A history of travel or stay in these endemic areas is important because long-dormant infection of the lungs can be reactivated during immunosuppression. For immunocompromised patients with severe disease, AmB remains the therapy of choice (see Table 12).

Fusariosis and pseudoallescheriosis can present as opportunistic pneumonias, very similar to aspergillosis and mucormycosis but cutaneous maculopapular lesions are more frequent and may produce necrotic ulcers. *Fusarium* and *Pseudoallescheria boydii* can be isolated from blood; both organisms are resistant to AmB. Fluconazole has been proposed for *Fusarium* infections.

C. Pneumonia Caused by Protozoans

P. carinii pneumonia (PCP) is an opportunistic infection in cancer patients with impaired cellular immunity, namely those with lymphoma, chronic leukemia, immunosuppressive therapy, and bone marrow transplantation. Presenting symptoms include dyspnea, fever, and dry cough; blood gases reveal hypoxemia. Chest radiograph classically shows diffuse interstitial pulmonary infiltrates, and pneumatoceles have been reported. Pneumothorax has been described increasingly in relation with pentamidine inhalation. Bronchoalveolar lavage is a safe and sensitive procedure for establishing the diagnosis (43). Overall, BAL represents a valuable approach to the diagnosis of pulmonary infiltration in neutropenic patients as shown in Table 13. *P. carinii* pneumonia in cancer patients is best treated with TMP-SMX at a daily dose of 20 mg/kg of TMP and 100 mg/kg of SMX in four divided doses, for a total duration of 14 days. Pentamidine at 4 mg/kg/d, diluted in 250 mL of 5% dextrose and infused over 60 minutes, constitutes an effective alternative to TMP-SMX, although the side effects are more severe and include arrythmia, hypotension, hypoglycemia, hypocalcemia, and azotemia. Aerosolized pentamidine has no systemic toxicity, but its use is decreasing because of a high rate of early relapse and a high frequency of extrapulmonary pneumocystosis. For mild and moderate PCP, oral administration of TMP-dapsone seems to be safe and effective. Relapse after a first episode of PCP is not uncommon in cancer patients and secondary prophylaxis may be indicated for patients who are supposed to remain severely immunosuppressed; this is the case after allogeneic bone marrow transplantation.

Rhodococcus equi is a pathogen of farm animals, causing suppurative pulmonary lesions in horses, pyometra in cattle, and suppurative adenitis in swine. Patients with severe deficiency in cellular immunity (e.g., those with lymphomas, transplant recipients, those with AIDS, or those receiving immunosuppressive therapy) and who are in contact with farm animals, are at risk of pneumonia with *R. equi*, which mimics mycobacterial infections with cavitary lesions in the upper lobes. The overall mortality rate is 20%. The organism is an intracellular parasite and should be treated with an antibiotic that can penetrate into cells. A combination of erythromycin and rifampicin seems to be the therapy of choice and long duration is recommended.

D. Viral Pneumonias

Cytomegalovirus pneumonia occurs in about 15% of bone marrow transplant recipients (44). The risk persists until day 120 after transplantation and is maximal around day 60. Seronegative recipients receiving bone marrow from seropositive donors are at high risk of CMV pneumonia. Cough, fever, and diffuse pulmonary infiltrates are the common presenting manifestations. Cytomegalovirus interstitial pneumonia may be part of a clinical syndrome, including pancytopenia, hepatitis, and gastrointestinal ulcerations. The mortality rate from established CMV pneumonia has decreased from 90% before the advent of ganciclovir to about 25%. The presence of CMV in a BAL specimen or a CMV-positive buffy coat obtained on day 35 after transplantation were significant factors associated with CMV pneumonia. These investigations are currently performed routinely on day 30 to 35 after bone marrow transplantation in most units, and recent studies suggest that ganciclovir should be given as soon as CMV is detected. Newer methods such as antigen detection and PCR have shortened significantly the delay of diagnosis in BAL; the testing of blood by these techniques is very specific but less sensitive than testing in BAL (45).

Ganciclovir is given at the dose of 5 mg/kg thrice daily IV for 2 weeks, followed by maintenance therapy with 5 mg/kg once daily, 5 days weekly until day 120. The CMV immunoglobulin continues to be used, although its efficacy for prophylaxis and treatment is controversial.

Adenovirus pneumonia was reported in 5% of bone marrow transplant recipients; usually, it is bilateral and interstitial, and pleural effusion has been described in 20% of cases. Disseminated adenovirus infections, with fatal hepatic necrois, has been described in cancer patients. Conjunctivitis may be a clue for the diagnosis. Adenovirus has also been associated with hematuria in bone marrow transplant recipients.

The HSV and herpes zoster-varicella (HZV) pneumonias have become rare in immunocompromised patients since the introduction of acyclovir. These pneumonias were mainly reported in allogeneic bone marrow transplant recipients; mucocutaneous lesions preceded the onset of pneumonia in more than 90% of cases. Focal or multifocal pneumonia can occur secondarily to contiguous spread of infection in patients with endotracheal intubation, and diffuse interstitial pneumonia was described. In one recent series that evaluated 73 immunocompromised patients with disseminated HZV infection in a comparative trial of acyclovir and vidarabine, pneumonia occurred only in one patient.

In immunocompromised patients, severe or fatal pneumonia can develop as a result of the respiratory syncytial virus (RSV), and mortality rate as high as 66% has been reported among bone marrow transplant recipients. Ribavirin seems to have a beneficial effect in the management of these patients if started before the onset of hypoxia. Ribavirin can also decrease the morbidity and mortality associated with influenza and parainfluenza infections.

IV. INFECTIONS OF THE DIGESTIVE TRACT

A. Infectious Diarrheas

The digestive tract, with its rapidly proliferating mucosa and its load of bacteria, is often the source of bacteremia in neutropenic patients. In addition, it is the natural site of a series of specific gastrointestinal infections, some of which are more common in cancer patients because of neutropenia, immunodepression, or both.

E. coli and *Salmonella* sp. are common causes of infectious diarrhea; the spectrum of clinical disease includes fever, nausea, vomiting, and abdominal cramps. Severe infection and death can occur in immunocompromised patients. Bacteremia has been reported in 30% of cancer patients with *Salmonella* infection, but in less than 5% of others with this infection. *Salmonella typhimurium* is an especially common cause of serious infection in cancer patients.

Aeromonas hydrophila has been described as a gastrointestinal pathogen in immunosuppressed patients with hematological malignancies or hepatic disease, especially in those who were neutropenic. Although *Aeromonas* enteritis is usually mild and self-limited, it can cause fulminant bloody diarrhea in immunocompromised patients.

Cancer patients are also at increased risk of *Clostridium difficile* colitis because antibiotic administration is common and because the higher rate of colonization in oncology units. *C. difficile* infection in cancer patients usually presents as a typical pseudomembranous colitis with severe diarrhea, abdominal pain, and fever. It usually responds promptly to vancomycin or metronidazole but can be fatal if untreated. *C. difficile* colitis has been described in cancer patients following chemotherapy without exposure to antibiotics.

Other bacteria are rarely reported as a cause of infectious diarrhea in cancer patients. Namely, *Mycobacterium tuberculosis* and *Mycobacterium avium-intracellulare*, which cause febrile hepatosplenomegaly, adenopathy, and abdominal pain in AIDS patients, are rarely seen in cancer patients.

Although the lower digestive tract is often involved in neutropenic patients in whom disseminated candidiasis develops symptoms suggestive of enteritis do not develop in most of these patients. Colonization of the digestive tract by *Candida* sp. most likely serves as the primary site for disseminated candidiasis; oral fungal prophylaxis reduces the frequency of *Candida* infections in neutropenic patients. Other fungi are only anecdotially reported in association with enteritis in cancer patients.

Cytomegalovirus is commonly associated with enteritis or ulceration of the digestive tract in immunosuppressed patients with AIDS; it is a rare cause of digestive tract disease in cancer patients but has been reported as a cause of gastroenteritis in bone marrow transplant recipients.

Similarly, parasitic infections such as giardiasis, cryptosporidiasis, isosporidiasis, strongyloidosis, or amebiasis, which are commonly seen in AIDS patients, have been rarely reported in cancer patients.

B. Infectious Mucositis

Thrush is a common complication in all kinds of debilitated patients, including those with cancer whether they are neutropenic or immunodepressed. It causes dysphagia or odynophagia. The infection may extend from the oral mucosa into the esophagus or upper respiratory tract, and often results in anorexia and weight loss from decreased food intake. Esophageal infection can be demonstrated by a radiograph of the esophagus and is confirmed by endoscopy and biopsy. The combination of oral candidiasis and esophageal symptoms is highly specific and sensitive for candidal esophagitis. Under these circumstances, an empirical trial of systemic therapy with ketoconazole or fluconazole may obviate the need for endoscopy in many patients. Esophagitis may be present without thrush and must be differentiated from lesions caused by HSV or CMV and reflux esophagitis; in these cases, endoscopic evaluation with biopsy is the definitive diagnostic procedure.

Some patients with candidal mucositis respond to topical antifungal therapy with nystatin or AmB, but most neutropenic or immunosuppressed patients require systemic therapy with AmB or one of the imidazoles (ketoconazole, fluconazole). Local therapy and, even more effectively, systemic therapy with imidazoles are active for the prevention of oral and esophageal candidal infection.

In case of documentation of a viral infection, acyclovir or ganciclovir are indicated respectively for HSV and CMV esophageal infections.

C. Noninfectious Causes of Diarrhea and Mucositis

Most malignancies can have a direct effect on the gastrointestinal system. Tumors of the gastrointestinal tract itself, including head and neck, esophageal, stomach, small bowel, or colorectal cancer, can cause problems of malnutrition, obstruction, ulceration, bleeding, or perforation. In addition to the gastrointestinal primary lesions, a number of tumors, including melanoma, breast cancer, ovarian cancer, lymphoma, and leukemia, can involve the gastrointestinal tract. Infiltration by these malignancies can cause the problems noted previously and can also be responsible for protein-losing enteropathies, malabsorption and secondary infections of the gastrointestinal tract such as perirectal abscesses with leukemia. In addition, chemotherapy, radiotherapy, surgery, and paraneoplastic syndromes can be responsible for gastrointestinal manifestations that can mimic infections.

D. Perianal Infections

The perianal area is a common site of bacterial infection, especially in patients with acute monocytic leukemia, during episodes of neutropenia. The main symptoms are pain and fever; the lesions usually spread rapidly and often progress to necrosis, leaving major sequelae if not treated early; bacteremia caused by *P. aeruginosa* or *E. coli* is often documented. Radiotherapy has been recommended but is usually ineffective. The role of surgery is controversial because extensive operative procedures are made difficult by concomitant thrombocytopenia. In most patients, therapy consists of broad-spectrum antibiotics and analgesics.

E. Neutropenic Enterocolitis: Typhlitis

Neutropenic enterocolitis, also termed *typhlitis*, is a rare but well-recognized gastrointestinal condition occurring during therapy of acute leukemia, lymphoma, aplastic anemia, and certain solid tumors. It is characterized by bowel wall inflammation and edema that can progress to necrosis, usually in the terminal ileum, cecum, or right colon. Profound neutropenia secondary to chemotherapy has been considered the hallmark of the disease and a major etiologic factor in its development; antitumor agents may also play a role in this disease.

Once the process begins, organisms invade the injured bowel wall, aggravate the damage, and invade the bloodstream; bacteremia caused by multiple gram-negative rods is frequent. The most common presenting signs and symptoms are fever, abdominal pain, and watery diarrhea. The abdomen is distended, tender, and radiographs demonstrate evidence of paralytic ileus with thickening of the bowel wall.

Care of these patients should be individualized. Nonoperative treatment with bowel rest, decompression, nutritional support, and broad-spectrum antibiotics is recommended initially. Operative intervention is recommended for those with perforation or those whose condition deteriorates. The overall mortality rate is very high, in excess of 50% (46).

F. Abdominal Surgery

The onset of abdominal pain in the setting of neutropenia can be due to a variety of intraabdominal processes whose complications surgeons are frequently called on to evaluate and treat.

Clear-cut guidelines do not exist for the treatment of acute abdominal pain in neutropenic patients. Pain usually can be diffuse or localized; it can be associated with nausea, diarrhea, vomiting, constipation, jaundice, or abdominal distention. Abdominal distention was associated with increased mortality rate in some series. No symptom or sign is pivotal in the decision for or against surgical intervention; clinical or radiological evidence of a surgically treatable disease or failure to respond to medical therapy for a presumed medically treatable disease should prompt surgical intervention, but the approach should be thorough to avoid needless operations. Otherwise, it is often recommended to provide conservative treatment because neutropenic enteropathy is responsible for the majority of cases. As indicated in Table 14, which has been established on the basis of several publications on abdominal pain in neutropenic patients, necrotizing enteropathy was diagnosed in 81 of 169 (48%) neutropenic patients with a painful acute abdomen. Hepatic disease, often related to drug administration, and severe constipation were each responsible for that presentation in 6% of the cases; the other causes represented a wide spectrum of diseases, of which none represented more than 5%.

Spontaneous intestinal and colonic perforation occurs more frequently in patients receiving corticosteroids with or without chemotherapy. Malignancy can be histologically documented at the site of perforation in about 50% of these patients.

Operation can be necessary for obstructing carcinomatosis of the gastrointes-

Table 14 Diseases Responsible for Surgical Intervention in Neutropenic Patients

	No.	Percent
Necrotizing enteropathy	81	48.0
Hepatic disease	11	6.5
Constipation-ileus	10	6.0
Appendicitis	7	4.0
Perforated colon	7	4.0
Perforated stomach	6	3.5
Cholecystitis	6	3.5
Gastric hemorrhage	4	2.3
Retroperitoneal hemorrhage	4	2.3
Neoplastic infiltration	4	2.3
Graft-versus-host disease	4	2.3
Perforated stomach	3	1.7
Peritonitis	3	1.7
Perforated ileum	2	1.2
Hemorrhage in tumor	2	1.2
Lymphadenitis	2	1.2
No disease	2	1.2
Esophagitis	2	1.2
Pneumonia	2	1.2
Incarcerated hernia	1	0.6
Hemorrhage in ileum	1	0.6
Hemorrhage in colon	1	0.6
Splenic infarction	1	0.6
Pseudomembranous colitis	1	0.6
Total	169	100

tinal, pancreatic, biliary, or urinary tract. In case of advanced disease, these operations do not always prevent recurrence of the obstruction; laparotomy is justified, if performance status is compatible with a reasonable quality of life.

V. NEUROLOGICAL MANIFESTATIONS

A. Opportunistic Infections of the Central Nervous System

Infections of the nervous system are rare in patients with cancer, accounting for about 1% of neurological events; however, it is important to recognize these complications because some may be successfully treated.

Table 15 Central Nervous System Infection in Patients with Cancer

Infection and usual causative agents	Clinical clues	Laboratory findings
Meningitis		
Streptococcus pneumoniae	Neutropenia, splenectomy, fever, ± nuchal rigidity, headache postsurgery (head and neck)	Minimal pleocytosis if neutropenic, gram-positive diplococci on smear, positive culture, positive CIE in CSF or urine, blood cultures positive, CSF protein ↑, glucose ↓
Neisseria meningitis	Neutropenia, splenectomy, fever, rash, headache, arthralgias, ± nuchal rigidity, rapid progression	Minimal pleocytosis, gram-negative diplococci on smear, positive culture, CIE positive in CSF, blood cultures positive, CSF protein ↑, glucose ↓
Pseudomonas aeruginosa *Enterobacteriaceae*	Neutropenia, leukemia, fever, headache, minimal neurologic findings, minimal defects in mentation or level of consciousness, ecthyma gangrenosum	Minimal pleocytosis, gram-negative rods on smear, positive culture of CSF and blood
Listeria monocytogenes	Immunosuppression, T-lymphocyte defects, ± CNS signs, fever, headache, ± nuchal rigidity, minimal personality change, cranial nerve palsy	Mononuclear or polymorphonuclear pleocytosis, CSF protein ↑, glucose ↓, or normal + Gram stain of CSF sediment (30%), positive CSF culture

Cryptococcus neoformans	Immunosuppression, low-grade fever, minimal nuchal reigidity, mild headache, ± cranial nerve palsy, personality change, insidius onset	Lymphocytic pleocytosis, positive CSF Gram stain or India ink preparation, positive culture (large volumes), positive latex agglutination in CSF or serum
Meningoencephalitis		
Toxoplasma gondii	Immunosuppression, lymphoma, meningoencephalitis ± focal signs, multiple organ involvement, rapid progression	Minimal pleocytosis (lymphocytes), IgM-IF specific antibody increase, Sabin Feldman dye test ≥ 1:1000
Varicella-zoster virus Herpes simplex virus	Immunosuppression, skin lesions	Brain biopsy positive, positive vesicle culture
Brain abscess		
Aspergillus and *Mucor* sp.	Neutropenia, immunosuppression, nasopharyngeal involvement, ± brain abscess, sudden onset of major neurologic fingings, postneurosurgery, pneumonia	Mild lymphocytic pleocytosis, CSF protein, glucose, ± culture
Nocardia asteroides	Immunosuppression, T-lymphocyte defects, pulmonary infection, subcutaneous abscesses, focal neurologic signs	Biopsy of brain abscess, culture at other sites of infection

Abbreviations: CIE, counter immunoelectrophoresis; CSF, cerebrospinal fluid; IF, immunofluorence; CNS, central nervous system.

The distribution of microorganisms causing neurological infections in patients with cancer is different from that found in the general population. The agents responsible for the infections of the nervous system in cancer are similar to those found in other pathological conditions in which immunity is depressed, suggesting that immunodepression is an important factor in the pathogenesis of nervous system infections in patients with malignant tumors. Another predisposing circumstance for central nervous system (CNS) infection is head and spine surgery.

The type of the underlying disease and its associated defect in host defence mechanisms allow, with a high degree of accuracy, prediction of the responsible organism of CNS infection. Table 15 summarizes the principal clinical features of CNS opportunistic agents. Neutropenia can predispose to bacterial meningitis with the usual pathogens (*S. pneumoniae, Neisseria meningitidis*) but also with gram-negative bacilli. This is a very rare event in that meningitis has not been documented in more than 2,000 consecutive patients with febrile neutropenia recently studied by the EORTC Cooperative Group. Bacteremia can usually be documented along with the meningitis during neutropenia. Diagnosis might be difficult, because neutropenic patients often lack the usual clinical signs and symptoms of infection because of the reduced inflammatory reaction. In severely neutropenic patients, pleocytosis within the cerebrospinal fluid (CSF) may be minimal. Therapy requires high doses of effective antimicrobials; third generation cephalosporins (ceftazidime, ceftriaxone) and imipenem penetrate well into the CSF; in case of gram-negative bacillary meningitis, intrathecal injection of aminoglycosides via lumbar puncture or intraventricularly might be considered.

In patients with cellular immunity defects, *Listeria monocytogenes, Toxoplasma gondii, C. neoformans*, and *N. asteroides* are opportunistic agents able to cause meningitis, meningoencephalitis, or brain abscesses. These infections are relatively rare and predominate in patients with Hodgkin's disease, non-Hodgkin's lymphomas, and chronic lymphocytic leukemia.

In granulocytopenic patients, *Aspergillus* sp., *Candida* sp., and mucorales should be added to the list of possible causative agents for neurological infection; however, the involvement of CNS is usually secondary to hematogenous dissemination or direct extension from the sinuses, especially in the case of aspergillosis and mucormycosis, and rarely presents as a meningitis.

Toxoplasma encephalitis, which is extremely common in AIDS patients, is rare in patients with neoplastic disease. The majority of these patients have hematological malignancies, mainly Hodgkin's disease. Reactivation of latent infection accounts for the majority of CNS toxoplasmosis cases during immunosuppression. The only change in CSF may be moderate elevation of protein; pleocytosis is often absent. The parasite can be demonstrated in centrifuged CSF by Giemsa staining, and it has been cultured on tissue monolayers used for viral isolation; this method has replaced the fastidious inoculation of specimens into mice. A four-fold increase in IgG antibody titers and demonstration of local production in the CSF of toxoplasma IgG antibodies are indicative of active disease. Cerebral CT scan usually demonstrates nodular ring-enhancing lesions, and magnetic resonance imaging can detect lesions not visualized by the CT scan. Stereotactic biopsy may be warranted in some circumstances. Therapy of CNS toxoplasmosis consists of oral administration of the combination pyrimethamine-sulfadiazine at 50 mg/d and 8 g/d, respectively. Mortality rate is about 70%. Other alternatives under evaluation include the association clindamycin-pyrimethamine or dapsone-pyrimethamine.

C. neoformans is another opportunistic agent that can cause infection of CNS in cancer patients. It is associated mainly with lymphoma. Demonstration of budding yeast in CSF by India ink preparation, isolation on culture, and detection of *Cryptococcus* antigen constitute the principal methods of diagnosis. Combined therapy of AmB (0.5 mg/kg/d) with 5-fluorocytosine (100–150 mg/kg) is the first choice in immunocompromised patients. Duration of therapy should be at least 6 weeks. Therapy with triazoles, such as fluconazole at 400 mg/d, is compa-

Table 16 Therapy of Neurological Opportunistic Infections

Agent	Therapy
Listeria monocytogenes	Ampicillin 3 g qid IV + gentamicin 1 mg/kg tid IV or TMP-SMX 480–2400 mg/d IV
Toxoplasma gondii	Pyrimethamine-sulfadiazine 50 mg–8 g/d PO for 5 weeks Alternatives: clindamycin-pyrimethamine or dapsone-pyrimethamine
Cryptococcus neoformans	Amphotericin B 0.7–1 mg/kg IV + 5-fluorocytosine 100 mg/kg/d Alternatives: Fluconazole 6–12 mg/kg/d orally or IV; itraconazole 5 mg/kg/d PO
JC virus	No therapy available
Aspergillus, Mucor	Amphotericin B 1 mg/kg; consider surgery if feasible
Herpes simplex virus	Acyclovir, 10 mg/kg IV every 8 h for 10–14 days Alternative therapy: vidarabine

rable to AmB therapy; early results with oral itraconazole, 200 mg/d, are also encouraging.

L. monocytogenes is a relatively frequent opportunistic pathogen encountered in cancer patients with central nervous system infection. It is a food-borne disease; dairy products, especially raw milk and soft cheeses, meat, eggs, and some vegetables have been incriminated as carriers. Meningitis, meningoencephalitis, and, less commonly, brain abscesses have been reported in immunocompromised patients. Bacteremia is usually present in patients with central nervous system infection. Because the organisms are present in small numbers in the CSF, direct Gram staining may be negative.

High-dose ampicillin alone or in combination with an aminoglycoside is usually recommended. Duration of therapy should be at least 2 weeks. Isolated reports have shown that TMP-SMX is also an effective therapy and may constitute a good alternative for patients allergic to penicillin. Mortality rate for patients with *L. monocytogenes* central nervous system infections varies from 30% to 62% (Table 16).

Progressive multifocal leucoencephalopathy (PML) is a demyelinating disease caused by the human polyomavirus JC virus (JCV). In cancer patients, PML has been mainly associated with Hodgkin's disease and chronic lymphocytic leukemia. The classic triad of hemianopsia, hemiparesis, and dementia, associated with subcortical hypodensities without contrast enhancement on CT scan, and the presence of IgG antibodies to JCV in a patient with cellular immunodeficiency should alert the physician to the possibility of PML. Brain biopsy is the most reliable and accurate method for the diagnosis. The prognosis is poor because no active antiviral drug is available (47).

B. Noninfectious Causes of CNS Disease in Cancer Patients

Neurological noninfectious complications are exceedingly common in cancer patients; CNS lesions can be documented at postmortem examination in about 30%

Table 17 Neurologic Complications in Cancer Patients and Their Possible Infectious Disease Counterparts

Complication	Infectious disease counterpart
Brain metastases	Brain abscesses, granulomas
Cerebrovascular diseases	Septic embolus, vasculitis
Meningeal carcinomatosis	Chronic meningitis (cryptococcal)
Epidural compression	Epidural abscess
Drug-induced encephalopathy	Encephalitis (PMLE, toxoplasmosis)
Paraneoplastic syndromes	Encephalitis (PMLE, toxoplasmosis)

of patients with cancer. As previously stated, infections represent only a small fraction of these events (±1%). The principal situations that can mimic neurological infectious diseases are metastatic disease, cerebrovascular disorders, meningeal carcinomatosis, epidural spinal compression, chemotherapy-induced encephalopathy, and paraneoplastic syndromes (Table 17).

REFERENCES

1. Mackowiak PA. Commentary: fever patterns. Infect Dis Clin Pract 1997; 6:308–309.
2. Pizzo PA, Armstrong D, Bodey G, et al. The design, analysis, and reporting of clinical trials on the empirical antibiotic management of the neutropenic patient. Report of a consensus panel. J Infect Dis 1990; 161:397–401.
3. EORTC International Antimicrobial Therapy Cooperative Group. Ceftazidime combined with a short or long course of amikacin for empirical therapy of gram negative bacteremia in cancer patients with granulocytopenia. N Engl J Med 1987; 317:1692–1698.
4. Cometta A, Calandra T, Gaya H, et al. Monotherapy with meropenem versus combination therapy with ceftazidime plus amikacin as empiric therapy for fever in granulocytopenic patients with cancer. Antimicrob Agents Chemother 1996; 40:1108–1115.
5. De Pauw BE, Deresinsky SC, Feld R, et al. Ceftazidime compared with piperacillin and tobramycin for the empiric treatment of fever in neutropenic patients with cancer. Ann Intern Med 1994; 120:834–844.
6. Awada A, Van der Auwera P, Meunier F, et al. Streptococcal and enterococcal bacteremia in patients with cancer. Clin Infect Dis 1992; 15:33–48.
7. EORTC International Antimicrobial Therapy Cooperative Group. Empiric antifungal therapy in febrile granulocytopenic patients. Am J Med 1989; 86:668–672.
8. Schmidt GM, Horak DA, Niland JC, et al. A randomized, controlled trial of prophylactic ganciclovir for cytomegalovirus pulmonary infection in recipients of allogeneic bone marrow transplants. 1991; 324:1005–1011.
9. Sakamaki H, Yuasa K, Goto H, et al. Comparison of cytomegalovirus (CMV) antigenemia and CMV in bronchoalveolar lavage fluid for diagnosis of CMV pulmonary infection after bone marrow transplantation. Bone Marrow Transplant 1997; 20: 143–147.
10. Knockaert DC, Vanneste LJ, Vanneste SB, et al. Fever of unknown origin in the 1980s: an update of the diagnosis spectrum. Arch Intern Med 1992; 152:51–55.
11. Pizzo AP, Robichaud KJ, Wesley R, et al. Fever in the pediatric and young adult patient with cancer: a prospective study of 1001 episodes. Medicine 1982; 61:153–165.
12. Luft FC, Rissing JP, White A. Infections or neoplasm as causes of prolonged fever in cancer patients. Am J Med Sci 1976; 272:65–74.

13. Klastersky J, Weerts D, Hensgens C. Fever of unexplained origin in patients with cancer. Eur J Cancer 1973; 9:649–656.
14. Chang JC, Gross HM. Neoplastic fever responds to the treatment of an adequate dose of naproxen. J Clin Oncol 1985; 3:552–558.
15. Wolff SM, Fauci AS, Dale DS. Unusual etiologies of fever and their evaluation. Annu Rev Med 1975; 26:277–281.
16. Talbot GH, Provencher M, Cassileth PA. Persistent fever after recovery from granulocytopenia in acute leukemia. Arch Intern Med 1988; 148:129–135.
17. Barton TD, Schuster MG. The cause of fever following resolution of neutropenia in patients with acute leukemia. Clin Infect Dis 1996; 22:1064–1068.
18. Vose JM, Armitage JO. Clinical applications of hematopoietic growth factors. J Clin Oncol 1995; 13:1023–1035.
19. American Society of Clinical Oncology. Recommendations for the use of hematopoietic colony-stimulating factors: evidence-based, clinical practice guidelines. J Clin Oncol 1994; 12:2471–2508.
20. Mitchell PLR, Morland B, Stevens MCG, et al. Granulocyte stimulating factor in established febrile neutropenia: a randomized study of pediatric patients. J Clin Oncol 1997; 15:1163–1170.
21. Maher DW, Lieschke GJ, Green M, et al. Filgrastim in patients with chemotherapy-induced febrile neutropenia. Ann Intern Med 1994; 121:492–501.
22. Schimpff SC. Growth factors and empiric therapy with antibiotics: should they be used concurrently? Ann Intern Med 1994; 121:538–539.
23. Talcott JA, Siegel RD, Findberg R, et al. Risk assessment in cancer patients with fever and neutropenia. A prospective, two-center validation of a prediction rule. J Clin Oncol 1992; 10:316–322.
24. Rubenstein E, Rolston K. Outpatient management of febrile episodes in neutropenic patients. Support Care Cancer 1994; 2:369–373.
25. Blay JY, Chauvin F, Le Cesne A, et al. Early lymphopenia after cytotoxic chemotherapy as a risk factor for febrile neutropenia. J Clin Oncol 1996; 14:636–643.
26. Klastersky J. Therapy of febrile neutropenia: an algorithm for current clinical attitudes taking into account cost benefit. Curr Opin Oncol. In press.
27. Messori A, Trippoli S, Tendi E. G-CSF for the prophylaxis of neutropenic fever in patients with small cell lung cancer receiving myelosuppressive antineoplastic chemotherapy: meta-analysis and pharmacoeconomic evaluation. J Clin Pharm Ther 1996; 21:57–63.
28. Viscoli C, Bruzzi P, Castagnola E, et al. Factors associated with bacteraemia in febrile, granulocytopenic cancer patients. Eur J Cancer 1994; 30A:430–437.
29. Reed WP. Intravenous access devices for supportive care of patients with cancer. Curr Opin Oncol 1991; 3:634–642.
30. Carde P, Cosset-Delaigue MF, Laplanche A, et al. Classical external indwelling central venous catheter versus totally implanted venous access systems for chemotherapy administration: a randomized trial in 100 patients with solid tumors. Eur J Cancer Clin Oncol 1989; 25:939–944.
31. Tomee JFC, Mannes GPM, van der Bij W, et al. Serodiagnosis and monitoring of *Aspergillus* infections after lung transplantation. Ann Intern Med 1996; 125:197–201.

32. Rex JH, Bennet JE, Sugar AM, et al. A randomized trial comparing fluconazole with amphotericin B for the treatment of candidemia in patients without neutropenia. N Engl J Med 1994; 331:1325–1330.
33. Anaissie EJ, Kontoyiannis DP, Huls C, et al. Safety plasma concentrations and efficacy of high-dose fluconazole in invasive mold infections. J Infect Dis 1995; 172: 599–602.
34. Sugar M, Hitchcock CA, Troke PF, et al. Combination therapy of murine invasive candidiasis with fluconazole and amphotericin B. Antimicrob Agents Chemother 1995; 39:598–601.
35. Mills V, Chopra R, Linch DC, et al. Liposomal amphotericin B in the treatment of fungal infections in neutropenic patients: a single-centre experience of 133 episodes in 116 patients. Br J Haematol 1994; 86:754–760.
36. Oppenheim BA, Herbrecht R, Kusne S. The safety and efficacy of amphotericin B colloidal dispersion in the treatment of invasive mycoses. Clin Infect Dis 1995; 21: 1145–1153.
37. Caillot D, Reny G, Solary E, et al. A controlled trial of the tolerance of amphotericin B infused in dextrose or in Intralipid in patients with hematologic malignancies. J Antimicrob Chemother 1994; 33:603–613.
38. Barry AL, Brown SD. In vitro studies of two triazoles antifungal agents (voriconazole [UK-109, 496] and fluconazole) against *Candida* species. Antimicrob Agents Chemother 1996; 40:1948–1949.
39. Martino P, Girmenia C. Are we making progress in antifungal therapy? Curr Opin Oncol 1997; 9:314–320.
40. Edwards JE, Bodey GP, Bowden RA, et al. International conference for the development of a consensus on the management and prevention of severe candidal infections. Clin Infect Dis 1997; 25:43–59.
41. Skrickova J, Mayer J, Vorlicek J. Pulmonary infiltrate etiology in leukemic patients with fever. *In*: Klastersky JA, ed. Febrile Neutropenia. New York: Springer Verlag, 1997.
42. Arnow PM, Sadigh M, Costas C, et al. Endemic and epidemic aspergillosis, hospital epidemiology, diagnosis, and treatment. J Infect Dis 1991; 164:998–1002.
43. Varthalitis I, Meunier F. *Pneumocystis carinii* pneumonia: the pathogen, the diagnosis and recent advances in management. Int J Antimicrob Agents 1991; 1:97–108.
44. Pannuti CS, Gingrich RD, Pfaller MA, et al. Nosocomial pneumonia in adult patients undergoing bone marrow transplantation: a 9-year study. J Clin Oncol 1991; 9:77–84.
45. Ibrahim A, Gautier E, Roittmann S, et al. Should cytomegalovirus be tested for in both blood and bronchoalveolar lavage fluid of patients at high risk of CMV pneumonia after bone marrow transplantation? Br J Haematol 1997; 98:222–227.
46. Wade DS, Nava HR, Douglass HO. Neutropenic enterocolitis. Clinical diagnosis and treatment. Cancer 1992; 69:17–23.
47. Major EO, Ameniya K, Tornatore CS, et al. Pathogenesis and molecular biology of progressive multifocal leukoencephalopathy, the JC virus-induced demyelinating disease of the human brain. Clin Microbiol Rev 1992; 5:49–73.

2

Fungal Infections

Ben E. De Pauw
University Hospital St. Radboud, Nijmegen, The Netherlands

I. INTRODUCTION

Fungi have only emerged as significant pathogens during the past 2 decades. Before the mid-1960s, accounts of fungal infections were mostly limited to sporadic case reports. During the past decade, there has been a dramatic increase in incidence of invasive fungal infections in patients who are not in an end stage of their underlying disease (1,2). Yeasts and molds rank among the 10 most frequently isolated pathogens, and approximately 7% of all febrile episodes can be attributed definitely to these microorganisms (3). Autopsy data show that 5% of patients with solid tumors, 10% to 15% of patients with lymphoma, and up to 20% of all patients with leukemia or those undergoing bone marrow transplantation have histological evidence of invasive fungal infections (1,4). Autopsy studies are of limited value in estimating the true prevalence of fungal infections because many patients who die are not examined and those who survive are also excluded. A reliable assessment is also confounded by empirical administration of intravenous amphotericin B in immunocompromised hosts, because patients may have received successful treatment without the diagnosis ever being confirmed.

If one takes into account the changes in the therapeutic approach of patients suffering from malignancies, it is hardly surprising that fungal infections have become a substantial obstacle in the treatment of patients with a malignant disease. Death resulting from fungal infection is a catastrophe for a potentially curable patient with cancer or leukemia. Most factors promoting invasive fungal infection are difficult or impossible to avoid. Never before were so many patients treated with irradiation as well as cytotoxic and immunosuppressive therapy. Moreover, with the technological advances in bone marrow processing and cryopreservation, and the ability to mobilize progenitor cells from the bone marrow into the peripheral blood, there has been a marked increase in the number of autologous bone marrow transplantations for both hematological malignancies and solid tumors.

II. RISK FACTORS

The relative incidence of the various fungal infections depends on geography as well as on medical practices and local conditions in a given hospital (5). *Candida* and *Aspergillus* species remain the prominent fungal pathogens among immunocompromised patients. In fact, every patient is steadily exposed to these environmental organisms. Fungal infections run a more severe course with early dissemination during neutropenia in comparison with patients with normal host defenses (Table 1).

Neutropenia is the principal predisposing factor for fungal infections (6). Bacteria are usually the initial cause of a fever during a chemotherapy-induced neutropenic episode but the modern, powerful antibiotics have virtually eliminated early death resulting from bacterial infections, thereby putting the patient at risk for other infectious complications. The broad-spectrum antibacterials used for this purpose suppress and alter the indigenous microbial flora, leading to increasing colonization by fungi over time. Thus, although fungal pathogens are infrequent causes of the initial febrile episode during neutropenia, they account for a large proportion of the superinfections.

Under normal circumstances, the intact epithelial surfaces of the gastrointestinal tract prohibit invasion by microorganisms and the mucociliary barrier of the respiratory tract prevents aspiration of fungal cells and spores; in contrast, dead or damaged tissue creates a nidus for infection. Many cancer chemotherapeutic agents cause ulceration of the pulmonary and gastrointestinal mucosa, thus facilitating colonization and invasion by molds and yeasts, as is witnessed by a high incidence of invasive fungal infections in bone marrow transplant recipients relative to those who received conventional cytoreductive chemotherapy (7,8). Permitted by the introduction of recombinant colony-stimulating factors as well as better antibacterial cover, doses of cytotoxic drugs have been escalated to optimize the chance for cancer control. Inevitably, these higher does of chemotherapeutic agents cause more damage to the mucosal barrier, resulting in impaired production of saliva, secretory IgA, mucus, and gastric acid, malabsorp-

Table 1 Risk Factors Associated with the Increased Incidence of Invasive Fungal Infections

More powerful antibiotics
Fewer early death from bacterial infections
Increased disturbance of commensal flora of the gastrointestinal tract
More aggressive chemotherapy and irradiation
Prolonged neutropenia
Enhanced mucosal damage
More malabsorption and malnutrition
More antacids
More fevers treated with broad spectrum antibacterials
More suppression of the cellular immunity
More effective chemotherapy
More patients treated for their malignancy
Inclusion of elderly patients and patients with history of a fungal infection
Fewer patients dying from their underlying disease
Increasing number of bone marrow transplantations
Stem cell transplantations for hematologic malignancies and solid tumors
Growing bone marrow banks: more matched, unrelated donor transplants and more graft-versus-host disease
More corticosteroids
More extensive abdominal surgery
Increased use of central venous catheters
Better diagnostic tools and increased awareness
Increased travel to regions with endemic mysoses
Continuing building activities in hospitals
More exposure to biodegrading material in composting devices and separate waste containers
Inadequate hygiene

tion, as well as decreased peristalsis (8). In case of concomitant neutropenia, any potential pathogen that has invaded the damaged tissues may gain easy access to the body and, subsequently, disseminate rapidly.

Although most *Candida* infections originate from endogenous organisms, nosocomial transmission of organisms has been documented beyond doubt (9). Inappropriate hygiene and long-standing venous access devices, with and without a subcutaneous tunnel tract, are major sources of fungal infections. The incidence of catheter-associated fungemia varies from 1% to 16% (10).

Building activities on the hospital premises, frequently mentioned as a risk factor (11), should not be considered a problem specific for a given hospital because nearly every hospital is constantly engaged in reconstructions. Relatively new risk factors are household composting devices and containers for biodegradable waste that, particularly during summer, can spread potentially dangerous amounts of fungal spores. Better supportive care has fostered the application of more intensive regimens to elderly individuals and patients with preexisting immunocompromising diseases such as diabetes mellitus, chronic obstructive pulmonary disease, and prior invasive fungal infection (12). Bone marrow transplantation with and without T-cell depletion has become accepted as a lifesaving option for many hematological malignancies, but the procedure is taking its toll. In a consecutive series of 1,186 patients who underwent bone marrow transplantation at the University of Minnesota Hospital between 1974 and 1989, a non-Candida fungal infection developed in 10% within 180 days after transplantation (13). Others have reported an incidence as high as 40% among recipients of sibling marrow (14). One should realize that, with the expansion of bone marrow registries, more unrelated donor transplantations will be performed with even more severe graft-versus-host disease and serious infectious complications. The vast majority of fungal infections will occur in allogeneic recipients as a consequence of additionally depressed cell-mediated immunity resulting from immunosuppressive agents given to prevent graft-versus-host disease. Moreover, during graft-versus-host disease cytotoxic T cells as well as the immunosuppressive agents used to control the disease may damage the important mucosal barriers. After marrow engraftment and healing of mucosa, the incidence of fungal infections diminishes accordingly until the cell-mediated immunity has fully recovered. This may require quite some time, especially when chronic graft-versus-host disease emanates in recipients of an allogeneic transplant.

III. CHANGES IN THE EPIDEMIOLOGY

It is generally acknowledged that the incidence of aspergillosis has increased (4), whereas that of *Candida* infections culminated in the late 1970s (Table 2). The rate of candidemia decreased by about 50% among patients with leukemia during the more recent period, and it doubled in patients with lymphoma and solid tumors (15). Furthermore, in 1984, 80% of *Candida* bloodstream infections were due to *Candida albicans*, whereas in the 1990s, non–*C. albicans* strains have become responsible for at least half of these infections (3,16). Both the decrease in the number of *Candida* infections and the shift toward non–*C. albicans* strains is presumably pertinent to the use of fluconazole for prophylaxis. After the introduction of fluconazole at the Johns Hopkins University Medical Center, the infection rate with *Candida krusei* and *Candida glabrata* apparently increased when compared with historical control subjects (17,18). Suppression of the predominant and virulent *C. albicans* created space for less aggressive and nonsusceptible organisms. However, this attractive, implicative hypothesis was not corroborated by several prospective, randomized multicenter studies on fluconazole prophylaxis (19,20). Therefore, other unknown mechanisms, such as a particular potential of non–*C. albicans* strains to exploit the deficits in host defense mechanisms imposed by aggressive chemotherapeutic regimens, cannot be excluded (8).

C. albicans continues to be one of the most frequently isolated species (3,16), followed by *C. tropicalis, C. glabrata*, and *Candida parapsilosis*; the latter is often encountered in association with central venous catheters (18,21). Over the past 10 years, new species have emerged, such as the aforementioned *C. krusei, Candida lusitaniae, Candida utilis*, and *Candida guillermondii* (17,22). Other yeasts such as *Trichosporon, Saccharomyces cerevisiae, Rhodotorula*, and *Malessezia furfur*, the organism responsible for pityriasis versicolor and folliculitis, have also been identified as the cause of septicemia in humans (23), with intravenous or peritoneal catheters being the major risk factors.

Histoplasmosis, coccidioidomycosis, blastomycosis, and paracoccidioidomycosis are referred to as the *endemic mycoses* because they used to be geographically confined to certain regions. Similarly, *Penicillium marneffei* was typically seen in Southeast Asia (24). However, as a result of rapid air travel, these infections can occur anywhere.

Other examples of extraordinary fungi in the immunocompromised patient are *Pseudallescheria* (25), *Fusarium* (23), and *Alternaria* sp. (26,27). These molds constitute a growing problem in neutropenic patients and bone marrow transplant recipients, just as does mucormycosis (28). Many of these infections follow inhalation, but some may originate from infected nails or cutaneous lesions adjacent to catheters.

IV. DIAGNOSIS AND CLINICAL FEATURES OF FUNGAL INFECTIONS

A. Invasive Aspergillosis

The most common initial presentation of invasive aspergillosis is unremitting fever accompanied by development of lung infiltrates despite broad-spectrum antibacterial treatment, typically after the second week of chemotherapy-induced neutropenia or bone marrow transplantation. In approximately 90% of cases, the lungs are the portal of entry, with nasal sinuses and the skin accounting for the remainder of cases.

Clinicians should suspect the diagnosis in a patient with pleuritic pain, hemoptysis, localized wheezing and rubbing, or radiographical evidence of a pleural effusion or localized pulmonary infiltrates. The symptoms, which are due to fungal invasion causing extensive necrosis and occlusion of small blood vessels, resemble those of pulmonary infarction. A distinct halo of low attenuation sur-

Table 2 Common Fungi and Trends in Their Incidence

Fungus	Trend	Clinical characteristics
Candida species		Superficial: beige plaques and local pain. Acute disseminated: hectic fever and chills, polymyalgia, polyarthralgia, not tender pinkish skin lesions, retinal exudates. Chronic disseminated: complaints of the organ involved; liver associated with increased alkaline phospatase, hepatosplenomegaly, distinct lesion on CT scan, abdominal discomfort, lethargy.
Candida albicans	−	
Candida glabrata	+++	
Candida krusei	++	
Candida tropicalis	=	
Candida parapsilosis	++	
Candida guillermondii	=	
Candida lusitaniae	=	
Trichosporon beigelii	+	Like acute disseminated candidiasis.
Saccharomyces cerevisiae	+	Like acute disseminated candidiasis.
Rhodutorula	+	Like acute disseminated candidiasis.
Malassezia furfur	+	Like acute disseminated candidiasis; folliculitis; hemorrhagic diathesis; pneumonitis.
Cryptococcus neoformans	=	Flu-like symptoms; skin lesions; central nervous system disease without meningismus.
Histoplasma capsulatum	+	Skin and mucosal lesions, cough with reticulonodular pulmonary infiltrates; headache.

Coccidioidomycosis	+	Pulmonary infection; no characteristic symptoms.
Paracoccidioidomycosis	=	No characteristic symptoms.
Blastomycosis	=	Pulmonary and cutaneous lesions; no characteristic symptoms.
Penicillium marneffei	+	Characteristic skin lesions and palatal papules; hepatosplenomegaly and lymphadenopathy.
Aspergillus species		Unremitting fever and pulmonary infiltrates during antibiotic therapy. Chest pain, pleural rub, pleural effusion, hemoptysis; halo and air crescent sign on chest radiograph and CT scan; clinical and radiologic sinusitis.
Aspergillus fumigatus	+++	
Aspergillus flavus	+	
Aspergillus niger	=	
Aspergillus nidulans	+	
Aspergillus terreus	+	
Aspergillus glaucus	=	
Aspergillus restrictus	=	
Fusariosis	++	Like aspergillosis, but more myalgia and gangrenous skin lesions.
Mucormycosis/Zygomycosis	++	Like aspergillosis, but rhinocerbral form more prominent and severe; serosanguinous nasal discharge.
Pseudallescheria boydii	+	Pneumonitis. Disseminated infections with and without septicemia; wound infections.
Alternariosis	+	Cutaneous lesions: noninvasive sinusitis.
Pneumocystis carinii	+	Dyspnea and diffuse interstitial pneumonitis.

Table 3 Value of Diagnostic Tools

	Blood culture	Clinical symptoms	Serology	Microscopy	Chest/sinus X-ray	CT scan	Ultrasound
Candida species	++	+	±	+	−	++	+
Trichosporon beigelii	+	−	−	+	−		
Saccharomyces cerevisiae	+	−	−				
Rhodutorula	+	−	−				
Malassezia furfur	+	±	−	+	+		
Cryptococcus neoformans	−	±	+++	++	+		
Histoplasma capsulatum	+	+	+++	+	+	+	
Coccidioidomycosis	−	−	++	++	+		
Blastomycosis	−	−	−	++	+	±	
Penicillium marneffei	−	+	−	++			
Aspergillus species	−	+	++	++	+++	++++	−
Fusariosis	+	+	−	+	++	++	−
Mucormycosis/Zygomycosis	−	+	−	++	+++	+++	−
Pseudallescheria boydii	+	−	−	+	++	+	−
Alternariosis	+	−	−	+	−	−	
Pneumocystis carinii	−	++	+++	++	+++	−	−

rounding the lesions and a so-called air crescent sign on a chest radiograph or computerized tomography (CT) scan are generally regarded as characteristic of aspergillosis (29,30). Isolation of an *Aspergillus* species from sputum is not a reliable means of confirming the diagnosis because no more than 25% of patients who are later shown to suffer from invasive aspergillosis have positive sputum cultures antemortem. On the other hand, the isolation of *Aspergillus* species from sputum or bronchoalveolar lavage specimens connotes either invasive infection or a high risk for developing infection in the near future and should never be dismissed (31). Infection of the paranasal sinuses may extend rapidly to the face, palate, orbits, and brain. Disseminated aspergillosis is usually a preterminal event.

B. Other Mold Infections

The clinical picture of mucormycosis or zygomycosis, fusariosis, and alternariosis is remarkably similar to that of aspergillosis. These thermotolerant fungi can be isolated ubiquitously in large numbers from soil, air, and decomposing organic debris. In mucormycosis, the rhinocerebral form is more prevalent and severe than in aspergillosis, featuring painful unilateral facial swelling, proptosis, and ophthalmoplegia, together with a serosanguinous nasal discharge. Severe myalgias, disseminated ecthyma gangrenosum-like skin lesions in 70% of patients, sinusitis, ocular symptoms, and multiorgan system involvement are distinctive symptoms of disseminated fusariosis. In alternariosis, cutaneous lesions are equally common. Smears or nasal scrapings or discharge are helpful in establishing a diagnosis, but biopsies or debridement of necrotic lesions is preferred. In the past, mucormycosis and fusariosis have probably been underreported because the histological demonstration of septated hyphae in pulmonary tissue can easily be interpreted as being due to *Aspergillus* sp. *Rhizopus arrhizus*, the causative agent in mucormycosis, can be distinguished morphologically from other molds by their characteristic broad, nonseptate filaments with right-angled branching, but cultures are essential for a definite discrimination. It is not extraordinary for blood cultures and biopsies of skin lesions to be positive; the latter may show a rather characteristic microscopic picture. *Pseudallescheria boydii* can be responsible for a wide range of clinical syndromes, encompassing esophagitis and pneumonitis, as well as disseminated infections with and without signs of sepsis.

C. Candidiasis

Candida sp. can cause superficial infections limited to the oropharynx and esophagus as well as major organ infections, disseminated disease, and candidemia. The attributable mortality rate from candidemia ranges from about 40% in patients with candidemia alone to more than 90% for those who have acute tissue invasion with or without fungemia (16).

Secondary bloodstream infections, which evolve from other infectious foci such as wounds, carry a much higher mortality rate than do primary, catheter-related infections. Sometimes, single positive blood cultures pose a diagnostic dilemma. In a patient with other evidence suggestive of candidiasis it would be considered indicative for a serious infection, whereas patients with one positive blood culture without clinical symptoms would be classified as having benign transient candidemia. The latter group should be followed up closely because a proportion of patients with apparently benign candidemia may later be seen with chronic disseminated candidiasis.

Some patients have sudden onset of fever, tachycardia, tachypnea, occasionally accompanied by chills, and hypotension during treatment with broad-spectrum antibacterials. Additional clinical clues that should lead to a suspicion of *Candida* infection include unexplained polymyalgia, polyarthralgia, and azotemia. In about 10% of patients with acute disseminated candidiasis, characteristic pinkish-purple, nontender subcutaneous nodules may arise anywhere on the body. Biopsy specimens should be cultured and meticulously screened histologically at multiple levels to establish a final diagnosis. Patients with esophagitis typically complain of a burning retrosternal pain that becomes worse on swallowing. Clinical symptoms of *Candida* ophthalmitis seldom occur in neutropenic patients because the lesions and complaints are the result of an inflammatory response of granulocytes.

Other patients show an insidious onset, in some cases owing to concurrent corticosteroids, which suppress fever; they feel initially relatively well until the infection progresses and organ failure becomes evident. Disseminated candidiasis may mimic a single organ infection, but in most cases a number of organs are affected. Primary *Candida* pneumonia is regarded as exceptional, whereas the frequency of pulmonary involvement in disseminated infection varies from 10% to more than 50% in different surveys. Chronic hepatic candidiasis is being recognized with increasing frequency (32). Typically, the patient has an irregular fever, hepatosplenomegaly, abdominal discomfort, and elevation of alkaline phosphatase levels after recovery from long-term myelosuppression and mucositis; an abdominal ultrasound or CT scan shows distinctive multiple abscesses in the liver and/or spleen, known as ''bull's eyes'' (33). Most patients require prolonged therapy before the infection resolves, but failure of antifungal therapy is not uncommon and the mortality rate may be 40%. Lethargy and disorientation may indicate infection of the central nervous system, but in fewer than 50% of such cases does examination of cerebrospinal fluid reveal yeast cells.

At least half of neutropenic patients in whom unequivocal evidence of invasive candidiasis develops never have had any positive blood culture. This may be due to an inadequate number of blood cultures or suboptimal procedures in the microbiology laboratory. Blood cultures need to be incubated for weeks rather than days in an oxygen replete environment.

D. Other Yeast Infections, Endemic Mycoses, and *Pneumocystis carinii*

The clinical signs and symptoms of infections by *Trichosporon* sp., *S. cerevisiae*, also known as baker's yeast, *Rhodotorula*, and *M. furfur* are in essence not different from those encountered in acute disseminated candidiasis. The diagnosis is seldom suspected until the organism is recovered from blood, urine, or a cutaneous lesion. In some patients with *Malassezia* infection, hemorrhagic diathesis or severe pneumonitis develops as a result of yeast cells infiltrating the lumen and walls of the pulmonary arteries. Cryptococcal infection can be found in transplant recipients and in other patients with a long-standing impaired cellular immunity, such as those with treatment-refractory Hodgkin's disease. Such infection classically presents with flulike symptoms, skin lesions, and/or central nervous system disease without meningeal signs or an altered state of consciousness. Antigen detection in the cerebrospinal fluid and the serum yields early, reliable information and offers an objective parameter to monitor therapy. In addition, magnetic resonance imaging or CT scan of the brain may show characteristic parenchymal lesions.

Coccidioidomycosis and blastomycosis are never recognized on the basis of characteristic clinical findings, which resemble those of candidiasis and cryptococcosis. Their diagnosis is dependent on serology, culture, or histopathology.

Histoplasmosis should be considered in transplant patients who are resident in midwestern and south-central parts of the United States. Typical presenting signs and symptoms are prolonged fever, skin and mucosal lesions, unexplained cough with reticulonodular radiographic findings progressing rapidly to an acute respiratory distress syndrome, and, less commonly, headache owing to central nervous system infection. Hypotension, respiratory, renal and/or hepatic failure, and coagulopathy have been reported in a minority of cases. Blood and/or bone marrow cultures are positive in more than 90% of patients with disseminated disease, and antigen assays appear promising to detect the disease in an early state of development.

Pneumocystis carinii, which is classified as a fungus, is the predominant cause of opportunistic interstitial pneumonia in transplant recipients. Patients complain of increasing dyspnea and fever, followed by malaise and nonproductive cough in association with chest radiography that typically reveals bilateral infiltrates or, occasionally, unilateral or asymmetric abnormalities.

E. Laboratory Methods and Imaging Techniques

The rapid accurate identification of fungal pathogens is extremely important in guiding appropriate therapy for mycotic infections. Only one-third of all invasive fungal infections confirmed at autopsy had been treated with any antifungal therapy (1). Partly because of the lack of normally functioning granulocytes, invasive fungal infections furnish minimal characteristic clinical symptoms and only trivial objective radiological or laboratory evidence of their presence.

The lysis centrifugation technique has improved the rate of positive blood cultures from about 60% to 85% to 90%, especially in cases of candidemia, offering an earlier detection as a bonus. In general, the yield of fungal cultures from sources other than blood, urine, or mucosa is low. It is virtually impossible to grow fungi from tissue biopsy specimens known to be infected on histological examination. Identification of fungi by morphological means is, therefore, of great value in the recognition of invasive fungal infections. Although most *Candida* sp., *Cryptococcus*, mucormycosis, and endemic mycoses can be recognized histologically with some confidence, it is nearly impossible to differentiate *Aspergillus* hyphae from other, more rare pathogenic molds.

Reliable serological tests are available for an accurate diagnosis of mycoses such as histoplasmosis, coccidioidomycosis, and cryptococcosis. Similar successes, however, have not been achieved in aspergillosis and candidiasis in neutropenic cancer patients. Even with the most sophisticated serological methods, antibodies are seldom found in immunocompromised patients. Hence, attention is concentrated on tests to detect products of the fungus rather than on the host response. The subject of most assays is galactomannan, an antigen present in the *Aspergillus* cell wall. An immunoassay showed a sensitivity of 70% to 80%, a specificity of 90%, a positive predictive value of 82%, and a negative predictive value of 85% (34). Increased titers of antigen could be detected before invasive aspergillosis was suspected in 30% of cases and before standard laboratory confirmation of infection in 46%. A sandwich enzyme-linked immunosorbent assay (ELISA) with an increased sensitivity for *Aspergillus* antigenemia proved highly predictive of invasive aspergillosis but its sensitivity remains low (35). Serial assays may increase the sensitivity because a single positive test result is seldom diagnostic, whereas increasing levels in sequential blood specimens from a neutropenic patient should raise suspicion and dictate further radiological investigations or therapeutic intervention. When identified in the bronchoalveolar lavage fluid, *Aspergillus* antigen is a reasonable indicator of invasive aspergillosis in neutropenic patients and ought to have the same value as the isolation of *Aspergillus*. An ELISA also produced encouraging results.

In contrast, the results of immunological tests for the diagnosis of disseminated candidiasis have generally been disappointing. Several attempts to detect antigens based on the recognition of mannan have been made, but mannan is only transiently present in the blood, resulting in a moderate sensitivity of 33% to 65% and a specificity of 100%. An ELISA detecting circulating enolase obtained positive results in 85% of patients with tissue-proven invasive candidiasis. However, only 52% of 122 samples were positive, which indicates that multiple samples must be collected for this test to be useful (36). Molecular biological techniques based on the polymerase chain reaction (PCR) have not been developed to a similar extent for fungal infection because the PCR is such a sensitive technique that it is difficult to use when the etiological agents exist as a pathogen in one patient and as a colonizer in another, as is the case in aspergillosis and, particularly, candidiasis (37). For the time being then, serological diagnosis of fungal infections can at best be considered an adjunct to other diagnostic procedures.

Chronic disseminated candidiasis can be identified on abdominal CT scans (32), and high-resolution CT scans of the chest and paranasal sinuses proved superior to conventional radiography in the diagnosis of aspergillosis. Appearance of a halo sign, which emerges before the typical cavitation, was highly indicative of early pulmonary disease in neutropenic patients (29). Moreover, serial chest CT scans were shown to facilitate early detection of suspicious lesions, leading to a reduction in time to diagnosis with eventually an increased overall survival rate resulting from early initiation of antifungal therapy (30). For the detection of early occult infections in patients with persisting unexplained fever, isotope scanning with labeled immunoglobulins is an interesting option (38).

V. PREVENTION OF FUNGAL INFECTIONS

A. Hygiene

The high incidence of fungal infection during hospitalization suggests nosocomial acquisition. Hand carriage and proximity are established risk factors for transmission of infections with *C. albicans* (9). Hence, hand disinfection by visitors, nurses, physicians, and other personnel is important, and its neglect will frustrate all other means of prevention. Furthermore, central venous catheters should be handled scrupulously, and gastric antacids should only be prescribed on very strict indication, because a low pH protects against colonization of the intestine by *Candida* species. Unnecessary use of antibacterials and corticosteroids should be avoided as should contact with soil and biodegrading materials, including separate waste containers and compost devices, to reduce exposure to spores. Patients should be placed in rooms protected by high-efficiency particulate air (HEPA) filters or laminar flow systems if high concentrations of spores are encountered in the hospital environment. Well-known sources of fungi, such as dried food and flowers, pepper, and medication cartons, must be eliminated.

B. Prophylaxis

Given the restrictions to diagnose a fungal infection in a stage beyond cure, chemoprophylaxis is a compelling option to many clinicians. However, this issue is far from straightforward and divides opinions of specialists in two extremes, ranging from those who believe the benefit far outweighs the costs and those who remain skeptical and eschew any form of prophylaxis. Only the value of trimethoprim-sulfamethoxazole as prophylaxis against *P. carinii* is generally recognized (39). The drug is fairly tolerated, is extraordinarily effective for this purpose, and provides protection against listeriosis and nocardiosis. Monthly pentamidine administration, either intravenously or by aerosol, may be seen as a substitute in case of intolerance or allergy. Confidence in prophylaxis for all other indications is based on opinion rather than on facts. Older studies and historical controls are inadequate for evaluating the efficacy of an antifungal chemoprophylactic regimen because the risk of infection varies considerably with time owing to changes in antitumor therapy, seasons, and building activities. Furthermore, centers that experience a high incidence of fatal fungal infection are those most interested in implementing a new prophylactic strategy and the discipline imposed by a clinical study often leads to better precautions (40).

Hematopoietic growth factors do not prevent neutropenia per se but can curtail its duration and, hypothetically, achieve a reduction in the incidence and severity of fungal infections. On the other hand, these factors add to the costs of care and, at present, there are no data to warrant their use for prophylactic purposes.

C. Oral Agents

The main target of orally administered antifungals is a reduction of the colonization grade of the gastrointestinal tract by yeasts (41). It seemed reasonable to speculate that the topically active, nonabsorbable antifungal agents would be able to reduce the yeast burden in the gut, thereby favorably influencing the incidence of invasive candidiasis. However, their efficacy in the prevention of disseminated mycoses is unimpressive. This trivializes the question of whether sucking troches, pastilles, or lozenges is better than swallowing suspension or tablets. Ketoconazole had frequent side effects and impaired absorption. While ketoconazole was able to reduce colonization by *C. albicans*, a fecal overgrowth with *C. glabrata* and *C. tropicalis* (42) was observed.

A prophylactic agent should be safe enough to permit its use during several weeks in patients who are susceptible to side effects of multiple other agents being administered simultaneously. With the advent of fluconazole, a new era in chemoprophylaxis commenced. A good safety profile and reliable absorption from the gastrointestinal tract made fluconazole an attractive agent for this purpose. Several prospective, randomized, double-blind, placebo-controlled trials with sufficient power were conducted to assess the role of fluconazole in the prevention of fungal infections in bone marrow recipients and patients with leukemia. The first study in 356 patients undergoing a bone marrow transplantation showed that fluconazole, at a dosage of 400 mg once daily, was effective in preventing superficial and disseminated candidiasis (19). Systemic fungal infection was documented in only 3% of fluconazole recipients compared with 16% in the placebo group. These results were corroborated in a second trial in which fluconazole additionally appeared to reduce empirical amphotericin B use as well as overall mortality rate (43). On the other hand, both studies showed a higher incidence of acute graft-versus-host disease in fluconazole recipients, which may be due to either more patients surviving in the fluconazole arm to acquire graft-versus-host disease or to interference with cyclosporine metabolism. Of note, there was no hematological toxicity, as demonstrated by equal time to engraftment in both arms. A retrospective study performed at the Detroit Medical Center indicated that a lower dosage of 100 to 200 mg daily may be equally efficacious (44).

The benefits of fluconazole are less conclusive in adults receiving remission induction therapy for acute leukemia (20,45). This might be related to the use of lower doses in some trials, although there was no obvious relationship between the dosage used and the results ultimately achieved (7), which indicates that a lower dose of fluconazole may suffice in many cases (20). Combining fluconazole with polyenes might be effective in preventing the aforementioned overgrowth with *C. krusei* and *C. glabrata*, but this has not been investigated and cannot be recommended with confidence.

Itraconazole has clinically worthwhile activity against *Aspergillus* sp. (46). However, in a prospective, double-blind randomized study in leukemic patients, 400 mg/d itraconazole neither reduced the incidence of documented and presumed *Aspergillus* infections nor influenced the perceived need for intravenous amphotericin B (47). These disappointing results might have been different had drug concentrations been monitored consistently during the trial and the dose of itraconazole adjusted accordingly. Itraconazole is poorly soluble in water and the resulting erratic absorption makes it an unreliable agent in acutely ill patients. A new formulation of itraconazole suspended in cyclodextrine solution appears to be better absorbed (48) but, so far, there are no conclusive reports on efficacy and tolerability of this formulation. Another concern about itraconazole is the induction of resistance to amphotericin B (49).

D. Amphotericin B Spray and Low Dose Intravenously

Local administration of amphotericin B by means of sprays or inhalations seemed to be an attractive idea to prevent colonization of the airways by molds. When compared with historical controls, the incidence of pulmonary aspergillosis was apparently lower in patients undergoing a bone marrow transplant procedure or patients who complied with remission induction therapy for hematological malignancy, but the overall mortality rate was not affected. The incidence of disseminated aspergillosis at centers conducting these studies was considerably higher before initiation of the trial than what has been reported in other surveys (50–52). A prospective, randomized study showed, disappointingly, that the aerosol of amphotericin B offered no statistically significant advantage with respect to the number of documented infections or overall survival rate (53). Furthermore, aerosols are badly tolerated by elderly patients and those with chronic obstructive lung disease, who constitute the population with the highest risk (52).

Intravenous administration of 0.1 to 0.25 mg/kg/d amphotericin B or 0.5 mg/kg three days a week has been tested in a prophylactic setting, principally in bone marrow transplant recipients, in an endeavour to reduce the toxicity of the drug while retaining its excellent antifungal activity. In two noncomparative (39,54) and a single small randomized study in bone marrow transplant recipients (55), the incidence of all fungal infections was shown to decrease from as high as 30% to 9% with low-dose amphotericin B prophylaxis. However, the improved survival rate was not directly attributable to the prevention of fungal infection, and the results from two controlled, randomized, prospective trials using conventional amphotericin B at a dose of 0.1 mg/kg/d (56) and liposomal amphotericin B (57), respectively, failed to support this claim. Overall, too few patients were included in these studies to allow a definite conclusion. To confuse things further, the prophylactic efficacy of fluconazole, which has no activity against *Aspergillus* sp., appeared to be similar to that of low-dose intravenous amphotericin B (58). Indeed, one may wonder how dosages of 0.2 mg/kg/d could be effective against organisms that might require as much as 1 mg/kg/d for treatment. Furthermore, the combination of conventional amphotericin B with the cyclosporine may induce renal toxicity, necessitating dosage adjustments of cyclosporine and increasing the risk of graft-versus-host disease.

E. Patients with Proven Infection

Patients in whom an invasive fungal infection has been diagnosed and who then undergo further cycles of chemotherapy or a bone marrow transplant are extremely at risk. Reactivations rates as high as 50% have been reported, mainly for aspergillosis and systemic candidiasis (17). When aspergillosis is confined to one or a few lung lesions, extirpation has been recommended before further bone marrow toxic therapy is given. Others should receive amphotericin B 1 mg/kg/d starting together with the next course of chemotherapy. This strategy of secondary prophylaxis has been shown to prevent recrudescence in most leukemic patients (59).

Provided that adequate serum levels can be ensured, itraconazole might be considered for bridging the period between two consecutive neutropenic episodes in patients who have acquired an invasive fungal infection (60,61). It is believed that the chronic form of disseminated candidiasis follows an acute infectious episode, but it may also convert into a fulminant infection when the patient's immune status deteriorates. In this setting, secondary prophylaxis with either fluconazole or intravenous amphotericin B is warranted (62,63).

F. Summary of Prevention

A recent meta-analysis has failed to show a convincing survival benefit as a result of prophylactically administered antifungal agents in patients with neutropenia (64). Nevertheless, it seems not unreasonable to try to protect patients who are at high risk (Fig. 1). There is no single agent that can be recommended as gold standard for all situations. Fluconazole, given at a dose of 150 to 400 mg/d, appears appropriate for patients with expected protracted and profound neutropenia and severe mucositis who are receiving broad-spectrum antibacterials (65)

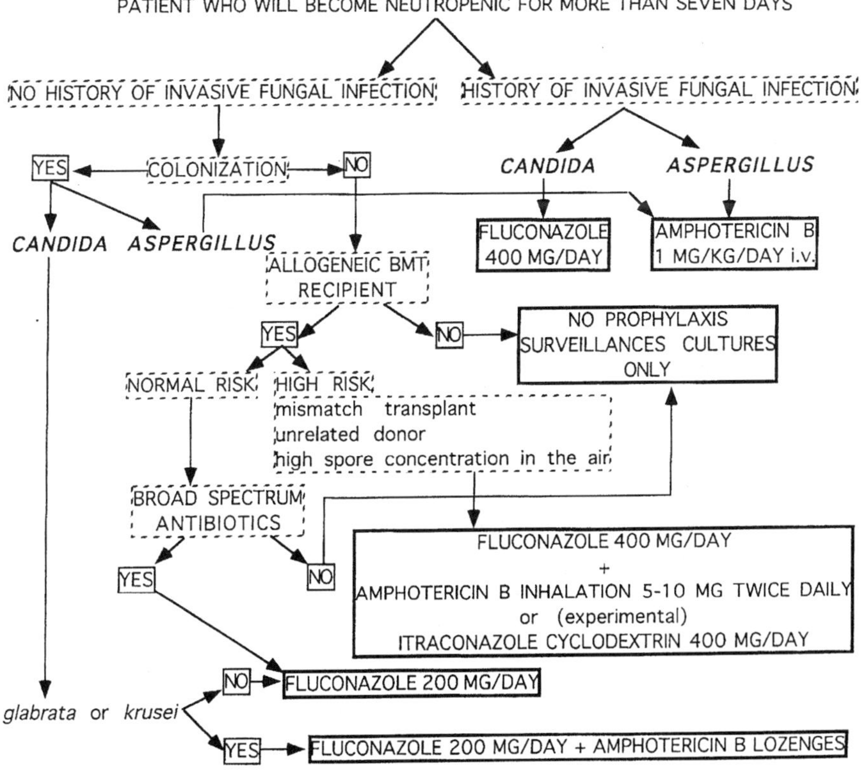

Figure 1 Algorithm for prophylaxis of fungal infections.

and for recipients of an allogeneic bone marrow transplant who are seropositive for cytomegalovirus and suffer from graft-versus-host disease (13). Fungal surveillance cultures may serve as an additional parameter to determine a subset of patients in whom invasive candidiasis is likely to develop (41). On the other hand, fungal surveillance cultures do not reliably predict systemic infection, with the exception of *C. tropicalis*, which has a relatively high likelihood of proceeding from colonization to infection (66). Patients who are colonized by fluconazole-resistant *Candida* sp., (i.e., *C. krusei* and *C. glabrata*) should be monitored closely, and early empirical therapy with amphotericin B should be initiated immediately as the signs and symptoms of systemic infection develop. The presence of *Aspergillus* sp. in the nasal cavity, sinuses, or bronchi is abnormal and has been found to be predictive of infection, although these findings vary with the spore burden in the air and may only reflect outbreaks in environments with a high spore concentration (31). Bone marrow transplant recipients might perhaps benefit from aerosolized amphotericin B of 10 to 20 mg/d in two or four divided doses and, possibly, there may soon be a role for itraconazole solution. Continuation of prophylaxis after recovery from neutropenia seems not to be indicated unless there is persistent and profound immunosuppression, such as in bone marrow transplant recipients with graft-versus-host disease. The potential for fungi to develop resistance during prophylaxis should be carefully assessed by obtaining fungal surveillance cultures regularly and testing all fungi isolated from patients for susceptibility.

VI. TREATMENT

A. Antifungal Drugs

1. Polyenes

Amphotericin B has the broadest spectrum of activity against fungi and is considered the principal antifungal agent for the treatment of systemic fungal infections in severely ill patients. There is no agreement on the therapeutic dose of amphotericin B desoxycholate; in most centers, a starting dosage of 1.0 mg/kg/d intravenously in a 1 to 4-hour infusion is used for most indications, including the prevailing cases with an unknown fungus as a causative pathogen. In view of the inherent toxicity, higher doses are only used in the treatment of refractory mycoses. Nephrotoxicity, reversible to some degree, is variable among patients and may be ameliorated by making certain that the patient is eunatremic (67). In less seriously threatened patients with an impaired kidney function and in those who receive concomitantly other possibly nephrotoxic drugs, a starting dosage of 0.7 mg/kg/d is recommended. This would suffice to control infections by certain fungal pathogens (Table 4). If the serum creatinine exceeds 250 μmol/L (or two times the baseline in children) during treatment, amphotericin B should be interrupted for 1 or 2 days to allow for recovery of the kidney function. Thereafter, amphotericin B has to be reinstituted at a dosage of 0.5 mg/kg/d, with daily increasing of the dose to the maximally tolerated level while monitoring the serum creatinine and/or potassium level. Many procedures have been suggested to mitigate the other side effects such as chills, fever, malaise, headache, nausea, or diarrhea, but there is no proof that any are helpful (67).

The inherent toxicity has fostered extensive research during the past 10 years, which has yielded lipid formulations of amphotericin B as safer alternatives to the standard deoxycholate preparation. Subsequently, the various products—amphotericin B lipid complex (Abelcet) (68–70), amphotericin B colloidal dispersion (Amphocil, Amphotec) (71,72), and liposomal amphotericin B (AmBisome) (73,74)—have been tested in many studies during the past 5 years. The new preparations cause amphotericin B to accumulate in the liver and spleen, whereas less is found in the kidney and serum relative to deoxycholate amphotericin B. Because individual pharmacological and chemical properties of these various preparations are fundamentally different, data generated by a trial on one of these drugs cannot be applied to the sister compounds. The rate of acute reactions seems to be lowest for AmBisome and highest for Amphocil, but all compounds are better tolerated than conventional amphotericin B, which suggests an improved therapeutic index (75). It is questionable whether higher dose will achieve superior results. Indeed, a recent trial by the European Organization for Research and Treatment of Cancer (EORTC) Invasive Fungal Infection Group (76) learned that a 1 mg/kg/d dosage of AmBisome was as effective as 4 mg/kg/d in treating invasive aspergillosis. However, until further data on other fungal infections are available, the use of dosages as low as 1 mg/kg/d for the initial treatment of acute fulminant fungal infections cannot be recommended because, in almost every model studied, deoxycholate amphotericin B was shown to be more efficacious than lipid-complexed amphotericin B on a milligram-per-kilogram basis. Moreover, there are limits to the safety of the lipid formulations in that decreases in creatinine clearance in conjunction with increased serum cyclosporine concentrations and low serum potassium have been found in transplant recipients (71). Nevertheless, it is of practical value to know that patients who would require amphotericin B urgently but do not tolerate the standard formulation can receive infusions of an alternative amphotericin B over 30 to 60 minutes without major discomfort. High costs are a major drawback of lipid-based amphotericin B, particularly if high dosages are being used (77). Theoretically, some costs may be recuperated because of the reduced number of expensive side effects such as nephrotoxicity, but the overall savings are probably marginal.

Amphotericin B deoxycholate dissolved in commercially available Intralipid at a dose of 1.2 mg/kg/d was suggested by French investigators as a cheaper

Table 4 Recommended Drugs for Invasive Fungal Infections

Infection	Amphotericin B deoxycholate	Amphotericin B lipid formulation	5-Flucytosine	Fluconazole	Itraconazole	Surgery useful
Candida species						
Candida albicans	0.7 mg/kg/day	3 mg/kg/day	4 dd 30 mg/kg	400–800 mg/day	400 mg/day	--
Candida glabrata	0.7 mg/kg/day	3 mg/kg/day	4 dd 30 mg/kg	800 mg/day	400 mg/day	--
Candida krusei	0.7 mg/kg/day	3 mg/kg/day	4 dd 30 mg/kg	xxx	400 mg/day	--
Candida tropicalis	0.7 mg/kg/day	3 mg/kg/day	4 dd 30 mg/kg	400 mg/day	400 mg/day	--
Candida parapsilosis	0.7 mg/kg/day	3 mg/kg/day	4 dd 30 mg/kg	400 mg/day	400 mg/day	--
Candida guillermondii	xxx	xxx	4 dd 30 mg/kg	400–800 mg/day	400 mg/day	--
Candida lusitaniae	xxx	xxx	4 dd 30 mg/kg	400–800 mg/day	400 mg/day	--
Trichosporon beigelii	1 mg/kg/day	5 mg/kg/day	xxx	800 mg/day	400 mg/day	--
Saccharomyces cerevisiae	0.7 mg/kg/day	3 mg/kg/day	xxx	400 mg/day	400 mg/day	--
Rhodutorula	0.7 mg/kg/day	3 mg/kg/day	xxx	400 mg/day	400 mg/day	--
Malassezia furfur	0.7 mg/kg/day	3 mg/kg/day	xxx	800 mg/day	400 mg/day	--
Cryptococcus neoformans	0.7 mg/kg/day	3 mg/kg/day	4 dd 30 mg/kg	400 mg/day	400 mg/day	--
Histoplasma capsulatum	0.7 mg/kg/day	3 mg/kg/day	xxx	xxx	200–400 mg/day	--
Coccidioidomycosis	0.7 mg/kg/day	3 mg/kg/day	xxx	400 mg/day	400 mg/day	--
Paracoccidioidomycosis	0.7 mg/kg/day	3 mg/kg/day	xxx	400 mg/day	200–400 mg/day	--
Blastomycosis	0.7 mg/kg/day	3 mg/kg/day	xxx	xxx	200–400 mg/day	--
Penicillium marneffei	0.7 mg/kg/day	3 mg/kg/day	xxx	800 mg/day	400 mg/day	--
Aspergillus species	1–1.25 mg/kg/day	3–5 mg/kg/day	xxx	xxx	800 mg loading dose foll. by 400 mg/day	±
Fusariosis	1.5 mg/kg/day	5 mg/kg/day	xxx	xxx	xxx	±
Mucormycosis/Zygomycosis	1.5 mg/kg/day	5 mg/kg/day	xxx	xxx	xxx	+
Pseudallescheria boydii	1.5 mg/kg/day	5 mg/kg/day	xxx	xxx	400 mg/day	+
Alternariosis	0.7 mg/kg/day	3 mg/kg/day		xxx	xxx	+
Geotrichum	xxx	xxx	xxx	xxx	400 mg/day	--

xxx = no activity and/or insufficient data.

alternative to the standard procedure against disseminated *Candida* infections in neutropenic patients but clinical experience is too limited to advocate its use in routine circumstances (78).

2. 5-Flucytosine

5-Flucytosine is a useful drug that is possibly synergistic when combined with amphotericin B against *Candida* species and *Cryptococcus* (79). Its spectrum encompasses *C. glabrata* and, in infections by this organism, it has been given as an adjunct to the triazoles. The recommended dosage, both orally and intravenously, is 100 to 150 mg/kg at 6 hourly intervals; serum concentrations should not exceed 100 mg/L. 5-Flucytosine has important limitations: when used alone, resistance ensues rapidly, and the drug is potentially toxic to the bone marrow, particularly at higher doses.

3. Azoles

The older azoles, clotrimazole and miconazole, are still successfully prescribed for superficial candidiasis. Twenty years ago, ketoconazole was promising in the treatment of yeast infections, but its toxicity and unreliable absorption tempered the initial enthusiasm. Fluconazole constitutes a far better option in the immunocompromised host. Even when used in high doses, it is the safest of all antifungal drugs and both its oral and intravenous formulations show good bioavailability. Clinically relevant interactions with cytochrome P450-associated drugs, including cyclosporine, have been observed. Absorption is not dependent on the presence of gastric acid and development of resistance during short-term use is not yet a problem. Widespread, long-term use of fluconazole may, however, shift the range of infecting organisms in a given center or ward toward less susceptible fungi. To circumvent this problem, some clinicians would combine fluconazole with intravenous amphotericin B, but currently there are no data to support this combination (80).

Itraconazole, in doses of 400 to 600 mg/d, is active against most *Candida* and *Aspergillus* species, as well as a wide array of other fungal pathogens. Toxicity is common with doses of more than 400 mg/d, although such doses probably would show the true potential of this drug in difficult-to-treat cases. Whether an initial loading dose of more than 800 mg/d followed by a lower dose over the next days would be tolerated by severely ill patients is unknown. Indeed, the unreliable absorption of the drug makes this compound less suitable in critical circumstances. The new cyclodextrin-based oral solution and intravenous preparation may obviate this problem, but hitherto these formulations have not been tested sufficiently. Other concerns about itraconazole include the possible induction or inhibition of hepatic enzymes by itraconazole and a propensity to increase intracellular levels of cytotoxic drugs, such as vincristine, which might enhance their therapeutic effects as well as toxicity (81). Prior or concurrent use of rifampicin, phenytoin, carbamazepine, and phenobarbital should be avoided (60,82), and transplant patients receiving cyclosporine who are to be given itraconazole should have an immediate cyclosporine dose reduction followed by frequent monitoring. There are theoretical considerations for possible antagonism of azoles and polyenes, but sequential use of the agents did not bear out this concern (60). This observation opens possibilities for starting treatment of critically ill patients with intravenous amphotericin B, which can be followed by oral itraconazole (83) when the patient is able to take oral medication reliably. There are no data on simultaneous administration of itraconazole with amphotericin B.

4. *New Agents*

Promising new agents like echinocandins, pneumocandins, pradimidicin, high-dose oral terbinafine, the newer azoles, voriconazole and SCH56592, and liposomal nystatin are under development and, at least some of them, will soon find their way into the therapeutic armamentarium. The first phase II study on the new azole voriconazole in 141 patients has already been reported and the results in the treatment of pulmonary aspergillosis are encouraging (84).

5. *Biological Response Modifiers*

Growth factors reduce the duration of neutropenia in both myelosuppressive and myeloablative chemotherapy, if neutropenia is defined as less than 500 granulocytes/mm^3. However, if neutropenia is defined by a granulocyte count of less than 100/mm^3, the duration of neutropenia is hardly influenced by the administration of growth factors. In profound neutropenia, growth factors should not be expected to stimulate cells that simply are not there. Consequently, the effect of growth factors on documented infections remains controversial. Data from placebo-controlled trials do not confirm a major impact on the incidence of fungal infections (85). Anaissie and colleagues found an original way to use hematopoietic growth factors. They pretreated healthy donors with growth factors and thereafter they harvested unequaled high numbers of white cells by means of leukapheresis and treated successfully some cases of therapy-refractory invasive mycoses (86).

The role of interleukins and interferons in the treatment of invasive fungal infections is still uncertain but results in animal studies warrant reasonable hope for the future (87).

B. Prognosis

The fatal outcome of a proven invasive fungal infection may well exceed 90%, particularly in cases with persisting neutropenia and unremitting underlying disease (88). To avoid this confrontation, most specialists prescribe systemic antifungal therapy to neutropenic patients who have continuing unexplained fever more than 5 days despite adequate broad-spectrum antibacterial treatment. This approach is based on two studies (89,90), which showed that a significantly lower number of systemic fungal infections was found at the end of neutropenia in patients who were given amphotericin B empirically. In the hope of improving the apparent success of this strategy, some centers initiate empirical antifungal therapy already after 3 days without there being any evidence that this might have any beneficial effect. In fact, starting too early leads to overtreatment and unnecessary toxicity in many patients. There are patients at high risk of an invasive fungal infection who will benefit from a very early institution of systemic antifungals. This pertains to the same patients who are the principal candidates for antifungal prophylaxis. If empirical treatment was restricted to this category of patients, it would constitute a preemptive rather than an empirical or prophylactic approach.

Until recently, it was assumed that amphotericin B was the only option for empirical treatment. However, in several randomized studies, empirical fluconazole, given at a dosage of 400 mg/d, proved at least as effective with respect to survival and far less toxic (91). These findings are remarkable and urge a reappraisal of the principle of empirical antifungal therapy since it was presumed that empirical antifungals aimed at early stages of mold infections and mold are not covered by flucohazole.

All empirical studies have enrolled too small numbers of patients to reach too uniform conclusions. Therefore, recommendations on the right time to start empirical antifungal therapy, the drugs to be used, and the appropriate duration are hard to formulate and, consequently, are rather based on individual perception than on scientifically valid evidence. Given its broad spectrum of activity, amphotericin B at a dosage of 1 mg/kg/d is still the drug of choice for empirical purposes; the lipid preparation should be reserved for patients who cannot tolerate the conventional formulation (92), and fluconazole should be reserved for cases with a low risk of invasive mold infections (91).

C. *Candida* Infections

1. *Superficial Candidiasis*

The diagnosis of superficial candidiasis has to be confirmed by means of microscopy or, preferably, by culture because, particularly in neutropenic patients, it is almost impossible to distinguish clinically between yeasts and other possibly causative organisms such as herpes virus and anaerobic bacteria. In general, patients should initially be given a topical antifungal agent, which should remain in contact with the lesions as long as possible (Table 5). This implicates that solutions, lozenges, or sucking pastilles should be prescribed. Clinical experience

Table 5 Antifungal Drugs for Superficial Candida Infections

Drug	Dose
Nystatin suspension	10^6U 5 times a day
Amphotericin suspension	200–400 mg 5 times a day
Amphotericin lozenges or pastilles	10 mg 4 times a day
Clotrimazole troches or suspension	5 mg 5 times a day
Miconazole suspension	100 mg 4 times a day
Fluconazole tablets or suspension	200 mg once daily

has shown that lack of compliance frequently necessitates systemic therapy for oropharyngeal and esophageal candidiasis. Patients should not be placed under too much pressure to take unpalatable medication to avoid confrontation with unreliable information on drug compatibility in unsuccessful cases or unnecessary guilt feelings. In contrast to the past, there is an attractive, tough, more expensive alternative. Fluconazole at a doses of 100 to 200 mg/d appears to be the drug of choice for this purpose.

2. Disseminated Candidiasis

Disseminated candidiasis, including candidemia, is often rapidly fatal if early therapy with antifungal drugs that have systemic activity is withheld. Because there are hardly any objective parameters to commence antifungal therapy at the most appropriate moment, the clinician has to rely on clinical impression and practical experience to make the decision of whether and when to begin treatment. Most authorities recommend antifungal therapy for patients with neutropenia and at least one positive blood culture for *Candida*. They are at extreme risk of having or of the imminent development of invasive candidiasis as is supported by autopsy evidence that many patients who die without any evidence of candidal infection during treatment for leukemia have organs that have been invaded by this fungus (1,93). Amphotericin B with or without 5-flucytosine is considered the standard therapy. It has been reported that 50% to 70% of patients, including those with *C. krusei* and *C. glabrata* infections, respond to this regimen. Similar response rates, at less toxicity, can be expected from the lipid formulations of amphotericin B. *C. lusitaniae* and *C. guilliermondii* may develop resistance to amphotericin B, such that an initially susceptible organism may become completely resistant during the course of therapy (22,94). Such patients and others with an invasive infection by susceptible *C. albicans* strains may benefit from fluconazole (Fig. 2) (63,93,95–97). A caveat is warranted about the use of fluconazole as a single agent in profound and prolonged neutropenia because under these circumstances superinfections by *Aspergillus* sp. may emerge (62,98).

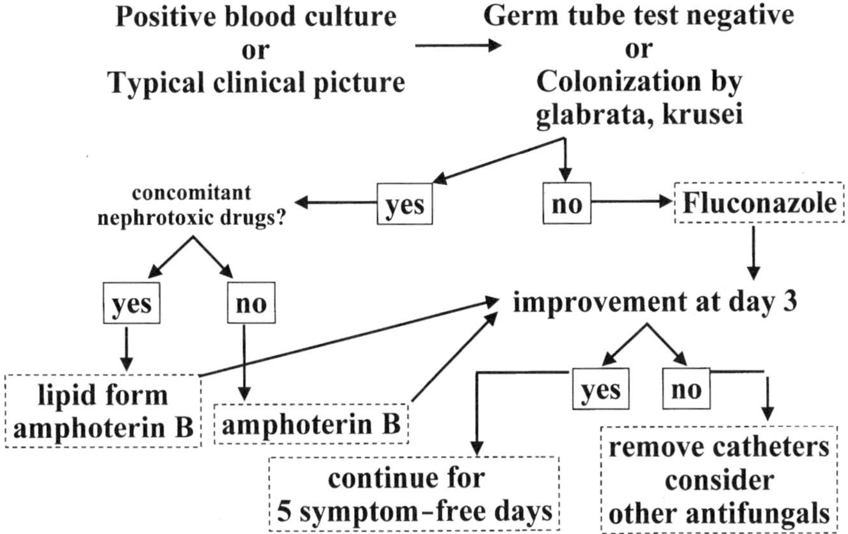

Figure 2 Algorithm for the treatment of acute candidiasis.

Given the variable susceptibilities of *Candida* sp. to fluconazole, an intravenous dosage of 800 mg/d may be considered as primary therapy for critically ill patients with hematogenous candidiasis. When the results of the cultures are available, the dose can be decreased to 400 mg/d and, depending on the clinical response, fluconazole can be given orally. Fluconazole and itraconazole are not of value in the treatment of a proven or presumed invasive fungal infection if they have been used as prophylactic agents in an adequate dosage, because it must be assumed that the offending pathogen is resistant to these drugs.

The current practice in cases of candidemia is to continue therapy at least until the resolution of granulocytopenia and fever. Whereas a short duration of therapy may be adequate for low-risk patients with candidemia, extended therapy is required for patients with extensive visceral involvement. Fluconazole and, theoretically, itraconazole provide the opportunity to manage these cases as well as chronic disseminated candidiasis in an outpatient setting, which is both convenient and less expensive (62,63,97).

3. Central Venous Line Infections

Retrospective studies in pediatric patients have suggested that removal of the central venous catheter, if present, is important to decrease the rate of complications of candidiasis (10). Conversely, another prospective study did not show any improved outcome of hematogenous candidiasis if a central venous catheter was pulled out promptly (96). Removal of a central venous catheter appears justified when a patient fails to respond to antifungal therapy within 96 hours, when candidemia persists for more than 48 hours, or when the tunnel tract is involved in the infection.

D. Aspergillus Infections

1. Amphotericin B

Conventional amphotericin B has been and remains, albeit imperfect, the standard therapy for invasive aspergillosis in neutropenic patients for 30 years. The target dose within the first day should be 1 mg/kg/d and the drug ought to be continued for at least 10 to 14 days. It is seldom possible to administer this dose to patients on cyclosporine or other potentially nephrotoxic therapy or to those with preexisting renal impairment. In these patients, the maximum tolerated dose should be explored by trial and error. Most cases of invasive aspergillosis are initially treated on a presumptive diagnosis because invasive diagnostic procedures are usually precluded by concomitant thrombocytopenia or hypoxemia. It is important that a definite diagnosis vigorously be pursued, even after treatment has commenced, and that infections by other pathogens such as actinomycosis, tuberculosis, and *Nocardia* be excluded. A questionable diagnosis nurtures uncertainty among attending physicians about the optimal therapeutic strategy, particularly if the patient is not responding optimally or if serious adverse events occur. A final diagnosis also carries an important prognostic value as well as implications for long-term treatment. Whereas the response rate of patients with persisting unexplained fever to systemically active antifungals is about 80% if neutropenia resolves, the successful outcome of documented invasive fungal infection may not, even under optimal circumstances, exceed 20% (88,98). This figure is influenced by the state of the underlying disease and possible recovery of the granulocytes. Fewer than 10% of bone marrow transplant recipients with invasive aspergillosis have survived. Especially, patients with disseminated disease or those with diffuse pulmonary disease fare worse than those with localized disease (13).

An arbitrary dose of total amphotericin B such as 1.5 to 3 g has been recommended repeatedly in the literature, but the notion that a particular dose of an antimicrobial agent might be appropriate regardless of weight of the patient and rate of delivery is unique in antimicrobial therapeutics and presumably ill-founded. This concept was perhaps based on the trivial observation that most patients with invasive fungal infections who had received less drug died. It is, however, questionable whether they died because they received an insufficient amount of amphotericin B or that the treatment course could not be completed because the patient had died of intractable disease. It is essential to see a clinical and preferably a radiological response before therapy is discontinued. On the other hand, in those in whom the criterion for commencing treatment was simply fever unresponsive to antibiotics without any evidence of invasive aspergillosis, treatment can be discontinued when the neutrophil count recovers. This also applies to those in whom the diagnosis becomes questionable during the further course of neutropenia despite initial features suspicious of invasive aspergillosis.

Lipid-based amphotericin B preparations have been used successfully in the treatment of invasive aspergillosis. However, their therapeutic niche in first line treatment is still difficult to assess because formal randomized comparisons with amphotericin B deoxycholate have never been performed. At first glance, the response rates appear superior but the vast majority of patients studied had been pretreated with amphotericin B deoxycholate (68–72,75).

2. *Surgery*

Surgery is indicated for cases in which localization of the lesions poses a direct threat of invasion of a major vessel, which can result in fatal hemorrhage, or for debridement of dead tissue after a period of antifungal therapy (99). Most units would reserve lung or lung segment resection for patients with a limited number of persisting shadows confined to one lobe who have to undergo subsequent bone marrow transplantation or more aggressive chemotherapy or to those with hemoptysis (100).

3. *Additional Options*

There is no reason to suppose that recovery from neutropenia would be any less important in contributing to a favorable outcome among patients receiving lipid-based amphotericin B.

The addition of rifampicin to amphotericin B in poorly responding patients is theoretically attractive because this combination is usually synergistic in vitro. However, rifampicin accelerates the activity of P450 enzyme system extensively and, in patients taking cyclosporine or corticosteroids, the underlying disease may flare or rejection may occur (82). The other agent that is being used for the treatment of invasive aspergillosis is itraconazole. A randomized study in neutropenic patients comparing itraconazole amphotericin B hinted at equivalence but did not reach a statistical endpoint (46). In a large open multicenter study of invasive aspergillosis performed by the Mycosis Study Group in the United States, 41% of patients showed a response by the end of therapy. In this study, all the patients were given a loading dose of 600 mg/d itraconazole for 4 days, followed by 400 mg/d thereafter (60). Unfavorable drug interactions led to failure in several patients, and the relapse rate in patients with continuing immunosuppression and a truncated course of therapy was high.

Another indication for itraconazole in the treatment of aspergillosis is infection that is resistant to amphotericin B because anecdotal responses of such cases to itraconazole have been described. Many highly immunocompromised patients require a longer duration of therapy than their period of hospitalization. For these cases, oral itraconazole after some days or weeks of amphotericin B therapy offers the opportunity of treatment on an outpatient basis (61,84).

E. Other Fungi

1. *Mucormycosis*

Localized mucormycosis is managed by aggressive surgical removal of all infected necrotic tissue, delay of further immunosuppressive therapeutic interventions when possible, and amphotericin B given at the maximum daily dose. Disseminated forms of mucormycosis are almost inevitably fatal (28). Although scanty data point to a possible usefulness of itraconazole and voriconazole, the bulk of the literature indicates that, for the time being, these compounds have no place in the treatment of infections caused by the *Mucorales*. The mainstay of antifungal therapy remains amphotericin B, but the result are disappointing in persistently neutropenic patients (28). A limited number of patients have received successful treatment with lipid-based forms of amphotericin B (68,71,75) or granulocyte transfusions obtained from growth factor-pretreated donors in combination with amphotericin B.

2. *Fusariosis*

Of all available agents, only amphotericin B seems to have marginal activity against *Fusarium*, and even this compound is not reasonably effective during neutropenia (23,101). There are some reports on successes achieved with liposomal amphotericin B (74) and amphotericin B lipid complex (68).

3. *Endemic Mycoses, Cryptococcosis, and Other Fungi*

Until recently, intravenous amphotericin B was considered the mainstay of therapy for disseminated histoplasmosis, including meningitis. Studies with the new triazoles have revealed that these agents, particularly itraconazole at a dose of 200 to 400 mg/d for approximately 1 year, are probably as effective, with success rates of 81%; the only failures occurred in the difficult-to-treat chronic cavitary form. Itraconazole proved highly efficacious against blastomycosis and has at least similar efficacy to fluconazole in coccidioidomycosis, sporotrichinosis, and paracoccidioidomycosis.

Cryptococcal disease, particularly cryptococcal meningitis, responds to both fluconazole and itraconazole, but amphotericin B with or without 5-flucytosine remains the first line choice for life-threatening cases (79).

Pseudallescheria is difficult to treat. In most cases, surgical debridement and excision of necrotic tissue should be performed in combination with prescription of systemically active antifungals. Although these organisms are often refractory to both amphotericin B and azoles, administration of itraconazole might be of benefit in some cases. The basis of the treatment of *Malassezia* infections is the withdrawal of the catheter and, in the absence of rapid improvement, intravenous amphotericin B. Experience with azole derivatives for this purpose is still limited. Despite occasional resistance, intravenous amphotericin B is the treatment of choice for systemic *Trichosporon beigelii* infections; in less acute situations, itraconazole may be considered as an appropriate alternative. If the infection is left untreated, 75% of patients will die of this infection. In patients with severe granulocytopenia, the rapid recovery of neutrophils is of utmost importance.

Alternariosis may emerge during prophylaxis with fluconazole. Therapy requires surgical excision and intravenous amphotericin B (26). *S. cerevisiae* and *Rhodotorula* have a low virulence. The infections usually resolve with the withdrawal of the catheter but some require additional treatment with intravenous amphotericin B or, alternatively, itraconazole and fluconazole. Intravenous amphotericin B also constitutes the first line therapy for *P. marneffei* with itraconazole and, to a far lesser extent, fluconazole as acceptable alternatives. Conversely, for *Geotrichum* infections, itraconazole appears to be the drug of choice in view of the unpredictable susceptibility to amphotericin B.

4. *Pneumocystis carinii*

The recommended dose of trimethoprim-sulfamethoxazole for *P. carinii* infections is 15 mg/kg/d in three or four divided doses for 14 to 21 days. Pentamidine at a dose of 4 mg/kg in a slow daily intravenous infusion over 1 to 2 hours is an accepted alternative for those who do not tolerate trimethoprim-sulfamethoxazole, the combinations of trimethoprim (20 mg/kg/d in four divided oral doses) with dapsone (100 mg/d as a single oral dose) and clindamycin (2400 mg/d in four divided intravenous doses) with primaquine (15 mg/d as a single oral dose) being less extensively tested options. For severe cases, adjunctive corticosteroids should be used at an initial dosage of 60 mg/d followed by tapering with improvement of the clinical condition.

VII. CONCLUSION

Factors such as the intensification of antitumor regimens, the expanded application of bone marrow transplantation to high-risk groups with attendant greater depth of immunodeficiency and prolonged delay in immune reconstitution, and the changing repertoire of fungi have led to an increased risk of fungal infections.

Clinicians need to be aware of the many issues involved in the diagnosis of fungal infections because problems in the management of these infections are more the consequence of diagnostic shortcomings than the lack of therapeutic options.

REFERENCES

1. Bodey GP, Bueltmann B, Duguid W, Gibbs D, Hanak H, Mall G, Martino P, Meunier F, Milliken S, Naoe S, Okudaira M, Scevola D, van't Wout J. Fungal infections in cancer patients: an international autopsy survey. Eur J Clin Microbiol Infect Dis 1992; 11:99–109.
2. Beck-Saqué CM, Jarvis WR, National Nosocomial Infections Surveillance Team. Secular trends in the epidemiology of nosocomial fungal infections in the United States, 1980–1990. J Infect Dis 1993; 167:1247–1251.
3. Fraser VJ, Jones M, Dunkel J, Storfer S, Medoff G, Dunagan WC. Candidemia in a tertiary care hospital: epidemiology, risk factors, and predictors of mortality. Clin Infect Dis 1992; 15:414–421.
4. Groll AH, Shah PM, Mentzel C, Schneider M, Just-Nuebling G, Hueber K. Trends in the postmortem epidemiology of invasive fungal infections at a university hospital. J Infect 1996; 33:23–32.
5. Wey SB, Mori M, Pfaller MA, Woolson RF, Wenzel RP. Risk factors for hospital-acquired candidemia. A matched case-control study. Arch Intern Med 1989; 149: 2349–2353.
6. Gerson SL, Talbot GH, Hurwitz S, Strom BL, Lusk EJ, Cassileth PA. Prolonged granulocytopenia: the major risk factor for invasive pulmonary aspergillosis in patients with acute leukemia. Ann Intern Med 1984; 100:345–351.
7. De Pauw BE. Practical modalities for prevention of fungal infections in cancer patients. Eur J Clin Microbiol Infect Dis 1997; 16:32–41.
8. Bow EJ, Loewen R, Cheang MS, Shore TB, Rubinger M, Schachter B. Cytotoxic therapy-induced D-xylose malabsorption and invasive infection during remission-induction therapy for acute myeloid leukemia in adults. J Clin Oncol 1997; 15: 2254–2261.
9. Burnie JP, Odds F, Lee W, Webster C, Williams JD. Outbreak of systemic *Candida albicans* in intensive care unit caused by cross infection. BMJ 1985; 290:746.
10. Lecciones JA, Lee JW, Navarro EE, Witebsky-FG, Marshall D, Steinberg SM, Pizzo PA, Walsh TJ. Vascular catheter-associated fungemia in patients with cancer: analysis of 155 episodes. Clin Infect Dis 1992; 14:875–883.
11. Dewhurst AG, Cooper MJ, Khan SM, Pallett AP, Dathan JRE. Invasive aspergillosis in immunosuppressed patients: potential hazard of hospital building work. BMJ 1990; 301:802–804.
12. Robertson MJ, Larssen RA. Recurrent fungal pneumonias in patients with acute nonlymphocytic leukemia undergoing multiple courses of intensive chemotherapy. Am J Med 1988; 84:233–239.
13. Morrison VA, Haake RJ, Weisdorf DJ. Non-candidal fungal infections after bone marrow transplantation: risk factors and outcome. Am J Med 1994; 96:497–503.

14. Goodrich JM, Reed EC, Mori M, Fisher LD, Skerrett S, Dandliker PS, Klis B, Counts GW, Meyers JD. Clinical features and analysis of risk factors for invasive candidal infection after marrow transplantation. J Infect Dis 1991; 164:731–740.
15. Bodey GP, Anaissie EJ. Opportunistic fungal infections: a major problem in immunocompromised patients. In: Richardson RG, ed. Opportunistic Fungal Infections: Focus on Fluconazole. New York: Royal Society of Medicine Services Limited 1989:1–16.
16. Meunier F, Aoun M, Bitar N. Candidemia in immunocompromised patients. Clin Infect Dis 1992; 14(suppl 1):S120–S125.
17. Wingard JR, Merz WG, Rinaldi MG, Johnson TR, Karp JE, Saral R: Increase in *Candida krusei* infection among patients with bone marrow transplantation and neutropenia treated prophylactically with fluconazole. N Engl J Med 1991; 325: 1274–1277.
18. Wingard JR, Merz WG, Rinaldi MG, Miller CB, Karp JE, Saral R. Association of *Torulopsis glabrata* infections in neutropenic bone marrow transplantation patients. Antimicrob Agents Chemother 1993; 37:1847–1849.
19. Goodman JL, Winston DJ, Greenfield RA, Chandrasekar PH, Fox B, Kaizer H, Shadduck RK, Shea T, Stiff P, Friedman DJ, Powderley WG, Silber JL, Horowitz H, Lichtin A, Wolff SN, Nangan KF, Silver SM, Weisdorf D, Ho WG, Gilver G, Buell D. A controlled trial of fluconazole to prevent fungal infections in patients undergoing bone marrow transplantation. N Engl J Med 1992; 326:845–851.
20. Menichetti F, Del Favero A, Martino P, Bucaneve G, Micozzi A, D'Antonio D, Ricci P, Carotenuto M, Liso V, Nosari AM, Barbui T, Fasola G, Mandelli F, The GIMEMA Infection Program. Preventing fungal infection in neutropenic patients with acute leukemia: fluconazole compared with oral amphotericin B. Ann Intern Med 1994; 120:913–918.
21. Wingard JR, Merz WG, Saral R. *Candida tropicalis*: a major pathogen in immunocompromised patients. Ann Intern Med 1979; 91:539–543.
22. Dick JD, Rosenguard BR, Merz WG, Stuart RK, Hutchins GM, Saral R. Fatal disseminated candidiasis due to amphotericin B-resistant *Candida guilliermondii*. Ann Intern Med 1985; 102:67–68.
23. Boutati EI, Anaissie EJ. *Fusarium*, a significant emerging pathogen in patients with hematologic malignancy: ten years' experience at a cancer center and implications for management. Blood 1997; 90:999–1008.
24. Supparatpinyo K, Chiewchanvit S, Hirunsri P, Uthammachai C, Nelson KE, Sirisanthana T. *Penicillium marneffei* infection in patients infected with human immunodefiency virus. Clin Infect Dis 1992; 14:871–874.
25. Mesnard R, Lamy T, Dauriac C, Le Prise PY. Lung abscess due to *Pseudallescheria boydii* in the course of acute leukaemia. Report of a case and review of the literature. Acta Haematol 1992; 87:78–82.
26. Morrison VA, Weisdorf DJ. *Alternaria*: A sinonasal pathogen of immunocompromised hosts. Clin Infect Dis 1993; 16:265–270.
27. Shearer C, Chandrasekar PH. Cutaneous alternariosis and regional lymphadenitis during allogeneic BMT. Bone Marrow Transplant 1993; 11:497–499.
28. Pagano L, Ricci P, Tonso A, Nosari A, Cudillo L, Montillo M, Cenacchi A, Pacilli L, Fabbiano F, Del Favero A, and the GIMEMA infection program (Gruppo Italiano

Malattie Ematologiche Maligne dell'Adulto). Mucormycosis in patients with haematological malignancies: a retrospective clinical study of 37 cases. Br J Haematol 1997; 99:331–336.

29. Kuhlman JE, Fishman EK, Siegelman SS. Invasive pulmonary aspergillosis in acute leukemia: characteristic findings on CT, the CT halo sign, and the role of CT in early diagnosis. Radiology 1985; 157:611–614.
30. Caillot D, Casasnovas O, Bernard A, Couaillier J-F, Durant C, Cuisenier B, Solary E, Pirard F, Petrella T, Bonnin A, Couillault G, Dumas M, Guy H. Improved management of invasive pulmonary aspergillosis in neutropenic patients using early thoracic computed tomographic scan and surgery. J Clin Oncol 1997; 15:139–147.
31. Yu VL, Muder RR, Poorsatter A. Significance of isolation of *Aspergillus* from the respiratory tract in diagnosis of invasive pulmonary aspergillosis. Results from a three-year prospective study. Am J Med 1986; 81:249–254.
32. Thaler M, Pastakia B, Shawker TH, O'Leary T, Pizzo PA. Hepatic candidiasis in cancer patients: the evolving picture of the syndrome. Ann Intern Med 1988; 108: 88–100.
33. Linker CA, DeGregorio MW, Ries CA. Computerized tomography in the diagnosis of systemic candidiasis in patients with acute leukemia. Med Pediatr Oncol 1984; 12:380–385.
34. Talbot HG, Werner MH, Gerson SL, Provencher M, Hurwitz S. Serodiagnosis of invasive aspergillosis in patients with hematological malignancy: validation of the *Aspergillus fumigatus* radio-immunoassay. J Infect Dis 1987; 155:12–27.
35. Verweij PE, Stynen D, Rijs AJMM, de Pauw BE, Hoogkamp-Korstanje JA, Meis JF. Sandwich enzyme-linked immunosorbent assay compared with Pastorex latex agglutination test for diagnosing invasive aspergillosis in immunocompromised patients. J Clin Microbiol 1995; 33:1912–1914.
36. Walsh TJ, Hathorn JW, Sobel JD, Merz WG, Sanchez V, Maret SM, Buckley HR, Pfaller MA, Schaufele R, Sliva C. Detection of circulating candida enolase by immunoassay in patients with cancer and invasive candidiasis. N Engl J Med 1991; 324:1026–1031.
37. Verweij PE, Latgé JP, Rijs AJMM, Melchers WJG, De Pauw BE, Hoogkamp-Korstanje JAA, Meis JFGM. Comparison of antigen detection and PCR assay using bronchoalveolar lavage fluid for diagnosing invasive pulmonary aspergillosis in patients receiving treatment for hematological malignancies. J Clin Microbiol 1995; 33:3150–3153.
38. Oyen WJG, Claessens RAMJ, Raemaekers JMM, de Pauw BE, van der Meer JW, Corstens FH. Diagnosing infection in febrile granulocytopenic patients with indium-111 labelled human immunoglobulin G. J Clin Oncol 1992; 10:61–68.
39. Hughes WT, Rivera GK, Schell MJ, Thornton D, Lott L. Successful intermittent chemoprophylaxis for *Pneumocystis carinii* pneumonitis. N Engl J Med 1987; 316: 1627–1632.
40. O'Donnell MR, Schmidt GM, Tegtmeier BR, Faucett C, Fahey JL, Ito J, Nademanee A, Niland J, Parker P, Smith EP, Snyder DS, Stein AS, Blume KG, Forman SJ. Prediction of systemic fungal infection in allogeneic marrow recipients: impact of amphotericin prophylaxis in high-risk patients. J Clin Oncol 1994; 12:827–834.

41. Martino P, Girmenia C, Venditti M, Girmenia C, Mandelli F. *Candida* colonization and systemic infection in neutropenic patients. Cancer 1989; 64:2030–2034.
42. Donnelly JP, Starke ID, Galton DAG, Catovsky D, Goldman JM, Darrell JH. Oral ketoconazole and amphotericin B for the prevention of yeast colonization in patients with acute leukaemia. J Hosp Infect 1984; 5:83–91.
43. Slavin MA, Osborne B, Adams R, Levenstein MJ, Schoch HG, Feldman AR, Meyers JD, Bowden RA. Efficacy and safety of fluconazole prophylaxis for fungal infections after marrow transplantation—a Prospective, randomized double blind study. J Infect Dis 1995; 171:1545–1552.
44. Alangaden G, Chandrasekar PH, Bailey E, Kaliq Y, and the Bone Marrow Transplantation Team. Antifungal prophylaxis with low-dose fluconazole during bone marrow transplantation. Bone Marrow Transplantation 1994; 14:919–924.
45. Winston DW, Chandrasekar PH, Lazarus HM, Goodman JL, Silber JL, Horowitz H, Shadduck RK, Rosenfeld CS, Ho WG, Islam MZ, Buell DN. Fluconazole prophylaxis of fungal infections in patients with acute leukemia. Results of a randomized placebo-controlled, double blind, multicenter trial. Ann Intern Med 1993; 118: 495–503.
46. Van't Wout JW, Novakova I, Verhagen CAH, Fibbe WE, De Pauw BE, Van der Meer JWM. The efficacy of itraconazole against systemic fungal infections in neutropenic patients: a randomized comparative study with amphotericin B. B J Infect 1991; 22:45–52.
47. Vreugdenhil G, Van Dijke BJ, Donnelly JP, Novakova IRO, Raemaekers JMM, Hoogkamp-Korstanje MAA, De Pauw B. Efficacy of itraconazole in the prevention of fungal infections among neutropenic patients with hematological malignancies and intensive chemotherapy. A double blind, placebo controlled study. Leuk Lymphoma 1993; 11:353–358.
48. Prentice AG, Warnock DW, Johnson SA, Phillips MJ, Oliver DA. Multiple dose pharmacokinetics of an oral solution of itraconazole in autologous bone marrow transplant recipients. J Antimicrob Chemother 1994; 34:247–252.
49. Schaffner A, Böhler A. Amphotericin B refractory aspergillosis after itraconazole: evidence for significant antagonism. Mycoses 1993; 36:421–424.
50. Conneally E, Cafferkey MT, Daly PA, Keane CT, McCann SR. Nebulized amphotericin B as prophylaxis against invasive aspergillosis in granulocytopenic patients. Bone Marrow Transplantation 1990; 5:403–406.
51. Jeffery GM, Beard MEJ, Ikram RB, Chau J, Allen JR, Heaton DC, Hart DNJ, Schousboe MI. Intranasal amphotericin B reduces the frequency of invasive aspergillosis in neutropenic patients. Am J Med 1991; 90:685–692.
52. Erjavec Z, Woolthuis GMH, De Vries-Hospers HG, Sluiter WJ, Daenen SMGJ, De Pauw BE, Halie MR. Tolerance and efficacy of amphotericin B inhalations for prevention of invasive pulmonary aspergillosis in haematological patients. Eur J Clin Microbiol Infect Dis 1997; 16:364–368.
53. Behre G, Schwartz S, Lenz K, Ludwig W-D, Wandt H, Schilling E, Heinemann V, Link H, Trittin A, Boenisch O, Treder W, Siegert W, Hiddemann W, Beyer J. Aerosol amphotericin B inhalations for the prevention of invasive pulmonary aspergillosis in neutropenic cancer patients. Ann Hematol 1995; 71:287–291.
54. Rousey SR, Russler S, Gottlieb M, Ash RC. Low-dose amphotericin B prophylaxis

against invasive *Aspergillus* infections in allogeneic marrow transplantation. Am J Med 1991; 91:484–492.
55. Riley DK, Pavia AT, Beatty PG, Petersen FB, Spruance JL, Stokes R, Evans TG. The prophylactic use of low-dose amphotericin B in bone marrow transplant patients. Am J Med 1994; 97:509–514.
56. Perfect J, Klotman ME, Gilbert CC, Crawford DD, Rosner GL, Wright KA, Peters WP. Prophylactic intravenous amphotericin B in neutropenic autologous bone marrow transplant recipients. J Infect Dis 1992; 165:891–897.
57. Tollemar J, Ringden O, Andersson S, Sundberg B, Ljungman P, Sparrelid E, Tyden G. Prophylactic use of liposomal amphotericin B (AmBisome) against fungal infections: a randomized trial in bone marrow transplant recipients. Transplant Proc 1993; 25:1495–1497.
58. Bodey GP, Anaissie EJ, Elting LS, Estey E, Obrien S, Kantarjian H. Antifungal prophylaxis during remission induction therapy for acute leukemia: fluconazole versus intravenous amphotericin B. Cancer 1994; 73:2099–2106.
59. Karp JE, Burch PA, Merz WG. An approach to intensive antileukemic therapy in patients with previous invasive aspergillosis. Am J Med 1988; 85:203–206.
60. Denning DW, Lee JY, Hostetler JS, Pappas P, Kaufmann CA, Dewsnup DH, Galgiani JN, Graybill JR, Sugar AM, Catanzaro A, Gallis H, Perfect JR, Dockery B, Dismukes WE, Stevens DA. NIAID mycosis study group multicenter trial of oral itraconazole therapy for invasive aspergillosis. Am J Med 1994; 97:135–144.
61. Nosari A, Cantoni S, Muti G, Cairoli R, Cipriani D, De Cataldo F. Itraconazole in leukemic patients with invasive aspergillosis (IA): impact on intensive chemotherapy completion. Eur J Haematol 1994; 53:183–185.
62. Anaissie E, Bodey GP, Kantarjian H, David C, Barnett K, Bow E, Defelice R, Downs N, File T, Karam G. Fluconazole therapy for disseminated candidiasis in patients with leukemia and prior amphotericin B therapy. Am J Med 1991; 91: 143–150.
63. De Pauw BE, Raemaekers JMM, Donnelly JP, Kullberg B-J, Meis JFGM. An open study on the safety and efficacy of fluconazole in the treatment of disseminated *Candida* infections in patients treated for a hematological malignancy. Ann Hematol 1995; 70:83–87.
64. Gøtzsche PC, Johansen HK. Meta-analysis of prophylactic or empirical antifungal treatment versus placebo or no treatment in patients with cancer complicated by neutropenia. BMJ 1997; 314:1238–1244.
65. Guiot HFL, Fibbe WE, Van't Wout JW. Risk factors for fungal infection in patients with malignant hematological disorders: implications for empirical therapy and prophylaxis. Clin Infect Dis 1994; 18:525–532.
66. Sanford GR, Merz WG, Wingard JR, Sarache P, Saral R. The value of surveillance cultures as predictors of systemic fungal infections. J Infect Dis 1980; 142:503–509.
67. Meyer RD. Current role of therapy with amphotericin B. Clin Infect Dis 1992; 14(suppl 1):S154–S160.
68. Lister J. Amphotericin B lipid complex (Abelcet) in the treatment of invasive mycoses: the North American experience. Eur J Haematol 1996; 56(suppl 57):18–23.
69. Walsh TJ, Hiemenz J, Seibel E, Anaissie EJ. Amphotericin B lipid complex in the

treatment of 228 cases of invasive mycosis. In: Program and Abstracts of the Thirty-Fourth Interscience Conference on Antimicrobial Agents and Chemotherapy, Orlando, USA. Washington, DC: American Society of Microbiology, 1994:(abstr M69) 247.

70. Mehta J, Kelsey S, Chu P, Powles R, Hazel D, Riley U, Evans C, Newland A, Trelaeven J, Singhal S. Amphotericin B lipid complex (ABLC) for the treatment of confirmed or presumed fungal infections in immunocompromised patients with hematologic malignancies. Bone Marrow Transplant 1997; 20:39–43.
71. Oppenheim BA, Herbrecht R, Kusne S. The safety and efficacy of amphotericin B colloidal dispersion in the treatment of invasive mycoses. Clin Infect Dis 1995; 21:1145–1153.
72. White MH, Anaissie EJ, Kusne S, Wingard JR, Hiemenz JW, Cantor A, Gurwith M, Du Mond C, Mamelok RD, Bowden RA. Amphotericin B colloidal dispersion vs. amphotericin B as therapy for invasive aspergillosis. Clin Infect Dis 1997; 24: 635–642.
73. Tollemar J, Andersson S, Ringden O, Tyden G. A retrospective clinical comparison between antifungal treatment with liposomal amphotericin B (AmBisome) and conventional amphotericin B in transplant recipients. Mycoses 1992; 35:215–220.
74. Ng TTC, Denning DW. Liposomal amphotericin B (AmBisome) therapy in invasive fungal infections. Evaluation of United Kingdom compassionate use data. Arch Intern Med 1995; 155:1093–1098.
75. Leenders ACAP, de Marie S. The use of lipid formulations of amphotericin B for systemic fungal infections. Leukemia 1996; 10:1570–1575.
76. Ellis M, Spence D, Meunier F, De Pauw BE, Bogaerts M, Van der Cam B, Doyen C, Marinus A, Colette L, Sylvester R, EORTC IFICG Brussels. (1996) Randomised multicentre trial of 1mg/kg (LD) versus 4mg/kg (HD) liposomal amphotericin B (Ambisome) (LAB) in the treatment of invasive aspergillosis (IA). In: Program and Abstracts of the Thirty-Sixth Interscience Conference on Antimicrobial Agents and Chemotherapy, New Orleans, USA. Washington, DC: American Society of Microbiology, 1996:(abstr LM39) 287.
77. Gutiérrez F, Wall PG, Cohen J. An audit on the use of antifungal agents. J Antimicrob Chemother 1996; 37:175–185.
78. Caillot D, Casasnovas O, Solary E, Chavanet P, Bonnotte B, Reny G, Entezam F, Lopez J, Bonnin A, Guy H. Efficacy and tolerance of of an amphotericin B lipid (Intralipid) emulsion on the treatment of candidaemia in neutropenic patients. J Antimicrob Chemother 1993; 31:161–169.
79. Bennet J, Dismukes W, Duma R, Medoff R, Sande M, Gallis H, Leonard J, Fields B, Bradshaw M, Haywood H, McGee ZA, Cate T, Cobbs C, Warner J. A comparison of amphotericin B alone and combined with flucytosine in the treatment of cryptococcal meningitis. N Engl J Med 1979; 301:126–131.
80. Sugar AM. Use of amphotericin B with azole antifungal drugs: what are we doing? Antimicrob Agents Chemother 1995; 39:1907–1912.
81. Vreugdenhil G, Raemaekers JMM, Van Dijke BJ, De Pauw BE. Itraconazole and multidrug resistance: possible effects on remission rate and disease-free survival in acute leukemia. Ann Hematol 1993; 67:107–109.
82. Tucker RM, Denning DW, Hanson LH, Rinaldi MG, Graybill JR, Sharkey PK,

Pappagianis D, Stevens DA. The interaction of azoles with rifampin, phenytoin and carbamazepine: *in vitro* and clinical observations. Clin Infect Dis 1992; 14: 165–174.

83. Caillot D, Casasnovas O, Solary E. Itraconazole as salvage therapy in invasive pulmonary aspergillosis occurring during amphotericin B therapy in neutropenic patients. Chemotherapy 1992; 38:50–51.
84. Denning DW, Del Favero A, Gluckman E, Rhunke M, Yonren S, Troke P, Sarantis N. The efficacy and tolerability of UK 109,496 (voriconazole) in the treatment of invasive aspergillosis (IA). Abtractbook 13th Congress of the International Society for Human and Animal Mycology. Salsomaggiore Terme, Italy, 1997:(abstr P552) 217.
85. Offner F. Hematopoietic growth factors in cancer patients with invasive fungal infections. Eur J Clin Microbiol Infect Dis 1997; 16:56–63.
86. Walsh TJ, De Pauw B, Anaissie E, Martino P. Recent advances in the epidemiology, prevention and treatment of invasive fungal infections in neutropenic patients. J Med Vet Mycol 1994; 32(suppl 1):33–51.
87. Kullberg BJ. Trends in immunotherapy of fungal infections. Eur J Clin Microbiol Infect Dis 1997; 16:51–55.
88. Verwey PE, Donnelly JP, Kullberg BJ, Meis JFGM, De Pauw BE. Amphotericin B versus amphotericin B plus 5-flucytosine: poor results in the treatment of proven mycoses in neutropenic patients. Infection 1994; 22:81–85.
89. Pizzo PA, Robichaud KJ, Gill FA, Witebsky FG. Empiric antibiotic and antifungal therapy for cancer patients with prolonged fever and granulocytopenia. Am J Med 1984; 72:101–107.
90. EORTC International Antimicrobial Therapy Cooperative Group. Empiric antifungal therapy in febrile neutropenic patients. Am J Med 1989; 86:668–672.
91. Viscoli C, Castagnola E, Van Lint MT, Moroni C, Garaventa A, Rossi MR, Fanci R, Menichetti F, Caselli D, Giacchino M, Congiu M. Fluconazole versus amphotericin B as empirical antifungal therapy of unexplained fever in granulocytopenic cancer patients: a pragmatic, multicentre, prospective and randomized trial. Eur J Cancer 1996; 32A:814–820.
92. Prentice HG, Hann IM, Herbrecht R, Aoun M, Kvalov S, Catovsky D, Pinkerton CR, Schey SA, Jacobs F, Oakhill A, Stevens RF, Darbyshire PJ, Gibson BES. A randomised comparison of liposomal versus conventional amphotericin B for the treatment of pyrexia of unknown origin in neutropenic patients. Br J Haematol 1997; 98:711–718.
93. Edwards JE, Bodey GP, Bowden RA, Büchner T, de Pauw BE, Filler SG, Ghannoum MA, Glauser M, Herbrecht R, Kauffman CA, Kohno S, Martino P, Meunier F, Mori T, Pfaller MA, Rex JH, Rogers TR, Rubin RH, Solomkin J, Viscoli C, Walsh TJ, White M. International conference for the development of a consensus on the management and prevention of severe candidal infections. Clin Infect Dis 1997; 25:43–59.
94. Merz WG. *Candida lusitaniae*: frequency of recover, colonization, infection, and amphotericin B resistance. J Clin Microbiol 1984; 20:1194–1195.
95. Anaissie EJ, Vartivarian SE, Abi-Said D, Uzun O, Pinczowski H, Kontoyiannis DP, Khoury P, Papadakis K, Gardner A, Raad II, Gilbreath J, Bodey GP. Flucona-

zole versus amphotericin B in the treatment of hematogenous candidiasis: a matched cohort study. Am J Med 1996; 101:170–176.

96. Anaissie EJ, Darouiche RO, Abi-Said D, Mera J, Gentry LO, Williams T, Kontoyiannis DP, Karl CL, Bodey GP. Management of invasive candidal infections: results of a prospective, randomized, multicenter study of fluconazole versus amphotericin B and a review of the literature. Clin Infect Dis 1996; 23:964–972.
97. Kaufman CA, Bradley SF, Ross SC, Weber DR. Hepatosplenic candidiasis: successful treatment with fluconazole. Am J Med 1991; 91:137–141.
98. Meis JF, Donnelly JP, Hoogkamp-Korstanje JA, De Pauw BE. *Aspergillus fumigatus* pneumonia in neutropenic patients during therapy with fluconazole for infection due to *Candida* species. Clin Infect Dis 1993; 16:734–735.
99. Denning DW, Stevens DA. Antifungal and surgical treatment of invasive aspergillosis: review of 2121 published cases. Rev Infect Dis 1992; 24:1147–1201.
100. McWhinney PHM, Kibbler CC, Hamon MD, Smith PO, Gandhi L, Berger LA, Walesby RK, Hoffbrand AV, Prentice HG. Progress in the diagnosis and management of aspergillosis in bone marrow transplantation: thirteen years experience. Clin Infect Dis 1993; 17:397–404.
101. Krcmery V, Jesenska Z, Spanik S, Gyarfas J, Nogova J, Botek R, Mardiak J, Sufliarsky J, Sisolakova J, Vanickova M, Kunova A, Studena M, Trupl J. Fungemia due to *Fusarium* spp in cancer patients. J Hosp Infect 1997; 36:223–228.

3

Management of Viral Infections

Pierre Reusser
University Hospital, Basel, Switzerland

I. INTRODUCTION

Immunodeficient cancer patients carry a substantial risk for serious viral disease. Both the underlying malignancy and the various cancer treatment modalities contribute to the immunosuppression that predisposes to viral reactivation and to more severe primary infection or reinfection (1). In addition, the transfusion of blood products, which is a frequent requirement in patients with neoplastic disorders, and the use of allogeneic bone marrow transplant (BMT) or peripheral blood stem cell transplant (PBSCT) increase the risk for transmission of viral agents (2–4). Patients who are particularly susceptible to diseases caused by viruses include those receiving treatment for leukemia or lymphoma and the recipients of allogeneic or autologous BMT and PBSCT (5–11).

Significant morbidity in immunocompromised cancer patients has been clearly demonstrated for several DNA and RNA viruses (Table 1). In general, DNA viruses are a more common cause of infection than RNA viruses, which may be related to their propensity to establish long-term latency following primary infection and to reactivate during periods of profound immunosuppression (1). In recent years, efficient strategies for the prevention and treatment of diseases caused by herpes simplex virus (HSV), varicella-zoster virus (VZV), and cytomegalovirus (CMV) in immunocompromised hosts were developed (1,7,12,13). Progress was primarily made possible by the introduction into clini-

Table 1 Viruses Causing Significant Morbidity in Immunodeficient Cancer Patients

DNA viruses	RNA viruses
Herpes simplex virus types 1 and 2	Respiratory syncytial virus
Varicella-zoster virus	Rhinovirus
Cytomegalovirus	Influenza virus types A, B, C
Epstein-Barr virus	Parainfluenza virus types 1 to 4
Human herpesvirus 6	Measles virus
Hepatitis B virus	Hepatitis A and C viruses
Adenovirus	Rotavirus
Polyomaviruses (JC, BK)	

Source: Ref. 12.

cal use of rapid and sensitive diagnostic techniques and of potent antiviral agents against these viruses (Fig. 1). This chapter reviews the current concepts and future prospects for the management of disease caused by HSV, VZV, and CMV, and it briefly discusses the challenging and mostly unresolved issue of treating other viral infections in cancer patients.

II. HERPES SIMPLEX VIRUS INFECTION

A. Frequency, Clinical Presentation, and Diagnosis

Most adult patients with malignancy are HSV seropositive and are thus at risk for reactivation of latent virus. In the absence of antiviral drug prophylaxis, HSV reactivation was documented in up to 80% of seropositive patients during induction chemotherapy for acute leukemia or in the first month after allogeneic BMT (7). Herpes simplex virus disease in cancer patients usually develops at mucocutaneous sites, including the orofacial region in 85% to 90% of cases and the genital area in 10% to 15%, and the diagnosis can often be made on clinical grounds alone (1,7). However, if severe mucositis is present, laboratory confirmation of oropharyngeal HSV infection may be required to substantiate the need for antiviral therapy. Another common manifestation of HSV infection is esophageal disease, which is present in about 10% of cancer patients who have symptoms of esophagitis (7,14). Infrequent presentations of HSV disease include pneumonia, encephalitis, hepatitis, adrenalitis, and bone marrow suppression (7,15–17).

Serological studies are not helpful in diagnosing active HSV infection among immunocompromised hosts, but they permit identification of patients at risk for HSV reactivation. Cell culture has been the standard method for identification of HSV in clinical specimens, and results are usually obtained within 48 hours

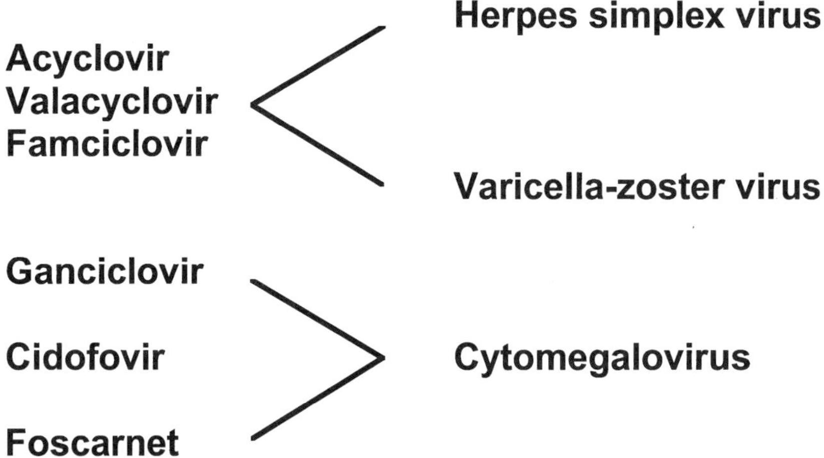

Figure 1 Antiviral drugs currently available for clinical use against herpesviruses. The drugs are grouped according to their main indications in the prevention and therapy of diseases caused by herpes simplex virus, varicella-zoster virus, and cytomegalovirus. Acyclovir is also used in high doses in the prevention of CMV infection after allogeneic bone marrow transplantation. (From Ref. 12.)

of cell inoculation. Antigen detection assays are more rapid, but their sensitivity decreases with more advanced stages of HSV lesions. Recently, the polymerase chain reaction (PCR) became available as a highly sensitive and specific technique for detection of HSV infection, and it has proved particularly useful in the diagnosis of HSV encephalitis (18,19).

B. Prevention and Therapy

Acyclovir has been extensively studied in immunodeficient hosts and is currently the drug of choice for both prophylaxis and therapy of HSV disease in patients with malignancy (12,20). Prophylactic acyclovir treatment is standard of care at many cancer centers for HSV seropositive patients receiving intensive chemotherapy or undergoing BMT and PBSCT. By contrast, antiviral prophylaxis is not warranted in HSV seronegative patients because their risk for HSV infection is very low. Recommended regimens for acyclovir prophylaxis and for therapy of established mucocutaneous or esophageal HSV disease are summarized in Table 2 (1,20). The therapy of HSV disease at other sites has not been systematically studied in cancer patients. Because of the often lethal outcome of HSV

Table 2 Prevention and Therapy of HSV Disease

Indication	Antiviral drug	Dosage and route	Duration
Prevention[a]			
Induction chemotherapy for acute leukemia	Acyclovir	250 mg/m^2 or 5 mg/kg q 12 h IV or	3–5 wk after initiation of chemotherapy or of conditioning regimen for BMT or PBSCT
Intensive chemotherapy/radiotherapy followed by autologous BMT or PBSCT		From 200 mg tid to 800 mg bid p.o.	
Therapy			
Mucocutaneous or esophageal disease	Acyclovir	250 mg/m^2 or 5 mg/kg q 8 h IV or 200–400 mg 5 times per day p.o.	7–10 d
Pneumonia, encephalitis	Acyclovir	500 mg/m^2 or 10 mg/kg q 8 h IV	10–14 d

[a] Only indicated in HSV seropositive patients.

Abbreviations: HSV, herpes simplex virus; BMT, bone marrow transplantation; PBSCT, peripheral blood stem cell transplantation; IV, intravenous; p.o., by mouth; bid, twice daily; tid, three times daily.

pneumonia and HSV encephalitis in immunodeficient hosts, high-dose intravenous acyclovir is recommended by some experts (see Table 2).

Valaciclovir and famciclovir, two additional antiviral agents with potent activity against HSV types 1 and 2 and against VZV, were recently licensed for clinical use in immunocompetent patients (21–23). Valaciclovir, a prodrug of acyclovir, and famciclovir, a prodrug of penciclovir, share a high oral bioavailability, which is up to five times higher than that of acyclovir and which permits less frequent dosing during therapy of HSV or VZV disease (24,25). Although both agents hold promise for the prophylaxis and therapy of HSV disease in immunocompromised cancer patients, results of investigations in this group need to be awaited before firm conclusions can be drawn.

C. Antiviral Drug Resistance

The emergence of resistant HSV strains that cause disease unresponsive to acyclovir in immunodeficent hosts is reported with increasing frequency (26). In a survey among centers of the European Group for Blood and Marrow Transplantation (EBMT), proven or suspected cases of HSV drug resistance were observed in 25% of the participating centers (27). In a large series, acyclovir-resistant HSV isolates were recovered from 14% of BMT recipients previously exposed to acyclovir but from none of the nontransplant cancer patients (28). Herpes simplex virus resistance occurs almost exclusively in patients receiving therapeutic antiviral regimens, and it does not seem associated with drug prophylaxis (26,29). If HSV disease is refractory to antiviral therapy, isolates should be tested for drug resistance (30). The most frequent mechanism of HSV resistance to acyclovir is deficient or altered activity of the viral thymidine kinase, resulting in reduced activation of acyclovir in HSV-infected cells (26,31,32). Foscarnet does not require intracellular activation and was used successfully as alternative systemic treatment in several cases of acyclovir-resistant HSV disease (Table 3) (27,33–35), but renal toxicity associated with foscarnet is of concern in patients, such as BMT recipients, who are exposed to other potentially nephrotoxic agents (36). If acyclovir-unresponsive HSV lesions are accessible, systemic drug treatment can be replaced by topical trifluridine solution or cidofovir gel (Table 3) (37,38).

III. VARICELLA-ZOSTER VIRUS INFECTION

A. Frequency, Clinical Presentation, and Diagnosis

Varicella (chickenpox) results from primary VZV infection and occurs in more than 90% of cases in children younger than 14 years of age. Chickenpox occurs in 2% to 3% of patients after BMT (39,40). Children with malignancy carry a

Table 3 Alternative Treatment for Herpesvirus Disease Resulting from Drug-Resistant Virus Strains

Virus	Resistance to	Alternative treatment regimens
HSV	Acyclovir	Intravenous foscarnet at 60 mg/kg bid or 40 mg/kg tid[a]
		Topical trifluridine 5% ophthalmic solution q 8 h[a]
		Topical cidofovir gel 0.3% or 1% once daily[a]
VZV	Acyclovir	Intravenous foscarnet at 60 mg/kg bid or 40 mg/kg tid[a]
CMV	Ganciclovir	Intravenous foscarnet
		Induction at 90 mg/kg q 12 h for 14 d
		Maintenance at 90 mg/kg once daily until recovery

[a] Until complete healing.
Abbreviations: HSV, herpes simplex virus; VZV, varicella-zoster virus; CMV, cytomegalovirus; bid, twice daily; tid, three times daily.

high risk for visceral dissemination of varicella. Without specific antiviral therapy, VZV pneumonia was observed in 32% of children with acute leukemia and in 19% of those with other cancers, and it was fatal in 7% of cases (41).

Herpes zoster (shingles) is due to reactivation of latent VZV and is particularly frequent in adults with lymphoreticular malignancy or leukemia. The incidence of zoster after allogeneic or autologous BMT ranges from 14% to 32% (5,39,40,42). In a series of 195 BMT recipients with herpes zoster, cutaneous dissemination developed in 23% and visceral involvement in 13%, and the fatality rate was 18%; median onset of zoster was at 5 months after BMT, and more than 85% of cases occurred within the first 9 posttransplant months (39).

Cutaneous chickenpox or herpes zoster can usually be diagnosed by clinical examination alone. Visceral organ involvement requires documentation of VZV in biopsy specimens by culture, histology, or PCR. For VZV pneumonia, detection of VZV in bronchoalveolar lavage (BAL) fluid may be used as substitute for lung biopsy.

B. Prevention and Therapy

Recommendations for the prevention and therapy of chickenpox and herpes zoster in immunodeficient cancer patients are summarized in Table 4. Prevention of chickenpox requires strict isolation from infectious individuals. A critical issue is that patients with chickenpox may be contagious up to 2 days before the onset

Table 4 Prevention and Therapy of VZV Disease

Indication	Antiviral drug	Dosage and Route	Duration	Other measures
Prevention				
Chickenpox				Strict isolation from infectious individuals VZV immunoglobulin IV if within 96 h of exposure Live attenuated VZV vaccine
Herpes zoster	Not recommended			Inactivated VZV vaccine?
Therapy				
Chickenpox, herpes zoster	Acyclovir	500 mg/m^2 or 10 mg/kg q 8 h IV or 800 mg 5 times per d p.o.	7–10 d	

Abbreviations: VZV, varicella-zoster virus; IV, intravenous; p.o., by mouth.

of skin rash, and isolation procedures are often too late in these instances (43). Cancer patients without a history of varicella who were exposed to infectious persons should receive intravenous VZV immunoglobulin if treatment is initiated within 96 hours of exposure (43). In addition, VZV seronegative children with malignancy can be safely vaccinated if they are at least 1 year away from induction chemotherapy (44,45). The live attenuated VZV vaccine used is given in two doses 3 months apart, and it is associated with a high degree of protection from breakthrough varicella infection and with a significant reduction of subsequent zoster compared to children who experience natural chickenpox (44–47).

The high incidence of herpes zoster after BMT led to placebo-controlled studies of long-term acyclovir prophylaxis in allogeneic BMT recipients (48,49). Prophylactic acyclovir abrogated VZV reactivation during the 6-month treatment period, but zoster developed in patients at the usual rate following completion of the prophylactic regimen (48,49). Thus, long-term acyclovir prophylaxis of herpes zoster is not advisable after BMT, because it only delays the occurrence of zoster and furthermore carries the potential for induction of VZV drug resistance (26). However, the severity of herpes zoster may be reduced by repetitive immunization with an inactivated VZV vaccine after BMT in patients who were VZV positive before transplantation (50).

For therapy of established chickenpox or herpes zoster in immunocompromised cancer patients, intravenous acyclovir is the current treatment of choice (see Table 4) (1,20,43). Despite limited data on the efficacy of oral acyclovir in patients with malignancy, it has also become common practice to treat localized zoster in cancer patients by use of oral acyclovir if oral intake of medication is possible (1). Preliminary results of a randomized comparison of oral acyclovir and famciclovir for therapy of localized zoster in various immunodeficent hosts (68% BMT recipients, 30% nontransplant cancer patients, and 2% solid organ transplant recipients) indicated equivalent efficacy and safety of both agents (51). Famciclovir in this trial was given at a dose of 500 mg three times daily for a total length of treatment of 10 days (51).

C. Antiviral Drug Resistance

Varicella-zoster virus resistance to antiviral drugs has mostly been documented in patients with the acquired immunodeficiency syndrome (AIDS) but does also occur in BMT recipients (26,27). Acyclovir-resistant VZV isolates show altered or deficient viral thymidine kinase function (52,53). Based on anecdotal reports, foscarnet may be used as therapeutic alternative if clinically refractory lesions are due to acyclovir-resistant VZV strains (see Table 3) (54).

IV. CYTOMEGALOVIRUS INFECTION

A. Diagnosis of CMV Infection and CMV Disease

The manifestations of CMV infection in immunocompromised hosts range from asymptomatic virus shedding to serious organ disease. In earlier studies, various definitions of CMV infection and CMV disease were used, which made comparison of results difficult. A common terminology was discussed at two recent consensus conferences, and the following agreements on definitions were reached (55,56).

The diagnosis of *CMV infection* requires the demonstration of CMV in clinical specimens by conventional tissue culture or rapid culture using confirmation by specific monoclonal antibodies, or by detection of the CMV lower matrix pp65 antigen in peripheral blood leukocytes. Positive PCR is valid if shown to correlate with culture-based detection of CMV. One exception is the PCR in cerebrospinal fluid in which this technique appears reliable, whereas virus cultures are insensitive. The diagnostic role of histology, immunochemistry, and in situ hybridization in tissue biopsies is less clear and requires further studies of the sensitivity and specificity of these methods. Because immunosuppressed cancer patients are often not able to mount a significant antibody response, the results of serological tests should not be used to define active CMV infection.

Diagnosis of *CMV disease* is made by documenting CMV in tissue specimens or in BAL fluid when CMV pneumonia is suspected, and detection of CMV must be associated with symptoms and/or signs from the affected organs.

B. Frequency and Clinical Presentation

Cytomegalovirus disease is a particularly frequent and serious problem in patients after BMT and PBSCT (1,10). In the absence of antiviral prophylaxis, the incidence of CMV infection when transplant donor or patient are CMV seropositive before transplantation is 60% to 70% in the first 3 months after allogeneic BMT (57). In one-third of allograft recipients and 10% to 20% of autograft recipients with evidence of CMV infection, CMV pneumonia develops, which, without specific therapy, is fatal in more than 80% of cases (6,57–59). Whereas CMV disease commonly affects the lungs and gastrointestinal tract following BMT and PBSCT, involvement of other organs appears to be infrequent.

The strongest predictor of CMV infection after allogeneic BMT is the pretransplant CMV seropositivity of the patient, which increases the risk of infection five-fold and suggests that reactivation of latent virus is an important source of CMV infection (60). Cytomegalovirus viremia is a major predisposing factor for CMV disease and was associated with a 5.5-fold risk for CMV pneumonia and a 3.2-fold risk for gastrointestinal disease among allograft recipients (60). Failure to reconstitute a CMV-specific $CD8^+$ cytotoxic T-lymphocyte (CTL) response after BMT or PBSCT is an additional important risk factor for CMV infection and CMV pneumonia (61–63).

There are only limited data on the importance of CMV infection in nontransplant cancer patients. In one study of adults receiving induction chemotherapy for acute leukemia, CMV infection occurred in 38% of patients and CMV disease in 15%, and the case-fatality rate was 42% (9).

C. Prevention and Therapy

1. *Therapy of CMV Pneumonia*

The therapy of established CMV pneumonia in BMT or PBSCT recipients remains a major challenge. The use of single agents, including ganciclovir and foscarnet, is ineffective (64,65). The best currently available treatment for CMV pneumonia after BMT and PBSCT consists of a combination of intravenous ganciclovir and high doses of intravenous immunoglobulin infusions, which was reported to result in survival rates of 31% to 84% early after completion of therapy (64,66–68). However, survival rate at 6 months after treatment of CMV pneumonia in these studies was only 22% to 40%, and nonleukemic deaths were often due to gram-negative septicemias and invasive fungal infections, which occurred at a higher rate than in BMT recipients in whom CMV pneumonia never developed. The therapeutic regimen currently used at the University Hospital in Basel is shown in Table 5. Because outcome of CMV pneumonia is still severe despite this combination therapy, major emphasis must be placed on the prevention of CMV disease in BMT and PBSCT recipients.

2. *Protection from Exposure to CMV*

Avoiding the acquisition of transfusion-transmitted virus is an important goal in the prevention of primary CMV infection after BMT and PBSCT. If both patient

Table 5 Therapy of CMV Pneumonia in BMT Recipients

Antiviral agent	Induction treatment	Maintenance treatment
Ganciclovir	5 mg/kg q 12 h IV for 14 d	5 mg/kg once a day IV for additional 30 d
Standard IV immunoglobulin	500 mg/kg every other day for 2 wk	500 mg/kg 2 times per wk for additional 4 wk

Regimen used in the BMT Unit at the University Hospital in Basel.
Abbreviations: CMV, cytomegalovirus; BMT, bone marrow transplantation; IV, intravenous.

and transplant donor are CMV seronegative, the exclusive use of screened seronegative or leukocyte-depleted blood products is a highly efficient approach to protection from primary CMV infection (2,3,69). This approach is of limited value, however, if the transplant donor is CMV seropositive, because virus can be transmitted by the graft (2).

3. Prophylaxis and Preemptive Treatment with Antiviral Drugs

Cytomegalovirus seropositive BMT and PBSCT recipients and those who are seronegative with a seropositive transplant donor are at risk of CMV infection by reactivation of latent virus present in the host or in the graft (2,57). With the introduction of potent antiviral drugs against CMV, two main strategies for the prevention of CMV infection and disease in these patients were developed. *Prophylactic treatment* is aimed at suppressing virus reactivation and is given to all patients regardless of the results of virological monitoring (70–72). Alternatively, *preemptive treatment* consists of initiating antiviral therapy only when active CMV infection is documented in order to prevent the development of CMV disease (73–75). Thus, with the preemptive treatment approach, the use of potentially toxic drugs against CMV, such as ganciclovir and foscarnet, is restricted to patients at highest risk for CMV disease. The results of selected prospective, controlled studies of the prophylaxis and preemptive drug treatment of CMV infection after allogeneic BMT are presented in Table 6 (70,71,73,75).

The prophylactic use of high-dose intravenous acyclovir in allogeneic BMT recipients is associated with improved survival when compared to untreated or placebo-treated control subjects but is only partially effective in preventing CMV disease (70,76). Among autograft recipients, acyclovir prophylaxis does not appear beneficial (77). Valaciclovir was recently evaluated for the prevention of CMV infection after allogeneic BMT in a multicenter controlled trial, but results have not been reported.

The antiviral agents ganciclovir and foscarnet have considerably more potent in vitro and in vivo activity against CMV than acyclovir. Prophylactic intravenous ganciclovir was assessed in two placebo-controlled studies of allograft recipients and resulted in marked reduction of CMV disease but was not associated with improved survival in either study (71,72). In contrast, preemptive ganciclovir treatment based on positive CMV cultures was associated with both a significantly decreased incidence of CMV disease and better survival after allogeneic BMT when compared with placebo treatment (73). However, 12% of patients screened for virus excretion in this trial, or 69% of those in whom CMV disease developed had CMV disease diagnosed before or coincident with first culture-based detection of CMV infection, and thus they did not benefit from preemptive antiviral therapy (73). Newer diagnostic techniques, such as the CMV antigenemia assay or the PCR in peripheral blood specimens, permit the detection of

Table 6 Prevention of CMV Disease After Allogeneic BMT Using Antiviral Drugs

Strategy	Antiviral drug	Dosage and route	Duration	Advantage	Disadvantage	Reference
Prophylaxis	Acyclovir	500 mg/m^2 q 8 h IV	From day 7 before to day 30 after BMT	CMV disease less frequent Survival benefit Low toxicity	Only partial protection from CMV disease	70
	Ganciclovir	5 mg/kg q 12 h IV for 5 days, then once daily	From engraftment until day 100 after BMT	CMV disease abrogated	Important toxicity (30% neutropenia requiring treatment modification) No survival benefit	71
Preemptive treatment						
Based on positive viral cultures from any site	Ganciclovir	5 mg/kg q 12 h IV for 7 days, then once daily	Until day 100 after BMT	CMV disease less frequent Survival benefit	12% of all patients screened, or 69% of those in whom CMV disease develops, without prior excretion of CMV	73
Based on positive PCR in blood leukocytes	Ganciclovir	5 mg/kg q 12 h IV for 14 days. If PCR still positive, 5 mg/kg once daily IV	Until PCR becomes negative	Early treatment Shorter duration of treatment Reduced toxicity Survival benefit	14% of patients require a second course of ganciclovir treatment	75

Abbreviations: CMV, cytomegalovirus; BMT, bone marrow transplantation; IV, intravenous; PCR, polymerase chain reaction.

CMV infection at an early stage when the systemic viral load is still low (75,78). The use of these highly sensitive and rapid screening methods might substantially reduce the proportion of patients in whom CMV disease develops without prior evidence of CMV infection, and could prolong the interval between detection of CMV infection and subsequent CMV disease. A first randomized comparison of PCR and viral cultures for initiation of preemptive ganciclovir therapy after allogeneic BMT showed a significantly shorter time to detection of CMV infection in PCR-monitored patients; earlier ganciclovir treatment in this group resulted in lower incidence of CMV disease and improved survival (75).

Ganciclovir use is associated with marked hematotoxicity in BMT recipients (71–73). Alternative agents with similar or better activity against CMV but fewer adverse effects are needed. In pilot studies, prophylactic foscarnet appeared to protect patients from CMV disease after BMT and was associated with transient renal dysfunction but only mild or absent hematotoxicity (36,79). Based on these studies, a randomized trial was conducted among centers of the EBMT comparing foscarnet and ganciclovir for preemptive therapy of CMV disease after allogeneic BMT or PBSCT, but results have not yet been reported. In this study, antiviral treatment was initiated upon detection of CMV by antigenemia assay or PCR in blood specimens, and was given for no longer than 4 weeks. In addition to reducing the likelihood of adverse events, antiviral therapy of shorter duration might be advantageous, because prolonged ganciclovir treatment impairs the reconstitution of CMV-specific $CD8^+$ CTL responses after BMT, thereby increasing the risk for late CMV disease (63).

Several novel compounds and modified formulations of known drugs with potent inhibitory activity against CMV were recently developed. Cidofovir is of particular interest because the long half-life of its active intracellular metabolite permits infrequent administration of the drug. Intravenous cidofovir was investigated for therapy of CMV retinitis in patients with AIDS, but the substantial renal toxicity observed precludes its use in transplant recipients who receive other potentially nephrotoxic drugs (80,81). Other agents, including lobucavir, compound 1263W94 and its analogue, and the new prodrug of ganciclovir, share a high oral bioavailability that is superior to that of presently available anti-CMV drugs. These agents might help to further improve the prevention of CMV disease after BMT and PBSCT (12).

4. *Immunotherapy*

The use of intravenous immunoglobulins in the prevention of CMV infection and CMV pneumonia after allogeneic BMT was investigated in several randomized, controlled trials that yielded conflicting results (for further discussion see Refs. 1 and 82). In view of the unclear benefit and of the important costs of immunoglobulin preparations, this approach to prevention of CMV infection and disease after BMT or PBSCT cannot be advocated without further studies.

Cytomegalovirus-specific T-cell immunity plays a pivotal role in the prevention and control of CMV infection after BMT and PBSCT (61–63). Restoration of the immune defense by the adoptive transfer of $CD8^+$ CTL clones specific for CMV appears safe after allogeneic BMT (83,84), and ongoing studies evaluate the antiviral efficacy of this treatment modality in allograft recipients (S. R. Riddell, personal communication, 1998).

D. Antiviral Drug Resistance

Cytomegalovirus disease associated with drug-resistant CMV strains and refractory to antiviral therapy is an increasing clinical problem in patients with AIDS, but it has infrequently been reported in BMT recipients (26,27,85–89). Most CMV isolates are resistant to ganciclovir, but cases of CMV resistance to foscarnet and to cidofovir have been described (86,89,90). For ganciclovir-resistant CMV disease, the use of intravenous foscarnet resulted in improvement or complete recovery in several cases and is a possible therapeutic alternative (see Table 3) (26,27). Broader use of susceptibility testing is needed to determine the incidence and clinical importance of CMV resistance to antiviral drugs after BMT and PBSCT. Future investigations should be facilitated by the introduction of more rapid and efficient techniques for detection of resistant CMV isolates (89,91,92). Moreover, new alternative treatment options need to be studied for patients with disease caused by drug-resistant CMV strains.

V. OTHER HERPESVIRUS INFECTIONS

A. Epstein-Barr Virus

Epstein-Barr virus (EBV) infection occurs in more than 90% of the normal population, and cancer patients are at risk for disease caused by EBV reactivation (93). After allogeneic BMT, EBV may cause B-cell lymphoproliferative disorder (LPD), particularly in patients who receive T-cell–depleted marrow grafts or anti-CD3 monoclonal antibodies for therapy of acute graft-versus-host disease (94,95). The overall actuarial incidence of EBV-associated LPD in a series of 2,475 allograft recipients was 0.6%, and the case-fatality rate was 87% (95).

Although acyclovir has inhibitory activity against EBV replication (93), its use for therapy of EBV-LPD in small series of BMT recipients had no detectable effect (94,95). A more promising approach to prophylaxis and treatment of EBV-related LPD after allogeneic BMT or PBSCT is the restoration of T-cell immunity by infusion of donor-derived leukocytes or EBV-specific CTL lines (96–98).

B. Human Herpesvirus 6

Human herpesvirus 6 (HHV-6) was discovered in 1986, and primary infection causes roseola (exanthema subitum) in early childhood. Except for BMT recipients, little is known about HHV-6 infection in cancer patients. The incidence of HHV-6 infection after BMT ranges from 38% to 60% (99). The frequency of HHV-6 infection as detected by PCR in blood leukocytes, throat washes, and urine is correlated with the severity of acute graft-versus-host disease in BMT recipients (100). Infection with HHV-6 after BMT was associated with interstitial pneumonia, bone marrow suppression, and encephalitis (101–105), but the causative role of HHV-6 for these disease manifestations requires further clarification.

Both ganciclovir and foscarnet show antiviral activity against HHV-6 in vitro, whereas acyclovir is less effective (99). Although the therapeutic efficacy of antiviral agents against HHV-6 has not been documented in controlled studies of transplant recipients, therapy of HHV-6–associated disease with intravenous ganciclovir or foscarnet is recommended by some experts if active infection was diagnosed by cell culture, shell-vial assay, PCR, or immunohistochemistry (99).

VI. COMMUNITY RESPIRATORY VIRUS INFECTION

The clinical importance of community respiratory viruses in immunocompromised patients with cancer has been increasingly recognized in recent years (8,11,106–109). In a prospective study of adult BMT recipients who were hospitalized with acute respiratory illness during two consecutive winter seasons, community respiratory viruses were isolated by culture from 67 (31%) of 217 patients (109). Forty-nine percent of these infections were due to respiratory syncytial virus (RSV), 18% each to influenza viruses and to picornaviruses, 9% to parainfluenza viruses, and 6% to adenovirus (109). Of 87 prospectively studied leukemic adults with acute respiratory disease, 9 (10%) had culture-proven RSV infection that was complicated by pneumonia in 6, with a mortality rate of 83% (108). Fatal respiratory failure was also reported to occur in one-third of patients after BMT who had parainfluenza virus infection involving the lower respiratory tract (8). Thus, community respiratory viruses are responsible for significant morbidity and mortality among both BMT recipients and leukemic patients in whom acute respiratory disease develops, and RSV infection appears to be particularly frequent.

Although rapid detection techniques are available for most community respiratory viruses, progress in the management of these infections is slow, which is, in part, related to the limited number of antiviral agents against these viruses and to the lack of data from controlled treatment trials in cancer patients. Ribavirin delivered by aerosol or administered intravenously was used for therapy of RSV infection in several patients after BMT (106,109,110). Aerosolized ribavirin was generally ineffective in patients with established RSV pneumonia and respiratory failure, but it might be beneficial if given early in the course of pneumonia or if administered preemptively when only the upper respiratory tract is involved (11,106,109). Ribavirin given intravenously was ineffective therapy of RSV pneumonia and was associated with acute hemolysis, raising concern about the safety of this route of ribavirin administration in BMT recipients (110). The combination of aerosolized ribavirin plus intravenous immunoglobulins containing high titers of RSV antibody could yield better results and deserves further study in cancer patients with RSV infection (11).

Amantadine and rimantadine are both effective in the therapy of influenza A virus infection in immunocompetent patients, but whether the prophylactic or therapeutic use of these agents is beneficial to immunodeficient cancer patients with influenza A infection is uncertain. Zanamivir, a new topical agent with potent activitiy against both influenza A and B viruses, was recently shown to be safe and to reduce symptoms of influenza virus infection in otherwise healthy adults when given by inhalation (111). Controlled clinical trials are needed to assess the use of zanamivir in cancer patients with influenza-like illnesses.

Because of the limited therapeutic options, emphasis must be placed on prophylaxis of respiratory virus infections in patients with malignancy. Infection control measures, including droplet precautions, prompt identification and isolation of infected patients, and prohibition of contact between patients and visitors or hospital staff with respiratory symptoms, result in significant reduction of nosocomial RSV infections in BMT recipients and patients with leukemia (112). Immunization with influenza virus vaccine of patients and hospital personnel before the influenza season has protective effects and is recommended for immunocompromised cancer patients (112,113). Other vaccines are under development and may help to further reduce the morbidity caused by community respiratory viruses among cancer patients in the future.

VII. VIRAL HEPATITIS

Although hepatitis A virus infection does not appear associated with serious disease in immunodeficient cancer patients, several reports indicate that both hepatitis B virus (HBV) and hepatitis C virus (HCV) may cause important morbidity in these patients (114–120).

Fulminant hepatitis caused by reactivation of HBV infection occasionally develops in patients treated for maligancy and is associated with reduction of immunosuppression (114,120). However, in two series of allogeneic BMT recipients, patients who were positive for HBV surface antigen before transplantation had no increase in severe liver disease during the posttransplant course, suggesting that BMT is not contraindicated in these patients (115,116). Because the risk of HBV infection varies greatly between different countries, active immunization with HBV vaccine should be given to BMT recipients in regions in which this vaccination is recommended to the general population (113).

Patients who test positive for antibodies to HCV after BMT carry a higher risk for chronic hepatitis than those who are seronegative (119). The PCR-based detection of HCV RNA in serum may be a more predictive test for liver disease after BMT than anti-HCV antibody testing. In a small series, PCR positivity for HCV RNA before BMT was associated with a significantly higher risk for posttransplant veno-occlusive disease, which was fatal in most cases (118). Treatment of HCV infection with interferon-α or other antiviral agents has not been systematically studied in immunocompromised cancer patients; thus, therapeutic recommendations cannot be made for this group.

VIII. POLYOMAVIRUS INFECTIONS

After BMT, the human polyomavirus BK is frequently reactivated and excreted in the urine and can cause hemorrhagic cystitis (121,122). JC virus, the etiological agent for progressive multifocal leucoencephalopathy (PML), is occasionally isolated from urinary specimens in BMT recipients, but PML is very rare in these patients (121,123). No antiviral agent was conclusively shown to be effective therapy of disease as a result of these viruses in cancer patients, and treatment remains largely supportive.

REFERENCES

1. Reusser P. Prophylaxis and treatment of herpes virus infections in immunocompromised cancer patients. Bailliere's Clin Infect Dis 1994; 1:523–544.
2. Bowden RA, Sayers M, Flournoy N, Newton B, Banaji M, Thomas ED, Meyers JD. Cytomegalovirus immune globulin and seronegative blood products to prevent primary cytomegalovirus infection after marrow transplantation. N Engl J Med 1986; 314:1006–1010.
3. Sayers MH, Anderson KC, Goodnough LT, Kurtz SR, Lane TA, Pisciotto P, Silberstein LE. Reducing the risk for transfusion-transmitted cytomegalovirus infection. Ann Intern Med 1992; 116:55–62.
4. Schreiber GB, Busch MP, Kleinman SH, Korelitz JJ, for the Retrovirus Epidemiology Donor Study. The risk of transfusion-transmitted viral infections. N Engl J Med 1996; 334:1685–1690.
5. Schuchter LM, Wingard JR, Piantadosi S, Burns WH, Santos GW, Saral R. Herpes

zoster infection after autologous bone marrow transplantation. Blood 1989; 74: 1424–1427.

6. Reusser P, Fisher LD, Buckner CD, Thomas ED, Meyers JD. Cytomegalovirus infection after autologous bone marrow transplantation: occurrence of cytomegalovirus disease and effect on engraftment. Blood 1990; 75:1888–1894.
7. Bustamante CI, Wade JC. Herpes simplex virus infection in the immunocompromised cancer patient. J Clin Oncol 1991; 9:1903–1915.
8. Wendt CH, Weisdorf DJ, Jordan MC, Balfour HH Jr, Hertz MI. Parainfluenza virus respiratory infection after bone marrow transplantation. N Engl J Med 1992; 326: 921–926.
9. Wade JC. Management of infection in patients with acute leukemia. Hematol Oncol Clin North Am 1993; 7:293–315.
10. Link H, Arseniev L, Ljungman P, Alessandrino EP, Amadori S, Bandini G, Beguin Y, Brinch L, Brunet S, Chopra R, Cordonnier C, De Witte T, Fauser A, Ferrant A, Garcia-Conde J, Juliusson G, Kubel M, Manna AT, Martinez-Rubio AM, Mundhenk P, Ordemann R, Ortega JJ, Potter M, Prentice HG, Raimondi R, Remez K, Reusser P, Rovira M, Russell J, Selleslag D, Uderzo C, Zaucha JM. Cytomegalovirus infections after allogeneic peripheral blood progenitor cell transplantation (PBPCT)—a survey of the infectious diseases working party of EBMT (abstr). Blood 1997; 90(suppl 1):544a.
11. Whimbey E, Englund JA, Couch RB. Community respiratory virus infections in immunocompromised patients with cancer. Am J Med 1997; 102(suppl 3A):10–18.
12. Reusser P. Current concepts and challenges in the prevention and treatment of viral infections in immunocompromised cancer patients. Support Care Cancer 1998; 6: 39–45.
13. Whitley RJ. Therapeutic approaches to varicella-zoster virus infections. J Infect Dis 1992; 166(suppl 1):S51–57.
14. Spencer GD, Hackman RC, McDonald GB, Amos DE, Cunningham BA, Meyers JD, Thomas ED. A prospective study of unexplained nausea and vomiting after marrow transplantation. Transplantation 1986; 42:602–607.
15. Ramsey PG, Fife KH, Hackman RC, Meyers JD, Corey L. Herpes simplex virus pneumonia. Clinical, virologic, and pathologic features in 20 patients. Ann Intern Med 1982; 97:813–820.
16. Ballen KK, Donadio D, Bouloux C, McCarthy P, Weinstein H, Antin JH. Herpes simplex virus and neutropenia following bone marrow transplantation. Transplantation 1992; 54:553–555.
17. Kaufman, Gandhi SA, Louie E, Rizzi R, Illei P. Herpes simplex virus hepatitis: case report and review. Clin Infect Dis 1997; 24:334–338.
18. Aurelius E. Johansson B, Sköldenberg B, Staland A, Forsgren M. Rapid diagnosis of herpes simplex encephalitis by nested polymerase chain reaction assay of cerebrospinal fluid. Lancet 1991; 337:189–192.
19. Lakeman FD, Whitley RJ, the National Institute of Allergy and Infectious Diseases Collaborative Antiviral Study Group. Diagnosis of herpes simplex encephalitis: application of polymerase chain reaction to cerebrospinal fluid from brain-biopsied patients and correlation with disease. J Infect Dis 1995; 171:857–863.

20. Whitley RJ, Gnann JW. Acyclovir: a decade later. N Engl J Med 1992; 327:782–789.
21. Beutner KR, Friedman DJ, Forszpaniak C, Andersen PL, Wood MJ. Valaciclovir compared with acyclovir for improved therapy for herpes zoster in immunocompetent adults. Antimicrob Agents Chemother 1995; 39:1546–1553.
22. Tyring S, Barbarash RA, Nahlik JE, Cunningham A, Marley J, Heng M, Jones T, Rea T, Boon R, Saltzman R, the Collaborative Famciclovir Herpes Zoster Study Group. Famciclovir for the treatment of acute herpes zoster: effects on acute disease and postherpetic neuralgia. A randomized, double-blind, placebo-controlled trial. Ann Intern Med 1995; 123:89–96.
23. Sacks SL, Aoki FY, Diaz-Mitoma F, Sellors J, Shafran SD, for the Canadian Famciclovir Study Group. Patient-initiated, twice-daily oral famciclovir for early recurrent genital herpes. JAMA 1996; 276:44–49.
24. Pue M, Benet LZ. Pharmacokinetics of famciclovir in man. Antiviral Chem Chemother 1993; 4(suppl 1):47–55.
25. Soul-Lawton J, Seaber E, On N, Wootton R, Rolan P, Posner J. Absolute bioavailability and metabolic disposition of valaciclovir, the L-valyl ester of acyclovir, following oral administration to humans. Antimicrobial Agents Chemother 1995; 39: 2759–2764.
26. Reusser P. Herpesvirus resistance to antiviral drugs: a review of the mechanisms, clinical importance, and therapeutic options. J Hosp Infect 1996; 33:235–248.
27. Reusser P, Cordonnier C, Einsele H, Engelhard D, Link H, Locasciulli A, Ljungman P, for the Infectious Diseases Working Party of the European Group for Blood and Marrow Transplantation (EBMT). European survey of herpesvirus resistance to antiviral drugs in bone marrow transplant recipients. Bone Marrow Transplant 1996; 17:813–817.
28. Englund JA, Zimmermann ME, Swierkosz EM, Goodmann JL, Scholl DR, Balfour HH Jr. Herpes simplex virus resistant to acyclovir. A study in a tertiary care center. Ann Intern Med 1990; 112:416–422.
29. Boivin G, Erice A, Crane DD, Dunn DL, Balfour HH Jr. Acyclovir susceptibilities of herpes simplex virus strains isolated from solid organ transplant recipients after acyclovir or ganciclovir prophylaxis. Antimicrob Agents Chemother 1993; 37:357–359.
30. Safrin S, Elbeik T, Mills J. A rapid screen test for in vitro susceptibility of clinical herpes simplex virus isolates. J Infect Dis 1994; 169:879–882.
31. Erlich KS, Mills J, Chatis P, Mertz GJ, Busch DF, Follansbee SE, Grant RM, Crumpacker CS. Acyclovir-resistant herpes simplex virus infections in patients with the acquired immunodeficiency syndrome. N Engl J Med 1989; 320:293–296.
32. Hill EL, Hunter GA, Ellis MN. In vitro and in vivo characterization of herpes simplex virus clinical isolates recovered from patients infected with human immunodeficiency virus. Antimicrob Agents Chemother 1991; 35:2322–2328.
33. Erlich KS, Jacobson MA, Koehler JE, Follansbee SE, Drennan DP, Gooze L, Safrin S, Mills J. Foscarnet therapy for severe acyclovir-resistant herpes simplex virus type-2 infections in patients with the acquired immunodeficiency syndrome (AIDS). An uncontrolled trial. Ann Intern Med 1989; 110:710–713.
34. Safrin S, Crumpacker C, Chatis P, Davis R, Hafner R, Rush J, Kessler HA, Landry

B, Mills J, and other members of the AIDS Clinical Trials Group. A controlled trial comparing foscarnet with vidarabine for acyclovir-resistant mucocutaneous herpes simplex in the acquired immunodeficiency syndrome. N Engl J Med 1991; 325:551–555.

35. Verdonck LF, Cornelissen JJ, Smit J, Lepoutre J, de Gast GC, Dekker AW, Rozenberg-Arska M. Successful foscarnet therapy for acyclovir-resistant mucocutaneous infection with herpes simplex virus in a recipient of allogeneic BMT. Bone Marrow Transplant 1993; 11:177–179.
36. Reusser P, Gambertoglio JG, Lilleby K, Meyers JD. Phase I-II trial of foscarnet for prevention of cytomegalovirus infection in autologous and allogeneic marrow transplant recipients. J Infect Dis 1992; 166:473–479.
37. Kessler HA, Hurwitz S, Farthing C, Benson CA, Feinberg J, Kuritzkes DR, Bailey TC, Safrin S, Steigbigel RT, Cheeseman SH, McKinley GF, Wettlaufer B, Owens S, Nevin T, Korvick JA, the AIDS Clinical Trials Group. Pilot study of topical trifluridine for the treatment of acyclovir-resistant mucocutaneous herpes simplex disease in patients with AIDS (ACTG 172). J Acquir Immune Defic Syndr 1996; 12:147–152.
38. Lalezari J, Schacker T, Feinberg J, Gathe J, Lee S, Cheung T, Kramer F, Kessler H, Corey L, Drew WL, Boggs J, McGuire B, Jaffe HS, Safrin S. A randomized, double-blind, placebo-controlled trial of cidofovir gel for the treatment of acyclovir-unresponsive, mucocutaneous herpes simplex virus infection in patients with AIDS. J Infect Dis 1997; 176:892–898.
39. Locksley RM, Flournoy N, Sullivan KM, Meyers JD. Infection with varicella-zoster virus after marrow transplantation. J Infect Dis 1985; 152:1172–1181.
40. Han CS, Miller W, Haake R, Weisdorf D. Varicella zoster infection after bone marrow transplantation: incidence, risk factors and complications. Bone Marrow Transplant 1994; 13:277–283.
41. Feldman S, Lott L. Varicella in children with cancer. Impact of antiviral therapy and prophylaxis. Pediatrics 1987; 80:465–472.
42. Christiansen NP, Haake RJ, Hurd DD. Early herpes zoster infection in adult patients with Hodgkin's disease undergoing autologous bone marrow transplant. Bone Marrow Transplant 1991; 7:435–437.
43. Straus SE, Ostrove JM, Inchauspé G, Felser JM, Freifeld A, Croen KD, Sawyer MH. Varicella-zoster virus infections. Biology, natural history, treatment, and prevention. Ann Intern Med 1988; 108:221–237.
44. Gershon AA, LaRussa P, Hardy I, Steinberg S, Silverstein S. Varicella vaccine: the American experience. J Infect Dis 1992; 166(suppl 1):S63–68.
45. White CJ. Varicella-zoster virus vaccine. Clin Infect Dis 1997; 24:753–763.
46. Gershon AA, Steinberg SP, the Varicella Vaccine Collaborative Study Group of the National Institute of Allergy and Infectious Diseases. Persistence of immunity to varicella in children with leukemia immunized with live attenuated varicella vaccine. N Engl J Med 1989; 320:892–897.
47. Hardy I, Gershon AA, Steinberg SP, LaRussa P, the Varicella Vaccine Collaborative Study Group. The incidence of zoster after immunization with live attenuated varicella vaccine. A study in children with leukemia. N Engl J Med 1991; 325: 1545–1550.

48. Ljungman P, Lönnqvist B, Ringdén O, Skinhöj P, Gahrton G, for the Nordic Bone Marrow Transplant Group. A randomized trial of oral versus intravenous acyclovir for treatment of herpes zoster in bone marrow transplant recipients. Bone Marrow Transplant 1989; 4:613–615.
49. Perren TJ, Powles RL, Easton D, Stolle K, Selby PJ. Prevention of herpes zoster in patients by long-term oral acyclovir after allogeneic bone marrow transplantation. Am J Med 1988; 85(suppl 2A):99–101.
50. Redman RL, Nader S, Zerboni L, Liu C, Wong RM, Brown BW, Arvin AM. Early reconstitution of immunity and decreased severity of herpes zoster in bone marrow transplant recipients immunized with inactivated varicella vaccine. J Infect Dis 1997; 176:578–585.
51. Ljungman P, for the FCV IC Study Group. Famciclovir (FCV) for the treatment of herpes zoster (HZ) in immunocompromised (IC) patients. 24th Annual meeting of the European Group for Blood and Marrow Transplantation (abstr). Courmayeur, Italy, March 22–26, 1998.
52. Talarico CL, Phelps WC, Biron KK. Analysis of the thymidine kinase genes from acyclovir-resistant mutants of varicella-zoster virus isolated from patients with AIDS. J Virol 1993; 67:1024–1033.
53. Boivin G, Edelman CK, Pedneault L, Talarico CL, Biron KK, Balfour HH Jr. Phenotypic and genotypic characterization of acyclovir-resistant varicella-zoster viruses isolated from persons with AIDS. J Infect Dis 1994; 170:68–75.
54. Safrin S, Berger TG, Gilson I, Wolfe PR, Wofsy CB, Mills J, Biron KK. Foscarnet therapy in five patients with AIDS and acyclovir-resistant varicella-zoster virus infection. Ann Intern Med 1991; 115:19–21.
55. Ljungman P, Griffiths P. Definitions of cytomegalovirus infection and disease. In: Michelson S, Plotkin SA, eds. Multidisciplinary Approach to Understanding Cytomegalovirus Disease. Amsterdam: Elsevier Science Publishers BV, 1993:233–237.
56. Ljungman P, Cordonnier C, de Bock R, Einsele H, Engelhard D, Grundy J, Link H, Locasciulli A, Prentice G, Reusser P, Ribaud P, for the Infectious Diseases Working Party of the EMBT. Immunisations after bone marrow transplantation: results of a European survey and recommendations from the Infectious Diseases Working Party of the European Group for Blood and Marrow Transplantation. Bone Marrow Transplant 1995; 15:455–460.
57. Meyers JD, Flournoy N, Thomas ED. Risk factors for cytomegalovirus infection after human marrow transplantation. J Infect Dis 1986; 153:478–488.
58. Wingard JR, Piantadosi S, Burns WH, Zahurak ML, Santos GW, Saral R. Cytomegalovirus infections in bone marrow transplant recipients given intensive cytoreductive therapy. Rev Infect Dis 1990; 12(suppl 7):S793–S804.
59. Enright H, Haake R, Weisdorf D, Ramsay N, McGlave P, Kersey J, Thomas W, McKenzie D, Miller W. Cytomegalovirus pneumonia after bone marrow transplantation. Risk factors and response to therapy. Transplantation 1993; 55:1339–1346.
60. Meyers JD, Ljungman P, Fisher LD. Cytomegalovirus excretion as a predictor of cytomegalovirus disease after marrow transplantation: importance of cytomegalovirus viremia. J Infect Dis 1990; 162:373–380.
61. Reusser P, Riddell SR, Meyers JD, Greenberg PD. Cytotoxic T lymphocyte re-

sponse to cytomegalovirus following human allogeneic bone marrow transplantation: pattern of recovery and correlation with cytomegalovirus infection and disease. Blood 1991; 78:1373–1380.

62. Reusser P, Attenhofer R, Hebart H, Helg C, Chapuis B, Einsele H. Cytomegalovirus-specific T-cell immunity in recipients of autologous peripheral blood stem cell or bone marrow transplants. Blood 1997; 10:3873–3879.
63. Li C-R, Greenberg PD, Gilbert MJ, Goodrich JM, Riddell SR. Recovery of HLA-restricted cytomegalovirus (CMV)-specific T-cell responses after allogeneic bone marrow transplant: correlation with CMV disease and effect of ganciclovir prophylaxis. Blood 1994; 83:1971–1979.
64. Reed EC, Bowden RA, Dandliker PS, Lilleby KE, Meyers JD. Treatment of cytomegalovirus pneumonia with ganciclovir and intravenous cytomegalovirus immunoglobulin in patients with bone marrow transplants. Ann Intern Med 1988; 109: 783–788.
65. Aschan J, Ringdén O, Ljungman P, Lönnqvist B, Ohlman S. Foscarnet for treatment of cytomegalovirus infections in bone marrow transplant recipients. Scand J Infect Dis 1992; 24:143–150.
66. Emanuel D, Cunningham I, Jules-Elysee K, Brochstein JA, Kernan NA, Laver J, Stover D, White DA, Fels A, Polsky B, Castro-Malaspina H, Peppard JR, Bartus P, Hammerling U, O'Reilly RJ. Cytomegalovirus pneumonia after bone marrow transplantation successfully treated with the combination of ganciclovir and high-dose intravenous immune globulin. Ann Intern Med 1988; 109:777–782.
67. Schmidt GM, Kovacs A, Zaia JA, Horak DA, Blume KG, Nademanee AP, O'Donnell MR, Snyder DS, Forman SJ. Ganciclovir/immunoglobulin combination therapy for the treatment of human cytomegalovirus-associated interstitial pneumonia in bone marrow allograft recipients. Transplantation 1988; 46:905–907.
68. Ljungman P, Engelhard D, Link H, Biron P, Brandt L, Brunet S, Cordonnier C, Debusscher L, deLaurenzi A, Kolb HJ, Messina C, Newland AC, Prentice HG, Richard C, Ruutu T, Tilg H, Verdonck L. Treatment of interstitial pneumonitis due to cytomegalovirus with ganciclovir and intravenous immune globulin: experience of European Bone Marrow Transplant Group. Clin Infect Dis 1992; 14:831–835.
69. Bowden RA, Slichter SJ, Sayers M, Weisdorf D, Cays M, Schoch G, Banaji M, Haake R, Welk K, Fisher L, McCullough J, Miller W. A comparison of filtered leukocyte-reduced and cytomegalovirus (CMV) seronegative blood products for the prevention of transfusion-associated CMV infection after marrow transplantation. Blood 1995; 86:3598–3603.
70. Meyers JD, Reed EC, Shepp DH, Thornquist M, Dandliker PS, Vicary CA, Flournoy N, Kirk LE, Kersey JH, Thomas ED, Balfour HH Jr. Acyclovir for prevention of cytomegalovirus infection and disease after allogeneic marrow transplantation. N Engl J Med 1988; 318:70–75.
71. Goodrich JM, Bowden RA, Fisher L, Keller C, Schoch G, Meyers JD. Ganciclovir prophylaxis to prevent cytomegalovirus disease after allogeneic marrow transplant. Ann Intern Med 1993; 118:173–178.
72. Winston DJ, Ho WG, Bartoni K, DuMond C, Ebeling DF, Buhles WC, Champlin RE. Ganciclovir prophylaxis of cytomegalovirus infection and disease in allogeneic

bone marrow transplant recipients. Results of a placebo-controlled, double-blind trial. Ann Intern Med 1993; 118:179–184.

73. Goodrich JM, Mori M, Gleaves CA, DuMond C, Cays M, Ebeling DF, Buhles WC, DeArmond B, Meyers JD. Prevention of cytomegalovirus disease after allogeneic marrow transplantation by early treatment with ganciclovir. N Engl J Med 1991; 325:1601–1607.
74. Schmidt GM, Horak DA, Niland JC, Duncan SR, Forman SJ, Zaia JA. A randomized, controlled trial of prophylactic ganciclovir for cytomegalovirus pulmonary infection in recipients of allogeneic bone marrow transplants. N Engl J Med 1991; 324:1005–1011.
75. Einsele H, Ehninger G, Hebart H, Wittkowski KM, Schuler U, Jahn G, Mackes P, Herter M, Klingebiel T, Löffler J, Wagner S, Müller CA. Polymerase chain reaction monitoring reduces the incidence of cytomegalovirus disease and the duration and side effects of antiviral therapy after bone marrow transplantation. Blood 1995; 86: 2815–2820.
76. Prentice HG, Gluckman E, Powles RL, Ljungman P, Milpied NJ, Fernandez Rañada JM, Mandelli F, Kho P, Kennedy L, Bell AR, for the European Acyclovir for CMV Prophylaxis Study Group. Impact of long-term acyclovir on cytomegalovirus infection and survival after allogeneic bone marrow transplantation. Lancet 1994; 343: 749–753.
77. Boeckh M, Gooley TA, Reusser P, Buckner CD, Bowden RA. Failure of high-dose acyclovir to prevent cytomegalovirus disease after autologous marrow transplantation. J Infect Dis 1995; 172:939–943.
78. Boeckh M, Bowden RA, Goodrich JM, Pettinger M, Meyers JD. Cytomegalovirus antigen detection in peripheral blood leukocytes after allogeneic marrow transplantation. Blood 1992; 80:1358–1364.
79. Bacigalupo A, Tedone E, van Lint MT, Trespi G, Lonngren M, Sanna MA, Moro F, Frassoni F, Occhini D, Gualandi F, Lamparelli T, Figari O, Benvenuto F, Raffo MR, Sogno G, Isaza A, Bernabo'Di Negro G, Felletti R, Hale G, Marbot AM. CMV prophylaxis with foscarnet in allogeneic bone marrow transplant recipients at high risk of developing CMV infections. Bone Marrow Transplant 1994; 13: 783–788.
80. Studies of Ocular Complications of AIDS Research Group in Collaboration with the AIDS Clinical Trials Group. Parenteral cidofovir for cytomegalovirus retinitis in patients with AIDS: the HPMPC peripheral cytomegalovirus retinitis trial. A randomized, controlled trial. Ann Intern Med 1997; 126:264–274.
81. Lalezari JP, Stagg RJ, Kuppermann BD, Holland GN, Kramer F, Ives DV, Youle M, Robinson MR, Drew WL, Jaffe HS. Intravenous cidofovir for peripheral cytomegalovirus retinitis in patients with AIDS. A randomized, controlled trial. Ann Intern Med 1997; 126:257–263.
82. Meyers JD. Prevention of cytomegalovirus infection after marrow transplantation. Rev Infect Dis 1989; 11(suppl 7):S1691–S1705.
83. Riddell SR, Watanabe KS, Goodrich JM, Li CR, Agha ME, Greenberg PD. Restoration of viral immunity in immunodeficient humans by the adoptive transfer of T cell clones. Science 1992; 257:238–241.
84. Walter EA, Greenberg PD, Gilbert MJ, Finch RJ, Watanabe KS, Thomas ED, Rid-

dell SR. Reconstitution of cellular immunity against cytomegalovirus in recipients of allogeneic bone marrow by transfer of T-cell clones from the donor. N Engl J Med 1995; 333:1038–1044.
85. Drew WL, Miner RC, Busch DF, Follansbee SE, Gullett J, Mehalko SG, Gordon SM, Owen WF Jr, Matthews TR, Buhles WC, DeArmond B. Prevalence of resistance in patients receiving ganciclovir for serious cytomegalovirus infection. J Infect Dis 1991; 163:716–719.
86. Knox KK, Drobyski WR, Carrigan DR. Cytomegalovirus isolate resistant to ganciclovir and foscarnet from a marrow transplant patient (letter). Lancet 1991; i: 1292–1293.
87. Slavin MA, Bindra RR, Gleaves CA, Pettinger MB, Bowden RA. Ganciclovir sensitivity of cytomegalovirus at diagnosis and during treatment of cytomegalovirus pneumonia in marrow transplant recipients. Antimicrob Agents Chemother 1993; 37:1360–1363.
88. Reusser P, Hostettler B, Attenhofer R. Ganciclovir-resistente Zytomegalievirus-Infektion: 2 Fälle mit unterschiedlicher klinischer Bedeutung. Schweiz Med Wochenschr 1996; 126:1779–1784.
89. Erice A, Gil-Roda C, Pérez JL, Balfour HH Jr, Sannerud KJ, Hanson MN, Bovin G, Chou S. Antiviral susceptibilities and analysis of UL97 and DNA polymerase sequences of clinical cytomegalovirus isolates from immunocompromised patients. J Infect Dis 1997; 175:1087–1092.
90. Dunn JP, MacCumber MW, Forman MS, Charache P, Apuzzo L, Jabs DA. Viral sensitivity testing in patients with cytomegalovirus retinitis clinically resistant to foscarnet or ganciclovir. Am J Ophthalmol 1995; 119:587–596.
91. Chou S, Erice A, Jordan MC, Vercellotti GM, Michels KR, Talarico CL, Stanat SC, Biron KK. Analysis of the UL97 phosphotransferase coding sequence in clinical cytomegalovirus isolates and identification of mutations conferring ganciclovir resistance. J Infect Dis 1995; 171:576–583.
92. Wolf DG, Smith IL, Lee DJ, Freeman WR, Flores-Aguilar M, Spector SA. Mutations in human cytomegalovirus UL97 gene confer clinical resistance to ganciclovir and can be detected directly in patient plasma. J Clin Invest 1995; 95:257–263.
93. Straus SE, Cohen JI, Tosato G, Meier J. Epstein-Barr virus infections: biology, pathogenesis, and management. Ann Intern Med 1993; 118:45–58.
94. Shapiro RS, McClain K, Frizzera G, Gajl-Peczalska KJ, Kersey JH, Blazar BR, Arthur DC, Patton DF, Greenberg JS, Burke B, Ramsay NKC, McGlave P, Filipovich AH. Epstein-Barr virus associated B cell lymphoproliferative disorders following bone marrow transplantation. Blood 1988; 71:1234–1243.
95. Zutter MM, Martin PJ, Sale GE, Shulman HM, Fisher L, Thomas ED, Durnam DM. Epstein-Barr virus lymphoproliferation after bone marrow transplantation. Blood 1988; 72:520–529.
96. Heslop HE, Brenner MK, Rooney CM. Donor T cells as therapy for EBV lymphoproliferation post bone marrow transplant. N Engl J Med 1994; 331:679–680.
97. Papadopoulos EB, Ladanyi M, Emanuel D, Mackinnon S, Boulad F, Carabasi MH, Castro-Malaspina H, Childs BH, Gillio AP, Small TN, Young JW, Kernan NA, O'Reilly RJ. Infusions of donor-leukocytes to treat Epstein-Barr virus-associated

lymphoproliferative disorders after allogeneic bone marrow transplantation. N Engl J Med 1994; 330:1185–1191.

98. Rooney CM, Smith CA, Ng CYC, Loftin S, Li C, Krance RA, Brenner MK, Heslop HE. Use of gene-modified virus-specific T lymphocytes to control Epstein-Barr-virus-related lymphoproliferation. Lancet 1995; 345:9–13.
99. Singh N, Carrigan DR. Human herpesvirus-6 in transplantation: an emerging pathogen. Ann Intern Med 1996; 124:1065–1071.
100. Wilborn F, Brinkmann V, Schmidt CA, Neipel F, Gelderblom H, Siegert W. Herpesvirus type 6 in patients undergoing bone marrow transplantation: serologic features and detection by polymerase chain reaction. Blood 1994; 83:3052–3058.
101. Carrigan DR, Drobyski WR, Russler SK, Tapper MA, Knox KK, Ash RC. Interstitial pneumonitis associated with human herpesvirus-6 infection after marrow transplantation. Lancet 1991; 338:147–149.
102. Carrigan DR, Kehl Knox K. Human herpesvirus 6 (HHV-6) isolation from bone marrow: HHV-6-associated bone marrow suppression in bone marrow transplant patients. Blood 1994; 84:3307–3310.
103. Cone RW, Hackman RC, Huang M-LW, Bowden RA, Meyers JD, Metcalf M, Zeh J, Ashley R, Corey L. Human herpesvirus 6 in lung tissue from patients with pneumonitis after bone marrow transplantation. N Engl J Med 1993; 329:156–161.
104. Drobyski WR, Dunne WM, Burd EM, Knox KK, Ash RC, Horowitz MM, Flomenberg N, Carrigan DR. Human herpesvirus-6 (HHV-6) infection in allogeneic bone marrow transplant recipients: evidence of a marrow-suppressive role for HHV-6 in vivo. J Infect Dis 1993; 167:735–739.
105. Drobyski WR, Knox KK, Majewski D, Carrigan DR. Brief report: fatal encephalitis due to variant B human herpesvirus-6 infection in a bone marrow-transplant recipient. N Engl J Med 1994; 330:1356–1360.
106. Harrington RD, Hooton TM, Hackman RC, Storch GA, Osborne B, Gleaves CA, Benson A, Meyers JD. An outbreak of respiratory syncytial virus in a bone marrow transplant center. J Infect Dis 1992; 165:987–993.
107. Whimbey E, Elting LS, Couch RB, Lo W, Williams L, Champlin RE, Bodey GP. Influenza A virus infections among hospitalized adult bone marrow transplant recipients. Bone Marrow Transplant 1994; 13:437–440.
108. Whimbey E, Couch RB, Englund JA, Andreeff M, Goodrich JM, Raad II, Lewis V, Mirza N, Luna MA, Baxter B, Tarrand JJ, Bodey GP. Respiratory syncytial virus pneumonia in hospitalized adult patients with leukemia. Clin Infect Dis 1995; 21:376–379.
109. Whimbey E, Champlin RE, Couch RB, Englund JA, Goodrich JM, Raad I, Przepiorka D, Lewis VA, Mirza N, Yousuf H, Tarrand JJ, Bodey GP. Community respiratory virus infections among hospitalized adult bone marrow transplant recipients. Clin Infect Dis 1996; 22:778–782.
110. Lewinsohn DM, Bowden RA, Mattson D, Crawford SW. Phase I study of intravenous ribavirin treatment of respiratory syncytial virus pneumonia after marrow transplantation. Antimicrob Agents Chemother 1996; 40:2555–2557.
111. Hayden FG, Osterhaus ADME, Treanor JJ, Fleming DM, Aoki FY, Nicholson KG, Bohnen AM, Hirst HM, Keene O, Wightman K, for the GG167 Influenza Study

Group. Efficacy and safety of the neuraminidase inhibitor zanamivir in the treatment of influenzavirus infections. N Engl J Med 1997; 337:874–880.

112. Raad I, Abbas J, Whimbey E. Infection control of nosocomial respiratory viral disease in the immunocompromised host. Am J Med 1997; 102(suppl 3A):48–52.
113. Ljungman P, Plotkin SA. Workshop on CMV disease; definitions, clinical severity scores, and new syndromes. Scand J Infect Dis 1995; (suppl 99):87–89.
114. Pariente EA, Goudeau A, DuBois F, Degott C, Gluckman E, Devergie A, Brechot C, Schenmetzler C, Bernuau J. Fulminant hepatitis due to reactivation of chronic hepatitis B virus infection after allogeneic bone marrow transplantation. Dig Dis Sci 1988; 33:1185–1191.
115. Locasciulli A, Bacigalupo A, Van Lint MT, Chemello L, Pontisso P, Occhini D, Uderzo C, Shulman HM, Portmann B, Marmont AM, Alberti A. Hepatitis B virus (HBV) infection and liver disease after allogeneic bone marrow transplantation: a report of 30 cases. Bone Marrow Transplant 1990; 6:25–29.
116. Reed EC, Myerson D, Corey L, Meyers JD. Allogeneic marrow transplantation in patients positive for hepatitis B surface antigen. Blood 1991; 77:195–200.
117. Kolho E, Ruutu P, Ruutu T. Hepatitis C infection in BMT patients. Bone Marrow Transplant 1993; 11:119–123.
118. Frickhofen N, Wiesneth M, Jainta C, Hertenstein B, Heymer B, Bianchi L, Dienes HP, Koerner K, Bunjes D, Arnold R, Kubanek B, Heimpel H. Hepatitis C-virus infection is a risk factor for liver failure from veno-occlusive disease after bone marrow transplantation. Blood 1994; 83:1998–2004.
119. Norol F, Roche B, Saint Marc Girardin M, Kuentz M, Desforges L, Cordonnier C, Duedari N, Vernant JP. Hepatitis C virus infection and allogeneic bone marrow transplantation. Transplantation 1994; 57:393–397.
120. Lee WM. Hepatitis B virus infection. N Engl J Med 1997; 337:1733–1745.
121. Arthur RR, Shah KV, Baust SJ, Santos GW, Saral R. Association of BK viruria with hemorrhagic cystitis in recipients of bone marrow transplants. N Engl J Med 1986; 315:230–234.
122. Apperley JF, Rice SJ, Bishop JA, Chia JC, Krausz T, Gardner SD, Goldman JM. Late-onset hemorrhagic cystitis associated with urinary excretion of polyomaviruses after bone marrow transplantation. Transplantation 1987; 43:108–112.
123. Myers C, Frisque RJ, Arthur RR. Direct isolation and characterization of JC virus from urine samples of renal and bone marrow transplant patients. J Virol 1989; 63:44–45.

4

New and Unusual Infections in Neutropenic Patients with Cancer: Concern About Antibiotic-Resistant Bacteria

Stephen H. Zinner
Brown University, Providence, Rhode Island

I. INTRODUCTION

Over the past three decades, considerable changes have occurred in the distribution of bacteria causing infection in febrile neutropenic patients with cancer. When the concept of empirical therapy for fever in these patients was introduced, bacteremia occurred in about 20% of febrile neutropenic episodes, and approximately 70% of these bloodstream infections were caused by gram-negative bacteria (predominantly *Escherichia coli, Klebsiella* sp., and *Pseudomonas aeruginosa*) and *Staphylococcus aureus*. The distribution of these organisms was so predictable that empirical therapy for febrile neutropenic patients directed against these organisms as introduced by Schimpff et al., readily became the accepted standard of care (1).

As has been well documented in the studies of the International Antimicrobial Therapy Cooperative Group (IATCG) of the European Organization for Research and Treatment of Cancer (EORTC), there has been a clear shift in these bacteremia-causing organisms so that currently 60% to 70% of single organism bacteremias are due to gram-positive cocci (Figure 1) (2,3).

Similar trends have been documented elsewhere and, of 320 isolates from 288 episodes of bacteremia in neutropenic patients in Barcelona, 200 (63%) were gram-positive organisms and 120 (37%) were gram-negative (4). In addition to infections with *S. aureus* and coagulase-negative staphylococci, infections caused

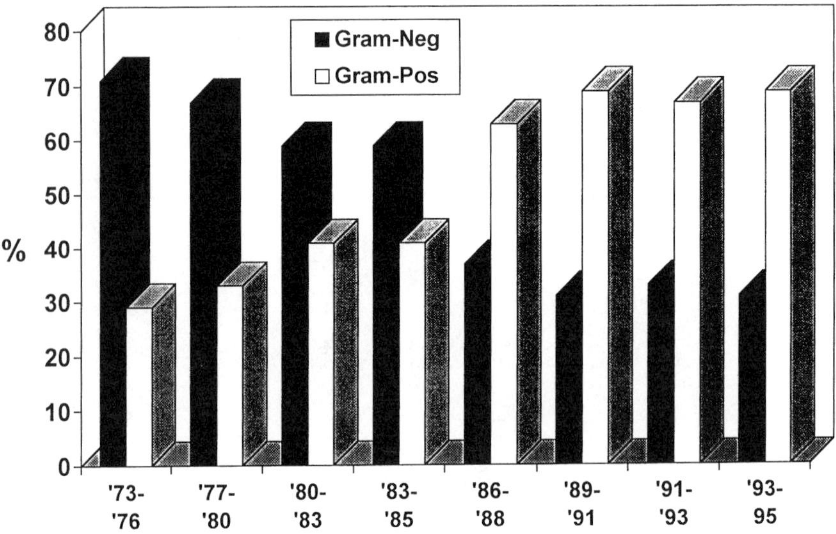

Figure 1 Changing frequency of gram-negative and gram-positive bacteria isolated in single organism bacteremias as reported from the International Antimicrobial Therapy Cooperative Group of the European Organization for Research and Treatment of Cancer.

by viridans streptococci, *Enterococcus* sp., and other streptococci in febrile neutropenic patients are much more common than they were 20 years ago.

Some of the factors believed responsible for the shift to a more gram-positive infecting flora include oral mucositis as a result of increasingly potent chemotherapeutic regimens including cytosine arabinoside, profound and prolonged neutropenia, increasing use of long-dwelling intravascular catheters, fluoroquinolone and trimethoprim-sulfamethoxazole prophylaxis, and sucralfate or H_2 blocker use (5). It is well known that fluoroquinolone prophylaxis has had a dramatic impact on decreasing the incidence of gram-negative rod bacteremia in neutropenic patients with cancer, but these antibiotics have not prevented bacteremias caused by gram-positive organisms (6,7) and may be contributing to the emergence of quinolone resistance in *E. coli* and other enteric organisms (8).

In the past two decades, the emergence of human immunodeficiency virus (HIV) infection and the acquired immunodeficiency syndrome (AIDS) has introduced an ever expanding list of new opportunistic pathogens. Not surprisingly, many of these organisms have made their way into the neutropenic population, because neutropenia is the most common alteration in host defenses in patients with cancer. This chapter reviews the changing array of infections in neutropenic and other immunocompromised patients with cancer and highlights infections caused by organisms that have been newly or recently associated with febrile neutropenic patients. It is likely that the future offers even more evidence of increasing pathogenicity of organisms once thought to be commensal or ''nonpathogenic.'' In the context of ever more immunosuppression in patients undergoing treatment for malignancies, no organism can be safely dismissed as a commensal, and physicians must increase their awareness of previously unencountered or unknown microbes. Of even greater concern is the appearance of more antimicrobial-resistant infections in these patients. Physicians face the incredible scenario of untreatable infections caused by previously susceptible and common organisms. These concerns are highlighted in this review.

II. "NEW" PATHOGENS IN NEUTROPENIC PATIENTS

A. Gram-Positive Organisms

Viridans streptococci were uncommon causes of bacteremia or sepsis in neutropenic patients two decades ago. More recently, these common oral organisms have been implicated in several series (Table 1). In a report from the IATCG, streptococcal species were responsible for 57 of 129 (44%) single-organism bacteremias (9). In 1990, eight cases of *Streptococcus mitis* bacteremia were reported from Dusseldorf (10). In all cases, patients had received prophylactic treatment with either trimethoprim-sulfamethoxazole or quinolones. Serious sepsis including the adult respiratory distress syndrome (ARDS) developed in most of these patients. Also, the pathophysiology of these infections has been described in two patients with *S. mitis* bacteremia from Ulm, Germany. These authors described increased levels of interleukin (IL)-6, tumor necrosis factor (TNF)-α, IL-1 receptor antagonist, and IL-2 receptors in these patients with α-hemolytic streptococcal shock syndrome. They also pointed out that shock or organ failure may develop after blood cultures have been sterilized with antibiotics (11). Table 2 lists suggested first time therapy choices for new pathogens in neutropenic patients.

Of serious concern for the neutropenic patient is the finding that antibiotic resistance in viridans streptococci is increasing. In a survey of 352 bacteremic α-hemolytic streptococci from 43 American centers, Doern et al. reported 13% penicillin resistance, 19% cefprozil resistance, and 17% ceftriaxone resistance (12). Only 4% of these strains were susceptible in vitro to cephalexin. Penicillin resistance was greater among strains of *S. mitis* and *Streptococcus salivarius* (16% and 17%, respectively) than among strains of *Streptococcus milleri*. Erythromycin resistance is also common and was present in more than 30% of these organisms. Other authors have reported penicillin resistance in 12% to 33% of organisms in the *S. milleri* group (13).

In another report, Alcaide et al. found that 34% of 410 strains of viridans

Table 1 Selected "New" Pathogens in Neutropenic Patients

Organism	Probable sources; infection site
Gram-positive	
Streptococcus mitis	Oropharynx; mucositis
Leuconostoc sp.	Oropharynx, skin; intravenous (IV) catheter infection
Enterococcus faecalis	Gastrointestinal (GI) tract; bacteremia
Corynebacterium jeikeium	Skin: axilla, chest; bacteremia, IV catheter infection
Stomatococcus mucilaginosus	Oropharynx; IV catheter, bacteremia
Lactobacillus sp.	Vagina, GI tract; bacteremia
Bacillus cereus	Skin; catheter infection, vesicular pustular eruption
Gram-negative	
Stenotrophomonas maltophilia	Cutaneous infection; catheter sepsis
Alcaligenes xylosoxidans	Catheter-related bacteremia
Capnocytophaga sp.	Oropharynx, GI tract; bacteremia
Chryseobacterium meningosepticum	Water; pneumonia, bacteremia
Burkholderia cepacia	IV solutions; catheter sepsis
Fusobacterium nucleatum	Oropharynx; bacteremia, nodular pneumonitis

group streptococci isolated from blood cultures were resistant to penicillin with minimum inhibitory concentrations (MICs) from 0.25 to 8 mg/L (14). Of the highly penicillin-resistant strains, 80% had cefotaxime and ceftriaxone MICs $\geq$ 2 mg/L. The clinical significance of these findings was emphasized in a report of three patients with penicillin-resistant *S. mitis* bacteremia following chemotherapy for childhood cancer. *S. mitis* meningitis was described in three children undergoing cytotoxic chemotherapy for central nervous system malignancy, two of whom died despite vancomycin treatment (15).

A recent review of viridans streptococcal bacteremia in neutropenic patients reported that *S. mitis* and *S. sanguis* II were most frequently isolated. ARDS, endocarditis, and septic shock were among the serious complications reported (16). A most disturbing case of vancomycin-resistant *S. mitis* bacteremia in a patient with leukemia under treatment with vancomycin and quinolone prophylaxis was reported from Slovakia (17).

Leuconostoc spp. are vancomycin-resistant, slow growing, fastidious gram-

Table 2 Suggested First Time Therapy

Organism	Therapeutic choices
Viridans streptococci	High-dose penicillin, vancomycin
Leuconostoc sp.	Clindamycin, aminoglycosides
Enterococcus faecium, vancomycin-resistant	Quinupristin/dalfopristin, chloramphenicol
Corynebacterium jeikeium	Vancomycin
Rhodococcus equi	Macrolides, vancomycin, clindamycin, aminoglycosides
Stomatococcus mucilaginosus	Vancomycin
Bacillus cereus	Vancomycin
Stenotrophomonas maltophilia	Trimethoprim-sulfamethoxazole,[a] fluoroquinolone,[a]
Alcaligenes xylosoxidans spp *xylosoxidans*	Ampicillin, pipercillin, imipenem, trimethoprim-sulfamethoxazole
Capnocytophaga sp.	Penicillin, clindamycin
Chryseobacterium meningosepticum	Trimethoprim-sulfamethoxazole, ciprofloxacin
Burkholderia cepacia	Antipseudomonal cephalosporins,[a] piperacillin,[a] trimethoprim-sulfamethoxazole
Fusobacterium nucleatum	Clindamycin, metronidazole
Fusarium solani	Amphotericin B

[a] If susceptible.

positive cocci that resemble viridans streptococci or enterococci when grown on blood agar. Although previously characterized as harmless commensals, *Leuconostoc* causes fever, intravenous catheter sepsis, bacteremia, abdominal pain, gastroenteritis or colitis, and even meningitis in the neutropenic patient (18). These organisms are resistant to both vancomycin and teicoplanin but are susceptible to clindamycin and aminoglycosides with intermediate susceptibility to penicillins and first generation cephalosporins.

Colonization and infection by vancomycin-resistant *Enterococcus* spp., especially *Enterococcus faecium* (VREF), are increasing throughout the world. There have been several comments in the recent literature about the serious potential for untreatable infections in neutropenic patients (19,20). Edmond et al. recently described an outbreak of VREF in an oncology unit in a tertiary care hospital in America where 10 of 11 patients were neutropenic with leukemia (21). A very high case-fatality rate was reported and more than 80% of the strains were identical, suggesting nosocomial spread. Predisposing factors included long-term therapy with many antibiotics.

Corynebacterium jeikeium is known to colonize the axillae, skin, and rectum in neutropenic patients, especially those who have received multiple antibiotics. These are nonhemolytic coccobacillary rods that form gray colonies with a metallic sheen on blood agar. They are important causes of sepsis, endocarditis, skin lesions, nodular pulmonary infiltrates, and catheter-related bacteremia in neutropenic patients (22). Effective therapy requires catheter removal and vancomycin. *Corynebacterium urealyticum* is a catalase-positive, urease-producing, gram-positive bacillus that recently has been reported to cause a necrotic soft tissue scrotal infection in a neutropenic patient (23). This organism is susceptible to vancomycin but is resistant to penicillins, aminoglycosides, penems, and ceftazidime.

Rhodococcus equi (formerly *Corynebacterium equi*) is a nonmotile, pleomorphic, gram-positive rod that may appear acid-fast when grown on Lowenstein-Jensen media. This organism causes suppurative pneumonitis, with abscess, effusion, or empyema in patients with AIDS and severe neutropenia. It is usually susceptible to chloramphenicol, macrolides, vancomycin, aminoglycosides, clindamycin, and sulfonamides but is often resistant to penicillin and first generation cephalosporins (24).

Stomatococcus mucilaginosus (formerly *Micrococcus mucilaginosus, Staphylococcus mucilaginosus*) is an oxidase-negative, catalase-variable, nonhemolytic, gram-positive coccus that produces slime and forms adherent gray mucoid colonies that do not grow on 5% NaCl. This organism is normally found in oral flora but has caused intravenous catheter associated sepsis in patients with profound neutropenia. Eight cases were reported from the Royal Free Hospital in London and these patients had received prophylactic trimethoprim-sulfamethoxazole or ciprofloxacin. Response to vancomycin is slow, and this fulminant infection may recur (25,26). In another report from St. Jude's Hospital, Memphis, TN, of eight children with cancer who had *S. mucilaginosus* bacteremia, septic shock and pneumonia occurred in 50%, and two had meningitis or central nervous system symptoms (27).

Lactobacillus spp. are known commensals in the vagina and may serve a protective role there in normal hosts. However, a recent report from France suggests that these organisms are emerging as pathogenic organisms in neutropenic patients (28). Patients had received ceftazidime plus vancomycin before their *Lactobacillus* infections but they responded to penicillin treatment and granulocyte recovery.

Another gram-positive rod, *Bacillus cereus*, is known to cause serious infection in neutropenic patients including pneumonia, catheter-associated sepsis, meningitis, and, in particular, wound infection and necrotizing fasciitis. Ten cases of infection in neutropenic patients were reported from St. Jude's Hospital in 1989 (29). *B. cereus* infections often present with a vesicle or pustule associated with erythema or a draining wound on the digit or limb, most frequently in spring and summer months. Cultures from these lesions are usually positive, but bacteremia is uncommon. This organism is resistant to penicillins, cephalosporins, and trimethoprim-sulfamethoxazole but is susceptible to vancomycin, clindamycin, aminoglycosides, chloramphenicol, and erythromycin; vancomycin is preferred therapy (29).

Clostridium difficile is well known as a cause of the toxin-mediated diarrhea and colitis associated with antibiotic use. Other clostridial species such as *Clostridium septicum* and *Clostridium tertium* have been reported to cause sepsis in neutropenic patients, especially those with bowel or hematological malignancies (30,31). A recent report describes a neutropenic patient with acute lymphoblastic leukemia in whom necrotizing enterocolitis, *C. septicum* bacteremia, rhabdomyolysis, and a meningeal vasculopathy developed (32). *C. tertium* bacteremia has been described as well as a cause of fever and gastrointestinal symptoms in neutropenic patients (33).

B. Gram-Negative Organisms

Although there has been a pronounced increase in the frequency of gram-positive organisms in infected neutropenic patients, gram-negative organisms remain important and are associated with considerably higher mortality rates. Several organisms have been newly associated with these patients, and disturbing trends in antimicrobial resistance are being seen.

In the past few years, cancer centers have identified more strains of *E. coli* that are resistant to fluoroquinolones. This trend was first described by Kern and colleagues from Ulm, where cancer center ofloxacin prophylaxis was routinely prescribed since 1988 (8). They reported an increase in cases of quinolone-resistant *E. coli* isolated from stools of leukemic patients from 69 to 327 per 10,000 discharges from 1988 to 1994. Moreover, cases of quinolone-resistant *E. coli* bacteremia increased from less than 0.5% to 4.5% over the same time interval. Cometta and colleagues also reported a dramatic increase in quinolone-resistant bacteremic *E. coli* strains from none in 1983 to 28% in 1993 cases of quinolone-resistant coagulase-negative staphylococci increased from none to 61% over the same time interval. This was associated with an increase in quinolone prophylaxis in neutropenic patients from 1.4% in 1983 to 45% in 1993 (34). In a subsequent study, these strains were found to be mostly clonally unrelated and diverse (35). Other studies also documented a similar increase in some centers in Europe (36,37).

Although recent meta-analyses support the use of fluoroquinolone prophylaxis because it reduces gram-negative rod bacteremia, the emergence of common bacteria such as *E. coli* that are resistant to these antibiotics suggests that this practice should be reevaluated. This is especially true in light of several reports of the use of fluoroquinolones as primary therapy of febrile neutropenic patients receiving treatment at home.

Serratia marcescens is a gram-negative organism that is not uncommonly isolated from blood cultures in nosocomial infections and it may cause serious septicemia in immunocompromised patients. Recently, a patient with autoimmune neutropenia and chronic gingivitis undergoing treatment with cyclosporin A was described with a lung abscess caused by *S. marcescens* (38).

Stenotrophomonas maltophilia (formerly *Xanthomonas maltophilia, Pseudomonas maltophilia*) is a gram-negative rod that is particularly concerning because of its relative lack of antibiotic susceptibility. *S. maltophilia* is frequently identified as a cause of nosocomial bacteremia and other infections. A cancer center in Slovakia described 31 patients with *S. maltophilia* bacteremia; risk factors for this infection included the presence of a central venous catheter, neutropenia, prophylactic quinolone therapy, or treatment with aminoglycosides, cephalosporins, or imipenem (39). A review from the M. D. Anderson Cancer Center, Houston, TX, described 17 cancer patients with *S. maltophilia* cutaneous and soft tissue infections (40). These patients were usually neutropenic and had metastatic cellulitis or ecthyma gangrenosum-like lesions that were described as mimicking disseminated fungal infections. Another case report described a patient with erythematous nonulcerated nodules with positive cultures for *S. maltophilia* (41).

In a report from Japan, 69 patients with cancer and hematological malignancies had *S. maltophilia* colonization of their respiratory tracts. Of these patients, the organism was responsible for pneumonia in 10, and all strains were susceptible to minocycline (42). These organisms may be susceptible to quinolones or trimethoprim-sulfamethoxazole, but in vitro susceptibility studies must be performed. Another recent report from Spain reported 26 patients with malignancies who were bacteremic as a result of infection with *S. maltophilia* and other glucose nonfermenting gram-negative bacilli including *Pseudomonas putida, Sphingomonas paucimobilis*, and *Alcaligines xylosoxidans*. Most of these patients had catheter-associated bacteremia, and response was associated with catheter removal and antibiotics, although two patients died as a result of the infection (43).

Alcaligenes xylosoxidans ssp. *xylosoxidans* is a nonfermenting peritrichous gram-negative bacillus formerly known as *Achromobacter xylosoxidans*. It was responsible for a nosocomial outbreak of catheter-associated bacteremia in 11 patients in an oncology unit in Essen, Germany (44). It was successfully eradicated by imipenem. This organism is resistant to aminoglycosides, cephalosporins, and tetracyclines but is sensitive to ampicillin, piperacillin, imipenem, and trimethoprim-sulfamethoxazole with intermediate susceptibility to quinolones.

Vibrio parahaemolyticus is a seawater-associated, gram-negative rod that may cause diarrhea or skin infections in normal hosts. It is not a common cause of infection in neutropenic patients, but an episode of bacteremia in a leukemic patient caused by this organism has been described. Apparently, the patient had lacerated a finger while preparing fresh squid and a paronychia, fever, hypotension, and hemolytic anemia subsequently developed. This organism was successfully eradicated with ceftazidime plus gentamicin, followed by oral trimethoprim-sulfamethoxazole (45).

Capnocytophaga sp. are normal members of the oral, gastrointestinal, and vaginal flora and were previously known as DF-1 or DF-2 (dysgonic fermenter). These gram-negative rods are capnophilic, facultatively anaerobic and grow on blood agar. They are catalase-, oxidase-, and indole-negative, but ferment glucose, sucrose, maltose, lactose, and mannose. *Capnocytophaga* sp. are identified as etiological agents of bacteremia in patients undergoing bone marrow transplantation, especially in the presence of severe oral pathology (46). They are susceptible to penicillin and clindamycin but are only variably susceptible to cephalosporins, imipenem, chloramphenicol, quinolones, and tetracycline. These organisms usually are resistant to aminoglycosides and trimethoprim. A recent case report of bacteremia with *Capnocytophaga sputigena* was due to an organism that was highly resistant to ampicillin, ureidopenicillins, cefazolin, cefuroxime, cefotaxime, and ceftazidime. This organism was also resistant to ciprofloxacin (47).

Chryseobacterium meningosepticum (formerly *Flavobacterium meningosepticum*) is a water-borne, gram-negative rod known to cause meningitis in neonates. Six cases of pneumonia and/or bacteremia were described in patients with leukemia or undergoing bone marrow transplantation at the University of California, San Francisco, hospital (48). This organism is resistant to cephalosporins, macrolides, clindamycin, vancomycin, and aminoglycosides but is susceptible to trimethoprim-sulfamethoxazole, ciprofloxacin, minocycline and rifampin.

Burkholderia cepacia (formerly *Pseudomonas cepacia*) is a biofilm-producing, gram-negative rod associated with central venous catheter sepsis. Recently contaminated heparin flush solutions were implicated in a cluster of 14 cases in an oncology unit (49). *B. cepacia* is usually resistant to imipenem, tobramycin, and ticarcillin but may be susceptible to pseudomonal active third generation cephalosporins, piperacillin, and trimethoprim-sulfamethoxazole.

Among the anaerobic gram-negative rods, *Fusobacterium nucleatum*, a beta-lactamase–producing organism, has been implicated in bacteremia and ulcerative pharyngitis and nodular pulmonary infiltrates (possibly resulting from septic emboli) in a neutropenic leukemic patient (50). The described patient responded to clindamycin plus metronidazole and the authors questioned the role of ureidopenicillins in selecting for this organism. Another report of three neutropenic patients with severe *F. nucleatum* infection was presented from The Netherlands, and severe mucositis was believed to be a risk factor (51).

Infections in neutropenic patients caused by *Bacteroides* sp. are not very common. However, over a 22-year observation, 13 such patients were described from a ''sterile unit'' in Japan. *Bacteroides fragilis* was most frequently associated with other organisms. Risk factors included prior antimicrobial use, cancer chemotherapy, neutropenia, thrombocytopenia, and hypoproteinemia (52). *Leptotrichia buccalis* was described as a cause of bacteremia in a series of patients with advanced cancer and leukemia at the National Cancer Institute (53). Most of these patients had severe oral and/or gastrointestinal mucosal ulceration. *L. buccalis* is resistant to vancomycin, quinolones, aminoglycosides, and macrolides but is susceptible to penicillins, cephalosporins, clindamycin, metronidazole, and tetracycline.

III. OTHER INFECTIONS

Recently, a large number of fungi have been newly associated with infections in neutropenic patients, including *Trichosporon beigelii, Trichosporon capitatum, Fusarium* sp., *Pseudallescheria boydii, Torulopsis pintolopesii, Candida krusei, Geotrichum candidum, Saccharomyces cerevisiae*, and *Pichia farinosa*, among many others. The general theme is that even relatively noninvasive organisms such as the dermatophytes may cause serious and widespread invasive infection in profoundly immunosuppressed and neutropenic patients. In a series from Brazil, 30 patients with fungal infections were described from among 313 episodes of febrile neutropenia. Predisposing factors included central venous catheters, profound and prolonged neutropenia, gram-positive bacteremia, corticosteroid use, and younger age (54).

Fusarium spp. are among the most serious and devastating fungal infections that present with painful necrotic skin nodules that may be vesicular and can result in disseminated infection, even though they had been considered as plant saprophytes incapable of causing infection in humans (55,56). However, patients with cancer and hematological malignancies may be seen with disseminated *Fusarium solani* infections that include tender erythematous papules with black necrotic centers (57). In normal hosts, this organism may cause onychomycosis, keratitis, endophthalmitis, or arthritis at the point of inoculation. In the immunocompromised host, it may cause fever, fungemia, myalgias, ocular symptoms, multiple organ involvement, and skin lesions, which may resemble ecthyma gangrenosum (58). Of particular note is that this organism is resistant to imidazoles and triazoles and is only, partially responsive to amphotericin B.

Many of the other fungi isolated from infections in neutropenic patients may be variably resistant to antifungal agents. For example, Wingard and colleagues have reported an increase in *Torulopsis glabrata* infections in patients who had been given fluconazole (59). Disseminated infection with *Acremonium strictum* has been reported in a neutropenic patient with positive fecal cultures and subsequent fungemia (60). These authors pointed out that hyphae and other adventitious forms could be seen with *Acremonium* infections as well as with *Fusarium*,

Paecilomyces, Scedosporium, and *Blastoschizomyces* species and that all of these could be confused with *Candida* sp. Many other fungal infections have been reported in febrile neutropenic patients as recently reviewed in several sources (54,59,61).

Still other infections may be caused by nontuberculous mycobacteria, *Bartonella henselae*, *Bartonella quintana*, and the microsporidia (62). A neuropenic patient with non-Hodgkin's lymphoma was recently described with *B. quintana* bacteremia. Successful treatment was attributed to cefotaxime, imipenem, and vancomycin therapy (63).

IV. DISCUSSION

As patients with cancer are subjected to ever increasingly potent and intensive chemotherapeutic regimens, it is imperative that efforts at preventing infection are maximized in these patients. Careful attention to infection control measures, including cooked food diets, appropriate use of prophylactic agents (which remain to be defined optimally), and prompt institution of empirical broad-spectrum antibiotic therapy, remain useful as guidelines in the management of neutropenic patients at risk of infection. It is also important for physicians to be aware of the potential for any organism to cause serious infection in these patients, even those organisms previously thought to be harmless commensals. Also, it is critically important for physicians to be aware of trends in infecting organisms and patterns of antimicrobial susceptibility and resistance in their environments. It is also imperative to carefully evaluate and study those new cephalosporins and quinolone antibiotics that are introduced for therapy.

The decision to institute antibacterial prophylaxis with fluoroquinolone antibiotics is controversial. Although several recent meta-analyses have supported the use of these agents in neutropenic patients because of their definitive reduction in gram-negative bacteremic episodes, a consistent benefit on the incidence or time to development of fever has not been found. Moreover, there is some evidence of increasing fluoroquinolone resistance among common bacteria within cancer centers, particularly in Europe. Certainly, if quinolones are being considered for primary therapy for febrile neutropenic patients (especially in outpatients), then serious concern about their prophylactic use must be raised.

The important lessons of the past two decades is that changes in bacterial ecology are unavoidable given the pressures of antibiotic use, increaseing immunosuppression, new use of invasive devices and procedures, and the changes in health care delivery. The physician must be especially vigilant regarding excess use of antibiotics and must encourage the strictest infection control practices in institutions that treat the most vulnerable patients.

REFERENCES

1. Schimpff SC, Satterlee W, Young VM, Serpick A. Empiric therapy with carbenicillin and gentamicin for febrile patients with cancer and granulocytopenia. N Engl J Med 1971; 284:1061–1065.
2. Cometta A, Zinner S, deBock R, et al. and the International Antimicrobial Therapy Cooperative Group of the European Organization for Research and Treatment of Cancer. Piperacillin-tazobactam plus amikacin versus ceftazidime plus amikacin as empiric therapy for fever in granulocytopenic patients with cancer. Antimicrob Agents Chemother 1995; 39:445–452.
3. Cometta A, Calandra T, Gaya H, et al., and the International Antimicrobial Therapy Cooperative Group of the European Organization for Research and Treatment of Cancer and The Gruppo Italiano Malattie Ematologiche Maligne Dell'adulto Infection Program. Monotherapy with meropenem versus combination therapy with ceftazidime plus amikacin as empiric therapy for fever in granulocytopenic patients with cancer. Antimicrob Agents Chemother 1996; 40:1108–1118.
4. Gonzalez-Barca E, Fernandez-Sevilla A, Carratala J, Granena A, Gudiol F. Prospective study of 288 episodes of bacteremia in neutropenic cancer patients in a single institution. Eur J Clin Microbiol Infect Dis 1996; 15:291–296.
5. Elting LS, Bodey GP, Keefe BH. Septicemia and shock syndrome due to viridans streptococci: a case-control study of predisposing factors. Clin Infect Dis 1992; 14: 1201–1207.
6. Zinner SH. Prophylactic uses of fluoroquinolone antibiotics. Infect Dis Clin Pract 1994; 3(suppl 3):S203–S210.
7. Cruciani M, Rampazzo R, Malena M, Lazzarini L, Todeschini G, Messori A, Concia E. Prophylaxis with fluoroquinolones for bacterial infections in neutropenic patients: a meta-analysis. Clin Infect Dis 1996; 23:795–805.
8. Kern WV, Andriof E, Oethinger M, Kern P, Hacker J, Marre R. Emergence of fluoroquinolone-resistant *Escherichia coli* at a cancer center. Antimicrob Agents Chemother 1994; 38:681–687.
9. European Organization for Research and Treatment of Cancer International Antimicrobial Therapy Cooperative Group and the National Cancer Institute of Canada-Clinical Trials Group. Vancomycin added to empirical combination antibiotic therapy for fever in granulocytopenic cancer patients. J Infect Dis 1991; 163:951–958.
10. Arning M, Gehrt A, Aul C, Runde V, Hadding U, Schneider W. Septicemia due to *Streptococcus mitis* in neutropenic patients with acute leukemia. Blut 1990; 61:364–368.
11. Engel A, Kern P, Kern WV. Levels of cytokines and cytokine inhibitors in the neutropenic patient with α-hemolytic streptococcus shock syndrome. Clin Infect Dis 1996; 23:785–789.
12. Doern GV, Ferraro MJ, Brueggemann A, Ruoff KL. Emergence of high rates of antimicrobial resistance among viridans group streptococci in the United States. Antimicrob Agents Chemother 1996; 40:891–894.
13. Bantar C, Fernandez Canigia L, Relloso S, Lanza A, Bianchini H, Smayevsky J.

Species belonging to the "*Streptococcus milleri*" group: antimicrobial susceptibility and comparative prevalence in significant clinical specimens. J Clin Microbial 1996; 34:2020–2022.

14. Alcaide F, Linares J, Pallares R, Garratala J, Benitez MA, Gudiol F, Martin R. In vitro activities of 22 beta-lactam antibiotics against penicillin-resistant and penicillin-susceptible viridans group streptococci isolated from blood. Antimicrob Agents Chemother 1995; 39:2243–2247.
15. Balkundi DR, Murray DL, Patterson MJ, Gera R, Scott-Emuakpor A, Kulkarni R. Penicillin-resistant *Streptococcus mitis* as a cause of septicemia with meningitis in febrile neutropenic children. J Pediatr Hematol Oncol 1997; 19:82–85.
16. Bochud PY, Calandra T, Francioli P. Bacteremia due to viridans streptococci in neutropenic patients: a review. Am J Med 1994; 97:256–264.
17. Krcmery V Jr, Spanik S, Trupl J. First report of vancomycin-resistant *Streptococcus mitis* bacteremia in a leukemic patient after prophylaxis with quinolones and during treatment with vancomycin (letter). J Chemother 1996; 8:325–326.
18. Handwerger S, Horowitz H, Coburn K, Kolokathis A, Wormser GP. Infection due to *Leuconostoc* species: six cases and review. Rev Infect Dis 1990; 12:602–610.
19. Chanock SJ, Pizzo PA. Infectious complications of patients undergoing therapy for acute leukemia: current status and future prospects. Semin Oncol 1997; 24:132–149.
20. Montecalvo MA, Shay DK, Patel P, Tacsa L, Maloney SA, Jarvis WR, Wormser GP. Bloodstream infections with vancomycin-resistant enterococci. Arch Intern Med 1996; 156:1458–1462.
21. Edmond MB, Ober JF, Weinbaum DL, Pfaller MA, Hwang T, Sanford MD, Wenzel RP. Vancomycin-resistant *Enterococcus faecium* bacteremia: risk factors for infection. Clin Infect Dis 1995; 20:1126–1133.
22. Van der Lelie H, Leversteinvanhall M, Mertens M, Vanzaanen HCT, Vanoers RHJ, Thomas BLM, Vondemborne AEGK, Kuijper EJ. *Corynebacterium* CDC group JK (*Corynebacterium jeikeium*) sepsis in haematological patients: a report of three cases and a systematic literature review. Scand J Infect Dis 1995; 27:581–584.
23. Saavedra J, Rodriguez JN, Fernandez-Jurrado A, Vega MD, Pascual L, Prados D. A necrotic soft-tissue lesion due to *Corynebacterium urealyticum* in a neutropenic child. Clin Infect Dis 1996; 22:851–852.
24. Harvey RI, Sunstrum JC. *Rhodococcus equi* infection in patients with and without human immunodeficiency virus infection. Rev Infect Dis 1991; 13:139–145.
25. Asher DP, Zbick C, White C, Fischer GW. Infections due to *Stomatococcus mucilaginosus*: 10 cases and review. Rev Infect Dis 1991; 13:1048–1052.
26. McWhinney PHM, Kibbler CC, Gillespie SH, et al. *Stomatococcus mucilaginosus*: an emerging pathogen in neutropenic patients. Clin Infect Dis 1992; 13:641–646.
27. Henwick S, Koehler M, Patrick CC. Complications of bacteremia due to *Stomatococcus mucilaginosus* in neutropenic children. Clin Infect Dis 1993; 17:667–671.
28. Fruchart C, Salah A, Gray C, Martin E, Stamatoullas A, Bonmarchand G, Lemeland JF, Tilly H. *Lactobacillus* species as emerging pathogens in neutropenic patients. Eur J Clin Microbiol Infect Dis 1997; 16:681–684.
29. Henrickson KJ, Shenep JL, Flynn PM, Pui C-H. Primary cutaneous *Bacillus cereus* infection in neutropenic children. Lancet 1989; 1:601–603.

30. Hassan H, Teh A. *Clostridium septicum* septicaemia in a patient with leukaemia. Singapore Med J 1994; 35:217–218.
31. Litam PP, Loughran TP Jr. *Clostridium septicum* bacteremia in a patient with large granular lymphocyte leukemia. Cancer Invest 1995; 13:492–494.
32. Crowley RS, Lembke A, Haroupian DS. Isolated meningeal vasculopathy associated with *Clostridium septicum* infection. Neurology 1997; 48:265–267.
33. Gosbell IB, Johnson CG, Newton PJ, Jelfs J. *Clostridium tertium* bacteremia: 2 cases and review. Pathology 1996; 28:70–73.
34. Cometta A, Calandra T, Bille J, Glauser MP. *Escherichia coli* resistant to fluoroquinolones in patients with cancer and neutropenia. N Engl J Med 1994; 330:1240.
35. Oethinger M, Conrad S, Kaifel K, Cometta A, Bille J, Klotz G, Glauser MP, Marre R, The International Antimicrobial Therapy Cooperative Group of the European Organization for Research and Treatment of Cancer, Kern WV. Molecular epidemiology of fluoroquinolone-resistant *Escherichia coli* blood stream isolates from patients admitted to European cancer centers. Antimicrob Agents Chemother 1996; 40:387–392.
36. Carratala J, Fernandez-Sevilla A, Tubau FE, Angeles-Dominguez M, Gudiol F. Emergence of fluoroquinolone-resistant *Escherichia coli* in fecal flora of cancer patients receiving norfloxacin prophylaxis. Antimicrob Agents Chemother 1996; 40: 503–505.
37. Kunova A, Trupl J, Krcmery V. Low incidence of quinolone resistance in gram-negative bacteria after five-years use of ofloxacin in prophylaxis during afebrile neutropenia. J Hosp Infect 1996; 32:155–156.
38. Mizota M, Kawakami K, Ijichi O, Takezaki T, Miyata K. *Serratia marcescens* lung abscess in a child with autoimmune neutropenia. Acta Paediatrica Japonica 1995; 37:377–380.
39. Krcmery V, Pichna P, Oravcova E, Lacka J, Kukockova E, Studena M, Grausova S, Stopkova K, Krupova I. *Stenotrophomonas maltophilia* bacteremia in cancer patients: report on 31 cases. J Hosp Infect 1996; 34:75–77.
40. Vartivarian SE, Papadakis KA, Palacios JA, Manning JT Jr, Anaissie EJ. Mucocutaneous and soft tissue infections caused by *Xanthomonas maltophilia*. A new spectrum. Ann Intern Med 1994; 121:969–973.
41. Burns RL, Lowe L. *Xanthomonas maltophilia* infection presenting as erythematous nodules. J Am Acad Dermatol 1997; 37:836–838.
42. Fujita J, Yamadori I, Xu G, Hojo S, Negayama K, Miyawaki H, Yamaji Y, Takahara J. Clinical features of *Stenotrophomonas maltophilia* pneumonia in immunocompromised patients. Respir Med 1996; 90:35–38.
43. Martino R, Martinez C, Pericas R, Salazar R, Sola C, Brunet S, Sureda A, Domingo-Albos A. Bacteremia due to glucose non-fermenting gram-negative bacilli in patients with hematological neoplasias and solid tumors. Eur J Clin Microbiol Infect Dis 1996; 15:610–615.
44. Knippschild M, Schmid EN, Uppenkamp M, Koenig E, Meusers P, Brittinger G, Hoeffken H-G. Infection by *Alcaligenes xylosoxidans* subsp. *xylosoxidans* in neutropenic patients. Oncology 1996; 53:258–262.
45. Dobroszycki J, Sklarin NT, Szilagy G, Tanowitz HB. *Vibrio parahaemolyticus* septicemia in a patient with neutropenic leukemia. Clin Infect Dis 1992; 15:738–739.

46. Bilgrami S, Bergstrom SK, Peterson DE, et al. *Capnocytophaga* bacteremia in a patient with Hodgkin's disease following bone marrow transplantation: case report and review. Clin Infect Dis 1992; 14:1045–1049.
47. Gomez-Garces JL, Alos JI, Sanchez J, Cogollos R. Bacteremia by multidrug-resistant *Capnocytophaga sputigena*. J Clin Microbiol 1994; 32:1067–1069.
48. Bloch KC, Nadarajah R, Jacobs R. *Chryseobacterium meningosepticum*: an emerging pathogen among immunocompromised adults. Medicine 1997; 76:30–41.
49. Pegues DA, Carson LA, Anderson RL, et al. Outbreak of *Pseudomonas cepacia* bacteremia in oncology patients. Clin Infect Dis 1993; 16:407–411.
50. Huyghebaert MF, Dreyfus F, Paul G, et al. Septicémie à Fusobacterium nucleatum, producteur de bêta-lactamase chez un sujet neutropénique. Ann Med Interne (Paris) 1989; 140:225–226.
51. Landsaat PM, van der Lelie H, Bongaerts G, Kuijper EJ. *Fuseobacterium nucleatum*, a new invasive pathogen in neutropenic patients? Scand J Infect Dis 1995; 27:83–84.
52. Funada H, Matsuda T. Bacteremia caused by the *Bacteroides fragilis* group in patients with hematologic diseases. Japan J Clin Oncol 1995; 25:86–90.
53. Weinberger M, Wu T, Rubin M, Gill VJ, Pizzo PA. *Leptotrichia buccalis* bacteremia in patients with cancer: report of four cases and review. Rev Infect Dis 1991; 13: 201–206.
54. Nucci M, Pulcherii W, Spector N, Bueno AP, Bacha PC, Caiuby MJ, Derossi A, Costa R, Morais JC, de Oliveira HP. Fungal infections in neutropenic patients. A 8-year prospective study. Rev Inst Med Trop Sao Paulo 1995; 37:397–406.
55. Nucci M, Spector N, Lucena S, et al. Three cases of infection with *Fusarium* species in neutropenic patients. Eur J Clin Microbiol Infect Dis 1992; 11:1160–1162.
56. Anaissie E, Bodey GP, Kantarjian H, et al. New spectrum of fungal infections in patients with cancer. Rev Infect Dis 1989; 11:369–378.
57. Bushelman SJ, Callen JP, Roth DN, Cohen LM. Disseminated *Fusarium solani* infection. J Am Acad Dermatol 1995; 32:346–351.
58. Martino P, Gastaldi R, Raccah R, Girmenia C. Clinical patterns of *Fusarium* infections in immunocompromised patients. J Infect 1994; 28(suppl 1):7–15.
59. Wingard JR, Merz WG, Rinaldi MG, Miller CB, Karp JE, Saral R. Association of *Torulopsis glabrata* infections with fluconazole prophylaxis in neutropenic bone marrow transplant patients. Antimicrob Agents Chemother 1993; 37:1847–1849.
60. Schell WA, Perfect JR. Fatal, disseminated *Acremonium strictum* infection in a neutropenic host. J Clin Microbiol 1996; 34:1333–1336.
61. Zinner SH. New and unusual infections in neutropenic patients. In: J Klastersky J, ed. Infectious Complications of Cancer. Boston: Kluwer Academic Publishers, 1995: 173–184.
62. Gentile G, Venditti M, Micossi A, et al. Cryptosporidiosis in patients with hematologic malignancies. Rev Infect Dis 1991; 13:842–846.
63. Rathbone P, Graves S, Miller D, Odorico D, Jones S, Hellyar A, Sinickas V, Grigg A. *Bartonella* (*Rochalimaea*) *quintana* causing fever and bacteremia in an immunocompromised patient with non-Hodgkin's lymphoma. Pathology 1996; 28:80–83.

5

Prevention of Infection in Cancer Patients

Stephen C. Schimpff

University of Maryland Medical System and University of Maryland School of Medicine, Baltimore, Maryland

I. INTRODUCTION

Implementing appropriate strategies to prevent infection in any immunocompromised patient begins with an assessment of the type of immune defects from which they suffer. This then helps define the types of infections that pose the greatest risk to that patient. The major types of immune defects that clinicians encounter can be divided into six broad categories: (1) granulocytopenia, (2) deficiencies of cellular immunity, (3) deficiencies of humoral immunity, (4) obstruction of a normal lumen by tumor or fibrosis, (5) central nervous system dysfunction, and (6) damage to normal anatomical barriers, such as the skin or mucosal surfaces (Table 1). Although approaches to preventing infection vary with each type of immune defect and the severity of the defect in a given patient four general approaches can be applied to all patients: (1) attempt to improve the patient's immune defects, (2) reduce acquisition of potential pathogens, (3) suppress organisms with which the patient is already colonized that are likely to cause infection later, and (4) reduce or avoid procedures that disrupt normal anatomical barriers (Table 2).

Table 1 Predisposing Factors to Infection in Cancer Patients

Granulocytopenia
Cellular immune deficiency
Humoral immune deficiency
Obstruction
Central nervous system dysfunction
Anatomical barrier damage

II. GRANULOCYTOPENIA

The risk of infection varies inversely with the absolute granulocyte count. Infection rates begin to increase between 500 and 1000 cells/μL and to increase markedly below 100 cells/μL with the majority of bacteremias occurring in this group (Fig. 1). The predominant infections seen early in the course of neutropenia are bacterial (Table 3). Gram-negative rods were formerly the major pathogens, but for a variety of reasons the numbers of gram-positive infections, particularly *Staphylococcus epidermidis* and α-hemolytic streptococci, have increased dramatically over the past two decades. Fungi, such as *Candida* spp, *Aspergillus flavus*, and *Aspergillus fumigatus*, also are important pathogens, particularly with more prolonged granulocytopenia and the use of broad-spectrum antibiotics. Efforts to prevent infection in these patients encompass each of the four approaches and are discussed here.

A. Improve Host Defense Mechanisms

Decreasing the duration and severity of neutropenia is the best approach to preventing infection; however, favorable responses to cytotoxic drugs are correlated with the ability to give maximum doses of chemotherapeutic agents, which result

Table 2 Basic Approaches to Infection Prevention

Augment immune function
Reduce organism acquisition
Suppress colonizing potential pathogens
Avoid and/or reduce disruption of natural barriers

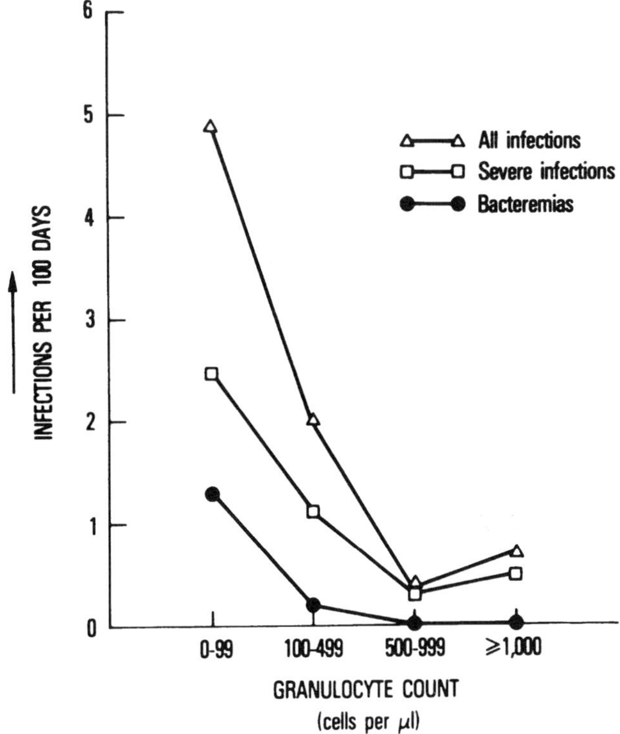

Figure 1 Incidence of infection in acute lymphocytic leukemia during induction therapy. (Modified from Ref. 74.)

in increased side effects, including bone marrow suppression. Early attempts focused on granulocyte transfusions. These have been shown in small controlled trials to prevent gram-negative bacteremia and to improve survival of infected patients with persistent neutropenia (1–4). Schiffer, in a review of granulocyte transfusions, suggests that some of the reasons for poor responses that caused this technique to be largely abandoned were the generally low doses of leukocytes used and the lack of attention to the problem of alloimmunization (5). Transfusions must be given on a daily basis, which places a great logistical strain on blood banks and taxes the donor pool. He describes good results using leukocytes from chronic myelogenous leukemia patients because high doses can be achieved and their content of early cells continue to divide for several days but have not caused problems with a graft-versus-host response. Another approach is to give

Table 3 Infections During Granulocytopenia

Common Sites:
Alimentary canal
Periodontitis/gingivitis
Pharyngitis
Esophagitis
Perianal lesions
Pneumonia
Skin lesions
Vascular access-related
Common Organisms:
Gram-negative
Escherichia coli
Pseudomonas aeruginosa
Gram-positive
Staphylococcus epidermidis
Staphylococcus aureus
α-hemolytic *Streptococcus* spp.
Yeast
Candida spp.
Fungi
Aspergillus flavus and *Aspergillus fumigatus*
Virus
Herpes simplex

The sites and organisms listed account for about 80% of infections during granulocytopenia.

a donor a colony-stimulating factor (CSF), giving rise to high leukocyte counts and peripheral progenitor cells. Another problem with leukocyte transfusions, which can be minimized with current techniques for screening donors, is that there is a risk of transmitting infections such as cytomegalovirus (CMV), other viruses, or more rarely, parasitic pathogens, such as toxoplasmosis. I recommend that granulocyte transfusions not be given on a prophylactic basis but that they should be considered as a treatment modality for patients with life-threatening infection who respond poorly to known appropriate antibiotics in the face of persistent neutropenia.

The cloning and expression of the recombinant myeloid CSFs, granulocyte CSFs (G-CSFs), and granulocyte-macrophage CSF (GM-CSF) have led to a whole new approach to chemotherapy-induced neutropenia. They can stimulate the recovery of neutrophil counts (6) and may have beneficial effects on phagocyte function (7). The usual approach to these cytokines has been to use them to allow more aggressive cancer chemotherapy, perhaps even avoiding the need for autologous bone marrow transplantation in some instances. The G-CSF and GM-CSF have been shown in randomized, double-blind, placebo-controlled trials to decrease the incidence of severe neutropenia, infection, antibiotic requirements, and period of hospitalization in patients receiving standard chemotherapy for small cell lung cancer (8). These cytokines have been used in the setting of bone marrow transplantation to speed recovery following engraftment. Peters and colleagues, working with breast cancer patients in autologous bone marrow transplantation (ABMT), have shown that GM-CSF begun immediately after marrow reinfusion led to a substantially shortened period of neutropenia (9). They later found that G-CSF gave similar results and that the period of absolute neutropenia, which had been unaffected by posttransplant CSF administration, could be shortened by infusion of peripheral blood progenitor cells. These cells are collected by leukopheresis before bone marrow transplantation after pretreatment with either GM- or G-CSF (10). This has led to fewer adverse events, including less time in the intensive care unit, a shorter hospital stay, and a reduction in total cost from about $100,000 to approximately $75,000 per transplant episode (W. P. Peters, personal communication, 1996). Decreased morbidity has also been seen using GM-CSF after ABMT for lymphoid neoplasias (11). This approach has become the standard of care with marrow or peripheral stem cell transplantation. In most cases, patients can undergo outpatient treatment.

Based on the available data, the following recommendations seem appropriate. First, G-CSF and GM-CSF are useful in the setting of autologous bone marrow and stem cell transplantation for reducing the nadir and the duration of granulocytopenia. Second, they are appropriate for patients receiving aggressive therapy that would be likely to cause more than a week of significant granulocytopenia. *Significant* is defined as less than 500 polymorphonuclear neutrophils (PMN) μL and perhaps a level of less than 200/μL, because almost all serious infections occur only in patients who have less than 200 PMN/μL (see Fig. 1).

Another approach to reducing the degree and duration of granulocytopenia is use of amifostine (originally known as WR-2721), a phosphorylated thiol developed by the United States Army as a protective agent in the event of nuclear warfare. Amifostine protects normal tissues from both radiation and chemotherapy yet it does not inhibit antitumor effect. Bone marrow stem cells are protected from chemotherapy and radiation therapy and, hence, can continue to produce new granulocytes. Because the colony stimulators are just that—stimulators of stem cell growth and division but not protectors—it may prove logical and effective to use both modalities at once (12).

B. Reduce Organism Acquisition

The concept is to reduce acquisition of new organisms, because it has been demonstrated that more than 50% of the infections in immunocompromised patients are caused by organisms acquired by the patient during hospitalization (13). The major routes of acquisition are the hands of health care workers, food, water, and the air. Hand washing is the most basic technique for preventing spread but it is frequently overlooked by health care workers. In one recent study of the efficacy of different hand washing agents in which the professional staff was observed the staff took advantage of only approximately 40% of hand washing opportunities (14). Although hand washing with any product is probably better than none, Doebbeling et al. found chlorhexidine significantly reduced nosocomial infections compared with the combined use of soap and alcohol. Chlorhexidine is currently the agent of choice and should be made readily available throughout hospital wards.

Gram-negative bacilli are acquired principally from food and, to a lesser degree, from water and hands. If the major cause of serious infection from acquired organisms is gram-negative rod infections, then the major sources must be dealt with, namely food and water. Remington and Schimpff have summarized the findings of others in an editorial entitled ''Please Don't Eat the Salads,'' in which they point out that a simple approach to a low microbial content diet can be effective (15). The importance of properly cooking meat was recently reemphasized by a large outbreak of disease secondary to Escherichia coli 0157:H7 in undercooked hamburger at a fast-food restaurant. *Candida* can also be acquired from food products including many fruits and unpasteurized fruit juices.

Most city water supplies are reasonably satisfactory as long as the faucet aerator at the end of the piping system has not become laden with organic debris that can support the growth of gram-negative rods, such as *Pseudomonas aeruginosa* or *Serratia marcescens*. Significant gram-negative contamination has also been linked to nosocomial sources, such as an ice machine.

Some bacterial pathogens, such as *Staphylococcus aureus* can be acquired via aerosol. In these cases, there is usually a point source, such as a patient with staphylococcal pneumonia, and the problem is best handled by isolating the source patient. *Aspergillus* can also be acquired via the air, and here the problem is more difficult because the spores are ubiquitous. Outbreaks have been associated with new construction or renovation, for example. In this situation care must be taken to ensure a clean air supply before beginning work. The old ''standard'' approach to reverse isolation, which generally included donning gowns, gloves, mask, and frequently booties and hats, with no attention to food, water, or air, was ultimately proved by Maki and colleagues to be of no utility (16). Laminar airflow rooms can be effective in ensuring adequate air filtration for patients at high risk of infection by airborne-related organisms such as *Aspergillus* (17). However, despite their utility, such measures require long-term isolation when simpler techniques may suffice. At the University of Maryland transplant unit, for example, there is a separate high-efficiency particulate air (HEPA) filtration system so that isolation is unnecessary. A portable laminar airflow unit was as effective as a wall unit in preventing infection in one study from Japan (18) and even placing air filtration devices in the patient's room can substantially reduce airborne organisms.

C. Suppression of Potential Pathogens

1. *Skin*

Cutaneous infections are common in granulocytopenic patients (see Chapter 21), particularly at sites where the skin has been interrupted by invasive procedures. It has been suggested that daily bathing with such agents as chlorhexidine may decrease the incidence of infection. The axilla and perianal area are at particularly high risk, and twice daily swabbing with povidone-iodine during the period of granulocytopenia has been shown to decrease infections (19); chlorhexidine should be equally effective.

2. *Periodontium*

Periodontal infections are frequent during periods of granulocytopenia (see Chapter 9). The oral mucosa is also a likely source of α-hemolytic streptococcal bacteremia. A program of professional and personal dental care before chemotherapy, with plaque removal, repair of any caries, and teeth extraction when necessary, as well as daily brushing and flossing, is prudent. Despite concerns to the contrary, pretherapy prophylaxis by a dental professional followed by regular brushing and flossing does not lead to bleeding or bacteremia but rather reduces acute flare-ups of chronic periodontitis during granulocytopenia (see Chapter 9).

3. *Oral Viral Infections*

Herpes simplex virus is latent in most adults and is commonly recognized as a severe oral or esophageal infection in the first 20 days following bone marrow transplantation (20). Acyclovir has been found to be nearly 100% effective as prophylaxis among these patients (21). Although severe herpes simplex oral infections are seen in patients with leukemia or other patients with cancer receiving intensive chemotherapy, it has been generally believed that the frequency and severity of infection are much less than in bone marrow transplant patients. However, patients with acute myelocytic leukemia receiving induction therapy have frequent herpes simplex oral infections (66% reactivation rates in seropositive patients), which, in turn, can be substantially prevented by the use of acyclovir (22). The oral infection frequently encountered has a bacterial component or even a component caused by *Candida albicans* or *Candida tropicalis*. This is similar to the observation of *Candida* esophagitis; that is, if one evaluates these patients early in their course, one finds that the initial lesion is often caused by herpes simplex, which, in turn, allows invasion by bacteria and then by *Candida*. Prevention of the initial viral lesion then helps to prevent the superinfection with bacteria and fungi.

4. Antibacterial Prophylaxis

Several different antibiotic strategies have been used to prevent bacterial infections. An early approach was to use a combination of oral nonabsorbable antibiotics, such as gentamicin, vancomycin, and nystatin (17). This was shown to reduce the incidence of infection, particularly gram-negative bacteremia; however, the regimens were expensive and poorly tolerated and resistant isolates were soon detected. Trimethoprim-sulfamethoxazole (TMP-SMX) was undergoing studies to prevent *Pneumocystis carinii* pneumonia and was coincidentally found to decrease the incidence of bacterial infection (23). The toxicities seen with TMP-SMX, such as prolongation of marrow suppression, development of resistant isolates, and possibly increased fungal infections, along with the lack of efficacy against *P. aeruginosa*, led to trials of the newly developed fluoroquinolones (norfloxacin, ciprofloxacin, pefloxacin, ofloxacin, and others) (24–26).

There are only a few double-blind, placebo-controlled trials, yet a meta-analysis suggests that fluoroquinolones can be effective in reducing gram-negative bacteremia but not gram-positive infection (27). Indeed, given alone, fluoroquinolones may increase the frequency of gram-positive bacteremias. As a result, oral penicillin needs to be added to fluoroquinolone prophylaxis in the neutropenic patient (28).

Perhaps of greatest concern is that physicians use these agents for patients at low or minimal risk of gram-negative bacteremia. Such patients simply do not need this type of prophylaxis, yet to use these drugs adds costs and, more importantly, adds to the likelihood of resistance development. Resistance by staphylococci, *P. aeruginosa*, and *E. coli* is steadily increasing (29).

However, it may be useful to use alimentary canal flora suppression for those patients at greatest risk of gram-negative bacteremia, namely those who will have prolonged (>10–14 days), profound (<100 PMN/μL) granulocytopenia. Addition of penicillin to a fluoroquinolone is necessary to prevent streptococcal bacteremia. Patients who are not expected to become profoundly granulocytopenic should not be routinely administered fluoroquinolones or any other antibacterial for that matter.

5. Antifungal Prophylaxis

Fungal infections remain a significant problem in neutropenic patients, and therapy of established disease is less than optimal. Therefore, several methods of prophylaxis have been investigated (30). Initial attempts focused on oral nonabsorbable polyenes, such as nystatin. Doses ranging from 2 to 30 million units/d produced disappointing results (31). Combining nystatin with oral amphotericin B did not add to its efficacy (32). Clotrimazole troches are effective in some groups but not in patients with leukemia, which probably means that they are not effective when in a combined setting of severe neutropenia and mucosal damage when antibiotic therapy has further shifted the oral flora toward yeasts (33). Flucytosine is not considered an option for prophylaxis because of bone marrow suppression (5-flucytosine is partially converted to 5-fluorouracil) and the rapid development of resistance (34).

Fluconazole, a new bistriazole, is well absorbed and widely distributed in the body and has a wide spectrum of antifungal activity. In neutropenic animal models of disseminated candidiasis, it works best when given before infection or very early in the course (35). In a randomized, double-blind placebo-controlled trial in bone marrow transplant patients, fluconazole clearly decreased the number of invasive fungal infections (36). There was no change in overall mortality rate; however, the mortality rate attributed to fungal infection was decreased in the fluconazole group. There was also a significant increase in the mean alanine aminotransferase level in the fluconazole patients. In this trial, there was a slight increase in the colonization with *Candida krusei* in the fluconazole group, and this organism was responsible for all three episodes of candidemia in the fluconazole group. Other researchers reported a marked increase in the number of infections with *C. krusei* when fluconazole prophylaxis was instituted in their bone marrow transplant patients (37). In adults undergoing chemotherapy for acute leukemia, fluconazole decreases colonization with *Candida* spp., except for *C. krusei*, and decreases superficial fungal infections (38). It is not clear that fluconazole or its cousin, itraconazole, significantly decrease the number of invasive fungal infections, the use of amphotericin B, or mortality. Nevertheless, it has the best track record of any oral antifungal to date and has become commonly used, usually in a dosage of 400 mg/d orally.

Systemic prophylactic amphotericin B has been advocated by some clinicians (39), but this has not been well studied. Perfect et al. (40) studied a regimen of 0.1 mg/kg/d of intravenous amphotericin B versus placebo in autologous bone marrow transplant patients. They found a decrease in candidal colonization but no differences in the number of fungal infections, number of patients advanced to high-dose amphotericin B, or overall mortality rate. More encouraging results have been reported by Rousey et al. (41) who observed a decrease in invasive aspergillosis, but historical controls were used, making these data less than ideal. At present, intravenous amphotericin B is not recommended as prophylaxis.

Amphotericin B administered as a nasal spray has been suggested as a logical approach to reducing *Aspergillus* sinusitis and perhaps pulmonary infection. The data to date do not support its use (42,43).

D. Reduce/Avoid Invasive Procedures

Using invasive diagnostic procedures and monitoring devices only when absolutely necessary and continuously reevaluating the need for such devices is the best way to avoid infectious complications. If urinary catheters are used, essentially all of them become colonized and represent a risk for infection. There is little in the way of specific care that prevents colonization, although maintaining a closed system is of some benefit.

Hickman and similar catheters frequently become colonized along the lumen, especially with *S. epidermidis*. They become encased in a glycocalyx, which not only stabilizes them but also reduces the ability of antimicrobials to reach them (44). Surprisingly, few of those colonized catheters actually progress to bacteremia; *S. epidermidis* bacteremia much more commonly originates from the alimentary canal than implanted catheters. Common infections, however, are at the entry site where skin organisms, especially *S. epidermidis*, invade locally. These can be treated with systemic therapy without removal of the catheter. Tunnel infections are rare but serious. One can sometimes cure them with the catheter still in place, but often the catheter must be removed to achieve resolution (44–46). Tunneled catheters are of great help to the patient, physician, and nurse, but a few basic actions must be taken to prevent infection. First, these catheters are placed in high-risk patients and should be placed only by highly skilled surgeons who do this procedure routinely; local complication rates are much higher otherwise. Second, the patient needs to be well educated in the care of the catheter, especially in aseptic technique. This reduces local, tunnel, and lumenal infections (45). To date, no effective prophylactic approach has been found to prevent lumenal colonization; the addition of vancomycin to the heparin solution has not been beneficial (46).

Infection prevention must be considered even when antibiotics are being used for treatment. Many antibiotics such as those commonly used for empirical therapy (e.g., ticarcillin, piperacillin) suppress the enteric mucosa because of their hepatoenteric circulation. This suppression reduces colonization resistance and makes it easier for an acquired organism to colonize. It has therefore been argued that, because anaerobes rarely cause infection during granulocytopenia, one should use agents for empirical therapy that do not suppress anaerobes (e.g., ceftazidime, which has no anaerobic activity, or imipenem, which has no hepatoenteric circulation). This is an intriguing concept well proven in animal models but never adequately investigated in clinical trials.

E. An Overview

Only the patient with prolonged profound granulocytopenia (e.g., bone marrow transplant, stem cell transplant, or therapy of acute leukemia) is at risk of the most serious infections, such as gram-negative or gram-positive bacteremia, candidemia, and invasive aspergillosis. Hence, only these patients should receive aggressive approaches such as antibacterial prophylaxis (e.g., fluoroquinolone and penicillin), oral absorbable antifungal prophylaxis (e.g., fluconazole or itraconazole), and/or colony stimulating factors (e.g., G-CSF, or GM-CSF). To give these agents to patients at lesser risk simply increases costs of care, leads to resistant organisms, adds to the patient's burden of pill-taking and toxicities, and has never been shown to be of realistic value. Equally important for the high-risk patient is thorough education of the risks of infection and what the patient can do to assist himself or herself. The patient must adhere to careful personal hygiene, must pay attention to whether others wash their hands before examination or catheter adjustment, and most strictly observe any prescribed prophylactic regimen. It is not adequate to simply write orders for drugs but not spend time educating the patient and family.

III. CELLULAR IMMUNE DYSFUNCTION

Defects in cellular immunity lead to infection with an entirely different array of pathogens than those seen with granulocytopenia. Typically, they are intracellular organisms and are found in patients with lymphomas or lymphocytic leukemias and after bone marrow transplantation in patients on long-term suppressive therapy, particularly those undergoing treatment for graft-versus-host disease. The organisms include those listed in Table 4 (47). The issues surrounding prevention can be approached in the same way as for those with granulocytopenia.

A. Improve Host Defenses

Currently, there are no methods of improving cellular immunity in general, analogous to techniques used for raising granulocyte counts. There have been attempts to transfer immune cells for specific diseases, such as CMV infection, but this is an exception. The use of vaccines is another possible approach. In general, live virus vaccines, such as yellow fever, oral polio, and oral typhoid vaccine, should be avoided in patients with cellular immune defects. The exception may be the Oka/Merck attenuated varicella vaccine (48). Primary varicella infection is associated with a high risk of morbidity and mortality in immunocompromised children and adults. The vaccine has been shown to protect both healthy children and children with acute leukemia in remission, although side effects were common in the immunocompromised patients (49–51). Ideally, the vaccine should be given before the most acute period of immunosuppression. This strategy can be applied to patients scheduled to undergo solid organ transplantation and bone marrow transplantation and perhaps lymphoma patients, but this luxury does not

Table 4 Infections in the Setting of Cellular Immune Dysfunction

Bacteria
Listeria monocytogenes
Salmonella spp.
Mycobacterium spp.
Nocardia asteroides
Legionella pneumophilia
Viruses
Varicella-zoster
Herpes simplex
Cytomegalovirus
Fungi
Cryptococcus neoformans
Histoplasma capsulatum
Coccidioides immitis
Protozoa
Pneumocystis carinii
Toxoplasma gondii
Helminth
Strongyloides stercoralis

exist in patients with newly diagnosed acute leukemia. It is unclear whether the vaccine will have an effect on reducing herpes zoster, a major problem for bone marrow transplant patients, postradiation lymphoma patients, and others.

B. Reduce Acquisition

With the recent increase in tuberculosis (TB) cases, particularly multidrug-resistant *Mycobacterium tuberculosis*, preventing infection is of paramount importance. Tuberculosis is transmitted by aerosol, with infection rates of 5% for contacts of smear-negative cases and reaching 80% for close contacts of smear-positive cases. Prevention of nosocomial transmission involves housing patients with respiratory infections on separate wards, providing respiratory isolation, controling ventilation systems, and possibly using ultraviolet lights to kill viable bacteria. As noted previously, *Aspergillus* is also transmitted via air, but the spores are ubiquitous and not transmitted via infected patients. Special care must be taken when any construction or renovation takes place: this can be the source of increased numbers of spores.

Disseminated toxoplasmosis can produce devastating neurological disease and death in immunocompromised patients. Transmission is via consumption of cysts found in infected tissue from virtually any animal or mature oocysts excreted in the stool of members of the cat family only. Transfusion of blood or leukocytes or organ transplantation can also transmit the disease. New infections can be prevented by avoiding contact with cat feces, thoroughly cooking all meat, washing hands after contact with raw meat, and washing all fruits and vegetables. Although there are few data, some clinicians recommend not using blood from seropositive donors for transfusion to immunosuppressed hosts (52).

It was recently demonstrated that epidemic listeriosis could be traced to contaminated foods (53); recent evidence has shown that the majority of sporadic cases are also food-borne (54,55). In a case-control study, an increased risk of infection was associated with soft cheeses, food from delicatessen counters, and eating undercooked chicken. The U.S. Centers for Disease Control, Food and Drug Administration, and Food Safety and Inspection Service recommend that high-risk individuals avoid soft cheeses (Mexican style, Brie, feta, Camembert, and blue-veined cheese), recook leftover or ready-to-eat foods, such as hot dogs, thoroughly before eating, and avoid or thoroughly cook foods from delicatessen counters (56). These recommendations are akin to the use of a low microbial, or cooked food, diet for neutropenic patients (15).

C. Suppression of Potential Pathogens

Treatment of some latent infections or antimicrobial prophylaxis can prevent disease in some circumstances. Isoniazid (INH) should be given for 12 months to patients with depressed cellular immunity and a positive purified protein derivative (PPD) test (defined as $\leq$ 5-mm induration in this population). Because cellular immune depression may lead to false-negative PPD results, a proxy may be needed, such as a Gohn (primary) complex on chest radiograph. If there has been contact with a known case or in cases of INH- or multidrug-resistant TB, an alternative agent, such as rifampin, or combination therapy may be appropriate. Few data show that any agent other than INH works for prophylaxis, and the approach to an individual patient should be based on sensitivities of the isolate from the index case and consultation with an expert in the field.

P. carinii pneumonia can be prevented by administration of trimethoprim-sulfamethoxazole (23). Alternative regimens include aerosolized pentamidine (although this is more expensive and has been associated with upper lobe and extrapulmonary disease in acquired immunodeficiency syndrome patients) and dapsone with or without trimethoprim. TMP-SMX has the additional advantage that it may provide prophylaxis against recrudescent toxoplasmosis in seropositive patients. Toxoplasmosis can be effectively prevented by a regimen of pyrimethamine and sulfadiazine, which has been recommended for the seronegative recipients of seropositive solid organs, such as hearts, in whom the risk of disease is very high.

Strongyloides stercoralis has the ability to complete its entire life cycle within the human host and can therefore produce a syndrome of hyperinfection affecting the gastrointestinal tract and lungs and even disseminate to the central nervous system and other sites. Disseminated disease carries a high mortality rate and is extremely difficult to treat. This can be easily prevented by treatment with thiabendazole for 3 days before beginning any immunosuppressive therapy. Suggested methods of diagnosis include stool samples, duodenal aspirates, and sputum Papanicolaou smears, but diagnosis can be difficult and it may be prudent to provide empirical treatment to any patient with a significant exposure history (e.g., patients with previous residence in Puerto Rico, Central America, or other high-risk areas).

Several members of the herpesvirus family—herpes simplex, varicella-zoster virus, and CMV—are important pathogens in this population. Herpes simplex virus infection can be prevented with acyclovir and varicella by use of the vaccine. There is no known prevention for herpes zoster. Cytomegalovirus is a difficult pathogen because of the high morbidity and mortality rates associated with invasive disease and its resistance to acyclovir. Autologous bone marrow transplant recipients who are seropositive or who receive seropositive marrow are at particularly high risk. Intravenous immunoglobulin may have some benefit. Ganciclovir (GCV), which does not require phosphorylation by viral thymidine kinase and is thus more active against CMV, lacks this enzyme (57). Two studies have shown that allogeneic bone marrow transplant patients who are followed up prospectively with surveillance cultures and then receive treatment with GCV have a significant decrease in the incidence of invasive CMV disease and death (58,59). One problem with this approach is that positive cultures do not develop in all patients before invasive disease. Two recent studies evaluated GCV given prophylactically to seropositive recipients of allogeneic bone marrow transplants (60,61). Both studies showed significantly decreased CMV infection and a decrease in incidence or severity of CMV disease. The study in which disease was significantly decreased also used acyclovir (for herpes simplex prophylaxis) during the period of neutropenia before engraftment. In all these studies, significant excess neutropenia was seen, which frequently required stopping the GCV and, in the study by Goodrich et al., was associated with an increase in bacterial infection (60). A phase I-II study of foscarnet shows it to be safe, except when given with cyclosporine and amphotericin B because of its nephrotoxicity, in BMT patients, and it appeared to prevent CMV infection and disease (62). It is clear that some type of prophylactic therapy for CMV is required in seropositive BMT patients. Because of the different toxicities of the therapies, it may be that the best approach combines ganciclovir before and after the transplantation with foscarnet given during the period of neutropenia. Another interesting approach being pursued by Riddell et al. at the Fred Hutchinson Cancer Research Center is the establishment of CMV immunity by the ''adoptive transfer'' of antigen-specific-

T-cells (63,64). The researchers isolated and propagated in vitro $CD8^+$ cytotoxic T cells from CMV-seropositive bone marrow donors and then showed that these can establish CMV immunity in BMT recipients. These data are exciting and may represent an approach for the future.

IV. HUMORAL IMMUNE DYSFUNCTION

Among cancer patients, humoral immune dysfunction is seen mainly in patients with multiple myeloma, chronic lymphocytic leukemia, and late after BMT in the course of chronic graft-versus-host disease. The main pathogens unique to this defect are encapsulated bacteria, such as *Streptococcus pneumoniae* and *Haemophilus influenzae*.

A. Improve Host Defense

Replacement with intravenous immunoglobulin has been shown to decrease the number of bacterial infections in IgG-deficient patients with chronic lymphocytic leukemia (65). In allogeneic bone marrow transplant patients, it decreases the incidence of interstitial pneumonia, bacterial infections, and acute graft-versus-host disease (66). However, a recent placebo-controlled study using intravenous immunoglobulin (IVI) for autologous bone marrow transplant patients showed no decrease in infection, and the IVI group had a significantly higher number of deaths caused by a higher incidence of hepatic veno-occlusive disease (67).

Capsular polysaccharide vaccines are available for *S. pneumoniae, Neisseria meningitidis* types A, C, Y, and W135, and a conjugated capsular vaccine is available for *H. influenzae* type B. There is little evidence, though, that they are effective because these patients do not respond with adequate, if any, normal antibody reaction.

B. Suppress Potential Pathogens

Long-term oral penicillin has been shown to decrease the incidence of bacterial infections in children with splenectomies. It should be used for patients with allogeneic BMT to reduce the frequency of infections caused by pneumococci.

Patients with multiple myeloma do not produce normal immunoglobulin and hence are at risk for infection with the encapsulated bacteria, although *S. pneumoniae* is by far the most frequent of these organisms to cause infection. Oral penicillin is the logical choice to prevent these infections. Once aggressive chemotherapy begins or autologous transplant occurs, the risk of granulocytopenia-related infections outweighs the frequency of pneumococcal infection. However, prophylaxis needs to be continued until the patient is in remission and producing normal antibody again.

V. OBSTRUCTION OF NATURAL PASSAGES

Solid tumors may impinge on the lumen of a variety of organs, such as bronchial obstruction by bronchogenic carcinoma, obstruction of the urinary tract secondary to cervical or prostatic carcinoma, eustachian tube by nasopharyngeal carcinoma, or biliary obstruction secondary to pancreatic or biliary duct carcinoma. In all of these examples, stasis leads to colonization and then infection with the normal flora found in the region of the obstruction. Relief of the obstruction via surgery, radiation therapy, mechanical stents, percutaneous drainage, or some combination of these is the key to treatment and prevention of infection in these patients. Many of these patients are debilitated, and they should also receive standard vaccinations, such as the influenza and pneumococcal vaccines.

VI. DAMAGE TO NORMAL ANATOMICAL BARRIERS

Damage to mucosal barriers is frequently seen with aggressive chemotherapy in which the normal mucosa of the gastrointestinal tract and respiratory tract is damaged. Here, meticulous hygiene and treatment or prevention of any concomitant infections, such as herpetic mucositis or candidiasis, are important.

Bridging normal defenses via the placement of intravenous, arterial, or urinary catheters or endotracheal tubes frequently leads to infection. The removal of any of these devices at the earliest possible time and meticulous care help prevent infection.

Normal barriers can also be interrupted secondary to nervous system dysfunction, leading to aspiration or incontinence of urine or feces. This may be caused by primary central nervous system tumors, metastatic disease to the brain or spinal cord, or paraneoplastic syndromes. Treatment of the underlying disease to try to reverse any dysfunction and meticulous nursing care may help prevent infection.

A. Bone Marrow Transplant

Patients who receive autologous bone marrow or peripheral stem cell transplants are principally at risk from granulocytopenia. Those who receive an autologous transplant, however, fall into nearly all of the aforementioned risk categories, namely, granulocytopenia caused by the conditioning agents; cellular immune dysfunction caused by the conditioning regimen and graft-versus-host disease and its therapy; humoral immune dysfunction caused by the conditioning regimen; infections associated with transfusions (e.g., hepatitis B, C, cytomegalovirus); and infections associated with vascular access devices (68).

Fig. 2 demonstrates the relative frequency of different types of infection and the general timeline of their occurrence in relationship to the time of transplantation (68). Table 5 reviews the specifics of the impaired defense mechanisms and their time course following transplantation (69).

A recent review of prophylactic measures (70) in bone marrow transplantation suggests the following:

1. Use quinolones and penicillin to reduce bacterial infection during granulocytopenia.
2. Use acyclovir to prevent herpes simplex virus infection during the engraftment period.
3. Use fluconazole to reduce colonization and infection with *Candida* sp. other than *C. krusei* and *Torulopsis glabrata* during the engraftment/granulocytopenic period.
4. Use trimethoprim-sulfamethoxazole to prevent *P. carinii* infection after engraftment and for a period of about 6 months.
5. Use TMP-SMX also to reduce the late bacterial infections that occur

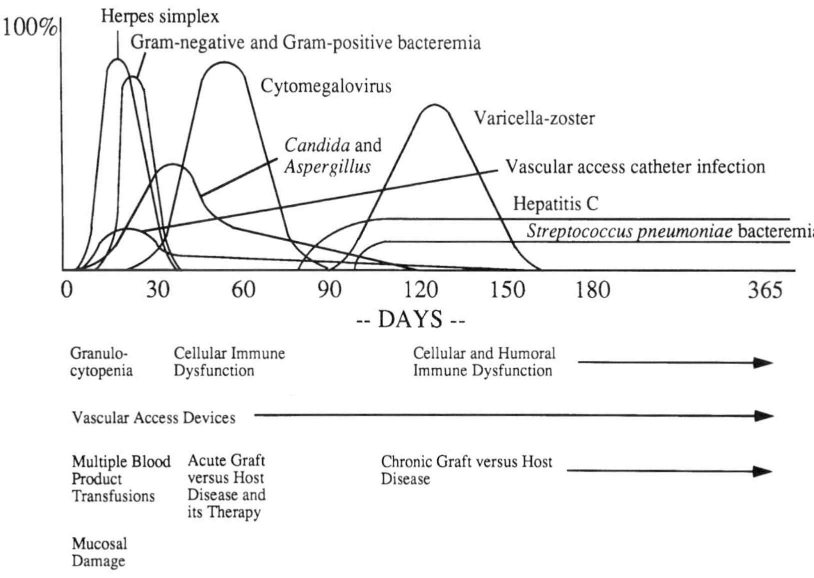

Figure 2 Infection in bone marrow transplantation—a model for examining predisposing factors to infection in cancer patients. (From Ref. 68.)

Table 5 Host Defenses Associated with Marrow Transplant Patients After Engraftment

Host defense system	Defect	Time of recovery[a]
Cell-mediated immunity	↓Numbers and function of nonspecific cytotoxic cells (NK cells, ADCC)	30 d
	↓ T cell numbers	120 d
	↓ CD4 (helper-inducer cells)	4–6 mo to 1 y
	↑ CD8 cells (cytotoxic suppressor cells) (↓ CD4 -CD8 ratio)	1–6 mo
	↓ Interleukin-2 production	100 d to 1 y
	↓ Blastogenic response in CD4 cells	2 y
	↓ Response to recall antigen	4 y
Humoral immunity	↓ IgG, IgM levels	30–160 d
	↓ IgA response to antigenic stimuli	180 d
	↓ Response to pneumococcal polysaccharide	180 d
Phagocytic defense		
Neutrophil function	↓ Chemotaxis	4 mo
Alveolar macrophage function		
	↓ Chemotaxis	>1 y
	↓ Phagocytosis	
	↓ Bactericidal, fungicidal activity	

[a] In the absence of graft-versus-host disease.
Abbreviations: NK, natural killer; ADCC, antibody-dependent cell-mediated cytotoxicity.
Source: Ref. 69.

Table 6 Prophylaxis for First Episode of Opportunistic Disease in HIV-Infected Adults and Adolescents

Pathogen	Indication	Preventive regimens (first choice)
Pneumocystis carinii	$CD4^+$ count $<200/\mu L$ *or* oropharyngeal candidiasis *or* unexplained fever for $\geq$ 2 wk	TMP-SMZ, 1DS po q.d. (AI); TMP-SMZ, SS po. q.d. (AI)
Mycobacterium tuberculosis		
Isoniazid-sensitive	TST reaction $\geq$5 mm or prior positive TST result without treatment or contact with case of active tuberculosis	Isoniazid, 300 mg po plus pyridoxine, 50mg po q.d. $\times$ 12 mo (AI) or isoniazid, 900 mg po b.i.w. plus pyridoxine, 50 mg po b.i.w. $\times$ 12 mo (BIII)
Isoniazid-resistant	Same; high probability of exposure to isoniazid-resistant tuberculosis	Rifampin, 600 mg po q.d. $\times$ 12 mo (BII)
Toxoplasma gondii	IgG antibody to *Toxoplasma* and $CD4^+$ count $<100/\mu L$	TMP-SMZ, 1 DS po q.d. (AII)
Mycobacterium avium complex	$CD4^+$ count $<50/\mu L$	Clarithromycin, 500 mg po b.i.d. (AI) *or* azithromycin, 1,200 mg po q.w. (AI)
Streptococcus pneumoniae	All patients	Pneumococcal vaccine, 0.5 mL IM $\times$ 1 (CD4+ $\geq 200/\mu L$, AII; CD4 + $<200/\mu L$, CIII)
Varicella zoster virus (VZV)	Significant exposure to chickenpox or shingles for patients who have no history of either condition or, if available, negative antibody to VZV	Varicella zoster immune globulin (VZIG), 5 vials (1.25 mL each) IM, administered $\leq$96 h after exposure, ideally within 48 h (AIII)
Hepatitis B virus	All susceptible (anti-HBc-negative) patients	Engerix B, 20 μg IM $\times$ 3 (BII); or Recombivax HB, 10 μg $\times$ 3 (BII)
Influenza virus	All patients (annually, before influenza season)	Whole or split virus, 0.5 mL IM/y (BIII)

Abbreviations: TST, tuberculin skin test; TMP-SMZ, trimethoprim-sulfamethoxazole; DS, double strength; SS, single strength; po, by mouth; q.d., per day; b.i.w., twice per week; qw, weekly; IM, intramuscularly.

Table 7 Prophylaxis for Recurrence of Opportunistic Disease (After Chemotherapy for Acute Disease) in HIV-infected Adults and Adolescents

Pathogen	Indication	Preventive regimens (first choice)
I. Recommended for life as standard of care		
Pneumocystis carinii	Prior *P. carinii* pneumonia	TMP-SMZ, 1 DS po q.d. (AI); TMP-SMZ 1 SS po q.d. (AI)
Toxoplasma gondii	Prior toxoplasmic encephalitis	Sulfadiazine 500–1,000 mg po q.i.d. *plus* pyrimethamine 25–75 mg po q.d. *plus* leucovorin, 10 mg po q.d. (AI)
Mycobacterium avium complex	Documented disseminated disease	Clarithromycin, 500 mg po b.i.d. (AI) *plus* one or more of the following: ethambutol, 15 mg/kg/d po (AII); rifabutin, 300 mg/d po (AII)
Cytomegalovirus	Prior end-organ disease	Ganciclovir, 5–6 mg/kg IV 5–7 d/w or 1,000 mg po t.i.d. (AI); *or* foscarnet, 90–120 mg/kg IV q.d. (AI); *or* cidofovir, 5 mg/kg IV q.o.w. (AI); *or* (for retinitis) ganciclovir sustained-released implant q 6–9 mo (AI)
Cryptococcus neoformans	Documented disease	Fluconazole, 200 mg po q.d. (AI)
Histoplasma capsulatum	Documented disease	Itraconazole, 200 mg po b.i.d. (AII)
Coccidioides immitis	Documented disease	Fluconazole, 400 mg po q.d. (AII)
Salmonella species (non-typhi)	Bacteremia	Ciprofloxacin, 500 mg po b.i.d. for several months (BII)
II. Recommended only if subsequent episodes are frequent or severe		
Herpes simplex virus	Frequent/severe recurrences	Acyclovir, 200 mg po t.i.d. *or* 400 mg po b.i.d. (AI)
Candida (oral, vaginal, or esophageal)	Frequent/severe recurrences	Fluconazole, 100–200 mg po q.d. (AI)

Abbreviations: TMP-SMZ, trimethoprim-sulfamethoxazole; DS, double strength; po, by mouth; q.d., per day; SS, single strength; q.i.d., four times per day; b.i.d., twice a day; d/w, days per week; IV, intravenously; t.i.d., three times per day; q.o.w., every other week.

from about the third month to the end of the first year in relation to chronic graft-versus-host disease and penicillin to reduce pneumococcal infection resulting from lessened humoral immunity.

No prophylactic agents are available for Epstein-Barr virus, BK-GC, or adenoviruses. Some clinicians would use acyclovir from months 2 to 6 to prevent herpes zoster infection, but high dosage is necessary with consequent side effects over a prolonged period in addition to a high cost factor. Finally, ganciclovir can be given to reduce CMV infection from the start of engraftment and continuing for about 6 months either in all seropositive patients (meaning many would receive prophylactic treatment unnecessarily with consequent toxicities and costs) or in those in whom evidence of pulmonary infection (i.e., positive bronchoalveolar lavage) develops before onset of interstitial pneumonia (requires lavage but substantially reduces the number of patients receiving prophylaxis) (59,71).

B. Prevention of Infection in Patients Infected with Human Immunodeficiency Virus

This textbook focuses on cancer, but many patients with the acquired immunodeficiency syndrome have cancers. In 1997, the U.S. Public Health Service and the Infectious Diseases Society of America published guidelines in a supplement to the Journal of Clinical Infectious Diseases (Tables 6 and 7) (72,73). The articles should be consulted for details (e.g., indications, alternative regimens).

REFERENCES

1. Alavi JB, Root RK, Djerassi I, et al. A randomized clinical trial of granulocyte transfusions for infection in acute leukemia. N Engl J Med 1977; 295:706–711.
2. Herzig RH, Herzig GP, Graw RG Jr, et al. Successful granulocyte transfusion therapy for gram-negative septicemia. A prospectively randomized controlled study. N Engl J Med 1977; 296:701–705.
3. Strauss RG, Connett JE, Gale RP, et al. A controlled trial of prophylactic granulocyte transfusions during initial induction chemotherapy for acute myelogenous leukemia. N Engl J Med 1981; 305:597–638.
4. Clift RA, Sanders JE, Thomas ED. Granulocyte transfusions for the prevention of infection in patients receiving bone-marrow transplants. N Engl J Med 1978; 298: 1052–1057.
5. Schiffer CA. Granulocyte transfusions: an overlooked therapeutic modality. Transfusion Med Rev 1990; 4:2–7.
6. Lieschke GJ, Burgess AW. Granulocyte colony-stimulating factor and granulocyte-macrophage colony-stimulating factor. N Engl J Med 1992; 327:99–106.

7. Roilides E, Walsh TJ, Pizzo PA, Rubin M. Granulocyte colony-stimulating factor enhances the phagocytic and bacterial activity of normal and defective human neutrophils. J Infect Dis 1991; 163:579–583.
8. Crawford J, Ozer H, Stoller R, et al. Reduction by granulocyte colony-stimulating factor of fever and neutropenia induced by chemotherapy in patients with small-cell lung cancer [see comments]. N Engl J Med 1991; 325:164–170.
9. Brandt SJ, Peters WP, Atwater SK, et al. Effect of recombinant human granulocyte-macrophage colony-stimulating factor on hematopoietic reconstitution after high-dose chemotherapy and autologous bone marrow transplantation. N Engl J Med 1988; 318:869–876.
10. Peters WP. Use of cytokines during prolonged neutropenia associated with autologous bone marrow transplantation (see comments) Rev Infect Dis 1991; 13:993–996.
11. Nemunaitis J, Rabinowe SN, Singer JW, et al. Recombinant granulocyte-macrophage colony-stimulating factor after autologous bone marrow transplantation for lymphoid cancer. N Engl J Med 1991; 324:1773–1778.
12. Capizzi RL, Schefler BJ, Schein PS. Amifostine-mediated protection of normal bone marrow from cytotoxic chemotherapy. Cancer 1993; 72:3495–3501.
13. Schimpff SC, Young VM, Greene WH, Vermeulen GD, Moody MR, Wiernik PH. Origin of infection in acute nonlymphocytic leukemia. Significance of hospital acquisition of potential pathogens. Ann Intern Med 1972; 77:707–714.
14. Doebbeling BN, Stanley GL, Sheetz CT, et al. Comparative efficacy of alternative hand-washing agents in reducing nosocomial infections in intensive care units. N Engl J Med 1992; 327:88–93.
15. Remington JS, Schimpff SC. Please don't eat the salads. N Engl J Med 1981; 304: 433–435.
16. Nauseef WM, Maki DG. A study of the value of simple protective isolation in patients with granulocytopenia. N Engl J Med 1981; 304:448–453.
17. Schimpff SC, Greene WH, Young VM, et al. Infection prevention in acute nonlymphocytic leukemia. Laminar air flow room reverse isolation with oral, nonabsorbable antibiotic prophylaxis. Ann Intern Med 1975; 82:351–358.
18. Hasegawa H, Horiuchi S. Application of simplified bioclean apparatuses for treatment of acute leukemia. Jpn J Clin Oncol 1983; 13(suppl 1):133–142.
19. Murillo J, Schimpff SC, Brouillet MD. Axillary lesions in patients with acute leukemia: evaluation of a preventive program. Cancer 1979; 43:1493–1496.
20. Wade JC, Newton B, McLaren C. Intravenous acyclovir to treat mucocutaneous herpes simplex virus infection after marrow transplantation. Ann Intern Med 1982; 96:265.
21. Wade JC, Newton B, Flourney N, et al. Oral acyclovir for prevention of herpes simplex reactivation after marrow transplantation. Ann Intern Med 1984; 100:823–828.
22. Bustamante CI, Wade JC. Herpes simplex virus infection in the immunocompromised cancer patient. J Clin Oncol 1991; 10:1903–1915.
23. Hughes WT, Kuhn S, Chaudhary S, et al. Successful chemoprophylaxis for *Pneumocystis carinii* pneumonitis. N Engl J Med 1977; 297:1419–1426.
24. Dekker AW, Rozenberg-Arska M, Verhoef J. Infection prophylaxis in acute leuke-

mia: a comparison of ciprofloxacin with trimethoprim-sulfamethoxazole and colistin. Ann Intern Med 1987; 106:7–12.
25. Karp JE, Merz WG, Hendricksen C, et al. Oral norfloxacin for prevention of gram-negative bacterial infections in patients with acute leukemia and granulocytopenia: a randomized, double-blind, placebo-controlled trial. Ann Intern Med 1987; 106: 1–7.
26. GIMEMA Infection Program. Gruppo Italiano Malattie Ematologiche Maligne dell'Adulto. Prevention of bacterial infection in neutropenic patients with hematologic malignancies. A randomized, multicenter trial comparing norfloxacin with ciprofloxacin. Ann Intern Med 1991; 115:7–12.
27. Cruciani M, Rampazzo R, Malena M, et al. Prophylaxis with fluoroquinolones for bacterial infections in neutropenic patients: a meta-analysis. Clin Infect Dis 1996; 23:795–805.
28. The International Antimicrobial Therapy Project Group of the EORTC. Reduction of fever and streptococcal bacteremia in granulocytopenic patients with cancer. JAMA 1994; 272:1183–1189.
29. Cometto A, Calandra T, Bille J, et al. *Escherichia coli* resistant to fluoroquinolones in patients with cancer and neutropenia (letter). N Engl J Med 1994; 330:1240–1241.
30. Klastersky J. Prevention and therapy of fungal infections in cancer patients. A review of recently published information. Support Care Cancer 1995; 3:393–401.
31. Wade JC, Schimpff SC, Hargadon MT, Fortner CL, Young VM, Wiernik PH. A comparison of trimethoprim-sulfamethoxazole plus nystatin with gentamicin plus nystatin in the prevention of infections in acute leukemia. N Engl J Med 1981; 304: 1057–1062.
32. Hann IM, Prentice HG, Corringham R, et al. Ketoconazole versus nystatin plus amphotericin B for fungal prophylaxis in severely immunocompromised patients. Lancet 1982; 1:826–829.
33. Owens NJ, Nightingale CH, Schweizer R, Schauer PK, Dekker PT, Quintiliani R. Prophylaxis of oral candidiasis with clotrimazole troches. Arch Intern Med 1984; 144:290–293.
34. Drouhet E, DuPont B. Evolution of antifungal agents: past present and future. Rev Infect Dis 1987; 9(suppl 1):S4–S14.
35. Walsh TJ, Lee J, Aoki S, et al. Experimental basis for use of fluconazole for preventive or early treatment of disseminated candidiasis in granulocytopenic hosts. Rev Infect Dis 1990; 12(suppl 3):S307–S317.
36. Goodman JL, Winston DJ, Greenfield RA, et al. A controlled trial of fluconazole to prevent fungal infections in patients undergoing bone marrow transplantation. N Engl J Med 1992; 326:845–851.
37. Wingard JR, Merz WG, Rinaldi MG, Johnson TR, Karp JE, Saral R. Increase in *Candida krusei* infection among patients with bone marrow transplantation and neutropenia treated prophylactically with fluconazole (see comments). N Engl J Med 1991; 325:1274–1277.
38. Winston DJ, Chandrasekar PH, Lazarus HM, et al. Fluconazole prophylaxis of fungal infections in patients with acute leukemia. Results of a randomized placebo-controlled, double-blind, multicenter trial. Ann Intern Med 1993; 118:495–503.

39. Tam JY, Blume KG, Prober CG. Prophylactic fluconazole and *Candida krusei* infections (letter). N Engl J Med 1992; 326:891.
40. Perfect JR, Klotman ME, Gilbert CC, et al. Prophylactic intravenous amphotericin B in neutropenic autologous bone marrow transplant recipients. J Infect Dis 1992; 165:891–897.
41. Rousey SR, Russler S, Gottlieb M, et al. Low-dose amphotericin B prophylaxis against invasive *Aspergillus* infections in allogeneic marrow transplantation. Am J Med 1991; 91:484.
42. Cushing D, Bustamante C, Devlin A. *Aspergillus* Infection Prophylaxis: Amphotericin-B Nose Spray, A Double-Blind Trial (abstr). Interscience Conference on Antimicrobial Agents and Chemotherapy 1991:737.
43. Jeffrey GM, Beard ME, Ikram RB, et al. Intranasal amphotericin B reduces the frequency of invasive aspergillosis in neutropenic patients. Am J Med 1991; 90: 685–692.
44. Tenney JH, Moody MR, Newman KA, et al. Adherent microorganisms on lumenal surfaces of long-term intravenous catheters: importance of *Staphylococcus epidermidis* in patients with cancer. Arch Intern Med 1986; 146:1949–1954.
45. Newman KA, Reed WP, Schimpff SC, et al. Hickman catheters in association with intensive cancer chemotherapy. Support Care Cancer 1993; 1:92–97.
46. Rackoff WR, Weiman J, Jakobowski, et al. A randomized, controlled trial of the efficacy of a heparin and vancomycin solution in preventing central venous catheter infections in children. J Pediatr 1995; 127:147–151.
47. Pizzo PA, Schimpff SC. Strategies for the prevention of infection in the myelosuppressed or immunosuppressed cancer patient. Cancer Treat Rep 1983; 67:223–234.
48. Gershon AA, LaRussa P, Hardy I, Steinberg S, Silverstein S. Varicella vaccine: the American experience. J Infect Dis 1992; 166(suppl 1):S63–S68.
49. Hardy IB, Gershon A, Steinberg S, LaRussa P. NIAID Collaborative Varicella Vaccine Study Group. The incidence of zoster after immunization with live attenuated varicella vaccine. A study in children with leukemia. N Engl J Med 1991; 325:1545–1550.
50. Gershon AA, Steinberg SP, LaRussa P, et al. Immunization of healthy adults with live attenuated varicella vaccine. J Infect Dis 1988; 158:132–137.
51. Weibel R, Neff BJ, Kuter BJ, et al. Live attenuated varicella virus vaccine: efficacy trial in healthy children. N Engl J Med 1984; 310:1409–1415.
52. Remington JS, McLeod R. Toxoplasmosis. In: Gorbach SL, Bartlett JG, eds. Infectious Diseases. 1st ed. Philadelphia: WB Saunders, 1992:1328–1342.
53. Linnan MJ, Mascola L, Lou XD, et al. Epidemic listeriosis associated with Mexican-style cheese. N Engl J Med 1988; 319:823–828.
54. Schuchat A, Deaver KA, Wenger JD, et al. Role of foods in sporadic listeriosis. I. Case-control study of dietary risk factors. JAMA 1992; 267:2041–2045.
55. Pinner RW, Schuchat A, Swaminathan B, et al. Role of foods in sporadic listeriosis. II. Microbiologic and epidemiologic investigation. JAMA 1992; 267:2046–2050.
56. Nightingale SL. Efforts to prevent foodborne listeriosis. JAMA 1992; 268:180.
57. Schmidt GM. Prophylaxis of cytomegalovirus infection after bone marrow transplantation. Semin Oncol 1992; 19:20–26.
58. Goodrich JM, Mori M, Gleaves CA, et al. Early treatment with ganciclovir to prevent

cytomegalovirus disease after allogeneic bone marrow transplantation. N Engl J Med 1991; 325:1601–1607.
59. Schmidt GM, Horak DA, Niland JC, Duncan SR, Forman SJ, Zaia JA. A randomized, controlled trial of prophylactic ganciclovir for cytomegalovirus pulmonary infection in recipients of allogeneic bone marrow transplants; The City of Hope-Stanford-Syntex CMV Study Group (see comments). N Engl J Med 1991; 324: 1005–1011.
60. Goodrich JM, Bowden RA, Fisher L, Keller C, Schoch G, Meyers JD. Ganciclovir prophylaxis to prevent cytomegalovirus disease after allogeneic marrow transplant. Ann Intern Med 1993; 118:173–178.
61. Winston DJ, Ho WG, Bartoni K, et al. Ganciclovir prophylaxis of cytomegalovirus infection and disease in allogeneic bone marrow transplant recipients. Results of a placebo-controlled, double-blind trial. Ann Intern Med 1993; 118:179–184.
62. Reusser P, Gambertoglio JG, Lilleby K, Meyers JD. Phase I-II trial of foscarnet for prevention of cytomegalovirus infection in autologous and allogeneic marrow transplant recipients. J Infect Dis 1992; 166:473–479.
63. Riddell SR, Watanabe KS, Goodrich JM, Li CR, Agha ME, Greenberg PD. Restoration of viral immunity in immunodeficient humans by the adoptive transfer of T cell clones. Science 1992; 257:238–241.
64. Riddell SR, Reusser P, Greenberg PD. Cytotoxic T cells specific for cytomegalovirus a potential therapy for immunocompromised patients. Rev Infect Dis 1991; 13(suppl 11):S966–S973.
65. Cooperative Group for the Study of Immunoglobulin in Chronic Lymphocytic Leukemia. Intravenous immunoglobulin for the prevention of infection in chronic lymphocytic leukemia. A randomized, controlled trial. N Engl J Med 1988; 319: 902–907.
66. Sullivan KM, Kopecky KJ, Jocom J, et al. Immunomodulatory and antimicrobial efficacy of intravenous immunoglobulin in bone marrow transplantation. N Engl J Med 1990; 323:705–712.
67. Wolff SN, Fay JW, Herzig RH, et al. High-dose weekly intravenous immunoglobulin to prevent infections in patients undergoing autologous bone marrow transplantation or severe myelosuppressive therapy. A study of the American Bone Marrow Transplant Group. Ann Intern Med 1993; 18:937–942.
68. Schimpff SC. Infection in bone marrow transplantation: a model for examining predisposing factors to infection in cancer patients. In: Schimpff SC, Klastersky J, eds. Infectious Complications in Bone Marrow Transplantation. Recent Results in Cancer Research 132. Heidelberg: Springer-Verlag, 1993:15–34.
69. Donowitz GR. Infections in bone marrow transplant recipients. In: Mandell GL, Douglas RG Jr, Bennett JE, eds. Principles and Practice of Infectious Diseases. Quarterly Update 12. New York: Churchill Livingstone, 1992:3–12.
70. Momin F, Chandrasekar PH. Antimicrobial prophylaxis in bone marrow transplantation. Ann Intern Med 1995; 123:205–215.
71. Schmidt GM. Treatment and prophylaxis of cytomegalovirus infection after bone marrow transplantation. In: Schimpff SC, Klastersky J, eds. Infectious Complications in Bone Marrow Transplantation. Recent Results in Cancer Research 132. Heidelberg: Springer-Verlag, 1993:161–174.

72. USPHS/IDSA Prevention of Opportunistic Infections Working Group. Preface to the 1997 USPHS/IDSA guidelines for the prevention of opportunistic infections in persons infected with human immunodeficiency virus. Clin Infect Dis 1997; 25(suppl 3):S299–S312.
73. USPHS/IDSA Prevention of Opportunistic Infections Working Group. 1997 USPHS/IDSA guidelines for the prevention of opportunistic infections in persons infected with human immunodeficiency virus: disease-specific recommendations. Clin Infect Dis 1997; 25(suppl 3):S313–S335.
74. Joshi JH, Schimpff SC. Infections in the compromised host. In: Mandell GL, Douglas RG Jr, Bennett JE, eds. Principles and Practice of Infectious Diseases. 2nd ed. New York: John Wiley & Sons, 1984:1664.

6

Bleeding and Coagulation Problems

M. Dicato, F. Ries, C. Duhem, and S. Rauh
Centre Hospitalier de Luxembourg, Luxembourg

I. INTRODUCTION

The time-honored coagulation cascade as an attempt to explain hemostasis by sequential conversion of clotting factors into their respective active proteins is at present considered inadequate. The complexity of multiple systems sequentially and simultaneously must be explained differently.

More emphasis is being placed on the role of tissue factor, endothelial exposure, and the cell surface thrombin binding thrombomodulin, which is converted into a protein C activator. Antithrombin III (ATIII), protein S, and especially protein C with thrombin interplay result in multiple feedback mechanisms of activation of classic clotting factors V and VIII and negative feedback mechanisms to thrombin itself.

Certainly not all mechanisms of procoagulant and anticoagulant activity are identified. For example, there has been a shift of emphasis in the explanation of thrombosis from the classic cascade and ATIII involvement to protein C and its activation by thrombin.

This understanding will probably allow us to predict not only propensity to thrombosis but also prophylaxis and treatment duration in common thrombotic events. The usual coagulation tests, such as prothrombin and (activated) partial thromboplastin time, do not detect abnormalities in these pathways. One recently published study revealed an autosomal dominant trait of resistance to activated protein C, responsible for nearly half of cases of venous thrombosis (1).

The early data on hypercoagulation in relation to resistance to activated Protein C, just described when the first edition of this book was published (1), have been amply verified and completed and need to be taken into account in oncology—as well as in medicine in general—due to their frequency in the Caucasian population. It has been appreciated that around half of all patients under 50 with a thromboembolic event have a mutation in the factor V (Arg 506 Glu). This mutation has also been generally called factor V Leiden. The prevalence of this mutation is around 7.5% of the general Caucasian population (i.e., an allele frequency of 3.75%). It is notable that in essential thrombocythemia, an entity with thromboembolic venous as well as arterial problems, the prevalence of the mutation has been the same as in a comparable normal population (1a).

It is important to have an understanding of this newly recognized and frequent condition as several risk situations—such as hormonal treatments, pregnancy, and abdominal or orthopedic surgery—markedly increase the risk of thromboembolic disease. There are no clear data yet available on patients on antioestrogens or on patients with the classical Trousseau phenomenon. With the wide spread use of tamoxifen and other similar drugs, the V Leiden prevalence needs to be taken into account. A simple standardized test, resistance to activated Prot C, is being performed routinely in an increasing number of clinical laboratories and should certainly be part of any work-up of a patient with a thromboembolic phenomenon, and especially in high risk situations. The clinician should make sure that the test being done in his laboratory is unaltered by anticoagulant therapy. If this test is found pathological, it pays to do a genetic test to confirm the mutation and, depending on the situation, to evaluate the patient's family. In the homozygote situation, the patient or family history will be obvious most of the time, with multiple TED phenomena known already. Interestingly, a case of an additional and expected (!) factor V mutation, called V Cambridge, has been described (1b).

Hyperhomocysteinemia has been of interest recently for several reasons: first, as a frequent and mostly unnoted cause of thrombophilia, and second, because of a fairly simple treatment possibility by folate supplementation (1c). Diagnosis by measuring the homocysteinemia, is fairly simple. Often the results are equivocal and a ''stress test'' needs to be done by giving a methionine overload and thereafter measuring the patient's homocystein level. As of now, routine tests are becoming available in many clinical laboratories, but, as above, the clinician should check with his correspondent laboratory about practical modalities. Studies are ongoing, and in the coming years more data regarding diagnostic and treatment modalities will become available.

Another remarkable event since the first edition of this book is the cloning of the hirudin gene and the recombinant production of hirudin and its analogs.

This protein derived from leeches has been extensively studied in cardiology, and although preliminary but promising data have become available on the usage of hirudin, the overall antithrombin, as an anticoagulant in general, is a possible improvement of therapy in heparin-induced thrombocytopenia (1d) and in DIC (1e).

Thromboembolic events are often multigenic and involving several simultaneous alterations in the same patient; an adequate work-up will need several or all of the possible involved factors to be determined. The financial and economic feasibility will determine what tests and in what sequence they should be obtained. Depending on the clinic, the ethnic background of the patient, and the personal and familial history, it would be logical to follow a sequence of tests according to available prevalence data and cost–benefit issues.

Normal hemostasis is a fine-tuned equilibrium between procoagulant and anticoagulant factors involving multiple interrelated cascades and spanning wide fields of clinical and laboratory medicine. Hemostatic problems in oncological patients are complex because they involve multiple physiological events simultaneously, including disease- or drug-induced bone marrow failure with pancytopenia, inadequate clotting factor production as a result of malnutrition or liver failure, drug-related hemostatic disorders, peripheral blood cell consumption, fibrinolysis, hypercoagulable states, infection, and many others, such as leukostasis and dysproteinemia.

Each of these aspects must be addressed separately and, at the same time, be integrated in a complex setting. Often, only one or a few aspects are apparent and others are clinically less obvious although part of the same general underlying mechanism. The leukemic patient with sepsis and severe pancytopenia often has the entire spectrum of bleeding problems and sometimes also disseminated intravascular coagulation. On the other hand, the solid tumor patient has (to a lesser extent) hemorrhagic, but more often thrombotic problems.

The availability of hematopoietic growth factors, high-dose chemotherapy, autologous bone marrow transplantation, and peripheral blood stem cell collection has increased the number of solid tumor patients who are liable to go into profound pancytopenia and who have the same management problems as the classic leukemic patient.

For more extensive biological details on coagulation and for technical details on transfusion, please refer to the classic hemostasis and transfusion medicine textbooks (e.g., Refs. 2 and 3). The specific neoplasia-related aspects and the more common problems of hemostasis are addressed in this chapter.

II. BLEEDING PROBLEMS

Hemorrhage is common in cancer patients. The awareness and the advent of preventive measures, however, have markedly decreased the incidence of hemorrhagic deaths in acute leukemia, for instance, from more than 60% to less than 10% over the past 40 years (4,5).

In leukemia and in intensive chemotherapy, profound pancytopenia is unavoidable. The anemia is easily alleviated by packed red blood cell transfusions. We have seen a shortening of the duration of severe neutropenia with the widely available granulocyte and granulocyte-macrophage colony-stimulating factors (GM-CSFs). For severe thrombocytopenia, platelet substitution is still necessary, but pharmacological means are undergoing clinical trials and will soon be widely available.

A. Thrombocytopenia

1. *Platelet Substitution*

Thrombocytopenia is an increasing problem as treatment for cancer has become more intensive over the past years and, even more, with the advent of cytokines and peripheral blood stem cell collection and support. For a short time, platelet substitution is successful, but in the long-term platelet support situation, induced alloimmunization is found in a substantial number of patients and its management is a difficult and unresolved issue. It is therefore important to avoid or at least decrease the incidence of induced alloimmunization and its consequence of refractoriness to platelet transfusion. Several aspects have been and still are explored in this field. Over the past years, several (6,7) but not all (8) studies have indicated that the use of single-donor platelet preparations and the practice of leukocyte depletion minimize alloimmunization. Older studies have suggested that there is a relation between the frequency rather than the amount of cellular blood exposure that induces HLA antibody formation (9).

Several studies have compared single-donor to random-donor platelets, and although there are contradictions, many physicians favor single-donor preparations with the hope of decreasing alloimmunization. The issue of selecting, especially in refractory patients, random, single, or HLA-matched donors is not settled, but non–HLA-matched donors are certainly easier to obtain—and at a lower cost—in most settings. One study (10) showed recently that, by using a cross-match assay that has become available over the past few years, an adequate prediction of refractoriness can be made, which is superior to HLA matching especially in alloimmunized patients. Previously, however, a randomized study comparing HLA-compatible to single-donor apheresis platelets showed no difference between the two groups (11). When feasible in our department, we favor random single-donor platelets, and most patients are able to provide a few donors—for example, family members.

Leukocyte depletion has been correlated in most studies with a decrease in alloimmunization, especially when using the lowest possible white blood cell

(WBC) contamination. The combined use of the more recent apheresis machines with better performing filters has decreased the amount of WBC contamination per platelet collection. Red blood cell substitution should also be as low as possible in leukocytes. Another potential clinical benefit of reduction in WBC in blood components is prevention of febrile reactions and cytomegalovirus (CMV) transmission. In one large study (12), no CMV transmission was noted in 184 patients with use of filters, but 75 of 303 control patients had positive CMV conversion. Filter use most likely will reduce other viral transfusions, including herpes, Epstein-Barr virus, hepatitis B and C, parvovirus B19, and human T-cell lymphotrophic virus types I and II. It follows that it is of paramount importance to avoid sensitization of patients by previous blood products.

Another approach to decrease alloimmunization is to use ultraviolet radiation (UVR) on platelets (13). Ultraviolet radiation decreases the ability of lymphocytes to stimulate or respond to mixed lymphocyte cultures, and UV-irradiated macrophages have been shown to have a poor antigen presentation. The UVR-treated platelets are able to shorten the bleeding time and improve the platelet count and have a hemostatic effect in thrombocytopenic situations. The light sources, the bags used, and the way the platelets are prepared are important. Because the existing data are encouraging, larger controlled studies should evaluate the appropriateness of this technique.

Another issue is to determine when platelets should be given. To correct a prolonged bleeding time in a profoundly thrombocytopenic but otherwise stable patient, a platelet count greater than 40,000/μL must be attained; however, bleeding problems in stable patients with a count between 20,000 and 40,000/μL are not frequent. Many clinicians use a threshold less than 20,000 to start platelet transfusion. The reference for this is a study by Gaydos et al. in 1962 (4). In that study, however, the authors could not establish a threshold above which there was no bleeding. A more recent study by Gmur et al. (5) provided a workable hypothesis using random single-donor platelets with the schedule outlined in Table 1.

An interesting study has been published recently comparing in patients being treated for acute myeloid leukemia, pooled platelet concentrates from random donors (controls), filtered pooled platelet concentrates from random donors, UVR pooled platelet concentrates from random donors, and, finally, filtered platelets obtained by apheresis from single random donors. The results of the three latter groups were similar regarding endpoints of refractoriness to platelet transfusions and development of alloimmunization (13a).

2. *Pharmacological Management of Thrombocytopenia*

The need for cytokines to reduce hematological chemotherapy toxicity is driven by the growing evidence that the dose intensity of administered cytotoxic agents

Table 1 Proposal for Single-Donor Platelet Transfusions

Morning platelet count ($\times 10^9$/L)	Prophylactic platelet transfusion, same day
0–5	In every case
6–10	If fresh minor hemorrhage, body temperature >38°C
11–20	Coagulation disorders and/or heparin, before bone marrow biopsy or spinal tap
>20	Major bleeding complications, before minor surgical procedures: biopsies, central venous catheters, arterial punction, others

may determine the effectiveness of some chemotherapy regimens. One approach to dose intensification is the administration of a single or several courses of high-dose chemotherapy with autologous peripheral blood stem cell (PBSC) rescue. An alternative way is the use of repeated, closely-timed courses of semi-intensive chemotherapy. G-CSF and GM-CSF have proven their ability to reduce chemotherapy-induced neutropenia and its complications. To a lesser extent erythropoietin (EPO) can reduce red blood cell transfusion requirements in defined cases of treatment related anemia.

Thrombocytopenia is a more intractable problem for which platelet transfusions into patients at risk of severe bleeding are the only current available solution as discussed in this chapter. Because, in clinical practice, even severe thrombocytopenia only rarely induces life-threatening complications, the efficacy of any thrombopoietic agent should not be evaluated only by the reduction in hemorrhagic deaths or in any severe bleeding episodes. More suitable clinical end points are a reduced demand for platelet transfusions, an acceleration of platelet recovery, and the respect of scheduled dose-intensity of chemotherapy, which often has an important influence on therapeutic success. However, after decades of active research, the megakaryocytic lineage-specific thrombopoietin (Tpo) has been recently cloned and recombinant molecules are currently under intense clinical investigation.

Before the ''Tpo Era,'' several candidate growth factors (GFs), have been largely evaluated for their ability to increase platelet counts after chemotherapy. In spite of the significant efficacy of some GFs on progenitor proliferation and/or megakaryocyte maturation in vitro, the results of most trials with Interleukin-3 (IL3), GM-CSF, the fusion protein PIXY, stem cell factor, EPO, and IL6 (alone or in combination) have been all disappointing in the clinical setting (14a–n). However, among non-Tpo GFs, IL11 deserves special attention. First isolated in 1990, IL11 was initially characterized as a hematopoietic GF with thrombopoietic activity through both progenitor proliferation and megakaryocytic maturation, but was subsequently proven to have pleiotropic effects on multiple tissues, including gut and brain.

In several recent randomized trials, RhIL11 was shown to have a significant thrombopoietic efficacy in patients treated for cancer (reduction of platelet nadir, acceleration of platelet recovery, reduction in platelet transfusion requirements) when given at a dose of 50 μg/kg/d for 12–14 days after chemotherapy (15a–c).

In most studies, the adverse effects of RhIL11, predominantly mild to moderate, were cardiovascular, including dyspnea, atrial arythmias, edema, increased pleural effusions, and conjonctival injection. These may be due to the ability of RhIL11 to increase plasma volume and cause hemodilution by stimulating renal sodium reabsorption. Moreover, RhIL11 did not seem to interfere with the hematopoietic effects of G-CSF, given in several trials in coadministration. RhIL11 with G-CSF did not slow the recovery of neutrophils nor increase the incidence of neutropenic fever when compared with the treatment with G-CSF alone.

Indeed, the treatment with RhIL11 seems to be effective in reducing acute or cumulative toxicity of chemotherapy on the platelet lineage at the price of modest side effects, in spite of its multiorgan activity. Now, the nearly simultaneous availability of recombinant TpO could hamper the development of RhIL11 as a thrombopoietic factor in the clinic. RhIL11 could be useful in settings where the recovery of the platelet lineage and the GI tract are simultaneously desirable after therapy-induced damage.

The greatest advance in the pharmacological management of thrombocytopenia comes from the isolation and the cloning of Tpo coding gene in 1994 (16a,b). The central role of the molecule in thrombopoiesis has been recently reviewed (16c). The cloning of Tpo gene resulted in the production of two recombinant molecules with broad in vitro megakaryocytic proliferative, maturational, and differentiation capabilities that have been tested in clinical trials. One product is the recombinant form of the naturally occurring Tpo (= RhTpo) whereas the other one is a pegylated version of a recombinant truncated Tpo called MK growth and development factor (MGDF). One measure of the impressive interest raised by the discovery of Tpo is noted in the rapid development of clinical trials with the two recombinant forms of the molecule.

Four phase I, randomized, dose-escalation clinical trials were recently published, leading to unanimous conclusions that Tpo has potent stimulatory effects on platelet production in patients with chemotherapy-induced thrombocytopenia and is devoid of any significant side effect (17–20). These studies were of similar design, utilizing either a single dose of RhTpo prior to chemotherapy (17) or a daily dose of PEG-RhuMDGF both prior to and following myelosuppressive treatment (18–20).

When given prior to chemotherapy, the administration of RhTpo or of PEG RhuMDGF led to profound dose-related stimulation of platelet production. When 1 μg/kg/d of PEG-RhuMDGF was given for 10 days, the platelet count climbed as high as $1.8 \times 10^6/mm^3$. Even a single SC dose of 2.4 μg/kg of RhTpo resulted in a doubling of the platelet count several days later. The kinetics of platelet production were carefully followed: the peak platelet count following a 7–10 day course of PEG-RhuMDGF did not occur for up to 12 days after cessation of therapy. This prolonged action of Tpo molecules is probably due to the 8–20 hour plasma half-life of these drugs and their effects on early aspects of hematopoiesis. In Tpo recipients, bone marrow megakaryocytes increased by as much as 80%, and when studied, platelet ultrastructure and function seemed to be unmodified.

The safety profile of Tpo molecules was excellent, without any significant change in patient vital signs, body temperature, or weight or bone pain or any organ dysfunction (21). In one study, 2 patients out of 84 treated patients developed either superficial or deep venous thrombosis, but those episodes could be related to their underlying disease (advanced malignancy) rather than Tpo treatment. There was no increase in frequency or thromboembolic episodes in subsequent studies (22). However, in three patients treated with the pegylated product, anti-TPO antibodies appeared and it seems that the company has stopped further development of the drug.

In contrast to the profound effect of Tpo in improving thrombocytemia following myelosuppressive therapy in animal models and in clinical trials its effectiveness after myeloablative treatments and stem cell transplantation seems to be less impressive. Two groups have reported that Tpo had no significant effect on the hematopoietic recovery of lethally irradiated mice or monkeys rescued with marrow transplant (23,24). The reasons for this discrepancy are unclear; possibly high-dose radiation may destroy stromal cells or other components essential for Tpo activity in vivo, which would be unaffected by moderately intensive chemotherapy. This could explain why irradiated mice transplantated with marrow cells from Tpo pretreated donor mice show an accelerated recovery of platelets and why post-transplant administration of Tpo had no further effect on this accelerated recovery. The same limited clinical activity of Tpo after myeloablative treatment with allo- or auto-stem cell transplantation rescue have been recently reported.

Another potential use for Tpo is to improve the quality of the stem cell product for transplantation. Indeed, despite its lineage-specific activity on mature cell development, administration of Tpo seems to result in a dose-dependent mobilization of multi-lineage progenitor cells able to reconstitute a normal, nonrestricted hematopoiesis when reinfused after high dose chemotherapy (26). This effect is comparable in magnitude to that previously noted with G-CSF. Moreover, combination of G-CSF and Tpo in the mobilization regimen appears to increase the CD34+ yield per apheresis and accelerate hematologic recovery when compared with G-CSF alone (27).

In addition to this potential application as stem cell mobilizer for auto- or allogenic transplantation, treatment of platelet donors with Tpo seems to result in increased apheresis yield and may decrease the number of procedures (28).

B. Disseminated Intravascular Coagulation

Disseminated intravascular coagulation (DIC) is a syndrome observed in various, usually severe disorders of many different fields, especially associated with major infection, tissue breakdown, and release from injured tissue of procoagulant material. The symptoms of DIC are caused by uncontrolled production by thrombin of fibrinogen and its degradation products (FDP) by plasmin. The relative balance between coagulation and fibrinolysis is disturbed, and an excess of each of its aspects is observed clinically, with exaggerated coagulation and thrombosis on the one hand and excessive fibrinolysis and bleeding on the other. The corresponding clinical picture in a given patient is thrombosis and bleeding at the same time. This leads to the consumption of clotting factors and proteinase inhibitors. Liver function is important in the clearance of thrombin and plasmin and the replacement of various consumed factors. The acute-phase reactants fibrinogen and α_2-antiplasmin induce additional excess bleeding and thrombosis, respectively. Because the clotting and fibrinolytic cascades are overfunctioning and FDPs have at the same time procoagulant and anticoagulant activity, most general laboratory tests of hemostasis are abnormal, with a prolonged prothrombin time, (partial) thromboplastin time, and thrombin time and the presence of FDPs. Measurement of the last is the most sensitive test, and the most widely used are the latex agglutination test and, more recently, the cross-linked FDP, D-dimer. Fibrinogen and platelets, being consumed, are usually decreased. In the occasional patient in whom mostly plasminogen activation is present, there may be a clinical picture of fibrinolysis with bleeding and the presence of FDPs and a low fibrinogen as a result of consumption but a normal platelet count with a low α_2-antiplasmin activity.

Disseminated intravascular coagulation can be observed as an acute clinical event when coagulation and fibrinolysis are activated by the massive release of procoagulant and fibrinolytic substances, as in acute leukemia. The clinical picture can be multifaceted, with thrombocytopenia secondary to bone marrow failure, increased platelet turnover in infection, tissue infiltration by cancer cells with release of tissue factors, poor liver clearance, and decreased production of clotting factors as a result of hepatic dysfunction.

On the other hand, in solid tumors, the pathophysiological events are less acute and massive, allowing the organism to adapt. The clotting aspects are clinically more apparent, with thrombosis caused by excess procoagulant activity and chronic DIC.

Because DIC is secondary to other pathophysiological events inducing activation of procoagulant and profibrinolytic activity, whenever possible the underlying cause should be treated and, along with it, the consumption coagulopathy as indicated. Blood component replacement for consumed and missing clotting factors can be done with frozen plasma. The addition of heparin is advocated by many clinicians, but its definitive value remains to be proven. Some patients have a clinical picture of bleeding and thrombocytopenia, and adjunct therapy with an anticoagulant may be hazardous. In patients with thrombosis, low-dose heparin can be given. In contrast, some may use antifibrinolytics, such as ε-aminocaproic acid or tranexamic acid, but these agents may induce thrombosis and can be considered in the patient with the ''bleeding'' type of DIC.

Low-grade or chronic DIC in cancer medicine usually presents as recurrent thrombosis and is discussed in another section of this chapter.

In acute promyelocytic leukemia, DIC is almost always present as a result of the massive release of profibrinolytic agents from the abnormal cells, the more so with chemotherapy, and hemorrhagic death has been drastically reduced by adjunct therapy with heparin (29). The differentiating agent tretinoin (retinoic acid) has also been successful in reducing this bleeding complication (30).

Liver failure is frequent in the patient with advanced cancer. Synthesis and clearance of hemostatic factors are decreased. Management of these patients is difficult and cannot be standardized because the clinical picture is various and rapidly changing. Intracranial bleeding is frequent, and antifibrinolytic agents may be useful.

Interesting preliminary data on recombinant hirudin analogs that have become available show promising results in DIC (6), however, the results of ongoing studies have to become available before these drugs can find a specific place in therapy. As of now they are at least as good, or better, than any other treatment of DIC.

C. Vitamin K Deficiency

Protracted anorexia leading to malnutrition is frequent in advanced cancer patients. The resulting vitamin K deficiency is a frequent finding in chronically hospitalized patients, and coagulation abnormalities are often observed (31). Vitamin K substitution is simple and should be given to these patients.

III. THROMBOSIS AND OTHER VASCULAR COMPLICATIONS

The relationship between cancer and thrombosis was first reported by Trousseau in 1868 (32). It has come to be recognized that disorders in hemostasis are frequent in patients with malignancy, with thromboembolic events preceding or following the diagnosis of cancer (33–35). In a study of 1400 patients with a diagnosis of venous thrombosis, 6% were found to have cancer (36), and thrombotic events can precede the diagnosis of cancer by months or even years. Occult cancer should always be suspected in patients with recurrent, migratory, superficial thrombosis, as well as in patients lacking classic risk factors for thrombosis (37–41). In approximately 15% of patients with malignancy, an episode of thrombosis develops (33,42,43). Thromboembolic problems are a major cause of morbidity and mortality in these patients (33,44). Many factors predispose the cancer patient to venous stasis and thrombosis; these include classic risk factors, such as prolonged periods of bed rest, infection, congestive heart failure, and vascular lesions by catheter manipulations, as well as cancer-specific problems, including cancer cell–related procoagulant activity, vascular compression and invasion by tumors, hyperviscosity problems, and chemotherapy-related and hormone therapy–related coagulopathy (33–35,42,43,45).

Thrombosis is considered to result from perturbations of three major interdependent components of the hemostatic system: blood flow, the vessel wall, and the composition of the blood itself. Thrombosis can be considered to represent hemostasis at the wrong time and in the wrong place in the circulation; this can occur when prothrombotic activity overwhelms the normal physiological antithrombotic mechanisms or when physiological antithrombotic systems are defective, with a variable impact on local and systemic factors.

A. Abnormalities of Blood Flow

Cancer patients are frequently confined to prolonged bed rest because of surgery, medical complications, or debilitating cancer, and immobilization can be considered a major risk factor for thrombosis. Venous stasis may cause a delayed clearance of activated coagulation factors, and interaction between platelets and vessel wall can be enhanced (46). Venous stasis may be localized in vascular compression by bulky tumor but may also be part of a general phenomenon in congestive heart failure precipitated by chronic illness or cardiotoxic chemotherapy. Additional problems, such as hypoxia, anemia, dehydration, and infection, may play a role. Hyperviscosity and leukostasis, specific problems impairing coagulation and microcirculation, occur primarily in monoclonal gammopathies and myeloproliferative disorders.

B. Abnormalities of the Vessel Wall

Apart from local compression by bulky tumor, direct tumor invasion of a vessel wall can contribute to enhance local thrombotic phenomena, primarily by interfering with the thromboresistant properties of the normal vessel wall and by the local release of procoagulant factors (47–50).

C. Platelets and Cancer

Secondary thrombocytosis is frequently found in cancer patients (51), but a direct relation between an increase in circulating platelets and an increased frequency of thrombosis is not clear.

Increased platelet-aggregating activity has been demonstrated in cell lines, human tumors, and tumor extracts (52–56). Mechanisms for increased platelet-aggregating activity include tumor-induced thrombin generation, ADP production, and activation of arachidonate metabolism (57–62) in normal platelets. In myeloproliferative disorders, abnormal platelets present increased as well as decreased aggregation.

D. Tumor Cell Procoagulant Activity

From the many published data about tumor cell procoagulant activity, only two factors appear to play a major role in the clinical setting: tissue factor and cancer procoagulant (34,45,63).

Tissue factor is the normal cellular activator of coagulation and has been found in many cancer cell lines and tumor tissue preparations. This factor is a receptor for factor VII and activated factor VII and is at the same time an activator site of unactivated factor VII. Tissue factor–factor VIIa complex is the real coagulation activator, leading to activation of factors IX and X. Factor Xa and factor Va together form a prothrombinase complex, generating thrombin and thus leading to conversion of fibrinogen to fibrin. Tissue factor appears to be an important activator of the coagulation system in malignant disease. A truncated tissue factor (a second soluble form) has also been described in malignancy with a possible relevance for hypercoagulability in cancer patients (63).

Cancer procoagulant is a proteinase from malignant cells that activates the coagulation system by directly activating factor X. This protein appears to be rather specific for undifferentiated cells; its expression is found in undifferentiated cancer cells, chorionic tissue, and undifferentiated fetal tissues and is repressed in normal tissue and differentiated cancer cells (63). Cancer procoagulant activity has been shown to parallel the course of leukemia, as measured on bone marrow aspirates, before, during, and after remission.

Coagulation activation can take place in at least two different environments, the extravascular, extracellular environment of the tumor and the vascular bed. In both systems, factor Xa can bind to membrane-bound Va and prothrombin and to the tumor cell or to platelets or macrophages to form the prothrombinase complex. Thrombin generation leads to the conversion of fibrinogen to fibrin, which can be formed either on the tumor cell membrane or at the vascular level. The net impact of the release of procoagulants from tumor is to facilitate intravascular activation of the coagulation system, leading to disseminated intravascular coagulation and deep vein thrombosis. At the same time, fibrin formation around tumor cells seems to play an essential role in cell growth support and adhesion, as well as in anti-immune defense.

E. Thrombogenic Abnormalities of the Endothelium

The normal vascular endothelium generates numerous molecules that regulate interactions of circulating blood cells and plasma factors. Maladaptive modulations of these endothelium-dependent regulatory pathways can occur in the context of local vascular injury as well as with diffuse infectious and inflammatory processes mediated by various toxins and cytokines (65–67).

Impaired endothelial expression of thromboprotective factors can be seen in various conditions. The most frequently affected factors are prostacyclin (prostaglandin I_2, PGI_2), nitrous oxide (endothelially derived relaxing factor), thrombomodulin, heparin-like glycosaminoglycans, tissue plasminogen activator (tPA), and endothelial ADPase. The production of some of these factors can be influenced by drugs (reduced PGI_2 production with anti-inflammatory drugs), by atherosclerotic lesions (reduced production of nitrous oxide and thrombomodulin), diffuse infravascular coagulation (inactivation complexing of heparin-like modules by platelet factor 4 secreted from activated platelets), infection, and inflammation (down-regulation of tPA production by IL-1, tumor necrosis factor [TNF], and endotoxins).

On the other hand, enhanced endothelial expression of prothrombotic factors can be found; the most frequently incriminated molecules are tissue factor, plasminogen activator 1 and 2, and von Willebrand's factor. Inflammation as mediated by several drugs, toxins, and cytokines can induce an increased release of some or all of these factors.

Finally, the stimulated endothelium expresses specific adhesion molecules that bind to receptors on stimulated peripheral leukocytes, further mediating inflammation. These adhesion molecules are E-selectin, P-selectin, intracellular adhesion molecules 1 and 2, vascular cell adhesion molecules, and leukocyte-activating cytokines, including IL-1, TNF, IL-8, and platelet-activating factor. Most of these factors are up-regulated by inflammatory stimuli, and some can interact directly with hemostasis (P-selectin-mediated platelet-neutrophil interactions) or indirectly after attachment and vascular transmigration of mononuclear cells that produce prothrombotic factors.

Several cancer-specific as well as nonspecific therapeutic interventions have been recognized as causing thrombotic complications in cancer patients, sometimes exacerbated by the underlying systemic prothrombotic state.

F. Intravenous Catheter

Cancer patients are frequently treated with infusion of various drugs, blood products, and intravenous feeding using diverse catheter systems and may have invasive investigations by arterial and venous catheterization. Venous thrombosis induced by catheters can be related to various physical, chemical, and microbial causes, including vascular injury from cannulation, use of hyperosmolar substances, microparticulate compounds, irritating action of certain drugs and electrolytes, and catheter infection (34). A relationship exists between the time an indwelling catheter is in place and the occurrence of thrombophlebitis (68). The incidence of thrombosis is also increased in the cannulation of small veins and veins with reduced blood flow (69). In this setting, the presence of a mediastinal tumor can predispose to subclavian or superior vena caval catheter-related thrombosis. Another predisposing factor is the type and schedule of chemotherapy (70). Subclavian vein thrombosis has been described in up to 40% of patients with long-term venous access by external Hickman catheters (71) and in 16% of patients with totally implanted systems (72). Thrombosis at this site may be difficult to recognize, sometimes being asymptomatic and sometimes announced only by nonspecific chest, neck, or shoulder pain; classic signs include venous dilatation and edema of the ipsilateral arm and venous collaterals in the pectoral and shoulder region. Venography provides a definitive diagnosis.

Catheter-related thrombophlebitis can best be prevented by avoiding the administration of concentrated, irritating solutions through peripheral veins, particularly in the case of a continuous infusion given over a few days. Removal of thrombogenic microparticulate components from infusion fluids by in-line filtration has been shown to reduce the incidence of infusion-related phlebitis and its further complications (73); small amounts of heparin may also be useful as a prophylactic measure (74). Aseptic techniques during catheter manipulations are necessary and attention should be paid to the use of less traumatizing catheters and needles.

G. Heparin

Heparin-associated immune thrombocytopenia (HIT) is recognized as a classic cause of arterial and venous thrombosis; as cancer patients are frequently treated with heparin, this problem may arise occasionally.

HIT typically occurs 5 or more days after the initiation of heparin therapy, independently of the dose (even after heparin flushes of a catheter) and is characterized by a 50% or greater decrease in platelet count. HIT is a severe immune-mediated drug reaction, the target antigen being the platelet factor 4 (PF4). The syndrome occurs when an antibody against a complex heparin PF4 develops. An enzyme immunoassay is able to reveal and measure this reaction, and is of current use as a diagnostic test.

When HIT is suspected, heparin treatment must be discontinued and local or systemic alternative measures for anticoagulation (avoiding coumarinics) and/or fibrinolysis should be considered, depending upon the clinical situation. As mentioned above, recombinant hirudin analogs, having a pure anti-thrombin effect, show promising results and have just become available in some countries.

Low molecular weight heparins (LMWHs), which are largely used as thrombosis prophylaxis in cancer patients, have significant reduced risk of triggering HIT. However, once HIT develops, LMWHs are also contraindicated because of their high degree of in vitro cross-reactivity (with the exception of Danaparoid) with the antibody responsible for HIT. Moreover, they can cause HIT in patients with a history of it (75).

H. Chemotherapy

Chemotherapeutic agents can induce venous thrombosis in the form of extremity thrombosis and of pulmonary emboli, even in the absence of bulky disease and without any cancer form specificity. In breast cancer trials, such observations have been reported in both adjuvant and metastatic settings although many elements (like addition of prednisone) are sometimes confounding.

In a randomized trial of one perioperative cycle of Fluorouracil, doxorubicine, and cyclophosphamide (FAC) versus observation alone (76), 27 of 1292 patients (2.1%) assigned to receive FAC developed thrombosis in comparison to 10 of 1332 (0.8%) assigned to receive surgery alone ($p = 0.004$). In this study, as in several others (77), the frequency of thromboembolism was higher among postmenopausal women when compared to premenopausal women (2.0% vs. 0.6%) (76). In those trials, the vast majority of thromboembolic events occurred in the period during which patients were receiving chemotherapy, suggesting that cytotoxic drugs may produce temporary changes in coagulation parameters, platelets, and/or vessel walls, which rapidly reverse after completion of the treatment.

The association of thrombotic thrombocytopenic purpura (TTP), hemolytic uremic syndrome (HUS), and cancer is well established but the relative contribution of chemotherapeutic agents and the underlying disease is not always clear. However, mitomycin-C has caused many cases of such thrombotic microangiopathy (78), while bleomycin, cisplatin, tamoxifen, and deoxycoformycin have been implicated in case reports, although their causal relationship may not have been obvious. The onset of this severe, life-threatening condition may be delayed with an interval ranging from 1 day to 7 months after chemotherapy and, when recognized, must be treated with plasma exchange, immunoabsorption columns, or immunosuppressive drugs.

Both thrombotic and hemorrhagic complications including CNS thrombosis have been reported after asparaginase therapy. This potent synthesis inhibitor can cause deficiencies of factors involved in the coagulation and fibrinolysis cascade like fibrinogen, von Willebrand factor, antithrombin III, and plasminogen. When such disorders are observed, only thrombotic events occur, transfusions of fresh frozen plasma can be helpful. Currently a randomized trial evaluating the benefit of prophylactic therapy with antithrombin III concentrates in children treated by L-asparaginase for acute lymphoblastic leukemia is ongoing (79).

Several vascular complications have been reported with cytotoxic agents: vasospasm, myocardial, and other infarction may occur in patients treated with fluorouracil, particularly with continuous IV infusion and independently of any underlying coronary disease (80). Cerebrovascular or peripheral ischemia can complicate cisplatin-containing treatments. Raynaud's phenomenon may develop after bleomycin, cisplatin, and/or vinca alcaloid combination regimens (81).

Veno-occlusive disease of hepatic vessels and in rare instances of pulmonary vessels is a classic and severe complication of very high dose chemotherapy and will be discussed in the bone marrow transplantation section of this book.

I. Hormone Therapy

High-dose estrogens and progestins, given as anticachectic treatment or as antitumorals for hormone-dependent cancers, have been clearly associated to thromboembolic and cardiovascular complications.

The antiestrogen tamoxifen (T) has been implicated as a thrombogenic agent in several reports. Tamoxifen is known to produce reduced levels of fibrinogen and marginally reduced levels of protein S and of antithrombin III, which may indeed increase the propensity for thrombosis (82,83).

However, there is a higher incidence of thromboembolic events for T given with concurrent chemotherapy when compared in randomized trials to T alone in the adjuvant setting (13.6% vs. 2.6% in Ref. 3).

IV. DIAGNOSIS AND TREATMENT OF THROMBOSIS

As a general principle, the approach to the diagnosis of thromboembolic disease should be the same in cancer patients as in the standard population. In cancer patients, the diagnosis can sometimes be less obvious, and the need for complete investigations must be discussed in every situation, according to the prognosis of the underlying disease and the possible therapeutic options.

A. Diagnosis

1. Deep Vein Thrombosis

Many authors recommend first line noninvasive investigations, such as impedance plethysmography, Doppler ultrasonography, or B-mode ultrasonography

(84–92), for diagnosis of deep vein thrombosis of the lower extremities, the most frequent thrombotic problem in cancer patients. All these techniques can be very useful for detection of proximal vein thrombosis, but calf vein thrombosis can be missed. A positive test with one of these techniques generally calls for further investigation with venography; this examination remains the diagnostic reference standard and can provide helpful information about an eventual embolic risk (93,94). A negative test with one of the noninvasive methods allows anticoagulant therapy to be withheld, but a second or even a third control may be needed.

Venography is superseding these other techniques, and we believe that it should be considered a first line investigation; the procedure can be coupled, if indicated, with the placement of an inferior vena caval filter (95).

2. Pulmonary Embolism

The clinical diagnosis of pulmonary embolism can be very difficult in cancer patients, dyspnea and chest pain being common manifestations of various origins, at least in patients with advanced disease or with thoracic involvement (96). In the postoperative cancer patient, these symptoms can have a more selective meaning, reducing the problems with the differential diagnosis. Overall, even if the clinical suspicion in favor of pulmonary embolism is low, it is potentially dangerous to exclude pulmonary embolism and its therapy on clinical grounds alone.

As a general approach, these patients should undergo chest radiography, electrocardiography, and arterial blood gas measurement and, as first line complementary investigation, a perfusion lung scan. If this test is strictly negative, anticoagulant therapy is withheld. In the case of one or several perfusion defects, ventilation lung scanning should be performed, looking for ventilation-perfusion mismatch (97–99). A high probability of embolism based on these tests is generally considered to confer sufficient evidence to justify anticoagulant therapy in the standard situation. If some doubt persists, or if there are relative contraindications for anticoagulation, confirmatory pulmonary angiography should be considered (100–102). Another approach in patients with high clinical suspicion of embolism but with doubtful lung scan results is to investigate first for evidence of deep vein thrombosis and to perform pulmonary angiography only if this investigation is negative. Evidence for deep vein thrombosis, on the other hand, is then considered sufficient for confirmation of pulmonary embolism on clinical grounds and allows initiation of anticoagulation or vena caval filter placement.

3. Upper Limb Vein Thrombosis

In cancer patients, upper extremity vein thrombosis can occur in the context of extrinsic compression or stenosis of the axillary or subclavian vein by tumor tissue or fibrosis, as well as in relation to catheter-related vessel wall trauma and stasis (103,104); finally, the thrombogenic and sclerosing effect of chemotherapy, as well as the irritative effects from parenteral nutrition, electrolytes, and various other drugs, can play a role (105a,b). Differential diagnosis must be made with arm swelling caused by lymphatic obstruction, particularly in the context of locoregional surgery, radiotherapy, and axillary tumor infiltration. Venography must be considered a first-line standard investigation. A locoregional contrast-enhanced computed tomographic (CT) examination can sometimes provide sufficient information and sometimes allows better visualization of an underlying neoplastic or fibrotic process.

4. *Migratory Superficial Thrombophlebitis (Trousseau's Syndrome)*

The clinical picture of migratory superficial thrombophlebitis is characterized by recurrent thrombophlebitis involving multiple superficial and unusual sites (including arms, forearms, and chest) in patients with absence of apparent predisposing factors (e.g., stasis and bed rest). Classically, this syndrome has been related to neoplasia, particularly pancreatic cancer (33). Spontaneous resolution of symptoms in involved areas over a few days has been described, as well as resistance to conventional anticoagulant therapy, particularly of the oral anticoagulant class (106).

5. *Nonbacterial Thrombotic Endocarditis*

Nonbacterial thrombotic endocarditis, a rare thrombotic complication characterized by aseptic endoluminal cardiac vegetations, has been described in a variety of nonmalignant diseases but is more common in patients with cancer, particularly in the context of mucin-producing adenocarcinomas. This complication may occur in patients with occult, localized neoplasms, as well as in patients with metastatic disease (107–109).

The clinical presentation is dominated by the occurrence of multiple emboli to the brain, spleen, kidney, and heart, leading to signs of infarction or ischemia of these and other peripheral organs (110). Heart murmurs are typically present, and some but not all of these patients have a history of damaged valves. The diagnosis can be confirmed by echocardiography and magnetic resonance imaging of the heart (111).

6. *Hepatic Vein Thrombosis and Portal Vein Thrombosis*

Hepatic vein thrombosis (Budd-Chiari syndrome) may be caused by a variety of underlying diseases, including malignancy (112–120); in cancer patients, this form of thrombosis is most notably associated with myeloproliferative disorders but has also been described in hepatoma and renal cell and adrenal carcinoma. In patients with myeloproliferative disorders, this syndrome can be the first manifestation of the disease and it may occur in the absence of pronounced erythrocytosis or thrombocytosis. The clinical presentation can be acute or insidious, generally including abdominal pain, hepatomegaly, and ascites; sometimes there is distention of superficial abdominal veins and splenomegaly secondary to portal hypertension; jaundice is rare, and liver function tests may be without diagnostic benefit. Liver echography with Doppler sonography, contrast-enhanced CT scanning, and magnetic resonance imaging are useful diagnostic tools. Venography by inferior vena caval and hepatic vein catheterization is the definitive diagnostic procedure.

Portal vein thrombosis may also occur acutely or insidiously; clinical signs include ascites (usually transient, present only during the acute phase), as well as splenomegaly and esophageal varices related to portal hypertension; bleeding of esophagogastric varices may be the first manifestation of this complication (115). Ultrasound examination is generally considered most helpful in establishing the diagnosis, followed by contrast-enhanced CT scan, magnetic resonance imaging, and portal venography.

B. Treatment

1. *General Considerations*

The first objective of treating patients with venous thromboembolic problems is to prevent death from pulmonary embolism; secondary objectives are to reduce morbidity from the acute event, reduce postphlebitic symptoms, and prevent thromboembolic pulmonary hypertension (116,117) and recurrence. The therapeutic approach to venous thromboembolism includes several therapeutic options: intravenous, subcutaneous, and oral anticoagulant therapy, thrombolysis, inferior vena caval interruption, and, more rarely, surgical thromboembolic deobstruction. The anticoagulant agents (IV heparin, subcutaneous low-molecular-weight heparin, and oral antivitamin K agents) serve primarily to prevent the extension and recurrence of established thrombosis and to prevent recurrent pulmonary embolism by interfering with the normal coagulation process. The thrombolytic agents (streptokinase, urokinase, and tissue plasminogen activator) have the potential for rapid thrombolysis of venous thrombi and pulmonary emboli of recent origin; these agents can be useful in the emergency setting or if there is a need for rapid symptomatic relief in non–life-threatening situations. Interruption of the inferior vena cava by different filter systems allows effective protection from pulmonary embolism; their placement must be considered in the case of high risk for potentially life-threatening embolism and if the use of anticoagulants or fibrinolytic agents is contraindicated.

2. *Heparin*

Heparin may be used for short-term as well as long-term anticoagulation in the therapeutic and prophylactic setting (118–122). The classic method of administration during the acute phase of deep vein thrombosis and thromboembolism is continuous intravenous infusion (119). A generally recommended program includes an initial bolus of 5,000 units of heparin intravenously, followed by an infusion of about 1,000–1,200 units/h; the subsequent dose is adapted to maintain a partial thromboplastin time at 1.5 to 2 times control (123). A recent trial demonstrated that the duration of initial heparin infusion can be shortened in most cases from 10 to 14 days to approximately 5 days if adequate oral anticoagulation is given simultaneously with heparin, at least in the standard patient population (124). In cancer patients, long-term outpatient subcutaneous heparin is frequently considered safer than therapy with oral anticoagulants, particularly in patients with cancer-related hypercoagulability and in patients with ongoing chemotherapy who are at risk for thrombocytopenia. Effective anticoagulation in cancer patients is not always possible, and complications may be more frequent than in the general population (125–127). Patients with liver metastasis or compromised liver function may have reduced synthesis of antithrombin III, implicating an inadequate response to heparin; hemorrhage can develop in other patients, especially at tumor-bearing sites (128).

The use of low-molecular-weight heparin (LMW heparin) may offer several advantages in the treatment and prophylaxis of cancer-related thrombosis, with the possibility for outpatient treatment without the need for laboratory monitoring and with a potentially reduced risk of hemorrhage (129,130). Most recently, randomized studies of LMW heparins compared with standard heparin therapy in deep venous thrombosis in the general population provided strong evidence that this therapeutic approach is safe and cost effective; more data are needed in the cancer patient (130).

3. *Oral Anticoagulant Therapy*

Most patients with deep vein thrombosis treated initially with heparin require continuing anticoagulant therapy to prevent early recurrence of thrombosis (131,132). Coumarinics, the most frequently used agents, have been shown to prevent these recurrences effectively, but their administration needs close laboratory monitoring, particularly until establishment of steady-state levels.

The prothrombin time (PT) test is the most common method for monitoring, being responsive to a reduction in three of the vitamin K–dependent clotting factors: factor II, factor VII, and factor X. Because factor VII has a short half-life, a rapid decrease in the prothrombin time can sometimes be observed, whereas the classic coagulation pathway is still unaffected. Because oral anticoagulants also affect some proteins with thrombolytic activity, such as protein C, whose half-life is short, a paradoxical state of hypercoagulability can sometimes be observed after 2 or 3 days of therapy, before effective reduction in factors II and X. This is why oral anticoagulation should always be given with a 4-day overlap of effective anticoagulation with heparin. To avoid long-term hospitalization, oral anticoagulants, if indicated, can be started within 24 hours of first heparin administration (124). The intensity and duration of oral anticoagulant therapy remain a matter of debate (133–135). For patients considered at risk for hemorrhage, a low to moderate reduction in the prothrombin time should not be exceeded; otherwise, it would be cautious to replace oral anticoagulants with low-dose subcutaneous heparin. As far as the duration of the treatment is concerned, recommendations vary markedly from 1 month to 1 year; for patients who have experienced a first episode of deep venous thrombosis, oral anticoagulation for 3 months can be considered a wise compromise, unless there is a high risk of recurrence with a persistent state of hypercoagulability (116).

Recurrent thrombophlebitis, particularly under oral anticoagulation, is not rare in cancer patients. If anticoagulation based on PT measurements has been suboptimal, oral anticoagulants can be reconsidered at a higher dose after initial heparin administration. If thrombophlebitis recurs despite a PT test in the therapeutic range, it seems wise to consider adjusted dose subcutaneous heparin or low-molecular-weight heparin as maintenance treatment. On rare occasions, further recurrences develop despite optimal anticoagulation by either method; in these patients, placement of an inferior vena caval filter must be considered, but ongoing anticoagulation may be needed to achieve symptomatic control of thrombosis.

4. *Thrombolytic Therapy*

Thrombolytic agents currently in use, such as streptokinase, urokinase, or tPA, act on the plasmin/plasminogen fibrinolytic system to induce fibrinolysis (136). Because plasmin also hydrolyzes fibrinogen, a systemic lytic state is also induced, correlated with a significant bleeding risk. Compared with the standard patient, supplementary risk factors must be considered in cancer patients: brain tumors and brain metastasis, pericardial metastases, tumor with tendency to bleed, active bleeding of any origin, and recent surgery or biopsy, all factors that contraindicate the use of fibrinolytic agents. Furthermore, cancer patients can have other hemostatic problems, including thrombocytopenia, abnormal platelet function, and disseminated intravascular coagulation, mostly as a result of their underlying disease or therapy. This explains why the use of thrombolytic agents in cancer patients is generally restricted to special settings, such as massive pulmonary embolism with shock or central venous catheter–related thrombosis in patients without specific contraindications (137).

The particular problem of central venous catheter occlusion caused by a clot, limited to the catheter tip, can generally be managed effectively and safely with low-dose local fibrinolysis. Streptokinase or urokinase (5,000–10,000 units) or 2 mg recombinant tPA diluted into a volume that will just fill the occluded catheter, instilled and left in place for 1 to 2 hour, usually restores catheter function (138,139); this procedure is very safe and can also be recommended for patients with profound thrombocytopenia. If the clot involves not only the catheter tip but the vessel wall as well, however, this technique is clearly insufficient and the risk of pulmonary embolism can only be avoided with standard anticoagulation or systemically effective fibrinolysis. Placement of the infusion catheter directly in the clot can allow effective resolution of these catheter-related clots, even at moderate dosage (urokinase at 500–2,000 U/kg/h) and with few bleeding complications. The median infusion duration for this method is 4 days, and results are best if the thrombus has been clinically present for less than 1 week and is not associated with signs of phlebitis (103).

V. HYPERVISCOSITY, LEUKOSTASIS, AND THROMBOCYTOSIS

A. Hyperviscosity

The hyperviscosity syndrome has been described mostly in monoclonal gammopathies and myeloproliferative disorders. In these conditions, increased blood viscosity induces specific signs and symptoms, most characteristically a triad of bleeding, visual disturbancies, and neurological deficits (140,141). The unique flow characteristics of blood can be altered by both cellular and soluble components. The measurement of viscosity is expressed relative to the viscosity of water and can be performed on whole blood but, in most laboratories, only on plasma or serum. The correlation between measured viscosity and the appearance of clinical symptoms and signs is generally considered rather weak, so that diagnosis depends mostly on clinical suspicion. Because hyperviscosity may lead to severe complications, including death, its diagnosis requires prompt therapeutic intervention.

1. Clinical Manifestations

The classic presentation of hyperviscosity includes bleeding, generally presenting with ecchymoses, epistaxis, and gingival and, more rarely, retinal and gastrointestinal hemorrhage. Visual disturbancies include vision loss, diplopia, and blurred vision. Fundoscopy can show a retinopathy with distended, tortuous, sausage-like appearing retinal veins, described as fundus paraproteinaemicus. The neurological picture includes headache, somnolence, stupor, coma, seizures, dizziness, vertigo, ataxia, hearing loss, and sometimes psychiatric presentations (142), and dyspnea.

According to the underlying disease, diverse laboratory abnormalities can be seen, including the presence of a monoclonal immunoglobulin, abnormal coagulation tests (143), pseudohyponatremia (144,145), pseudohypoglycemia (146), cryoglobulinemia (147), plasma hyperviscosity (148), rouleaux formation, increased packed cell volume, and abnormal platelet aggregation tests (142).

According to the soluble or cellular origin of hyperviscosity, two large categories can be discussed: monoclonal gammopathies and polycythemia vera.

2. *Monoclonal Gammopathies*

The prototype of a malignant disease that induces hyperviscosity is Waldenström's macroglobulinemia, with an incidence of about 10% to 30% at presentation (142). Hyperviscosity results from high monoclonal IgM concentration and IgM polymer formation. A bleeding diathesis is frequently present, as are visual and neurological disturbancies. The correlation between absolute IgM level and the degree of hyperviscosity is rather weak and can be a result of the individually variable tendency of the IgM to polymerize and of interactions of the monoclonal protein with other plasma proteins (142).

In multiple myeloma, hyperviscosity has been described in 3% to 4% of IgG myeloma and 5% to 10% of IgA myeloma. The symptoms are similar to those described for macroglobulinemia, but hemorrhage is more common in IgA than IgG myeloma with hyperviscosity.

For some monoclonal immunoglobulins the concentration-viscosity relation may be linear; for others, high viscosity can even occur with a nonlinear relationship at low concentration: this is typically the case for IgG_3 and IgA, which can act as macromolecules as a result of in vivo polymerization (149–153).

Apart from hyperviscosity, monoclonal proteins may interact with coagulation proteins to induce bleeding. Inhibitor activity to factors V, VII, and VIII and the prothrombin complex has been described, as has reduction in several coagulation factors (143).

Treatment of hyperviscosity and bleeding diathesis of monoclonal gammopathy can be managed with prompt plasmapheresis in the emergency situation, followed by disease-specific cytotoxic therapy (154,155). Plasmapheresis should always be performed if the symptoms or signs of hyperviscosity are present and should be considered if the risk is high, as with significant increases in monoclonal IgM, IgA, and IgG_3. The volume and frequency of plasma exchange depend on the clinical situation. Plasma exchange (up to 6 Ls) may be necessary during the first day in the acute situation, but generally a 3- to 4-L exchange is sufficient. A lower volume maintenance program once or twice a week can prevent recurrence while waiting for the effect of the primary, cytotoxic therapy. Because the distribution volume of IgM is lower (80% intravascular) than that of IgG and IgA (40% intravascular), smaller volumes of exchange (2–3 L/d) may provide effective relief of symptoms in Waldenström's macroglobulinemia. With automated apheresis machines, cellular elements are returned and volume replaced with plasma substitutes. Substitution including fresh frozen plasma may be preferable, particularly if a bleeding diathesis is present (156).

3. *Polycythemia Vera*

Hyperviscosity caused by increased packed cell volume as occurs in polycythemia vera typically presents with thrombotic complications affecting both the arterial and venous systems (157–159). Arterial thrombosis is predominant at the cerebrovascular and peripheral microvascular level, with signs and symptoms including headache, confusion, vertigo, and stroke, as well as occlusive signs involving fingers and toes, sometimes leading to gangrenous lesions. In the venous circulation, thrombotic complications include superficial and deep venous thrombosis, Budd-Chiari syndrome, and thrombosis of splenic and portal veins.

The role of the frequently elevated platelet count as the pathophysiological cause of these complications in polycythemia vera remains controversial. The essential goal of therapy in the acute situation of polycythemia-related hyperviscosity is to reduce the packed red cell volume by therapeutic bleeding. In patients with symptoms of hyperviscosity, thrombosis, bleeding, or signs of congestive heart failure, with hematocrit values above 0.6, immediate therapeutic apheresis should be performed to lower the hematocrit to below 0.55 to 0.6. If venisection (phlebotomy) is poorly tolerated, the blood loss can be replaced with physiological solutions. Therapeutic phlebotomy inducing an iron-deficiency state constitutes at the same time standard therapy of the disease and is generally preferable to cytotoxic drugs and radioactive phosphorus because of a reduced risk of leukemogenesis (160–162).

B. Leukostasis

The leukostasis syndrome, mostly discussed in the context of hyperviscosity syndromes, is generally not caused by an increase in whole blood viscosity and should be considered a separate entity (163). Leukostasis occurs in hyperleukocytic leukemias, more commonly in myelocytic than lymphocytic forms. The classic leukostasis syndrome includes dyspnea with respiratory insufficiency, mental status changes with confusion and stupor, visual abnormalities, and a potential for central nervous system hemorrhage (163–165).

These manifestations are caused by the formation of leukocyte aggregates and thrombi, vascular invasion, microcirculation hyperviscosity, and vascular stasis. The syndrome has been mostly described with chronic myelocytic leukemia and acute leukemias, being very rare in chronic lymphocytic leukemia, even at very high lymphocyte counts.

Although no absolute white blood cell level can predict the occurrence of symptoms, patients with granulocyte counts greater than 100,000/mL and lymphocyte counts above 750,000/mL are considered at risk (163).

The optimal therapy for leukostasis should be prompt leukapheresis, a decrease in the white cells by 30% to 40% generally leading to reversal of the symptoms (166). This can be achieved, on average, with a single procedure. In the acute setting, leukapheresis has an advantage over chemotherapy in giving a quick result without supplemental risk of tumor lysis syndrome or urate nephropathy. It allows the introduction of cytotoxic therapy after initial diagnostic work-up and patient preparation with allopurinol and adequate hydration. Red blood cell transfusion before reduction of the white count should be avoided because of the risk of hyperviscosity (163).

C. Thrombocytosis

Although thrombocytosis is common in cancer patients, symptomatic thrombocytosis is generally limited to patients with myeloproliferative diseases, including essential thrombocythemia, polycythemia vera, chronic myelocytic leukemia, myelofibrosis, and ''overlap'' myeloproliferative syndromes (167–169). Significant, potentially dangerous thrombocytosis is generally limited to platelet counts above 1,000,000/mm^3, but in some patients complications can occur below these values. Thrombocytosis can present with thrombotic as well as bleeding problems. Bleeding complications are classically of the platelet-vascular type, involving cutaneous and mucosal hemorrhage. Thrombotic complications include deep vein thrombosis and pulmonary embolism but more characteristically also include hepatic vein and portal vein thrombosis, erythromelalgia with burning pain in the extremities, and signs of digital ischemia as well as neurological complications related to cerebrovascular ischemia. Recurrent spontaneous abortions and fetal growth retardation have also been described, probably related to multiple placental infarctions. These complications are recognized with increasing frequency when the platelet count is above 1,000,000/mm^3. Overall, however, the correlation between the degree of thrombocytosis and the risk of hemostatic complications is weak, and indications for therapy according to the platelet count are controversial.

In general, there is little rationale for chronic cytoreductive therapy in asymptomatic patients; however, treatment should be considered in patients with recurrent hemostatic complications, particularly if typical cerebrovascular or digital thrombotic events occur.

If a rapid decrease in the platelet count appears necessary, platelet apheresis should be considered. As far as cytoreductive chemotherapy is concerned, hydroxyurea is probably the most useful agent, providing effective long-term control generally without severe marrow toxicity or serious side effects.

Recombinant interferon-α is also highly effective, generally safe, and rapidly acting at a daily dose of 3×10^6 units subcutaneously, but long-term maintenance therapy is necessary if recurrence of uncontrolled thrombocytosis with related symptoms must be avoided. Side effects are rather frequent and occasionally severe enough to necessitate treatment discontinuation (170,171).

Anagrelide, an orally administered, nonmutagenic drug, has been found to induce a selective platelet reduction in thrombocythemia, probably by suppression of megakaryocytopoiesis with concomitant functional antiplatelet activity. This drug has been shown to be highly effective, even in patients refractory to other treatment modalities, at a dose of 0.5 to 1 mg four times daily (172).

The use of aspirin and other antiplatelet drugs in thrombocytosis remains controversial and should not be recommended indiscriminately. Because these patients sometimes have abnormal platelet function with bleeding tendencies, serious bleeding complications can be precipitated. On the other hand, patients with recurrent thrombotic complications, particularly of the digital and cerebrovascular ischemia type, will probably benefit from aspirin in combination with platelet-lowering therapy. The decision to use antiplatelet drugs should therefore be made on an individual basis, depending on the clinical situation, with periodic reassessment according to the evolution of the disease.

REFERENCES

1. Svensson PJ, Dahlback B. Resistance to activated protein C as a basis for venous thrombosis. N Engl J Med 1994; 330:512–522.

1a. Dicato M, Knauf-Huebel D, Schroell B, et al. The Factor V Leiden mutation (arg 506 Gin) is not an additional risk factor for thromboembolic disease in essential thrombocythemia (ET). Blood 1998; 92(suppl 1):118b.

1b. Williamson D, Brown K, Luddington R, et al. Factor V Cambridge: a new mutation ($Arg^{306} \rightarrow Thr$) associated with resistance to activated Protein C. Blood 1998; 91: 1140–1144.

1c. Eichinger S, Stumpflen A, Hirschl M, et al. Hyperhomocysteinemia is a risk factor of recurrent venous thromboembolism. Thromb Haemost 1998; 80:566–599.

1d. Warkentin T, Ching H, Greinacher A. Heparin-induced thrombocytopenia: towards consensus. Thromb Haemost 1998; 24(1):53–59.

1e. Riewald M, Riess H. Treatment options for clinically recognized disseminated intravascular coagulation. Thromb Haemost 1998; 24(1):53–59.

2. Colman RW, Hirsch J, Marder VJ, Salzman EW. Hemostasis and Thrombosis, Philadelphia: JB Lippincott, 1993.

3. Mollison PL, Engelfriet CP, Contreras M. Blood Transfusion in Clinical Medicine. Oxford: Blackwell, 1994.

4. Gaydos LA, Freireich EJ, Mantel N. The quantitative relation between platelet count and hemorrhage in patients with acute leukemia. N Engl J Med 1962; 266: 905–909.

5. Gmur J, Burger J, Schanz U, et al. Safety of stringent prophylactic platelet transfusion policy for patients with acute leukemia. Lancet 1991; 338:1223–1226.

6. Sintnicolaas K, Vriesendorp HM, Sizoo W, et al. Delayed alloimmunization by random single donor platelet transfusions. Lancet 1981; 1:750–753.

7. Gmur J, Von Felten A, Osterwalder B, et al. Delayed alloimmunization using ran-

dom single donor platelet transfusions: a prospective study in thrombocytopenic patients with acute leukemia. Blood 1983; 62:473–479.
8. Dutcher JP, Schiffer CA, Aisner J, et al. Long-term follow-up of patients with leukemia receiving platelet transfusions: identification of a large group of patients who do not become alloimmunized. Blood 1981; 58:1007–1011.
9. Ferrara GB, Tosi RM, Azzolina G, et al. HLA unresponsiveness induced by weekly transfusions of small aliquots of whole blood. Transplant 1974; 17:194–198.
10. Friedberg RC, Donnelly SF, Boyd JC, et al. Clinical and blood bank factors in the management of platelet refractoriness and alloimmunization. Blood 1993; 81: 3428–3434.
11. Messerschmidt G, Makuch R, Appelbaum F, et al. A prospective randomized trial of HLA-matched versus mismatched single donor platelet transfusions in cancer patients. Cancer 1988; 62:795–801.
12. Klein HG, Dzik WH, Strauss RG, et al. Leukocyte-reduced blood component therapy. ASH Education Program, Denver, CO, 1992:76–85.
13. Pamphilon DG, Potter M, Cutts M, et al. Platelet concentrates irradiated with ultraviolet light retain satisfactory in vitro storage characteristics and in vivo survival. Br J Haematol 1990; 75:240–244.
13b. The Trail to Reduce Alloimmunization to Platelets Study Group. Leukocyte reduction and ultraviolet B irradiation of platelets to prevent alloimmunization and refractoriness to platelet transfusions. New Engl J Med 1997; 337(26):1861–1868.
14a. Hoffmann R. Regulation of megakaryocytopoiesis. Blood 1989; 74:1196–1202.
14b. Postmus PE, Gietma JA, Damsa O, et al. Effects of recombinant interleukin-3 in patients with relapsed small-cell lung cancer treatment with chemotherapy: dose-finding study. J Clin Oncol 1992; 10:1131–1140.
14c. D'Hondt V, Weynants P, Humblet Y, et al. Dose-dependent interleukin-3 stimulation of thrombopoiesis and neutropoiesis in patients with small-cell lung cancer before and following chemotherapy. J Clin Oncol 1993; 11:2063–2071.
14d. Biesma B, Willemse PHB, Mulder NH, et al. Effects of interleukin-3 after chemotherapy. Blood 1992; 80:1141–1148.
14e. Lindemann A, Ganser A, Herman F, et al. Biologic effects of recombinant human interleukin-3 in vivo. J Clin Oncol 1990; 9:2120–2127.
14f. Brugger M, Frisch J, Schultz G, et al. Sequential administration of interleukin-3 and granulocyte-macrophage stimulating factor following standard-dose combination chemotherapy with etoposide, ifosfamide, and cisplatin. J Clin Oncol 1992; 9:1452–1459.
14g. Vadhan-Raj S, Rapadopoulos N, Burgess A, et al. PIXY 321 (GMCSF/IL3 fusion protein) chemotherapy induced multilineage myelosuppression in patients with sarcoma. Blood 1992; 80 (suppl 1, abstract 987):2490.
14h. Jarubowski A, Raptis G, Gilewski T, et al. A phase I/II trial PIXY 321 (PIXY) in patients with metastatic breast cancer receiving doxorubicin and thiotepa. Blood 1992; 80 (suppl 1, abstract 342):88a.
14i. Bridell RA, Bruno E, Cooper RJ, et al. Effect of c-kit ligand on in vitro human megakaryocytopoiesis. Blood 1991; 78:2854–2859.
14j. Demetri G, Costa J, Hayes D, et al. A phase I trial of recombinant methionyl human stem factor (SCF) in patients with advanced breast carcinoma pre- and post-chemo-

therapy (CHEMO) with cyclophosphamide (C) and doxorubicin (A) (abstract). Proc ASCO 1993; 12:367.

14k. Weber J, Yang JC, Topalian SL, et al. Phase I trial of subcutaneous interleukin-6 in patients with advanced malignancies. J Clin Oncol 1993; 11:499–506.

14l. Gameren MM, Velenga E, Willemse PHB, et al. The effects of recombinant interleukin-6 on in vivo hematopoiesis in cancer patients. Blood 1992; 80 (suppl 1, abstract 985):249a.

14m. Demetri GD, Samuels B, Gordon M, et al. Recombinant human interleukin-6 (IL-6) increases circulating platelet counts and C-reactive protein levels in vivo: initial results of a phase I trial in sarcoma patients with normal hematopoiesis. Blood 1992; 80 (suppl 1, abstract 344):88a.

14n. Paul SR, Bennett F, Calvetti JA, Leary AC, Siblgy B, et al. Molecular cloning of a cDNA encoding interleukin 11, a novel stromal cell-derived lymphopoietic and hematopoietic cytokine. Proc Natl Acad Sci USA 1990; 87:7512–7516.

15a. Du X, Williams DA. Interleukin-11: review of molecular, cell biology and clinical use. Blood 1997; 89(11):3897–3908.

15b. Tepler I, Elias L, Smith JW, et al. A randomized placebo controlled trial of recombinant human interleukin-11 in cancer patients with severe thrombocytopenia due to chemotherapy. Blood 1996; 87(9):3607–3614.

15c. Isaacs C, Robert NJ, Bailey FA, et al. Randomized placebo-controlled study of recombinant human interleukin-11 to prevent chemotherapy-induced thrombocytopenia in patients with breast cancer receiving dose intensive cyclophosphamide and doxorubicin. J Clin Oncol 1997; 15(11):3368–3377.

16a. De Sauvage AJ, Hass PE, Spencer SD, et al. Stimulation of megakaryocytopoiesis and thrombopoiesis by the c-mpl ligand. Nature 1994; 369:533.

16b. Bartley TD, Bogenberger J, Hunt P, et al. Identification and cloning of a megakaryocyte growth and development factor, that is a ligand for the cytokine receptor mpl. Cell 1994; 77:1177.

16c. Eaton DL, De Sauvage AFJ. Thrombopoietin. The primary regulator of megakaryocytopoiesis and thrombopoiesis. Exp Hematol 1997; 25:1–7.

17. O'Malley CJ, Rasko JEJ, Basser RL, et al. Administration of regulated recombinant human megakaryocyte growth and development factor to humans stimulates the production of functional platelets that show no evidence of in vivo activation. Blood 1996; 88(9):3288–3293.

18. Fanucchi M, Glaspy J, Crawford J, et al. Effects of polyethylene glycol-conjucated recombinant human megakaryocytic growth and development factor on platelet counts after chemotherapy for lung cancer. N Engl J Med 1997; 336(6):404–409.

19. Basser RL, Rasko JEJ, Clarke R, et al. Randomized, blind, placebo-controlled phase I trial of pegylated-controlled human megakaryocyte growth and development factor with filgastrim after dose intensive chemotherapy in patients with advanced cancer. Blood 1997; 89(9):3118–3128.

20. Vadhan-Raj S, Murray LJ, Buejo-Ramos C, et al. Stimulation of megakaryocyte and platelet production by a single dose of recombinant human thrombopoietin in patients with cancer. Ann Int Med 1997; 126(9):673–681.

21. Nasch R, Kurzrock R, Dipersio J, et al. Safety and activity of recombinant human

thrombopoietin (rhTPO) in patients (pts) with delayed platelet recovery (DPR). Blood 1997; 90 (suppl 1):1151 (abstr).
22. Vredenburg J, Glaspy J, Bolwell B, et al. The incidence of thrombotic and embolic events in controlled trials with breast cancer (CA) patients (pts) undergoing high dose chemotherapy (HDC) with the stamp I regimen and autologous peripheral blood progenitor cells (PBPC) transplantation. Blood 1997; 90 (suppl 1):972 (abstr).
23. Neelis KJ, Wognum AW, Eaton D, et al. Preclinical evaluation of thrombopoietin in rhesus monkeys. Blood 1995; 86(S1):256 (abstr).
24. Fibbe WE, Heemskerk DPM, Laterveer L, et al. Accelerated reconstitution of platelets and erythrocytes after syngenic transplantation of bone marrow cells derived from TPO pretreated donor-mice. Blood 1995; 86:3308.
25. Bolwell B, Vredenburg J, Overmoyer B, et al. Safety and biologic effect of pegylated recombinant human megakaryocyte growth and development factor (PEG-rhu-MGDF) in breast cancer patients following autologous peripheral blood progenitor cell transplantation (PBPC). Blood 1997; 90 (suppl 1):756 (abstr).
26. Rasko JE, Basser RL, Mansfield R, et al. Multilineage mobilization of peripheral blood progenitor cells in humans following administration of PEG-rhu-MGDF. Br J Haematol 1997; 97:871–880.
27. Somio G, Sniecinski I, Brent J, et al. Recombinant human thrombopoietin (rhTPO) in combination with G-CSF is safe and effective as peripheral blood cell (PBPC) mobilizer. Blood 1997; 90 (suppl 1):2513 (abstr).
28. Kuter D, McCullough J, Romo J, et al. Treatment of platelet (PLT) donors with pegylated recombinant human megakaryocyte growth and development factor (PEG-rhu-MDGF) increases platelet increments in recipients of PTL transfusions. Blood 1997; 90(suppl 1):2579 (abstr).
29. Hoyle CF, Swirsky DM, Freedman L, et al. Beneficial effect of heparin in the management of patients with APL. Br J Haematol 1988; 68:283.
30. Dombret H, Scrobohaci ML, Ghorra P, et al. Coagulation disorders associated with acute promyelocytic leukemia: corrective effect of all trans-retinoic acid treatment. Leukemia 1993; 7:2–9.
31. Alperin JB. Coagulopathy caused by vitamin K deficiency in critically ill, hospitalized patients. JAMA 1987; 258:1916–1919.
32. Trousseau A. Phlegmasia alba dolens. Clin Med Hotel-Dieu Paris (London: New Sydenham Society) 1868; 3:695–727.
33. Sack GH, Levin J, Bell WR. Trousseau's syndrome and other manifestation of disseminated coagulopathy in patients with neoplasms: clinical pathophysiologic and therapeutic features. Medicine (Baltimore) 1977; 56:1–37.
34. Luzzato G, Schafer AI. The prethrombotic state in cancer. Semin Oncol 1990; 17: 147–159.
35. Rickles FR, Edwards RL. Activation of blood coagulation in cancer. Blood 1983; 62:14–31.
36. Lieberman JS, Borrero J, Urdaneta E, Wright IS. Thrombo-phlebitis and cancer. JAMA 1961; 177:542–545.
37. Aderka D, Brown A, Zelikovski A, Pinkhas J. Idiopathic deep vein thrombosis in an apparently healthy patient as a premonitory sign of occult cancer. Cancer 1986; 57:1846–1849.

38. Goldberg RJ, Seneff M, Gore J. Occult malignant neoplasm in patients with deep vein thrombosis. Arch Intern Med 1987; 147:251–253.
39. Griffin MR, Stanson AW, Brown ML, et al. Deep venous thrombosis and pulmonary embolism. Risk of subsequent malignant neoplasm. Arch Intern Med 1987; 147:1907–1911.
40. Monreal M, Latoz E, Casals A, et al. Occult cancer in patients with deep venous thromboembolism. A systematic approach. Cancer 1991; 67:541–545.
41. Prandoni P, Lensing AWA, Büller HR, et al. Deep-vein thrombosis and the influence of subsequent symptomatic cancer. N Engl J Med 1992; 327:1128–1133.
42. Sun NCJ, McAfee WM, Hum GJ, et al. Hemostatic abnormalities in malignancy, a prospective study of one hundred eight patients. Am J Clin Pathol 1979; 71:10–16.
43. Soong BC, Miller SP. Coagulation disorders in cancer. Fibrinolysis and inhibitors. Cancer 1970; 25:867–874.
44. Ambrus JL, Ambrus CM, Pickren JW. Causes of death in cancer patients. J Med 1975; 6:61–64.
45. Patterson WP, Ringenberg QS. The pathophysiology of thrombosis in cancer. Semin Oncol 1990; 17:140–146.
46. Shattil SS. Diagnosis and treatment of recurrent venous thromboembolism. Med Clin North Am 1984; 68:577–600.
47. Hedderich GS, O'Connor RJ, Reid EC, et al. Caval tumor thrombus complicating renal cell carcinoma: a surgical challenge. Surgery 1987; 102:614–619.
48. Ritchey ML, Kinard R, Novick DE. Adrenal tumors: involvement of the inferior vena cava. J Urol 1987; 138:1134–1136.
49. Prichett TR, Lieskowsky G, Skinner DG. Extension of renal cell carcinoma into the vena cava: clinical review and surgical approach. J Urol 1986; 135:460–464.
50. Sharifi R, Ray P, Schade SG, et al. Inferior vena cava thrombosis. Unusual presentation of testicular tumor. Urology 1988; 32:146–150.
51. Levin J, Conley CL. Thrombocytosis associated with malignant disease. Arch Intern Med 1964; 114:497–500.
52. Karpatin S, Pearlstein E. Role of platelets in tumor cell metastases. Ann Intern Med 1981; 95:636–641.
53. Marcum JM, McGill M, Bastida E, et al. The interaction of platelet, tumor cells, and vascular subendothelium. J Lab Clin Med 1980; 96:1046–1053.
54. Gasic GJ, Gasic TB, Galanti N, et al. Platelet-tumor cell interactions in mice. The role of platelets in malignant disease. Int J Cancer 1973; 11:704–718.
55. Grignani G, Jamieson GA. Platelets in tumor metastasis: generation of adenosine diphosphonate by tumor cells is specific but unrelated to metastatic potential. Blood 1988; 71:844–849.
56. Bastida E. The metastatic cascade: potential approaches for the inhibition of metastasis. Semin Thromb Hemost 1988; 14:66–72.
57. Gordon SG, Franks JJ, Lewis B. Cancer procoagulant A: a factor X activating procoagulant from malignant tissue. Thromb Res 1975; 6:127–137.
58. Curatolo L, Colucci M, Cambini AL, et al. Evidence that cells from experimental tumours can activate coagulation factor X. Br J Cancer 1979; 40:228–233.
59. Bastida E, Ordinas A, Escolar G, et al. Tissue factor in microvesicles shed from

U87MG human gliblastoma cells induces coagulation, platelet aggregation, and thrombogenesis. Blood 1984; 64:177–184.
60. Bastida E, Ordinas A, Jamieson GA. Differing platelet aggregating effects by two tumor cell lines: absence of a role for platelet-derived ADP. Am J Hematol 1981; 11:367–378.
61. Mohanty D, Hilgard P. A new platelet aggregating material (PAM) in an experimentally induced rat fibrosarcoma. Thromb Haemost 1984; 51:192–195.
62. Honn KV, Busse WD, Sloane BF. Prostacyclin and thromboxanes. Implications for their role in tumor cell metastasis. Biochem Pharmacol 1983; 32:1–11.
63. Gordon S. Cancer cell procoagulants and their implications. Hematol Oncol Clin North Am 1992; 6:1359–1374.
64. Scates MS. Diagnosis and treatment of cancer-related thrombosis. Hematol Oncol Clin North Am 1992; 6:1329–1339.
65. Pober JS, Cotran RS. Cytokines and endothelial cell biology. Physiol Rev 1990; 70:427.
66. Harker LA, Mann FG. Thrombosis and cardiovascular disorders. In: Fuster V Verstreate M, eds. Thrombosis and Fibrinolysis. Philadelphia: WB Saunders, 1992:1–26.
67. Huber AR, Kinckel S, Todd RF III, Weiss SJ. Regulation of transendothelial neutrophil migration by endogenous interleukin-8. Science 1991; 254:99–101.
68. Bennegard K, Curelaru I, Gustavsson B, et al. Material thrombogenicity in central venous catherization. Comparison between uncoated and heparin-coated, long antebrachial, polyethylene catheters. Acta Anaesthesiol Scand 1982; 26:112–120.
69. Sketch MH, Cale M, Mohiuddin SM, et al. Use of percutaneously inserted venous catheters in coronary care units. Chest 1972; 62:684–689.
70. Lokich JJ, Becker B. Subclavian vein thrombosis in patients treated with infusion chemotherapy for advanced malignancy. Cancer 1983; 52:1586–1589.
71. Lazarus HM, Lowder JN, Herzig RH. Occlusion and infection in Broviac catheters during intensive cancer therapy. Cancer 1983; 52:2342–2348.
72. Lokich JJ, Bothe A Jr, Benotti P, et al. Complications and management of implanted venous access catheters. J Clin Oncol 1985; 3:710–717.
73. Falchuck KH, Peterson L, McNeil BJ. Microparticulate induced phlebitis. Its prevention by in-line filtration. N Engl J Med 1985; 312:78–92.
74. Daniell HW. Heparin in the prevention of infusion phlebitis. JAMA 1973; 226: 1317–1321.
75. Warkentin TE, Levine MN, Hirsch J, et al. Heparin-induced thrombocytopenia in patients treated with low molecular weight heparin or unfractionated heparin. N Engl J Med 1995; 332:1330–1335.
76. Clahsen PC, Van de Velde CJM, Julien JP, et al. Thromboembolic complications after perioperative chemotherapy in women with early breast cancer: a European organization for research and treatment of cancer breast cooperative group study. J Clin Oncol 1994; 12:1266–1271.
77. Pritchard KI, Paterson AHG, Paul NA, et al. Increased thromboembolic complications with concurrent tamoxifen and chemotherapy in a randomized trial of adjuvant therapy for women with breast cancer. J Clin Oncol 1996; 10:2731–2737.
78. Mazzuconi MG, Gugliotta L, Leone G, et al. Antithrombin III infusion suppresses

the hypercoagulable state in adult acute lymphoblastic leukemia patients treated with a low dose escherichia coli L-asparaginase; A Gimmema study. Blood Coagul Fibrinol 1994; 5:23–28.
79. Nowak-Goettl U, Kuhn N, Wolff JE, et al. Inhibition of hypercoagulation by antithrombin substitution in E. coli L-asparaginase-treated children. Eur J Haematol, 1996; 56:35–38.
80. Freeman N, Costanza M. 5-Fluorouracil associated cardiotoxicity. Cancer 1988; 61:36–45.
81. Adoue D, Arlet P. Bleomycin and Raynaud's phenomenon. Ann Int Med 1984; 100:770–777.
82. Anger AL, Mackie MJ. Effects of tamoxifen on blood coagulation. Cancer 1998; 61:1316–1319.
83. Jones AL, Powles TJ, Treleaven JC, et al. Haemostatic changes and thromboembolic risk during tamoxifen in normal women. Br J Cancer 1992; 66:744–747.
84. Forbes CD, Lowe GDO. Clinical diagnosis. In: Hirsh J, ed. Venous Thrombosis and Pulmonary Embolism. Diagnostic Methods. Vol. 18. New York: Churchill Livingstone, 1987:9–19.
85. Hull R, Raskob G, Leclerc J, et al. The diagnosis of clinically suspected venous thrombosis. Clin Chest Med 1984; 5:439–456.
86. Hull R, van Aken WG, Hirsh J, et al. Impedance plethysmography using the occlusive cuff technique in the diagnosis of venous thrombosis. Circulation 1976; 53: 696–700.
87. Wheeler HB, Pearson D, O'Connell D, et al. Impedance plebography: technique, interpretation end results. Arch Surg 1972; 104:164–169.
88. Huisman HV, Buller HR, ten Cate CJ, et al. Serial impedance plethysmography for suspected deep venous thrombosis in outpatients. The Amsterdam general practioner study. N Engl J Med 1986; 314:823–825.
89. Hull R, Hirsh J, Carter C, et al. Diagnostic efficacy of impedance plethysmography for clinically suspected deep vein thrombosis: a randomized trial. Ann Intern Med 1985; 102:21–28.
90. Sigel B, Felix WR, Popky LG, et al. Diagnosis of lower limb venous thrombosis by Doppler ultrasound technique. Arch Surg 1972; 104:174–179.
91. Strandness DE, Sumner DS. Ultrasonic velocity detector in the diagnosis of thrombophlebitis. Arch Surg 1972; 104:180–183.
92. Lensing AWA, Prandoni P, Brandjes D, et al. Detection of deep vein thrombosis by real-time B-mode ultrasonography. N Engl J Med 1989; 320:342–345.
93. Rabinov K, Paulin S. Roentgen diagnosis of venous thrombosis in the leg. Arch Surg 1972; 104:134–144.
94. Bettmann MA. Contrast phlebography. In: Hirsh J, ed. Venous Thrombosis and Pulmonary Embolism. Diagnostic Methods. Vol. 18. New York: Churchill Livingstone, 1987:20–32.
95. Calligaro KD, Bergen WS, Hant MJ, et al. Thromboembolic complications in patients with advanced cancer: anticoagulation versus Greenfield filter placement. Ann Vasc Surg 1991; 5:186–189.
96. Bell WR, Simon TL, Demets DL. The clinical features of submassive and massive pulmonary emboli. Am J Med 1977; 62:355–360.

97. Hull R, Hirsh J, Carter C, et al. Diagnostic value of ventilation-perfusion in patients with suspected pulmonary embolism and abnormal perfusion lung scans. Chest 1985; 88:819–828.
98. Denardo G, Goodwin DA, Ravisini R, et al. The ventilatory lung scan in the diagnosis of pulmonary embolism. N Engl J Med 1974; 282:1334–1336.
99. Williams O, Lyall J, Vernon M, et al. Ventilation-perfusion lung scanning for pulmonary emboli. BMJ 1974; 1:600–602.
100. Hull R, Hirsh J, Carter C, et al. Pulmonary angiography, ventilation lung scanning, and venography for clinically suspected pulmonary embolism with abnormal perfusion lung scan. Ann Intern Med 1983; 98:891–899.
101. Bookstein JJ, Silver TM. The angiographic differential diagnosis of acute pulmonary embolism. Radiology 1974; 110:25–33.
102. Grollman JH, Gyepes MT, Helmer E. Transfemoral selective bilateral pulmonary arteriography with a pulmonary-artery-seeking catheter. Radiology 1970; 96:202–204.
103. Fraschini G, Jadeja J, Lawson M, et al. Local infusion of urokinase for the lysis of thrombosis associated with permanent central venous catheters in cancer patients. J Clin Oncol 1987; 5:672–678.
104. Hung SS. Deep vein thrombosis of the arm associated with malignancy. Cancer 1989; 64:531–535.
105a. Montemurro P, Lattanzio A, Chetta G, et al. Increased in vitro and in vivo generation of procoagulant activity (tissue factor) by mononuclear phagocytes after intralipid infusion in rabbits. Blood 1985; 65:1391–1395.
105b. Harrell RM, Sibley R, Vogelzang N. Renal vascular lesions after chemotherapy with vinblastine, bleomycin and cisplatin. Am J Med 1982; 73:429–433.
106. Bell WR, Starksen NF, Tong S, et al. Trousseau's syndrome. Devastating coagulopathy in the absence of heparin. Am J Med 1985; 79:423–430.
107. Deppish LM, Fayemi AO. Nonbacterial thrombotic endocarditis. Clinicopathological correlations. Am Heart J 1976; 92:723–729.
108. Ondrias F, Slugen I, Valach A. Malignant tumors and embolizing paraneoplastic endocarditis. Neoplasma 1985; 32:135–140.
109. Min KW, Gyorkey F, Sato C. Mucin producing adenocarcinomas and nonbacterial thrombotic endocarditis. Cancer 1980; 45:2374–2382.
110. Guinn GA, Ayala A, Liddicoat J. Clinical and therapeutic considerations in nonbacterial thrombotic endocarditis. Chest 1973; 64:26–28.
111. Gomes AS, Lois JF, Child JS, et al. Cardiac tumors and thrombus: evaluation with MR imaging. AJR AM J Roentgenol 1987; 149:895–899.
112. Mitchell MC, Boitnott JK, Kaufman S, et al. Budd-Chiari syndrome: etiology, diagnosis and management. Medicine (Baltimore) 1982; 61:199–218.
113. Valla D, Casadevall N, Lacombe C, et al. Primary myeloproliferative disorder and hepatic vein thrombosis. A prospective study of erythroid colony formation in vitro in 20 patients with Budd-Chiari syndrome. Ann Intern Med 1985; 103:329–334.
114. Murphy FB, Steinberg HV, Shires GT, et al. The Budd-Chiari syndrome: an overview. AJR AM J Roentgenol 1986; 147:9–15.
115. Sherlock S, Extrahepatic portal venous hypertension in adults. Clin Gastroenterol 1985; 14:1–19.

116. Levine M, Hirsh J. The diagnosis and treatment of thrombosis in the cancer patient. Semin Oncol 1990; 17:160–171.
117. Scates SM. Diagnosis and treatment of cancer-related thrombosis. Hematol Oncol Clin North Am 1992; 6:1329–1339.
118. Salzman EW, Deykin D, Shapiro RM, et al. Management of heparin therapy. N Engl J Med 1975; 292:1046.
119. Hull RD, Raskob GE, Hirsh J, et al. A double-blind randomized trial of intravenous versus subcutaneous heparin in the initial treatment of proximal-vein thrombosis. N Engl J Med 1986; 315:1109–1114.
120. Galzier RL, Crowell EB. Randomized prospective trial of continuous or intermittent heparin therapy. JAMA 1976; 236:1365–1367.
121. Mant MJ, O'Brien BD, Thong KL, et al. Hemorrhagic complications of heparin therapy. Lancet 1977; 1:1133–1135.
122. Wilson JR, Lampman J. Heparin therapy: a randomized prospective study. Am Heart J 1979; 97:155–158.
123. Basu D, Gallus A, Hirsh J, et al. A prospective study of the value of monitoring heparin treatment with the active partial thromboplastin time. N Engl J Med 1972; 287:324–327.
124. Gallus AS, Jackman J, Mills W, et al. Safety and efficacy of warfarin started early after submassive venous thrombosis or pulmonary embolism. Lancet 1986; 2: 1293–1296.
125. Levine MN, Hirsh J. Hemorrhagic complications of anticoagulant therapy. Semin Thromb Hemost 1986; 12:39–57.
126. Levine MN, Raskob G, Hirsh J. Hemorrhagic complications of long-term anticoagulant therapy. Chest 1989; 95(suppl):26–36.
127. Chian A, Woodruff RK. Complications and failure of anticoagulation in the treatment of venous thromboembolism in patients with disseminated malignancy. Aust N Z J Med 1992; 22:119–122.
128. Choucair AK, Silver P, Levin VA. Risk of intracranial hemorrhage in glioma patients receiving anticoagulant therapy for venous thromboembolism. J Neurosurg 1987; 66:357–358.
129. Frickler JP, Vergues Y, Schach R, et al. Low dose heparin versus low molecular weight heparin in the prophylaxis of thromboembolic complications of abdominal oncological surgery. Eur J Clin Invest 1988; 18:561–567.
130. Hull RD, Pineo GF. Treatment of venous thromboembolism with low-molecular weight heparins. Hematol Oncol Clin North Am 1992; 6:1095–1104.
131. Hull RD, Delmore T, Genton E, et al. Warfarin sodium versus low-dose heparin in the long-term treatment of venous thrombosis. N Engl J Med 1979; 301:855–858.
132. Lagerstedt CI, Olsson CT, Fagher BO, et al. Need for long-term anticoagulant treatment in symptomatic calf-vein thrombosis. Lancet 1985; 1:515–518.
133. Hirsh J, Poller L, Deykin D, et al. Optimal therapeutic range for oral anticoagulants. Chest 1989; 95(suppl):5–11.
134. Hull R, Hirsh J, Jay R, et al. Different intensities of oral anticoagulant therapy in the treatment of proximal-vein thrombosis. N Engl J Med 1982; 307:1676–1681.
135. Holmgren K, Andersson G, Fagrell B, et al. One month versus six months therapy

with oral anticoagulants after symptomatic deep vein thrombosis. Acta Med Scand 1985; 218:279–284.
136. Sasahara AA, St Martin CC, Henkin J, Barker WM. Approach to the patient with venous thromboembolism: treatment with thrombolytic agents. Hematol Oncol Clin North Am 1992; 6:1141–1160.
137. Gray W, Bell W. Fibrinolytic agents in the treatment of thrombotic disorders. Semin Oncol 1990; 17:228–237.
138. Atkinson JB, Baguall HA, Gomperts E. Investigational use of tissue plasminogen activator (t-PA) for occluded central venous catheters. J Parenter Enter Nutr 1990; 14:310–311.
139. Haire WD, Atkinson JB, Stephens LC, Kotaluk GD. Urokinase (UK) vs recombinant tissue plasminogen activator (R-TPA) in thrombosed central venous catheters (CVCs): a double-blind randomized controlled clinical trial. (Proc ASCO abstract 1485). J Clin Oncol 1993; 12:431.
140. Fahey JL, Barth WF, Solomon A. Serum hyperviscosity syndrome. JAMA 1965; 192:120–123.
141. Patterson WP, Caldwell CH, Doll DC. Hyperviscosity syndromes and coagulopathies. Semin Oncol 1990; 17:210–216.
142. Somer T. Rheology of paraproteinaemias and the plasma hyperviscosity syndrome. Baillieres Clin Haematol 1987; 1:695–723.
143. Lackner H. Hemostatic abnormalities associated with dysproteinemias. Semin Hematol 1973; 10:125–133.
144. Nanji AA, Blank DW. Pseudohyponatremia and hyperviscosity. J Clin Pathol 1983; 36:834–835.
145. Vader HL, Vink CLJ. The influence of viscosity on dilution methods: its problems in the determination of serum sodium. Clin Chim Acta 1975; 65:379–387.
146. Haibach H, Wright DL, Bailey LE. Pseudohypoglycemia in a patient with Waldenström's macroglulinemia, an artifact of hyperviscosity. Clin Chem 1986; 32:1239–1240.
147. Meltzer M, Franklin EC. Cryoglobulinemia: a study of twenty-nine patients. IgG and IgM cyroglobulins and factors affecting cryoprecipitability. Am J Med 1966; 40:828–836.
148. Pruzanski W, Watt JG. Serum viscosity and hyperviscosity syndrome in IgG multiple myeloma. Ann Intern Med 1972; 77:853–860.
149. Crawford J, Cox EB, Cohen HJ. Evaluation of hyperviscosity in monoclonal gammapathies. Am J Med 1985; 79:13–22.
150. Lindsley H, Teller D, Noonan B, et al. Hyperviscosity syndrome in multiple myeloma. A reversible concentration-dependent aggregation of the myeloma protein. Am J Med 1973; 54:682–688.
151. Preston FE, Cooke KB, Foster ME, et al. Myelomatosis and the hyperviscosity syndrome. Br J Haematol 1978; 38:517–530.
152. Chandy KG, Stockley RA, Leonard RCF, et al. Relationship between serum viscosity and intravascular IgA polymer concentration in IgA myeloma. Clin Exp Immunol 1981; 46:653–661.
153. Alker U, Hansson UB, Lindstrom FD. Factors affecting IgA related hyperviscosity. Clin Exp Immunol 1983; 51:617–623.

154. Powles R, Smith C, Kohn J, et al. Method of removing abnormal protein rapidly from patients with malignant paraproteinaemias. BMJ 1971; 2:664–667.
155. Buskard NA, Galton DAG, Goldman JR, et al. Plasma exchange in the long-term management of Waldenström's macroglobulinemia. Can Med Assoc J 1977; 117: 135–137.
156. Bensinger WI. Plasma exchange in the management of hematologic malignancies. In: Wiernik PH, Canellos GP, Kyle RA, et al, eds. Neoplastic Diseases of the Blood. New York: Churchill Livingstone, 1985:1013–1023.
157. Pearson TC. Rheology of the absolute polycythemias. Baillieres Clin Hematol 1987; 1:637–664.
158. Barabas AP, Offen DN, Meinhard EA. The arterial complications of polycythaemia vera. Br J Surg 1973;60:183–187.
159. Kremer M, Lambert CD, Lawton N. Progressive neurological deficits in primary polycythemia. BMJ 1972; 3:216–218.
160. Gerson SL, Lazzarus HM. Hematopoietic emergencies. Semin Oncol 1989; 16: 532–542.
161. Berk PD, Goldberg JD, Donovan PB, et al. Therapeutic recommendations in polycytemia vera based on polycytemia vera study group protocols. Semin Hematol 1986; 23:132–143.
162. Berk PD, Goldberg JD, Silverstein MN, et al. Increased incidence of acute leukemia in polycytemia vera associated with chlorambucil therapy. N Engl J Med 1981; 304:441–447.
163. Lichtman MA, Heal J, Rowe JM. Hyperleukocytic leukaemia: rheological and clinical features and management. Bailliere's Clin Haematol 1987; 725–746.
164. Vernant JP, Brun B, Mannoni P, et al. Respiratory distress of hyperleucocytic granulocytic leukemias. Cancer 1979; 44:264–268.
165. Lichtman MA, Rowe JM. Hyperleucocytic leukemia: rheologic, clinical and therapeutic considerations. Blood 1982; 650:279–283.
166. Schiffer CA. Therapeutic cytapheresis. In: Wiernik P, Canellos GP, Kyle RA, et al, eds. Neoplastic Diseases of the Blood. New York: Churchill Livingstone, 1985: 999–1012.
167. Miters AJ, Schafer AI. Thrombocytosis and thrombocytemia. Hematol Oncol Clin North Am 1990; 4:157–178.
168. Pearson TC. Primary thrombocytemia: diagnosis and management. Br J Haematol 1991; 78:145–148.
169. Schafer AI. Essential thrombocytemia. Prog Hemost Thromb 1991; 10:69–96.
170. Gisslinger H, Chot A, Scheithauer W, et al. Interferon in essential thrombocytemia. Br J Haematol 1991; 79(suppl 1):42–47.
171. Sacchi S, Tabilio A, Leoni P, et al. Interferon alpha-2b in the long-term treatment of essential thrombocytemia. Am J Hematol 1991; 63:206–209.
172. Anagrelide Study Group. Anagrelide, a therapy for thrombocythemic states: an experience in 577 patients. Am J Med 1992; 92:69–76.

7

Bone Marrow Transplantation

D. Bron
Institut Jules Bordet, Université Libre de Bruxelles, Brussels, Belgium

I. INTRODUCTION

Bone marrow transplantation (BMT) is an accepted form of therapy with increasing indications in a variety of malignant diseases, genetic disorders, and aplastic anemia.

Morbidity and mortality within the first 100 days is substantial, particularly following allogeneic BMT. The possibility that this therapeutic procedure might induce toxic death is of particular concern when survival of the patients without BMT may be considerably longer (i.e., chronic myeloid leukemia in first year of chronic phase). Patients undergoing such treatment suffer from prolonged marrow aplasia, significant nonmarrow toxicities, profound immunosuppression, and unique complications such as graft-versus-host diseases (GVHD). This requires maximum supportive care including close monitoring of clinical and laboratory parameters to anticipate or detect as early as possible potential complications. In addition, this requires the dedication and expertise of the medical and nursing team.

This chapter focuses on the prevention, treatment, and follow-up of early and late complications of patients undergoing BMT. Topics such as prevention of bacterial and fungal infections, use of cytokines, use of antiemetics, and oral care are discussed elsewhere in this book.

II. SIDE EFFECTS OF CONDITIONING

A. Cytotoxic Drug Toxicity

High-dose cyclophosphamide (CY) chemotherapy is used for its antineoplastic and immunosuppressive effects in preparation for BMT. A unique cardiotoxicity is associated with high-dose CY. Manifestations of CY cardiotoxicity range from an asymptomatic pericardial effusion with reduction in electrocardiographic voltage to a myopericarditis and congestive heart failure (CHF), which may be fatal. Braverman et al. have prospectively studied the incidence, risk factors, and course of cardiotoxicity following high-dose CY administration (1). The CY toxicity is thought to be due to toxic endothelial damage followed by extravasation of toxic metabolites with resultant myocyte damage and interstitial hemorrhage and edema. Microthrombosis leading to further ischemic damage may be responsible for more serious cardiotoxicity that leads to death. Braverman reports 35% of baseline fractional shortening. The risk of cardiotoxicity is directly related to the dose, and the authors suggest fractionating high-dose CY to reduce cardiotoxicity, as reported in animal models, without losing the therapeutic efficacy. Prior radiation therapy has not been found to predispose the patient to cardiotoxicity in at least three studies. Increased toxicity related to prior administration of anthracyclines remains questionable. Only a history of clinical CHF or a baseline ejection fraction less than 50% was an independent predictor of cardiotoxicity.

The administration of high-dose CY is also associated with hemorrhagic cystitis. This complication is uncommon but its treatment is difficult. A recent randomized study suggests that bladder irrigation does not prevent hemorrhagic cystitis, (2) but mesna (2. mercapto-ethane sulfonate) administration is mandatory (10–20 mg/kg/4 h for 24 h beyond the last dose of CY). The treatment of hemorrhagic cystitis includes bladder irrigation (1 L/h) with water, saline, or Alun (10 g/L) and correction of clotting abnormalities.

Busulfan has been associated with seizures during its administration or shortly thereafter. Because it is known that high blood levels of busulfan can persist for 24 to 48 hours after the end of oral busulfan administration, antiseizure prophylaxis should include phenytoin for at least 48 hours after the last dose (3).

B. Mucositis

Mucositis is a frequent complication of BMT conditioning but severity of these lesions may be reduced by the administration of acyclovir, suggesting an important role of herpes simplex virus in the development of oral mucositis. Pathogenesis of these lesions could be related to the increased tumor necrosis factor (TNF)-α serum levels observed after BMT. Ciprofloxacin, a drug that interferes with TNF-α transcription, has been reported to enhance hematopoietic recovery and improve survival in a murine model (4). About 90% of allogeneic transplant patients suffer from mucositis that is sufficiently painful as to require opioid analgesics in continuous infusion.

C. Hemolytic-Uremic Syndrome

Renal dysfunction and hemolytic-uremic syndrome have been recognized as a rare but serious complication of allogeneic transplantation (5). Hemolytic-uremic syndrome occurs as early as 30 days and as late as 2 years after BMT. Recommendation to treat this hemolytic-uremic syndrome is discontinuation of cyclosporin A, high doses of steroids, and ≥3 L/d plasma exchange. Prognosis is poor but patients with less severe hemolysis (lactate dehydrogenase [LDH] < 1,000 U/L) appear to have a better outcome (6).

III. GRAFT-VERSUS-HOST DISEASE

Graft-versus-host disease remains a significant problem following allogeneic BMT. The risk of significant grade II to IV GVHD is associated with increasing age and any combination other than a female-to-female donor-to-recipient pair. Other less important risks are associated with female donors who are immunized and donors who are cytomegalovirus (CMV) positive (7). The essential requirements for the development of GVHD are:

1. The graft must contain immunologically competent cells.
2. The recipient must express relevant transplantation antigens that are capable of immunologically stimulating donor cells.
3. The recipient must be immunologically deficient, that is, incapable of mounting an immune response.

These requirements are present not only after allogeneic transplantation but also after transplantation of solid organs containing lymphoid tissue and after transfusion of nonirradiated blood products, particularly in immunocompromised patients. Under certain circumstances, GVHD has been demonstrated after autologous or syngeneic BMT.

The pathogenesis of this reaction is currently understood as a two-step process with, first, an activation of donor T cells by recipient tissue antigens and, second, a secretion of cytokines (TNF-α, interferon [IFN]-γ, interleukin [IL]-1, IL-2) by activated donor T lymphocytes, which attack the recipient's skin, liver, and intestinal tract (8).

Acute GVHD generally develops within 2 to 8 weeks after marrow transplantation. Clinical manifestations include fever, skin rash, jaundice, diarrhea, vomiting, and, in some hyperacute cases, capillary damage and fluid retention. Patients may have mild bilirubin abnormalities but marked transaminase eleva-

Table 1 Grading of Graft-Versus-Host Disease

Skin desquamation (%)	Gastrointestinal tract	Liver	Grade
<50	—	—	I
>50	Diarrhea (<500 mL)	↑ Bilirubin (<20 μM)	II
>50	Diarrhea (<1.5 L)	↑ Bilirubin (>20 μM)	III
>50	Diarrhea (>1 L) Ileus	↑ Bilirubin (>20 μM) ↑ AST, ALT	IV

Abbreviations: AST, aspartate aminotransferase; ALT, alanine aminotransferase.

tions. Although not universally accepted, the Seattle classification is the most common grading system (Table 1). A severity index for grading a GVHD was developed by the International Bone Marrow Transplantation Registry (IBMTR), grouping patients with patterns of organ involvement associated with similar risk of transplant related mortality and treatment failure. Four categories have been established (A to D) and proposed as a revised acute GVHD severity grading index to enhance interpretation of clinical trials (9).

The clinical picture may suggest the diagnosis of GVHD but only skin or rectal biopsies can assess the diagnosis; liver biopsy is also needed to differentiate GVHD from veno-occlusive disease or toxic or viral hepatitis (Table 2).

A. Prevention of Acute Graft-Versus-Host Disease

There have been many advances in the prevention of acute GVHD but cyclosporine with methotrexate (Table 3) remains the most effective combination in decreasing the incidence of GVHD (10,11). FK506 in combination with methotrexate appears equally active in preventing acute GVHD but comparative studies are still warranted (12). However, with the expanded use of matched unrelated

Table 2 Differential Diagnosis of Jaundice Early After Transplantation

	Veno-occlusive disease	Acute graft-versus-host disease	Hepatitis
Days after bone marrow transplantation	0–25	>15	0–100
Bilirubin	↑-↑↑	↑↑	↑-↑↑
Transaminases	0-↑	↑↑	↑↑↑
Alkaline phosphatase	↑	↑	↑↑
Weight gain	+++	+	−

Table 3 Most Popular Regimen for Prophylaxis of Acute Graft-Versus-Host Disease

Day	Cyclosporine[a]	Methotrexate[b]
−1	5 mg/kg/d intravenously (IV)	
+1	5 mg/kg/d IV	15 mg/m^2 IV
+3	5 mg/kg/d IV	10 mg/m^2 IV
+6	5 mg/kg/d IV	10 mg/m^2 IV
+11	5 mg/kg/d IV	10 mg/m^2 IV
+35	2 × 5 mg/kg/d po	
+180	Stop	

[a] Cyclosporin A dose adjusted on levels in the serum.
[b] 50% if bilirubin >2 mg/dL, 25% if bilirubin >3 mg/dL, 0% if bilirubin >5 mg/dL.

as well as mismatched related donors, the increased incidence and severity of GVHD poses a new clinical challenge. Future strategies will include sequential therapies directed at blocking endogenous cytokines followed by blocking alloreactive donor cells and immunological advances such as the induction of tolerance (10).

T-cell depletion of the marrow using anti–T-cell antibodies is an effective way to reduce acute and chronic GVHD but at the price of a higher relapse rate. Therefore, experimental approaches with delayed T-cell reinfusion are under investigation to maintain the graft-versus-leukemia effect with a minimal GVHD.

One of the seeming contradictions is the lower incidence of acute GVHD after allogeneic peripheral blood transplantation, although a large number of mature T cells and natural killer cells are transplanted. It appeared that granulocyte colony-stimulating factor (G-CSF)-mobilized peripheral blood stem cells polarized donor T-cell to type 2 cytokine production (IL-4, IL-10), favoring tolerance rather than GVHD (more related to IL-2 and IFN-γ by type I helper cells). This th1 → th2 shift in the initial response of donor T cells offer a new approach to the prevention of GVHD. Finally, another promising approach is the use of a suicide gene in donor T lymphocytes (13).

B. Treatment of Acute Graft-Versus-Host Disease

Therapy of acute GVHD should be aggressive because response correlates with survival when grade ≥ II GVHD develops. First line therapy should be steroids, usually 1–2 mg/kg/d of intravenous (IV) methylprednisolone for 7–10 days and tapered slowly according to the clinical and biological improvement. Some centers start with 1 g/m^2 × 3/d followed by rapid consecutive taper over 30 days.

Fifty percent to 80% of patients respond to this treatment. In case of resistance, the second line of therapy is polyclonal antithymocyte globulins (5–10 mg/kg IV for 5–7 days) (14). Other antibody therapy directed against T lymphocytes or their cytokines is still under investigation. FK506—as continuous infusion—has also been reported to be effective in steroid-resistant acute GVHD (15).

C. Treatment of Chronic Graft-Versus-Host Disease

Chronic GVHD occurs to some extent in approximately 40% of recipients in allogeneic BMT. Chronic GVHD differs from acute GVHD in its pathogenesis, target organs, and clinical presentations, which are summarized in Table 4. T cells in chronic GVHD react in an autoimmune fashion against histocompatibility alloantigens of the host. These T cells release cytokines and stimulate collagen production. Although this may be associated with a beneficial graft-versus-leukemia effect under certain circumstances, it generally leads to significant morbidity and mortality. Much of the management of these patients consists of symptomatic therapy of the associated skin disease, Sjögren's syndrome (16), and severe immunosuppression with infectious complications (17).

It is generally recommended to treat chronic GVHD with steroids, but in the case of thrombocytopenia, a poor prognostic factor, cyclosporine should be added (18). In case of severe chronic GVHD resistant to steroids and cyclosporine, then azathioprine should be tried. Recent papers report contradictory results with thalidomide (19,20). For the treatment of drug-resistant cutaneous GVHD, a combination of 8-methoxypsoralen and ultraviolet A was tested in 11 patients; six complete and five partial responses were observed (Table 5) (21,22).

Table 4 Clinical Features of Chronic Graft-Versus-Host Disease

Skin muscle	Sclerosis, depigmentation, alopecia, contractures with restriction of movement
Liver	Jaundice caused by biliary obstruction, liver failure, cirrhosis
Exocrine glands	Sicca syndrome, ocular damage, anhydria
Gastrointestinal tract	Ulceration, malabsorption, weight loss, pancreatic insufficiency
Lungs	Bronchiolitis, recurrent chest infections, pneumothorax
Blood cell count	Cytopenia by decreased marrow production or autoimmune destruction

Table 5 Management of Graft-Versus-Host Disease

Prevention	
ex vivo	T-cell depletion of donor marrow
	Irradiation of blood products
in vivo	Cyclosporine (12 mg/kg/d)
	Methotrexate (10 mg/m^2 days 1, 3, 6)
	Steroids (prednisone, 2 mg/kg/d)
	Antithymocyte globulins (5 mg/kg $\times$ 5 d)
Treatment	
Acute	Steroids
	Antithymocyte globulins
	Anti-CD2, anti-CD5
	Anti-IL-2
	Anti-TNF
Chronic	Steroids
	Cyclosporine
	Azathioprine
	Thalidomide

IV. LIVER DYSFUNCTION

Hepatic dysfunction frequently occurs after BMT and various causes such as veno-occlusive disease, graft-versus-host disease, infections, drug injury, or parenteral nutrition must be distinguished. Time of onset, duration, treatment, and prognosis are different for each diagnosis.

A. Veno-occlusive Disease

Veno-occlusive disease (VOD) is a consequence of toxic injury to the liver resulting from the high-dose chemotherapy, and radiotherapy used to condition the patient. It is the most common life-threatening complication of conditioning regimen-related toxicity and it is clinically suspected if jaundice, weight gain, and painful hepatomegaly develop in the first 2 weeks after BMT (23). The incidence of VOD is lower in autologous BMT as compared to allogeneic BMT and this led to speculation of immunological mechanisms involved in the pathogenesis of VOD.

Pathogenesis is not fully understood but the toxic concentration of active metabolites of antineoplastic agents in centrolobular zone of the liver sinusoids may lead to obstruction of small intrahepatic venules resulting from edematous, injured, and necrotic hepatocytes. It is believed that release of (TNF-α) potentiates cytotoxicity and activates coagulation, leading to more severe obstruction of hepatic sinusoids and venules. This can cause a shift of fluid containing sodium and albumin from the intravascular to the extravascular space; the clinical picture then consists of edema, ascites, abdominal pain, hepatomegaly, and impaired liver function with icterus. In severe cases with prolonged liver dysfunction, renal insufficiency may develop secondary to pre-renal failure. In patients receiving cyclosporine, prostacylin release from endothelial cells is reduced, which may facilitate capillary thrombosis.

A number of contradictions exist among published risk factors from different institutions. McDonald et al. have stratified the potential risk factors for development of VOD into three areas: (1) pretransplant factors, (2) marrow conditioning and type of transplant, and (3) clinical course factors.

Among pretransplant factors, elevated SGOT above the upper normal limit is one of the strongest risk factors for VOD, and the increased risk is proportionate to the degree of SGOT elevation. In most series, the causes of pretransplant hepatitis are primarily non-A, non-B hepatitis, more likely hepatitis C. In the multivariate analysis of McDonald and colleagues (72), an additional risk is related to septicemia and/or the use of broad-spectrum antibiotics (including vancomycin and amphotericin B). It could be that persistent fever requiring the use of these drugs reflects increased level of TNF-α involved in the pathogenesis of VOD. Other pretransplant risk factors include status of the disease, positive CMV serology, heavy pretreatment with chemotherapy, and older age. However, some of these factors have not been confirmed in recent studies.

Conditioning regimen is the major risk for VOD when more intensive cytoreductive regimens are administered. The administration of high-dose busulfan is often incriminated in the increased risk of VOD (24). However, the rate of VOD varies greatly after conditioning with busulfan and cyclophosphamide. This marked variability has come to be better understood by pharmacological data: the apparent volume of distribution and clearance rate was twice as high in children, possibly accounting for the higher risk in adult patients who received doses calculated per body weight (16 mg/kg). The hepatotoxicity of total body irradiation (TBI) is sharply increased because the TBI dose is increased despite the use of fractionated schedules.

Jaundice, hepatomegaly, fluid retention, and ascites may be nonspecific findings and a liver biopsy can be useful to distinguish VOD from acute GVHD and infection of the liver. Because patients are generally severely thrombocytopenic, a transvenous liver biopsy should be used instead of percutaneous liver biopsy, which carries an increased risk of hemorrhage. However, these clinical manifestations early after transplantation are highly suggestive of VOD; ascites and significant weight gain are usually not seen in drug-induced hepatotoxicity. Acute GVHD usually appears after the first 2 weeks without ascites.

Thirty percent of patients first seen with VOD ultimately die of hepatorenal

Table 6 Management of Veno-Occlusive Disease

Prevention
Low molecular weight heparin (7500 UI/d CIV)
Heparin (100 U/kg CIV)
Prostaglandin E_1 (0.5 mg/d/CIV)
Treatment
Electrolyte balance surveillance
Fluid restriction with preservation of renal perfusion
Maintenance of osmotic pressure (albumin)
Tissue plasminogen activator (0.05 mg/kg/h IV (4 h) × 4 d)
Defibrotide (10–20 mg/kg CIV)

CIV = continuous introveinous.

failure. Therefore, several prophylactic options have been proposed (Table 6). The spectacular results observed with pentoxifylline (2 g/d), a TNF-α blocker, have not been confirmed in randomized studies. Another option has been reported by Attal and colleagues in a randomized study comparing continuous infusion of low-dose heparin (100 U/kg/d) starting with conditioning regimen until day 30 and no prophylactic treatment. The heparin-treated group was significantly superior ($p < 0.01$) to the control group. The effect was achieved without an increased risk of bleeding (25). A randomized trial with low molecular weight heparin has also confirmed this reduced incidence of VOD (26). Prophylactic infusion of prostacyclin may also be effective but side effects such as fluid retention and painful extremities are limiting toxicities.

The treatment of VOD is limited to symptomatic measures: a restriction of sodium intake to achieve a negative sodium balance. Total volume of perfusion should be reduced but renal perfusion must be maintained. Albumin (up to four times 25 g IV/d) is useful to maintain the osmotic pressure. Hemoglobin should be maintained at a level of ≥ 10 g/dL to provide sufficient oxygen to hepatocytes and renal tubular cells. Spironolactone is recommended if serum creatinine is normal. Administration of low-dose tissue plasminogen activator or defibrotide can reverse bilirubin elevation in some patients but experience with these approaches are limited (27). Drugs such as cyclosporine, methotrexate, sedatives, and analgesics need dose adjustment or discontinuation.

B. Acute and Chronic Graft-Versus-Host Disease

The hepatotoxicity of acute GVHD is probably the result of both cellular attack (by T lymphocytes) and cytokines, such as TNF and IFN. In most patients, some degree of skin or intestinal involvement by acute GVHD is present concurrently. Usually, transaminases and serum bilirubin are moderately increased. Acute liver failure with ascites, coagulation disorders, and encephalopathy is uncommon. In some cases, liver biopsy is required to make the diagnosis. The treatment of GVHD is described previously in this chapter.

Most patients with chronic GVHD show some degree of hepatic involvement: the main targets of chronic GVHD of the liver are the small interlobular bile ducts. A biopsy is often needed to exclude other pathological conditions. Rarely, hepatic failure and cirrhosis are observed. About half of the patients remain free of chronic GVHD after immunosuppressive drug withdrawal.

C. Infections

The most common infections of the liver in BMT recipients are of viral origin: hepatitis B or C, CMV, varicella-zoster virus (VZV), and herpes simplex virus (HSV). With new screening tests, the role of transfusion in this risk is very small (28). Fungal infections such as candidiasis should also been excluded (29–31).

V. PREVENTION OF VIRAL INFECTIONS

Viral opportunistic infections and primarily CMV infections represent a major infectious problem in transplanted patients. However, significant progress has been made in identifying risk factors for prevention and treatment of CMV infection. In addition to pneumonitis, retinitis, and hepatitis, CMV has been associated with a delay in the recovery of platelets after allogeneic and autologous BMT (32,33). However, CMV is rarely a life-threatening complication in autologous BMT and, in this setting, CMV prophylaxis is not recommended.

Several centers have reported that screened (CMV negative) blood products can prevent CMV infection in seronegative recipients with seronegative donors; this aspect is discussed in Chapter 5 (34). Several recent studies have also demonstrated that leukocyte-depleted blood products can prevent CMV infection in CMV-negative patients (35,36). Even in patients receiving the marrow from a CMV-positive donor, leukocyte-depleted blood products could reduce the incidence of CMV infection (37). Intravenous immunoglobulin (IVIG) was also studied in CMV-seronegative BMT recipients and was found to be ineffective in prevention (38).

For CMV-positive recipients, two approaches have been widely studied: (1) immunoprophylaxis with high doses of (IVIG) and (2) antiviral drug prophylaxis using acyclovir or ganciclovir.

A. High-Dose IgG Immunoglobulins

There are several reasons to support immunoprophylaxis in the prevention of CMV infection, for example, hyperimmune immunoglobulins have proven useful in the prevention of various viral infections, such as hepatitis, varicella, and rubella. Other rational bases derive from animal data showing that hyperimmune immunoglobulins can protect immunosuppressed or newborn mice against CMV-induced interstitial pneumonia. Also, after allogeneic BMT, patients with higher antibody response to CMV antigens have been reported to have a better outcome (39).

At least five controlled studies have shown a decrease in the incidence of interstitial pneumonia, whereas the incidence of CMV infection is not always significantly reduced. In addition, in a large comparative study reported by the Seattle-group, several other advantages of the treatment with IVIG have been pointed out: a reduced risk of GVHD, a reduced incidence of bacterial septicemia, a reduced number of pneumonitis cases. The mechanism of action of IVIG is not fully elucidated. It does increase the circulating level of specific anti-CMV (and antibacteria) immunoglobulins with cytotoxic and neutralizing activities. It is also likely that the increase of IgG level in the serum and respiratory tract decreases the risk of infectious problems including CMV. The reduced incidence of GVHD could be related to antilymphocyte antibodies or to a blockade of FC receptors on CD8 lymphocytes involved in the process of GVHD. A relationship exists between CMV infection and acute GVHD, and a reduced incidence of GVHD could probably have an indirect effect in the prevention of CMV infection (40,41).

A promising immunological approach is being investigated in phase I trials: adoptive immunotherapy using T-cell clones obtained from seropositive donors. It has been shown that transplanted patients with a specific anti-CMV T-cell response have a better outcome than patients unable to have such a cytolytic T-cell response (42).

Although the role of IVIG in CMV prophylaxis is still debated and not recommended for this specific indication, the other beneficial effects of IVIG have led many centers to adopt this immunoprophylaxis using 500 mg/kg weekly for the first 100 days and monthly up to the end of immunosuppressive drug therapy. Also, in CMV interstitial pneumonia, better outcome has been observed when IVIG (three times a week) are combined with GCV treatment.

B. Antiviral Drugs Prophylaxis and Preemptive Treatment

The first convincing study was reported by Meyers in 1990 using acyclovir at the dose of 500 mg/m^2 every 8 hours from day 7 to day 30 in seropositive allogeneic transplanted patients. In this series, the incidence of both CMV infections and interstitial pneumonia was reduced (43). However, acyclovir is not the optimal antiviral drug and ganciclovir, which slows the replication of CMV, is a better candidate for CMV prophylaxis. At least one study has indicated that prophylactic ganciclovir (5 mg/kg/12 h $\times$ 14 ds) can completely prevent CMV pneumonia in seropositive recipient or seropositive donor (44), but myelosuppression is the limiting toxicity for half of the patients. Therefore, recent strategies using ganciclovir as preemptive therapy after two consecutive positive tests on buffy coat cells using polymerase chain reaction (PCR) technique or CMV antigenemia are more rational approaches for seropositive patients or seronegative recipients with a seropositive donor (45,46).

More recently, the new antiviral drug, foscarnet, has gained interest because of its anticytomegalovirus activity by inhibition of CMV DNA polymerase. This drug has been shown to be effective in some cases of ganciclovir-resistant CMV and is less toxic for the marrow. This drug should be used with caution in patients with renal failure.

VI. GRAFT FAILURE

Graft failure can manifest itself as primary engraftment failure or as initial engraftment followed by secondary graft loss. Graft failure may or may not be associated with reappearance of recipient cells, but an active host response to the graft is often involved in allogeneic BMT (47). In the setting of autologous BMT, other causes are involved in the process of graft failure.

Definition of graft failure is not universally settled; however, when granulocyte count is not sustained at $>200/\mu L$ by day 28, graft failure is thought to be present. Graft failure is confirmed when marrow biopsy reveals an empty or a poor marrow without myeloid, erythroid, or megakaryocytic precursors.

In the patient receiving HLA identical donor graft, failure is mostly observed in patients with aplastic anemia who had been multiply transfused and who were thus sensitized to minor histocompatibility antigens of the donor. Experience in patients whose initial graft was rejected has indicated that cyclophosphamide (4×50 mg/kg) and anti thymocyte globulins (ATG) (3×30 mg/kg) allowed for sustained engraftment. This approach has been applied for the first conditioning regimen with encouraging results. Another approach to reducing graft failure is to increase the immunosuppression of the recipient by drug or irradiation (total body or total lymphoid irradiation). The best approach for patients with aplastic anemia is to do transplantation early while they are still untransfused. When blood products are necessary, leukocyte depletion of the transfusion product reduces the risk of sensitization. Recent reports in dogs suggest that irradiation of blood products with ultraviolet light could abrogate the sensitizing ability of the blood product (48). This observation deserves further investigation in humans.

In histoincompatible transplants, graft failure is more common even after TBI-containing regimens. Severe GVHD is more likely to develop in these patients and aggressive attempts to prevent GVHD using T-cell depletion has reduced the risk of GVHD but increased the incidence of graft failure. Other approaches to overcoming this problem include the use of monoclonal antibodies (anti-HLA class II, anti-LFA 1) and ATG. However, although the engraftment is facilitated, the regimen-related toxicity is increased.

Autologous BMT is a successful therapeutic approach with increasing indications. Autologous marrow is often damaged by prior treatments or cryopreservation and the rate of hemopoietic recovery appears to be dependent upon the number of $CD34^+$ stem cells and of colony-forming units (CFUs) as determined in vitro by the CFU-GM assay. In the case of ''purged'' marrow, it is always recommended to store a second unmanipulated backup marrow for rescue.

Several ongoing investigations aimed at improving recovery after autologous BMT are promising. Hematopoietic stem cells circulating in the peripheral blood have been shown to be capable of complete hematopoietic reconstitution, and data in humans demonstrate that recovery is faster than with marrow cells (49,50). This recovery is further accelerated if the patient is pretreated with recombinant myeloid growth factors before harvesting of the peripheral blood stem cells (51). Another interesting area of research is the ''positive purging'' or the isolation of very early hemopoietic precursors characterized by CD34 antigen.

Late decreases in peripheral blood counts in patients following marrow transplantation can be due to a variety of causes. Suppression by cotrimoxazole may be one cause, and the drug should be avoided or combined with folinic acid. Cytomegalovirus infection often leads to a decrease in blood counts, which is usually reversible after successful treatment of the CMV. Although rare, accidental administration of unirradiated blood products in the immunosuppressive posttransplant period can result in the establishment of transfusion-associated GVHD and consequent marrow aplasia. Isolated thrombocytopenia may occur in the setting of chronic GVHD, representing a poor risk factor.

Isolated anemia can be due to renal dysfunction, to persistent parvovirus B19 infection, or to the result of ABO incompatible marrow graft. In this latter situation, persistent host B lymphocytes can produce isoagglutinins that react with donor red cells and lead to persistent hemolytic anemia.

VII. CYTOKINES

High-dose chemoradiation therapy used before autologous or allogeneic BMT is intensively myelosuppressive and immunosuppressive, and frequently results in severe and life-threatening infections. Hematopoietic growth factors (HGFs) have the potential to accelerate hematopoietic recovery after BMT and, by shortening the period of pancytopenia, they are likely to reduce infections and bleeding complications. On the other hand, cytokines and particularly recombinant human interleukin-2 (IL-2) may have clinical applications in the acceleration of immune recovery and some antitumoral benefit in malignant hemopathies.

A. Hematopoietic Growth Factors

Several HGFs are currently available for clinical use: erythropoietic (EPO), granulocyte-colony-stimulating factor (G-CSF), granulocyte-macrophage colony-stimulating factor (GM-CSF), macrophage colony stimulating factor (M-CSF), and interleukin-3 (IL-3). Interleukin-11 (IL-11), thrombopoietin (TPO), and stem cell factor (SCF) are currently under investigation.

Several groups have reported increases in EPO levels parallel to hemoglobin levels in autologous BMT (52). In allogeneic BMT, several authors have shown impaired or deficient production of EPO, and an inappropriate response of EPO levels to anemia has been detected (53). An uncontrolled trial has shown that EPO is capable of accelerating erythroid engraftment in allogeneic BMT and this observation is now confirmed by a recent randomized prospective study. An earlier appearance of reticulocytes and a diminished need of red blood cell transfusions were observed in patients given EPO (54). Of note, the treated group received also significantly fewer platelet transfusions, but this requires further study.

Because there was a concern of provoking GVHD in allogeneic BMT, many of the studies have been conducted in autologous or syngeneic BMT (55). In a prospective, placebo-controlled trial of GM-CSF after autologous BMT for lymphoid malignancies, Nemunaitis et al.(56) reported significantly fewer infections, days of fever, and days of antibiotic use in patients receiving GM-CSF compared to those in the placebo control group. There was a trend toward earlier neutrophil recovery to 1,000/mm^3 in the GM-CSF treated group. Red blood cell recovery was not different from the control group but platelet recovery was accelerated, with fewer bleeding complications in the GM-CSF treated group. Additionally, patients given GM-CSF had fewer days with mucositis and less interstitial pneumonia.

Granulocyte CSF has been extensively studied in the setting of high-dose chemotherapy allogeneic and autologous BMT. Using 5 to 10 μg/kg/d, neutrophil recovery was significantly accelerated in G-CSF treated patients. These patients had fewer days of fever, antibiotic therapy, and oral mucositis. Recovery of platelets and erythroblasts was not different (57). Granulocyte CSF is better tolerated than GM-CSF with only mild myalgia in some patients receiving higher dosages.

Preliminary data are available with IL-3 and M-CSF after BMT. They suggest that the duration of severe granulocytopenia may be reduced by M-CSF (58) and platelet recovery may be accelerated by IL-3.

In the setting of allogeneic BMT, G- and GM-CSF have been used with caution because of an increased risk of GVHD. Clinical trials did not demonstrate an increased incidence of GVHD or graft failure but an accelerated recovery of neutrophils. The incidence of GVHD and relapse rate was similar compared to historical control subjects (59).

Human growth factor accelerates hematopoietic recovery after autologous and allogeneic BMT without increasing the incidence of graft failure of GVHD and is recommended after transplantation (60).

B. Interleukin-2

The rationale for the use of IL-2 after marrow transplantation is based on several experimental observations. First, freshly isolated leukemia and lymphoma cells have previously been shown to be sensitive to lysis by IL-2–induced lymphocyte-activated killer (LAK) cells in vitro. Moreover, IL-2 responsive LAK precursors (natural killer [NK] cells) have been identified in the peripheral blood of patients as early as 3 weeks after high-dose chemotherapy and marrow infusion. Soiffier and colleagues have recently shown that IL-2 can be continuously administered for prolonged periods after autologous and allogeneic BMT (61). At low dose (2×10^5 U/m^2/d), all patients showed an increase in the number of NK cells in their peripheral blood. Moreover, the sensitivity of these NK cells to further activation by IL-2 in vitro was markedly enhanced while patients were receiving IL-2 in vivo. In this report, toxicity was minimal but the dose used is generally one-tenth of the dose administered by others (62–64) who reported thrombocytopenia, capillary leak syndrome, and so on. This lower dose allows a longer period of administration (>3 mo). Another noteworthy feature is the absence of GVHD in the Soiffier series, although with higher dose, Favrot et al. reported a severe GVHD after allogeneic BMT. This can be accounted for by a specific stimulation of NK cells without a change in T-cell number and, in these cases, a T-cell depletion of the marrow. Because NK cells are more likely involved in the graft-versus-leukemia effect of the marrow, this IL-2 stimulation of NK cells might be beneficial to the patients in terms of relapse rate. In this setting, large randomized studies are still warranted (65,66).

VIII. LONG-TERM FOLLOW-UP

Marrow transplantation is associated with a number of long-term complications that may not manifest themselves for months after the BMT. They result from immunological abnormalities, structural damage secondary to the conditioning regimen, and recurrence of underlying disease (67).

A. Infectious Problems and Vaccination Policy

Late infectious complications are more frequently seen in allogeneic BMT as opposed to autologous BMT and are far more frequent in patients with chronic GVHD (68). After discharge from the hospital, most patients are maintained on cotrimoxazole prophylaxis for 6 to 12 months or as long as immunosuppressive treatment is needed. Both bacterial (encapsulated organisms) and *Pneumocystis carinii* are effectively prevented by this prophylaxis and, in case of intolerance to sulfonamides, penicillin and inhaled pentamidine can be administered.

After allogeneic BMT, patients require revaccination and, because it is unlikely to have an adequate antibody and T-cell immune response during the first year, it is generally recommended to revaccinate at 12 months with diphtheria and tetanus toxoid, 23-valent pneumococcal vaccine, 4-valent meningococcal vaccine, and HIB protein conjugate vaccine. Tetanus toxoid antibody levels can be controlled 6 to 8 weeks after vaccination. Killed poliomyelitis (Salk) vaccine should also be administered 1 to 2 years after transplantation. Measles, mumps, and rubella vaccines, which are live viruses, should not be administered to allograft recipients with chronic GVHD. They can be given 2 years after transplantation but their real necessity in BMT setting is still debated. Booster vaccines for pneumococcal, meningococcal, and Hib antigens are recommended at 24 months (Table 7) (69).

Viral infections, generally caused by reactivation of latent endogenous virus either in the host or the donor cells, are frequent; VZV recurrence may be expected in the majority of patients who were seropositive for VZV before transplantation, generally occurring within the first 9 months after BMT but sometimes as late as 18 to 24 months. Such patients should be given acyclovir (10 mg/kg/8 h for 10 d). Adenovirus, HSV, and CMV infections generally occur within the first 4 months after transplantation.

Table 7 Recommended Immunizations After Bone Marrow Transplantations

At 1 year	Diphtheria, tetanus
	Salk poliovirus (inactivated)
	H-influenzae (Hib)
	Influenza
	Hepatitis B
At 2 years	Repeat diphtheria, tetanus
	Repeat inactivated poliovirus
	Pneumococcal (23 valent vaccine)
	Meningococcal vaccine
	Measles, mumps, rubella[a]
Repeat every year	Influenza

[a] To be avoided in case of immunosuppressive drugs or chronic GVHD.

B. Hormonal Surveillance

Endocrine function is impaired in a significant number of patients after marrow transplantation. Asymptomatic, well-compensated hypothyroidism occurs in up to two-thirds of patients after transplantation. This complication appears to be primarily limited to patients who have received irradiation in their conditioning. It is reasonable to evaluate patients on a yearly basis with thyroid-stimulating hormone (TSH) levels as well as routine thyroid function tests.

Growth retardation may be seen in children both because of a direct effect on the growth plates of the bone by radiation therapy and, in some cases, because of growth hormone abnormalities induced by central nervous system irradiation.

Patients with total body irradiation have a generally greater than 95% incidence of development of infertility secondary to ovarian failure or azoospermagenesis. Chemotherapy alone may recover hormonal function, but it is particularly dependent upon age, with the majority of women younger than 25 years old having return of menstruation and normal follicle-stimulating hormone and luteinicing hormone levels. About two-thirds of men given chemotherapy alone have return of sperm production.

C. Osteoporosis and Aseptic Necrosis

Osteoporosis is a recognized complication of steroid therapy and is frequent after treatment for graft-versus-host disease. A recent important study compared intermittent etidronate therapy versus placebo in the prevention of steroid-induced osteoporosis and found a reduced loss of vertebral and trochanteric bone in the etidronate group (70). Aseptic necrosis develops in 4% of allotransplanted patients after a period ranging from 2 to 130 months; this complication is correlated with steroid treatment for GVHD and requires replacement of the hip in 88% of the cases (71).

D. Secondary Tumors

Secondary malignancies have been relatively infrequent (35/2,000 patients in the Seattle experience). Some secondary non-Hodgkin's lymphomas may arise in the setting of Epstein-Barr virus–associated lymphoproliferative disease. This complication, which can occur early after transplantation, is most frequent in heavily immunosuppressed individuals, particularly those receiving T-cell depleted marrow from an unrelated or mismatched donor. Such B-cell proliferations (oligo or polyclonal) can be rapidly progressive and fatal. As in solid organ transplant settings, reduction or stopping of immunosuppression can result in spontaneous regression. Other therapeutical approaches, such as anti-B monoclonal antibodies, high-dose immunoglobulins, and interferon-α, have been proposed but remain experimental.

REFERENCES

1. Braverman AC, Antin JH, Plappert MT, et al. Cyclophosphamide cardiotoxicity in bone marrow transplantation: a prospective evaluation of new dosing regimens. J Clin Oncol 1991; 9:1215–1223.
2. Atkinson K, Biggs JC, Golovsky D, et al. Bladder irrigation does not prevent haemorrhagic cystitis in bone marrow transplant recipients. Bone Marrow Transplant 1991; 7:351–354.
3. De La Camara R, Tomas JF, Figuera A, et al. High dose busulfan and seizures. Bone Marrow Transplant 1991; 7:363–364.
4. Kletter Y, Riklis I, Shalit I, et al. Enhanced repopulation of murine hematopoietic organ in sublethally irradiated mice after treatment with ciprofloxacin. Blood 1991; 78:1685–1691.
5. Rabinowe SN, Soiffer RJ, Tarbell NJ, et al. Hemolytic-uremic syndrome following bone marrow transplantation in adults for hematologic malignancies. Blood 1991; 77:1837–1844.
6. Llamas P, Romero R, Cabrera R, et al. Management of thrombotic microangiopathy following allogeneic transplantation: what is the role of plasma exchange? Bone Marrow Transplant 1997; 20(4):305–306.
7. Weysdorf D, Hakke R, Blazar B, et al. Risk factors for acute graft-versus-host disease in histocompatible donor bone marrow transplantation. Transplantation 1991; 5:1197–1203.
8. Marcellus DC, Vogelsang GB. Graft-versus-host disease. Curr Opin Oncol 1997; 9(2):131–138.
9. Rowlings PA, Przepiorka D, Klein JP, et al. IBMTR severity index for grading acute graft-versus-host disease: retrospective comparison with Glucksberg grade. Br J Haematol 1997; 97(4):855–864.
10. Lazarus HM, Vogelsang GB, Rowe JM. Prevention and treatment of acute graft-versus-host disease: the old and the new. A report from the Eastern Cooperative Oncology Group (ECOG). Bone Marrow Transplant 1997; 19(6):577–600.
11. Erer B, Polchi P, Lucarelli G, et al. CsA-associated neurotoxicity and ineffective prophylaxis with clonazepam in patients transplanted for thalassemia major. Bone Marrow Transplant 1996; 18(1):157–162.
12. Nash RA, Pineiro LA, Storb R, et al. FK506 in combination with methotrexate for the prevention of graft-versus-host disease after marrow transplantation from matched unrelated donors. Blood 1996; 88(9):3634–3641.
13. Cohen JL, Boyer O, Salomon B, et al. Prevention of graft-versus-host disease in mice using a suicide gene expressed in T lymphocytes. Blood 1997; 89(12):4636–4645.
14. Ruutu T, Niederwieser D, Gratwohl A, et al. A survey of the prophylaxis and treatment of acute GVHD in Europe: a report of the European Group for Blood and

Marrow Transplantation (EBMT). Chronic Leukaemia Working Party of the EBMT. Bone Marrow Transplant 1997; 19(8):759–764.
15. Ohashi Y, Minegishi M, Fujie H, et al. Successful treatment of steroid-resistant severe acute GVHD with 24-h continuous infusion of FK506. Bone Marrow Transplant 1997; 19(6):625–627.
16. Singhal S, Powles R, Treleaven J, et al. Pilocarpine hydrochloride for symptomatic relief of xerostomia due to chronic graft-versus-host disease or total-body irradiation after bone-marrow transplantation for hematologic malignancies. Leuk Lymph 1997; 24(5-6):539–543.
17. Sullivan KM, Agura E, Anasetti C, et al. Chronic graft-versus-host disease and other late complications of bone marrow transplantation. Semin Hematol 1991; 28:250–259.
18. Sullivan KM, Witherspoon RP, Storb R, et al. Alternating-day cyclosporine and prednisone for treatment of high-risk chronic graft-v-host disease. Blood 1988; 72: 555–561.
19. Chao NJ, Parker PM, Niland JC, et al. Paradoxical effect of thalidomide prohylaxis on chronic graft-vs-host disease. Biol Blood Marrow Transplant 1996; 2(2): 86–92.
20. Vogelsang GB, Farmer ER, Hess AD, et al. Thalidomide therapy of chronic graft versus host disease. N Engl J Med 1992; 326:1055–1058.
21. Dall'Amico R, Rossetti F, Zulian F, et al. Photopheresis in paediatric patients with drug-resistant chronic graft-versus-host disease. Br J Haematol 1997; 97(4):848–854.
22. Eppinger T, Emninger G, Steinert M, et al. 8-methoxypsoralen and UVA therapy for cutaneous GVHD. Transplantation 1990; 50:807–811.
23. Bearman SI. The syndrome of hepatic veno-occlusive disease after marrow transplantation. Blood 1995; 85(11):3005–3020.
24. Ozkaynak MF, Weinberg K, Kohn D, et al. Hepatic veno-occlusive disease post-bone marrow transplantation in children conditioned with busulfan and cyclophosphamide: incidence, risk factors, and clinical outcome. Bone Marrow Transplant 1991; 7:467–474.
25. Attal M, Huguet F, Rubie H, et al. Prevention of hepatic veno-occlusive disease after bone marrow transplantaion by continuous infusion of low-dose heparin: a prospective, randomized trial. Blood 1992; 79:2834–2840.
26. Or R, Nagler A, Shpilberg O, et al. Low molecular weight heparin for the prevention of veno-occlusive disease of the liver in bone marrow transplantation patients. Transplantation 1996; 61(7):1067–1071.
27. Bearman SL, Lee JL, Baron AE, et al. Treatment of hepatic venocclusive disease with recombinant human tissue plasminogen activator and heparin in 42 marrow transplant patients. Blood 1997; 89(5):1501–1506.
28. Schreiber GB, Busch MP, Kleinman SJ, et al. The risk of transfusion-transmitted viral infections. N Engl J Med 1996; 334:1685–1690.
29. Andstrom EE, Ringden O, Remberger M, et al. Safety and efficacy of liposomal amphotericin B in allogeneic bone marrow transplant recipients. Mycoses 1996; 39(5-6):185–193.
30. Jantunen E, Ruutu P, Niskanen L, et al. Incidence and risk factors for invasive fungal

infections in allogeneic BMT recipients. Bone Marrow Transplant 1997; 19(8):801–808.
31. Trigg ME, Morgan D, Burns TL, et al. Successful program to prevent *Aspergillus* infections in children undergoing marrow transplantation: use of nasal amphotericin. Bone Marrow Transplantat 1997; 19(1):43–47.
32. Reusser P, Fisher LD, Buckner CD, et al. Cytomegalovirus infection after autologous bone marrow transplantation: occurrence of cytomegalovirus disease and effect on engraftment. Blood 1990; 75:1888–1894.
33. Verdonck LF, De Gast GC, Van Heugten HG, et al. Cytomegalovirus infection causes delayed platelet recovery after bone marrow transplantation. Blood 1991; 78: 844–848.
34. Miller WJ, McCullough J, Balfour HH Jr, et al. Prevention of cytomegalovirus infection following bone marrow transplantation: a randomized trial of blood product screening. Bone Marrow Transplant 1991; 7:227–234.
35. Bowden RA, Slichter SJ, Sayers MH, et al. Comparison of filtered leukocyte-reduced and cytomegalovirus (CMV) seronegative blood products for prevention of transfusion-associated CMV infection after marrow transplant. Blood 1995; 86:3598.
36. Landaw EM, Kanter M, Petz LD. Safety of filtered leukocyte-reduced blood products for prevention of transfusion-associated cytomegalovirus infection. Blood 1996; 87(11):4910–4919.
37. De Witte T, Schattenberg A, Van Dijk BA, et al. Preventing of primary cytomegalovirus infection after allogeneic bone marrow transplantation by using leukocyte-poor random blood products from cytomegalovirus-unscreened blood-bank donors. Transplantation 1990; 50:964–968.
38. Ruutu T, Ljungman P, Brinch L, et al. No prevention of cytomegalovirus infection by anti-cytomegalovirus hyperimmune globulin in seronegative bone marrow transplant recipients. The Nordic BMT Group. Bone Marrow Transplant 1997; 19(3): 233–236.
39. Bron D, Lagneaux L, Delforge A, et al. Prevention of CMV-induced myelosuppression by anti-CMV antibodies: an in vitro model. Exp Hematol 1991; 19:132–135.
40. Bron D, Klastersky J. Immunoprophylaxis of cytomegalovirus infections in transplanted patients. Eur J Cancer Clin Oncol 1989; 25, 9:1365–1368.
41. Sullivan KM, Kopecky K, Jocom J, et al. Immunomodulatory and antimicrobial efficacy of intravenous immunoglobulin in bone marrow transplantation. N Engl J Med 1990; 323:705–712.
42. Reusser P, Riddell SR, Meyers JD, et al. Cytotoxic T-lymphocyte response to cytomegalovirus after human allogeneic bone marrow transplantation: pattern of recovery and correlation with cytomegalovirus infection and disease. Blood 1991; 78: 1373–1380.
43. Meyers JD, Reed EC, Shepp DH, et al. Acyclovir for prevention of cytomegalovirus infection and disease after allogeneic marrow transplantation. N Engl J Med 1988; 318:70–75.
44. Atkinson K, Downs K, Golenia M, et al. Prophylactic use of ganciclovir in allogeneic bone marrow transplantation: absence of clinical cytomegalovirus infection. Br J Haematol 1991; 79:57–62.
45. Goodrich J, Mori M, Gleaves C, et al. Early treatment with ganciclovir to prevent

cytomegalovirus disease after allogeneic bone marrow transplantation. N Engl J Med 1991; 325:1601–1607.
46. Schmidt GM, Horak DA, Niland JC, et al. A randomized, controlled trial of prophylactic ganciclovir for cytomegalovirus pulmonary infection in recipients of allogeneic bone marrow transplants. N Engl J Med 1991; 325:1601–1607.
47. Klumpp TR. Immunohematologic complications of bone marrow transplantation. Bone Marrow Transplant 1991; 8:159–170.
48. Pamphilon DH, Alnaqdy AA, Wallington TB. Immunomodulation by ultraviolet light: clinical studies and biological effects. Immunol Today 1991; 12:119–123.
49. Lopez M, Mortel O, Pouillart P, et al. Acceleration of hemopoietic recovery after autologous bone marrow transplantation by low doses of peripheral blood stem cells. Bone Marrow Transplant 1991; 7:173–181.
50. Pavletic ZS, Bishop MR, Tarantolo SR, et al. Hematopoietic recovery after allogeneic bone stem-cell transplantation compared with bone marrow transplantation in patients with hematologic malignancies. J Clin Oncol 1997; 15(4):1608–1616.
51. Kotasek D, Sepherd KM, Sage RE, et al. Factors affecting blood stem cell collections following high-dose cyclophosphamide mobilization in lymphoma, myeloma and solid tumors. Bone Marrow Transplant 1992; 9:11–17.
52. Bosi A, Vannucchi AM, Grossi A, et al. Serum erythropoietin levels in patients undergoing autologous bone marrow transplantation. Bone Marrow Transplant 1991; 7:421–425.
53. Beguin Y, Clemons GK, Oris R, et al. Circulating erythropoietin levels after bone marrow transplantation: inappropriate response to anemia in allogeneic transplants. Blood 1991; 77:868–873.
54. Steegmann JL, Lopez J, Otero MJ, et al. Erythropoietin treatment in allogeneic BMT accelerates erythroid reconstitution: results of a prospective controlled randomized trial. Bone Marrow Transplant 1992; 10:541–546.
55. Brandt SJ, Peters WP, Atwater SK, et al. Effect of recombinant granulocytemacrophage colony-stimulating factor on hematopoietic reconstitution after high-dose chemotherapy and autologous bone marrow transplantation. Blood 1988; 318:869–876.
56. Nemunaitis J, Rabinowe SN, Singer JW, et al. Recombinant granulocytes-macrophage colony-stimulating factor after autologous bone marrow transplantation for lymphoid cancer. N Engl J Med 1991; 324:1773–1778.
57. Taylor KM Cd, Jagannath S, Spitzer G, et al. Recombinant human granulocyte colony-stimulating factors hastens granulocyte recovery after high-dose chemotherapy and autologous bone marrow transplantation in Hodgkin's disease. J Clin Oncol 1989; 7:1791–1799.
58. Nemunaitis J, Meyers JD, Buckner CD, et al. Phase I trial of recombinant human macrophage colony-stimulating factor (rhM-CSF) in patients with invasive fungal infections. Blood 1991; 78:907–913.
59. Masaoka T, Takaku F, Kato S, et al. Recombinant human granulocyte colony-stimulating factor in allogeneic bone marrow transplantation. Exp Hematol 1989; 17: 1047–1050.
60. Update of recommendations for the use of hematopoietic colony-stimulating factors: evidence-based clinical practice guidelines. Adopted by the ASCO (1996). J Clin Oncol 1996; 14(6):1957–1960.

61. Soiffier RJ, Murray C, Cochran K, et al. Clinical and immunological effects of prolonged infusion of low-dose recombinant interleukin-2 after autologous and T-cell-depleted allogeneic bone marrow transplantation. Blood 1992; 79:517–526.
62. Blaise D, Olive D, Stoppa AM, et al. Hematologic and immunologic effects of the systemic administration of recombinant interleukin-2 after autologous bone marrow transplantation. Blood 1990; 76:1092–1099.
63. Favrot MC, Floret D, Negrier S, et al. Systemic interleukin-2 therapy in children with progressive neuroblastoma after high dose chemotherapy and bone marrow transplantation. Bone Marrow Transplant 1989; 4:499.
64. Higuchi CM, Thompson JA, Peterson FB. Toxicity of immunomodulatory effects of interleukin-2 after autologous bone marrow transplantation for hematologic malignancies. Blood 1991; 77:2561–2568.
65. Klingemann HG, Philipps GL. Immunotherapy after bone marrow transplantation. Bone Marrow Transplant 1991; 8:73–81.
66. Weinthal JA. The role of cytokines following bone marrow transplantation: indications and controversies. Bone Marrow Transplant 1996; 18(3):S10–S14.
67. Gallardo D, Ferra C, Berlanga JJ, et al. Neurologic complications after allogeneic bone marrow transplantation. Bone Marrow Transplant 1996; 18(6):1135–1139.
68. Roy V, Ochs L, Weisdorf D. Late infections following allogeneic bone marrow transplantation: suggested strategies for prophylaxis. Leuk Lymph 1997; 26(1-2): 1–15.
69. Centers for Disease Control. Update and adult immunization: recommendations of the immunization Practices Advisory Committee. MMWR 1991; 40(12):13–15.
70. Adachi JD, Bensen WG, Brown J, et al. Intermittent etidronate therapy to prevent corticosteroid induced osteoporosis. N Eng J Med 1997; 337:382–387.
71. Socie G, Cahn JY, Carmelo J, et al. Avascular necrosis of bone after allogeneic bone marrow transplantation: analysis of risk factors for 4388 patients by the Société Française de Greffe de Moelle (SFGM). Br J Haematol 1997; 97(4):865–870.
72. McDonald GB, Sharma P, Matthens DE, et al. Veno-occlusive disease of the liver after bone marrow transplantation: diagnosis, incidence and predisposing factors. Hematology 1984; 4:116–121.

8

Management of Nausea and Vomiting

Maurizio Tonato and Fausto Roila
Policlinico Hospital, Perugia, Italy

I. INTRODUCTION

In 1983, Coates et al. published a patient survey showing that vomiting and nausea were respectively the first and second most distressing side effects of cancer chemotherapy (1).

In the following years, a better understanding of the pathophysiology of chemotherapy-induced emesis and the introduction of the 5-HT3 antagonists in clinical practice determined a significant increase in complete protection from nausea and vomiting. In this review, progress is reported and practical guidelines for the prevention of chemotherapy-induced emesis are suggested.

Emesis is characterized by three components: vomiting, nausea, and retching, which are often, but not always, related to each other. Three types of chemotherapy-induced emesis can be distinguished: acute emesis, which occurs in the first 24 hours after chemotherapy administration; delayed emesis, which has been arbitrarily defined as the emesis beginning 24 hours after chemotherapy administration and which can persist up to 6 or 7 days; and anticipatory emesis, which can occur before a subsequent cycle of chemotherapy in patients with a previous history of acute and delayed emesis from chemotherapy.

II. PREVENTION OF EMESIS INDUCED BY CISPLATIN

A. Acute Emesis

In 1981, Gralla et al. were the first to demonstrate that high-dose intravenous (IV) metoclopramide was significantly more efficacious than placebo and prochlorperazine in the prevention of cisplatin-induced acute emesis (2). These results have since been confirmed by several subsequent studies and complete protection from acute emesis in 20% to 40% of patients was obtained.

In the following years, the addition to high-dose metoclopramide of other antiemetic drugs, first steroids (in particular dexamethasone and methylprednisolone) and then diphenhydramine or lorazepam, substantially increased antiemetic activity; complete protection from acute emesis in about 60% of patients was obtained (3).

Several problems remained to be solved: (1) Even with the metoclopramide combinations, 30% to 40% of patients still suffered from acute emesis; (2) Tolerability of the metoclopramide combinations was not completely satisfactory; (3) Sedation, diarrhea, nervousness, and especially extrapyramidal reactions in about 3% of patients were reported. Complete protection from vomiting significantly decreased in the subsequent cycles of chemotherapy.

The development and the marketing of the 5-HT3 receptor antagonists (in particular, ondansetron, granisetron, tropisetron, and dolasetron) has represented an important improvement for the prevention of chemotherapy-induced emesis. In fact, 5-HT3 receptor antagonists achieved complete protection from acute emesis induced by cisplatin in 40% to 60% of patients in different studies (3). Their combination with dexamethasone increased substantially the complete protection from acute emesis—up to 70% to 90% of patients (3). Furthermore, they are well tolerated; the most frequent adverse effects are headache (10%–20% of patients) and constipation (5%–10%). Therefore, to identify the optimal antiemetic prophylaxis, a combination of a 5-HT3 receptor antagonist plus dexamethasone had to be compared with a combination of high-dose metoclopramide.

At present, two large, double-blind studies have shown that ondansetron plus dexamethasone are more efficacious and tolerable than high-dose metoclopramide plus dexamethasone and diphenhydramine or lorazepam (Table 1) (4,5). Furthermore, the efficacy of this combination persists, at least for vomiting, over the first three cycles of chemotherapy (4–6). Therefore, a combination of a 5-HT3 antagonist plus dexamethasone should be considered the antiemetic of choice for the prevention of cisplatin-induced acute emesis.

B. Delayed Emesis

The antiemetic treatment of choice for the prevention of cisplatin-induced delayed emesis has so far been considered a combination of orally administered

Table 1 5-HT3 Receptor Antagonists plus Dexamethasone Versus Metoclopramide Combinations in Cisplatin-Treated Patients

Study	No. patients	Antiemetics	CP (%)	Results	Ref.
DB	289	OND 0.15 mg/kg IV × 3 + DEX 20 mg IV	78.7	OND + DEX → MTC + DEX + DIP	4
		MTC 3 mg/kg IV × 2 + DEX 20 mg IV + DIP 50 mg IV	59.5		
DB	237	OND 8 mg IV + DEX 20 mg IV	73.0	OND + DEX → MTC + DEX + LOR	5
		MTC 3 mg/kg IV × 2 + DEX 20 mg IV + LOR 1.5 mg/m^2 IV	56.0		

Abbreviations: DB, double-blind; OND, ondansetron; DEX, dexamethasone; MTC, metoclopramide; DIP, diphenhydramine; LOR, lorazepam; CP, complete protection from acute emesis.

metoclopramide (0.5 mg/kg four times daily) plus dexamethasone (8 mg twice on days 2 and 3, and 4 mg twice on days 4 and 5). This combination has been shown to be superior with respect to dexamethasone alone and to placebo (7,8). However, despite this combination, about 50% of patients still suffer from delayed nausea and vomiting, suggesting the need for greater benefit (9).

The 5-HT3 receptor antagonists used alone showed, at best, only moderate activity against delayed emesis (10). Their combination with dexamethasone, however, seems to increase antiemetic efficacy with respect to the 5-HT3 receptor antagonist alone (11). Therefore, to identify the optimal antiemetic prophylaxis, a double-blind trial was carried out in 322 patients, comparing on days 2 through 4 after cisplatin chemotherapy oral ondansetron (8 mg twice) with oral metoclopramide (20 mg every 6 h), both associated with intramuscular dexamethasone (8 mg twice on days 2 and 3, and 4 mg twice on day 4) (12).

Patients received the same intravenous prophylaxis for acute emesis: ondansetron 8 mg and dexamethasone 20 mg. Complete protection from delayed vomiting and nausea was not significantly different and was achieved by 62% and 43.7%, respectively, of patients given ondansetron and by 60% and 53.7%, respectively, of those receiving metoclopramide. The multifactorial analysis showed that patients who vomited in the first 24 hours achieved the lowest complete protection from delayed emesis. In these patients, ondansetron offered better complete protection from delayed vomiting than metoclopramide (28.6% versus 8.8%). Both treatments were well tolerated. Therefore, because of its lower cost, the combination of metoclopramide plus dexamethasone remains the treatment of choice for the prevention of cisplatin-induced delayed emesis. The combination of ondansetron plus dexamethasone is a valid alternative regimen that should be preferred in patients who do not tolerate metoclopramide and in those who suffer from acute vomiting.

III. PREVENTION OF EMESIS INDUCED BY MODERATELY EMETOGENIC CHEMOTHERAPY

A. Acute Emesis

Intravenous cyclophosphamide, doxorubicin, epirubicin, and carboplatin used alone or in combination are considered moderately emetogenic chemotherapeutic drugs. High and repeated doses of dexamethasone (8 mg IV before chemotherapy plus 4 mg orally starting contemporarily and repeated every 6 hours four times) or methylprednisolone (40–125 mg IV or intramuscularly [IM] for three times starting 30 minutes before chemotherapy and every 6 hours) induce about 60% to 80% complete protection from acute vomiting (3). Contrasting results have been achieved in studies that have compared the efficacy of repeated doses of corticosteroids and metoclopramide. In some studies, corticosteroids have been shown to be superior or equivalent to repeated low doses of metoclopramide and they were always found to be better tolerated (3).

The various 5-HT3 receptor antagonists have been studied in comparative trials with a variety of antiemetic drugs. When used alone, they have been shown to have superior antiemetic activity with respect to metoclopramide (13–19), alizapride (20,21), or phenothiazines (22–24) (sometimes combined with a single high dose of dexamethasone before chemotherapy). The percentage of complete protection from vomiting varied among studies from 50% to 70%. When compared with high and repeated doses of dexamethasone, the 5-HT3 receptor antagonists showed, in two studies, similar efficacy in the control of acute vomiting and nausea (Table 2) (25,26). Furthermore, one of these studies demonstrated that the combination of granisetron plus dexamethasone was significantly superior with respect to dexamethasone alone and granisetron alone (complete protection from acute vomiting in 93%, 71%, and 72%, respectively) (26). Therefore, there is clear evidence that, when used at appropriate dose and schedule, corticosteroids are at least as efficacious as the 5-HT3 receptor antagonists, but the most effective therapy is a combination of the two classes of drugs. In conclusion, even in the prevention of acute emesis induced by moderately emetogenic chemotherapy, a combination of a 5-HT3 receptor antagonist plus dexamethasone is the most efficacious antiemetic treatment.

Table 2 5-HT3 Receptor Antagonists Versus Dexamethasone in Patients Receiving Moderately Emetogenic Chemotherapy

Study	No. patients	Chemotherapy	Antiemetics	CP (%)	Results	Ref.
DB OX	112	CTX ± DOX ± VP16	OND 4 mg IV + 4 mg-orally every 6 hours	73	OND = DEX	25
			DEX 8 mg IV + 4 mg orally every 6 hours	66		
DB	428	CBDCA or CTX or DOX or EPI	GRAN 3 mg IV	72	GRAN + DEX → GRAN = DEX	26
			DEX 8 mg IV + 4 mg orally every 6 h	71		
			GRAN + DEX as above	93	GRAN = DEX	

Abbreviations: CP, Complete protection from acute vomiting; DB, double-blind; XO, crossover; OND, ondansetron; GRAN, granisetron; DEX, dexamethasone; CTX, cyclophosphamide; DOX, doxorubicin; CBDCA, carboplatin; EPI, epirubicin.

B. Delayed Emesis

Evidence for the efficacy of any antiemetic therapy in the prevention of delayed emesis induced by moderately emetogenic chemotherapy is sparse. Often it has been inferred by studies that are difficult to interpret because the patient groups did not receive the same antiemetic in the first 24 hours and this could have influenced the extent of nausea and vomiting beyond 24 hours.

Recently, two well-conducted studies have been published. In the first, 302 patients given IV single-dose dexamethasone plus ondansetron in the first 24 hours were randomized to receive oral ondansetron 8 mg b.i.d. or placebo on days 2 to 5. Complete protection from delayed emesis was significantly superior with ondansetron (60%) with respect to placebo (42%) (27). In the second study, 92 patients were submitted to IV granisetron plus single-dose dexamethasone in the first 24 hours. They were randomized to receive oral dexamethasone (4 mg b.i.d.) or placebo on days 2 to 5. Complete protection from vomiting was significantly superior with dexamethasone (56%) with respect to placebo (33%) (28).

The latter study was not blind and, in both studies, patients did not receive the optimal antiemetic prevention of acute emesis (dexamethasone was administered as a single intravenous dose before chemotherapy). This treatment would have determined a greater percentage of complete protection from acute emesis that would have significantly reduced the incidence of delayed emesis. In fact, a recent study carried out in patients monitored for three consecutive cycles of chemotherapy without receiving any antiemetic prophylaxis for delayed emesis showed that the incidence of delayed vomiting or moderate to severe nausea was low in patients who did not have acute vomiting or acute moderate-severe nausea; instead, it is substantial in patients who did (29).

Therefore, patients having no acute vomiting or no acute moderate to severe nausea may not need any antiemetic prophylaxis for delayed vomiting or nausea, whereas patients with a history of acute vomiting or moderate-severe acute nausea should always undergo treatment for delayed emesis. In this case, dexamethasone or ondansetron can be used. Well-conducted, double-blind, comparative trials are necessary to identify the best prophylaxis of delayed emesis induced by moderately emetogenic chemotherapy.

IV. PREVENTION OF ACUTE EMESIS INDUCED BY LOW AND REPEATED DOSES (20–40 mg/m^2/d for 3–5 d) OF CISPLATIN

The emetogenic potential of cisplatin is dose related and, therefore, low and repeated doses may require different antiemetic treatment. Six comparative studies have evaluated the antiemetic efficacy of the 5-HT3 receptor antagonists in this group of patients. In a double-blind study, ondansetron was shown to be superior to high-dose intravenous metoclopramide and was also less toxic (30).

In two studies, one open and the other single-blind, granisetron showed an antiemetic efficacy similar to high-dose intravenous metoclopramide or alizapride combined with dexamethasone (31,32).

Finally, in three studies, the combination of ondansetron plus dexamethasone (and chlorpromazine in one study) was shown to be superior to ondansetron alone (33) and to the combination of alizapride (34) or high-dose metoclopramide (35) with dexamethasone. Therefore, there is adequate evidence that a combination of a 5-HT3 receptor antagonist with dexamethasone is clearly more efficacious and better tolerated than regimens containing metoclopramide or alizapride, and more efficacious with respect to the 5-HT3 receptor antagonist used alone.

V. PREVENTION OF ACUTE EMESIS INDUCED BY ORAL CMF

Oral cyclophosphamide, methotrexate, and fluorouracil (CMF) is a widely used chemotherapy treatment, mainly in breast cancer patients. However, the control of nausea and vomiting induced by 14-day oral cyclophosphamide at doses of 100 mg/m^2/d, as used in the standard CMF regimen, has been evaluated only recently.

Oral ondansetron in a randomized, double-blind, placebo-controlled trial in 82 patients, at a dosage of 8 mg three times daily for 14 days, gave significantly greater complete protection from vomiting (60%) compared with placebo (35%) (36). However, in a double-blind, randomized study in 165 patients in which ondansetron (8 mg three times daily orally for 7 d) was compared to dexamethasone (10-mg single dose intravenously on day 1) plus metoclopramide (10 mg three times daily orally for 7 d), there was no statistically significant difference in efficacy between the two regimens, except for significantly less nausea during the first 24 hours after chemotherapy in patients receiving the metoclopramide combination regimen (37).

Therefore, a combination of dexamethasone plus metoclopramide should be considered the treatment of choice. A 5-HT3 receptor antagonist is a valid alternative regimen in patients who do not tolerate the combination, but it is much more expensive.

VI. WHAT IS THE OPTIMAL DOSE, ROUTE, AND SCHEDULE OF THE 5-HT3 RECEPTOR ANTAGONISTS?

The IV route is the most frequently used modality of administration of the 5-HT3 antagonists for the prevention of cisplatin-induced acute emesis, even if preliminary data suggest that the oral route may be equivalent to intravenous administration (38–40). Furthermore, a single intravenous dose before cisplatin is sufficient for all 5-HT3 antagonists.

Instead, the optimal IV doses have been evaluated in several trials, but contrasting data have resulted. This is the reason for the different single doses approved in various countries; that is, 8 mg of ondansetron and 3 mg granisetron in Europe and 32 mg and 1 mg, respectively, in the United States.

For ondansetron, despite a study (41) that reported that a 32-mg dose was superior to an 8-mg one, other double-blind dose-finding studies and comparative trials versus granisetron demonstrated that an 8-mg single intravenous dose achieved results similar to a 32-mg one (42–44).

For granisetron, a dose of 10 μg/kg (1 mg) seems to be optimal, considering that dose levels of 2 or 5 μg/kg achieved inferior results and that the slightly higher complete protection from vomiting obtained with 40 μg/kg is clinically insignificant (45–48).

For tropisetron, dose-finding studies and a comparative trial with ondansetron suggest that a single intravenous dose of 5 mg is as effective as a 10-, 20-, and 40-mg dose (49,50).

For dolasetron, two large double-blind studies showed that a 1.8-mg/kg single dose is similar to a 2.4-mg/kg dose (51,52) and can be considered the dose of choice. Several studies comparing efficacy and tolerability of the intravenously administered 5-HT3 receptor antagonists in the prevention of acute emesis have been published. No significant differences were shown and, therefore, the choice among them should be based only on the acquisition cost of the optimal doses that varies among countries and even among institutions within a country (53).

Both intravenous and oral administration of 5-HT3 antagonists have been used for the prevention of acute emesis induced by moderately emetogenic chemotherapy. A total oral daily dose of 12 to 16 mg of ondansetron seems to be optimal. This can be administered as a single dose before chemotherapy (54) or divided into two (55,56) or three (57,58) daily doses.

For granisetron, a total daily dose of 2 mg as a single oral administration before chemotherapy or as 1 mg twice daily is the most appropriate (59,60). No double-blind dose ranging studies of oral tropisetron have yet been published and, therefore, no recommendations can be made.

Finally, the optimal single oral dose of dolasetron has not been clearly identified. The three double-blind studies carried out in patients submitted to moderately emetogenic chemotherapy showed contrasting results (61–63). A single oral dose of 100 to 200 mg can be recommended.

No dose-finding studies of the 5-HT3 antagonists on the prevention of delayed emesis induced by cisplatin and moderately emetogenic chemotherapy have been published, and neither have dose-finding studies on the prevention of low and repeated doses of cisplatin.

VII. RESCUE ANTIEMETIC TREATMENT

Antiemetic failure is the presence of any vomiting and/or moderate-severe nausea (mild nausea, by definition, does not interfere with normal daily life) after chemotherapy administration.

Two different problems should be considered:

1. What is the rescue treatment for patients with emesis despite an optimal antiemetic prophylaxis both for acute and delayed emesis?
2. What is the best antiemetic prophylaxis in subsequent cycles of chemotherapy in patients failing with a standard regimen at previous cycle?

In the first case, an efficacious rescue medication should reduce the persistence of vomiting/moderate-severe nausea with respect to placebo. In such studies, some methodological problems should be solved. How long should the antiemetic response be evaluated after rescue medication? When, after rescue, should the response be evaluated? (Is another emetic episode immediately after rescue administration a failure or is it not?) Only a properly designed trial can permit definitive conclusions on the efficacy of the various treatments used in clinical practice (e.g., another dose of a 5-HT3 receptor antagonist, a different 5-HT3 receptor antagonist, high-dose metoclopramide combinations).

However, no similar studies have been published, probably also because, if one uses a different definition of failure (i.e., more than two emetic episodes), the number of patients to follow up to have a sufficient number of eligible patients for the study is high (in the order of thousands).

In the second case, few trials have investigated patients with refractory emesis defined as emesis in the previous cycle of chemotherapy, but without emesis before the subsequent cycle of chemotherapy (no anticipatory emesis). In two randomized trials, metopimazine improved the efficacy of ondansetron (64) and of ondansetron plus methylprednisolone (65) in patients with refractory emesis, but more data are needed before firm conclusions can be drawn.

VIII. CONCLUSION

Important progress has been made in the control of chemotherapy-induced emesis. At present, 80% and 90% of patients submitted to cisplatin and moderately emetogenic chemotherapy, respectively, have obtained complete protection from acute emesis with a combination of a 5-HT3 receptor antagonist plus dexamethasone. This combination is the antiemetic of choice also for the prevention of emesis induced by low and repeated doses of cisplatin. Complete protection from vomiting during the 4 to 5 days of cisplatin chemotherapy is achieved in about 55% to 60% of patients. Instead, in the prevention of emesis induced by oral CMF, a combination of intravenous dexamethasone on day 1 and day 8 plus 14-day oral metoclopramide is the regimen of choice.

A combination of oral dexamethasone plus metoclopramide/dexamethasone alone is the best choice for the prevention of delayed emesis induced by cisplatin/moderately emetogenic chemotherapy. Complete protection from vomiting on days 2 to 5 has been achieved in about 60%/60% of patients in both therapies.

In the prevention of delayed emesis, the 5-HT3 antagonists should be used only in patients failing to respond or who do not tolerate the antiemetic of choice.

The aforementioned are the results obtained in randomized clinical trials in the past 15 years. Therefore, it was important to verify if the achieved progress modified patient's perceptions of chemotherapy-induced nausea and vomiting.

In two recently published studies, carried out in 155 and 197 patients, respectively, the patients scored vomiting as the third and the fifth most distressing side effect of chemotherapy (66,67). Nausea again scored the first place in both studies.

This demonstrates that, albeit a reduction in incidence and intensity of nausea and vomiting has been achieved, especially in the first 24 hours after chemotherapy, from the patient's point of view, this does not translate into a better tolerance of chemotherapy for the following reasons:

1. There may be a lack of correlation between the frequency and/or severity of symptoms and the level of distress expressed by patients (i.e., for a patient, 10 days of minor nausea may be more distressing than 1 day of severe vomiting).
2. The 5-HT3 receptor antagonists have improved the prevention of acute nausea and vomiting rather than the prevention of delayed nausea and vomiting (in one of the two studies, 57% of patients suffered from delayed nausea).
3. Several antiemetic trials evaluated the efficacy during the first cycle only. It is known, however, that in the subsequent cycles, there is, at least for nausea, a decrease in complete protection. This may influence the patient's perception of the whole treatment period.
4. In clinical practice, as has been demonstrated recently by a study of the Italian Group for Antiemetic Research (68), the use of antiemetic drugs is far from being optimal. In fact, about 25% of patients submitted to cisplatin and 58% of those receiving moderately emetogenic chemotherapy did not receive the standard 5-HT3 receptor antagonists plus dexamethasone combination. Furthermore, this study showed that 50% of patients given cisplatin did not receive any antiemetic prophylaxis for delayed emesis.

In conclusion, despite the progress obtained, the optimal control of chemotherapy-induced nausea and vomiting requires more studies.

REFERENCES

1. Coates A, Abraham S, Kaye SB, Sowerbutts T, Frewin C, Fox RM, Tattersall MHN. On the receiving end: patients' perception of the side effects of cancer chemotherapy. Eur J Cancer Clin Oncol 1983; 19:203–208.
2. Gralla RJ, Itri LM, Pisko SE. Antiemetic efficacy of high-dose metoclopramide: randomized trials with placebo and prochlorperazine in patients with chemotherapy-induced nausea and vomiting. N Engl J Med 1981; 305:905–909.
3. Roila F, Tonato M, Ballatori E, Del Favero A. Comparative studies of various antiemetic regimens. Support Care Cancer 1996; 4:270–280.
4. Italian Group for Antiemetic Research. Ondansetron + dexamethasone versus metoclopramide + dexamethasone + diphenhydramine in prevention of cisplatin-induced emesis. Lancet 1992; 340:96–99.
5. Cunningham D, Dicato M, Verweij J, Crombez R, de Mulder P, du Bois A, Stewart A, Smyth J, Selby P, van Straelen D, Parideans R, McQuade B, McRae J. Optimum antiemetic therapy for cisplatin induced emesis over repeat courses: ondansetron plus dexamethasone compared with metoclopramide, dexamethasone plus lorazepam. Ann Oncol 1996; 7:277–282.
6. Italian Group for Antiemetic Research. Difference in persistence of efficacy of two

antiemetic regimens on acute emesis during cisplatin chemotherapy. J Clin Oncol 1993; 11:2396–2404.
7. Kris MG, Gralla RJ, Tyson LB, Clark RA, Cirrincione C, Groshen S. Controlling delayed vomiting: double-blind, randomized trial comparing placebo, dexamethasone alone, and metoclopramide plus dexamethasone in patients receiving cisplatin. J Clin Oncol 1989; 7:108–114.
8. Moreno I, Rosell R, Abad A, Barnadas A, Carles J, Ribelles N, Solano V, Font A. Comparison of three protracted antiemetic regimens for the control of delayed emesis in cisplatin-treated patients. Eur J Cancer 1992; 28A:1344–1347.
9. The Italian Group for Antiemetic Research. Cisplatin-induced delayed emesis: pattern and prognostic factors during three subsequent cycles. Ann Oncol 1994; 5:585–589.
10. Navari RM, Madajewicz S, Anderson N, Tchekmedyian NS, Whaley W, Garewal H, Beck TM, Chang AY, Greenberg B, Caldwell KC, Huffman DH, Gould JR, Carron G, Ossi M, Anderson EM. Oral ondansetron for the control of cisplatin-induced delayed emesis: a large, multicenter, double-blind, randomized comparative trial of ondansetron versus placebo. J Clin Oncol 1995; 13:2408–2416.
11. Gridelli C, Ianniello GP, Ambrosini G, Mustacchi G, Pedicini T, Farris A, Jacobelli S, Rossi G, Boni C, D'Aprile M, De Lena M, Di Carlo A, Bonsignori M, Silingardi V, Catalano G, Mosconi M, Olivieri A, Bianco AR. Ondansetron vs ondansetron plus dexamethasone in the prophylaxis of delayed emesis over three courses of cisplatin chemotherapy: results of a double-blind randomised study. Proc Am Soc Clin Oncol 1996; 15:545.
12. The Italian Group for Antiemetic Research. Ondansetron versus metoclopramide, both combined with dexamethasone, in the prevention of cisplatin-induced delayed emesis. J Clin Oncol 1997; 15:124–130.
13. Bonneterre J, Chevallier B, Metz R, Fargeot P, Pujade-Lauraine E, Spielmann M, Tubiana-Hulin M, Paes D, Bons J. A randomized double-blind comparison of ondansetron and metoclopramide in the prophylaxis of emesis induced by cyclophosphamide, fluorouracil and doxorubicin or epirubicin chemotherapy. J Clin Oncol 1990; 8:1063–1069.
14. Kaasa S, Kvaloy S, Dicato MA, Ries F, Huys JV, Royer E, Carruthers L, International Emesis Study Group. A comparison of ondansetron with metoclopramide in the prophylaxis of chemotherapy-induced nausea and vomiting: a randomized, double-blind study. Eur J Cancer 1990; 26:311–314.
15. Marschner NW, Adler M, Nagel GA, Christmann D, Fenzl E, Updhyaya B. Double-blind randomized trial of the antiemetic efficacy and safety of ondansetron and metoclopramide in advanced breast cancer patients treated with epirubicin and cyclophosphamide. Eur J Cancer 1991; 27:1137–1140.
16. Soukop M, McQuade B, Hunter E, Stewart A, Kerr D, Khanna S, Smith J, Coleman R, Cunningham D, Powles T, Davidson N, Hutcheon A, Green J, Slater A, Rustin G, Carney D. Ondansetron compared with metoclopramide in the control of emesis and quality of life during repeated chemotherapy for breast cancer. Oncology 1992; 49:295–304.
17. Anderson H, Thatcher N, Howell A, Logan K, Sage T, de Bruijn KM. Tropisetron compared with a metoclopramide-base regimen in the prevention of chemotherapy-induced nausea and vomiting. Eur J Cancer 1994; 30A:610–615.

18. Fauser A, Bleiberg H, Chevallier B, Favre R, Fabbro M, Claverie N, Hahne W. A double-blind randomized comparative trial of IV dolasetron vs IV metoclopramide in prevention of emesis in moderately emetogenic chemotherapy. Proc Am Soc Clin Oncol 1995; 14:530.
19. Campora E, Giudici S, Merlini L, Rubagotti A, Rosso R. Ondansetron and dexamethasone versus standard combination antiemetic therapy. Am J Clin Oncol (CCT) 1994; 17:522–526.
20. Clavel M, Bonneterre J, D'Allens H, French Ondansetron Study Group. Oral ondansetron in the prevention of chemotherapy-induced emesis in breast cancer patients. Eur J Cancer 1995; 31A:15–19.
21. De Nigris A, Paladini G, Giosa F, Sfeir C, Pagan MG, Maltoni C. Tropisetron (Navoban) compared with alizapride in the control of emesis induced by cyclophosphamide-containing regimens. Eur J Cancer 1994; 30A:1902–1903.
22. Palmer R, Moriconi W, Cohn J, Ryan T, Fitts D, Gruben D, Friedman C. A double-blind comparison of the efficacy and safety of oral granisetron with oral prochlorperazine in preventing nausea and emesis in patients receiving moderately emetogenic chemotherapy. Proc Am Soc Clin Oncol 1995; 14:528.
23. Marty M, on behalf of the Granisetron Study Group. A comparative study of the use of granisetron, a selective 5-HT3 antagonist, versus a standard antiemetic regimen of chlorpromazine plus dexamethasone in the treatment of cytostatic-induced emesis. Eur J Cancer 1990; 26(suppl 1):28–32.
24. Warr D, William A, Fine S, Wilson K, Davis A, Erlichman C, Rusthoven J, Lofters W, Osoba D, Laberge F, Latreille J, Pater J. Superiority of granisetron to dexamethasone plus prochlorperazine in the prevention of chemotherapy-induced emesis. J Natl Cancer Inst 1991; 83:1169–1173.
25. Jones AL, Hill AS, Soukop M, Hutcheon AW, Cassidy J, Kaye SB, Sikora K, Carney DN, Cunningham D. Comparison of dexamethasone and ondansetron in the prophylaxis of emesis induced by moderately emetogenic chemotherapy. Lancet 1991; 338: 483–487.
26. The Italian Group for Antiemetic Research. Dexamethasone, granisetron, or both for the prevention of nausea and vomiting during chemotherapy for cancer. N Engl J Med 1995; 332:1–5.
27. Kaizer L, Warr D, Hoskins P, Latreille J, Lofters W, Yau J, Palmer M, Zee B, Levy M, Pater J. Effect of schedule and maintenance on the antiemetic efficacy of ondansetron combined with dexamethasone in acute and delayed nausea and emesis in patients receiving moderately emetogenic chemotherapy: a phase III trial by the National Cancer Institute of Canada Clinical Trials Group. J Clin Oncol 1994; 12: 1050–1057.
28. Koo WH, Ang PT. Role of maintenance oral dexamethasone in prophylaxis of delayed emesis caused by moderately emetogenic chemotherapy. Ann Oncol 1996; 7:71–74.
29. The Italian Group for Antiemetic Research. Delayed emesis induced by moderately emetogenic chemotherapy: do we need to treat all patients? Ann Oncol 1997; 8: 561–567.
30. Sledge GW, Einhorn L, Nagy C, House K. Phase III double-blind comparison of intravenous ondansetron and metoclopramide as antiemetic therapy for patients receiving multiple-day cisplatin-based chemotherapy. Cancer 1992; 70:2524–2528.

31. Bremer K, on behalf of the Granisetron Study Group. A single-blind study of the efficacy and safety of intravenous granisetron compared with alizapride plus dexamethasone in the prophylaxis and control of emesis in patients receiving 5-day cytostatic therapy. Eur J Cancer 1992; 28A:1018–1022.
32. The Granisetron Study Group. The antiemetic efficacy and safety of granisetron compared with metoclopramide plus dexamethasone in patients receiving fractionated chemotherapy over 5 days. J Cancer Res Clin Oncol 1993; 119:555–559.
33. Fox SM, Einhorn LH, Cox E, Powell N, Abdy A. Ondansetron vs ondansetron, dexamethasone and chlorpromazine in the prevention of nausea and vomiting associated with multiple-day cisplatin chemotherapy. J Clin Oncol 1993; 11:2391–2395.
34. Nicolai N, Mangiarotti B, Salvioni R, Piva L, Faustini M, Pizzocaro G. Dexamethasone plus ondansetron versus dexamethasone plus alizapride in the prevention of emesis induced by cisplatin-containing chemotherapies for urological cancers. Eur Urol 1993; 23:450–456.
35. Rath U, Upadhyaya BK, Arechavala E, Böckmann H, Dearnaley D, Droz JP, Fossa SD, Henriksson R, Auliteky WE, Jones WG, Weissbach L, Paska W, Freeman A. Role of ondansetron plus dexamethasone in fractionated chemotherapy. Oncology 1993; 50:168–172.
36. Buser KS, Joss RA, Piquet D, Aapro MS, Cavalli F, Haeflinger JM, Jungi WF, Bauer J, Obrist R, Brunner KW, Weber T, Verity L, Butcher M. Oral ondansetron in the prophylaxis of nausea and vomiting induced by cyclophosphamide, methotrexate and 5-fluorouracil (CMF) in women with breast cancer. Results of a prospective, randomized double-blind, placebo-controlled study. Ann Oncol 1993; 4:475–479.
37. Levitt M, Warr D, Yelle L, Rayner HL, Lofters WS, Perrault DJ, Wilson KS, Latreille J, Potvin M, Warner E, Pritchard KI, Palmer M, Zee B, Pater JL. Ondansetron compared with dexamethasone and metoclopramide as antiemetics in the chemotherapy of breast cancer with cyclophosphamide, methotrexate and fluorouracil. N Engl J Med 1993; 328:1081–1084.
38. Gralla RJ, Popovic W, Strupp J, Culleton V, Preston A, Friedman C. Can an oral antiemetic regimen be as effective as intravenous treatment against cisplatin: results of a 1054-patient-randomized study of oral granisetron versus IV ondansetron. Proc Am Soc Clin Oncol 1997; 16:52a.
39. Krzakowski M, Graham E, Goedhals L, Pawlicki M, Yelle L, Joly F. Control of acute cisplatin-induced nausea and emesis using a once daily oral treatment regimen of ondansetron plus dexamethasone. Eur J Cancer 1997; 33:(suppl 8):19.
40. Kris MG, Pendergrass KB, Navari RM, Grote TH, Nelson AM, Thomas V, Ferguson BB, Allman DS, Pizzo BA, Baker TW, Fernando IJ, Chernoff SB. Prevention of acute emesis in cancer patients following high-dose cisplatin with the combination of oral dolasetron and dexamethasone. J Clin Oncol 1997; 15:2135–2138.
41. Beck TM, Hesketh PJ, Madajewicz S, Navari RM, Pendergrass K, Lester EP, Kish JA, Murphy WK, Hainsworth JD, Gandara DR, Bricker LJ, Keller AM, Mortimer J, Galvin DV, House KW, Bryson JC. Stratified, randomised, double-blind comparison of intravenous ondansetron administered as a multiple-dose regimen versus two single-dose regimens in the prevention of cisplatin-induced nausea and vomiting. J Clin Oncol 1992; 10:1969–1975.

42. Seynaeve C, Schuller J, Buser K, Porteder H, Van Belle S, Sevelda P, Christmann D, Schmidt M, Kitchener H, Paes D, De Mulder PHM, on behalf of the Ondansetron Study Group. Comparison of the antiemetic efficacy of different doses of ondansetron given as either a continuous infusion or a single intravenous dose, in acute cisplatin-induced emesis. A multicentre, double-blind, randomised, parallel group study. Br J Cancer 1992; 66:192–197.
43. Ruff P, Paska W, Goedhals L, Pouillart P, Rivière A, Vorobiof D, Bloch B, Jones A, Martin C, Brunet R, Butcher M, Forster J, McQuade B, on behalf of the Ondansetron and Granisetron Emesis Study Group. Ondansetron compared with granisetron in the prophylaxis of cisplatin-induced acute emesis: a multicentre double-blind, randomized, parallel group study. Oncology 1994; 51:113–118.
44. Italian Group for Antiemetic Research. Ondansetron versus granisetron, both combined with dexamethasone, in the prevention of cisplatin-induced emesis. Ann Oncol 1995; 6:805–810.
45. Navari RM, Kaplan HG, Gralla RJ, Grunberg SM, Palmer R, Fitts D. Efficacy and safety of granisetron, a selective 5-hydroxytryptamine-3 receptor antagonist, in the prevention of nausea and vomiting induced by high-dose cisplatin. J Clin Oncol 1994; 12:2204–2210.
46. Rivière A, on behalf of the Granisetron Study Group. Dose finding study of granisetron in patients receiving high-dose cisplatin chemotherapy. Br J Cancer 1994; 69: 967–971.
47. Soukop M, on behalf of the Granisetron Study Group. A dose-finding study of granisetron, a novel antiemetic, in patients receiving high-dose cisplatin. Support Care Cancer 1994; 2:177–183.
48. Navari R, Gandara D, Hesketh P, Hall S, Mailliard J, Ritter H, Friedman C, Fitts. D, on behalf of the Granisetron Study Group. Comparative clinical trial of granisetron and ondansetron in the prophylaxis of cisplatin-induced emesis. Clin Oncol 1995; 13:1242–1248.
49. Van Belle SJP, Stamatakis L, Bleiberg H, Cocquyt VFJ, Michel J, De Bruijn KM. Dose-finding study of tropisetron in cisplatin-induced nausea and vomiting. Ann Oncol 1994; 5:821–825.
50. Marty M, Kleisbauer J-P, Fournel P, Vergnenegre A, Carles P, Loria-Kanza Y, Simonetta C, De Bruijn KM, the French Navoban Study Group. Is Navoban (tropisetron) as effective as Zofran (ondansetron) in cisplatin-induced emesis? Anti-Cancer Drugs 1995; 6:15–21.
51. Hesketh P, Navari R, Grote T, Gralla R, Hainsworth J, Kris M, Anthony L, Khojasteh A, Tapazoglou E, Benedict C, Hahne W, for the Dolasetron Comparative Chemotherapy-induced Emesis Preventive Group. Double-blind, randomized comparison of the antiemetic efficacy of intravenous dolasetron mesylate and intravenous ondansetron in the prevention of acute cisplatin-induced emesis in patients with cancer. J Clin Oncol 1996; 14:2242–2249.
52. Thant M, Pendergrass K, Harman G, Modiano M, Martin L, Du Bois D, Cramer M, Hahne W. Double-blind, randomised study of the dose-response relationship across five single doses of IV dolasetron mesylate for the prevention of acute nausea and vomiting after cisplatin chemotherapy. Proc Am Soc Clin Oncol 1996; 15: 533.

53. Roila F, Ballatori E, Tonato M, Del Favero A. 5-HT3 receptor antagonists: differences and similarities. Eur J Cancer 1997; 33A:1364–1370.
54. Kaizer L, Warr D, Hoskins P, Latreille J, Lofters W, Yau J, Palmer M, Zee B, Levy M, Pater J. Effect of schedule and maintenance on the antiemetic efficacy of ondansetron combined with dexamethasone in acute and delayed nausea and emesis in patients receiving moderately emetogenic chemotherapy: a phase III trial by the National Cancer Institute of Canada Clinical Trials Group. J Clin Oncol 1994; 12: 1050–1057.
55. Beck TM, York M, Chang A, Navari R, Harvey WH, Meshad M, Griffin D, Wentz A, for the S3A-376 Study Group. Oral ondansetron 8 mg twice daily is as effective as 8 mg three times daily in the prevention of nausea and vomiting associated with moderately emetogenic cancer chemotherapy. Cancer Invest 1997; 15:297–303.
56. Dicato M. Oral treatment with ondansetron in an outpatient setting. Eur J Cancer 1991; 27(suppl 1):518–519.
57. Cubeddu LX, Pendergrass K, Ryan-T, York M, Burton G, Meshad M, Galvin D, Ciociola AA, Ondansetron Study Group. Efficacy of oral ondansetron, a selective antagonist of 5-HT3 receptors, in the treatment of nausa and vomiting associated with cyclophosphamide-based chemotherapies. Am J Clin Oncol (CCT) 1994; 17: 137–146.
58. Beck TM, Ciociola AA, Jones SE, Harvey WH, Tchekmedyian NS, Chang A, Galvin D, Hart E, Ondansetron Study Group. Efficacy of oral ondansetron in the prevention of emesis in outpatients receiving cyclophosphamide-based chemotherapy. Ann Intern Med 1993; 118:407–413.
59. Bleiberg HH, Spielmann M, Falkson G, Romain D. Antiemetic treatment with oral granisetron in patients receiving moderately emetogenic chemotherapy: a dose-ranging study. Clin Ther 1995; 17:38–51.
60. Ettinger DS, Eisenberg PD, Fitts D, Wilson-Lynch K, Yocom K. A double-blind comparison of the efficacy of two dose regimens of oral granisetron in preventing acute emesis in patients receiving moderately emetogenic chemotherapy. Cancer 1996; 78:144–151.
61. Rubenstein EB, Gralla RJ, Hainsworth JD, Hesketh PJ, Grote TH, Modiano MR, Khojasteh A, Kalman LA, Benedict CR, Hahne WF. Randomized, double-blind, dose-response trial across four oral doses of dolasetron for the prevention of acute emesis after moderately emetogenic chemotherapy. Cancer 1997; 79:1216–1224.
62. Fauser AA, Duclos B, Chemaissani A, Del Favero A, Cognetti F, Diaz Rubio E, Cortes Funes H, Conte PF, Dressler H. Therapeutic equivalence of single oral doses of dolasetron mesylate and multiple doses of ondansetron for the prevention of emesis after moderately emetogenic chemotherapy. Eur J Cancer 1996; 32A:1523–1529.
63. Grote TH, Pineda LF, Figlin RA, Pendergrass KB, Hesketh PJ, Karlan BY, Reeves JA, Porter LL, Benedict CR, Hahne W, on behalf of the Oral Dolasetron Dose Response Study Group. Oral dolasetron mesylate in patients receiving moderately emetogenic platinum-containing chemotherapy. Cancer J Sci Am 1997; 3:45–51.
64. Herrstedt J, Sigsgaard T, Boesgaard M, Jensen TP. Dombernowsky P. Ondansetron plus metopimazine compared with ondansetron alone in patients receiving moderately emetogenic chemotherapy. N Engl J Med 1993; 328:1076–1080.

65. Lebeau B, Depierre A, Giovannini M, Rivière A, Kaluzinski L, Votan B, Hèdouin M, d'Allens H, French Ondansetron Study Group. The efficacy of a combination of ondansetron, methylprednisolone and metopimazine in patients previously uncontrolled with a dual antiemetic treatment in cisplatin-based chemotherapy. Ann Oncol 1997; 8:887–892.
66. Griffin AM, Butow PN, Coates AS, Childs AM, Ellis PM, Dunn SM, Tattersall MHN. On the receiving end V: patient perceptions of the side effects of cancer chemotherapy in 1993. Ann Oncol 1996; 7:189–195.
67. de Boer-Dennert M, de Wit R, Schmitz PIM, Djontono J, Beurden V, Stoter G, Bverveij J. Patient perceptions of the side-effects of chemotherapy: the influence of 5-HT3 antagonists. Br J Cancer 1997; 76:1055–1061.
68. The Italian Group for Antiemetic Research. Transferability to clinical practice of the results of controlled clinical trials: The case of antiemetic prophylactic treatment for cancer chemotherapy-induced nausea and vomiting. Ann Oncol 1998; 9:759–765.

9

Oral Care for the Cancer Patient

C. Daniel Overholser
University of Maryland at Baltimore, Baltimore, Maryland

I. INTRODUCTION

The primary objective in the treatment of a patient with cancer is the eradication of the disease. Over the past 2 decades, tremendous strides have been made in the diagnosis and treatment of these patients. However, intensive radiation and/or chemotherapy protocols disrupt the integrity and function of the tissues of the oral cavity. Complications such as mucosal ulceration, xerostomia, bleeding, and infections can cause significant morbidity and may compromise the systemic treatment of the patient. With proper oral evaluation before systemic treatment, most of the complications can be minimized or prevented.

II. RADIATION THERAPY

When upper mantle radiation therapy is planned for the treatment of the patient with head and neck cancer, consideration must be given to the numerous complications of this form of cancer treatment. These include mucositis, xerostomia, infection, trismus, altered taste, radiation caries, and osteoradionecrosis. Most of these adverse sequelae can be prevented or at least diminished through a preoperative dental consultation (1). Dental evaluation should occur during the admission work-up of the patient to develop the best treatment plan for that patient. The amount and portals of radiation, the urgency of the radiation therapy, prognosis of therapy, and oral health of the patient must all be considered when deciding on the most appropriate dental treatment plan for the patient. The oral health status to be evaluated includes the severity of dental caries and periodontal disease, the estimated compliance of the patient in performing thorough oral hygiene procedures, and the need and extent of oral surgical procedures. Surgical procedures should be performed at least 2 weeks before the onset of radiation therapy. Prevention of osteoradionecrosis is of utmost importance. Secondarily, the reduction or elimination of other side effects such as mucositis, radiation caries, and trismus is attempted. The prevention protocol for the side effects of radiation therapy is summarized in Table 1.

A. Mucositis

Mucositis, inflammation of the mucous membranes, is a common reaction to radiation therapy. It is first seen 1 to 2 weeks after initiation of therapy and presents as an erythematous patch. The mucosal epithelium becomes thin as a result of the killing of the rapidly dividing basal layer mucosal cells. Between 1000 cGy and 3000 cGy areas begin to desquamate and eventually develop into frank ulcerations. These ulcerations are extremely painful, may become secondarily infected, and often force interruption of the radiation therapy.

Table 1 Prevention Protocol for Patients Receiving Radiation Therapy

Protocol	Timing
A. Prior to radiation therapy	3 weeks prior
1. Dental consultation Examination, radiographs, treatment plan	
2. Oral surgery	3 weeks prior
3. Dental care (custom mouth trays for fluoride delivery; restorative, endodontics oral hygiene instructions, periodontics, diet counseling)	Prior to radiation therapy
B. During radiation therapy	Weekly
1. Oral hygiene reinforcement	
2. Fluoride therapy (1% neutral fluoride)	Daily
3. Dietary management	Weekly
C. Postirradiation therapy	
1. Oral evaluation	Monthly
2. Fluoride therapy (0.4% stannous fluoride)	Daily for 6 mo

Normal oral mucosa acts as a barrier against chemicals that are ingested and more importantly against the ever present oral microorganisms. The disruption of the mucosal barrier thus leads to secondary infection, increased pain, delayed healing, and decreased nutritional intake.

Prevention of radiation mucositis is difficult. Occasionally, stents can be constructed to prevent the irradiation of uninvolved tissues. The use of multiple ports and fractionation of the therapy into smaller doses over a longer period of time often reduces the severity. Teeth with sharp edges, fractured restorations, and ill-fitting prosthesis can damage the soft tissues and lead to further interruption of mucosal barriers. Correction of these problems before radiation therapy can diminish these complications.

Treatment of mucositis is symptomatic (2). Topical application of anesthetics such as dyclonine hydrochloride, Viscous Xylocaine 2%, or benzocaine HCL help to reduce severity of the pain. A mouth rinse of Kaopectate and diphenhydramine often provides relief to many patients (3). Kamillosan Liquidem (Asta Pharma, AG, Frankfurt, Germany) has been reported to diminish the severity of mucositis (4). Kamillosan Liquidem is a solution prepared from the camomile plant and contains chamazulene, levomenol, polyins, and flavonids. The study was uncontrolled and the drug, therefore, needs further evaluation. Rinsing with water, ice chips, saline, and bicarbonate all have been used to somewhat alleviate discomfort. Kaopectate, sucralfate, and Orabase are agents that coat the ulcers and provide relief to some patients. Management of mucositis is summarized in Table 2. If the patient is unable to eat a normal diet, food can be processed through a blender, and diet supplements can be used. Occasionally, a nasogastric tube must be placed to assist in proper nutrition. The patient should attempt to

Table 2 Management of Oral Mucositis

Topical Anesthetics
Viscous Xylocaine 2%
Dyclonine
Diphenhydramine
Benzocaine
Rinses
Water, saline
Ice chips
Bicarbonate
Kamillosan Liquidem
Coating Agents
Kaopectate
Sucralfate
Orabase

perform normal oral hygiene procedures to help prevent secondary infection. A mixture of salt and baking soda can be used to gently cleanse the hard and soft tissues of the mouth if normal oral hygiene becomes too difficult. When secondary infections occur, culture and sensitivity tests should be performed to determine the appropriate antibiotic to be used. An effective agent to treat superficial candidal infections is nystatin pastilles, 200,000 U four times a day. The tablet is held in the mouth until it dissolves, which allows sufficient contact time for the drug to be effective. Clotrimazole is also effective in managing these infections. Other secondary infections can be managed with the indicated systemic antibiotic.

B. Salivary Changes

Radiation to the salivary glands produces atrophy of the acini, fibrosis, and ultimately a decrease in the production of saliva. This decreased secretion is first seen 1 to 2 weeks after the initiation of the radiotherapy. If all the major salivary glands are in the field, the decrease in saliva can be dramatic. Additionally, the saliva produced is increased in viscosity, which contributes to food retention and increased plaque formation. This increase in viscosity is likely due to the more deleterious effects of the radiation on the serous portion of the salivary glands. Because saliva is necessary for bolus formation and deglutition, these xerostomic patients have difficulty in managing a normal diet. Normal saliva also has bacteriostatic properties that are compromised in these patients, which may help to account for the increase in plaque formation and bacterial colonization. Unless aggressive measures are taken, rampant dental caries will result. Radiation-induced xerostomia is often irreversible, but partial return of salivary flow is seen, especially in younger patients (5).

Preventing salivary gland dysfunction is primarily dependent on shielding the major glands from the field of radiation. On occasion, shields can be constructed to assist in this. The use of pilocarpine during radiation therapy reduces the severity of the resulting dysfunction and is useful in the partial restoration of function of the glands in previously irradiated patients (6–8). Often the use of sugar-free chewing gum can act as a stimulant for salivary flow. Finally, a number of agents appear useful to ameliorate the symptoms. These include saliva substitutes (Moi-Stir 10, Mouthkote, Salivart Synthetic Saliva), proper hydration, and ice chips.

C. Radiation Caries

A rampant form of dental caries (dental decay) that sometimes follows radiation therapy is called *radiation caries*. It usually develops in the cervical region of the teeth adjacent to the gingiva. It often affects many teeth and proceeds to envelop the teeth quickly. Originally, it was thought to be a direct result of the radiation, but it is secondary to the damage done to the salivary glands. Radiation caries is initiated by dental plaque, but its rapid progress is due to changes in saliva. In addition to the diminution in the amount of saliva, both the salivary pH and buffering capacity are diminished, which decreases the anticaries activity of saliva. The oral flora also changes with xerostomia, which also may lead to the increase in caries activity.

Prevention of radiation caries can be accomplished by improved oral hygiene, chlorhexidine rinses, daily applications of topical fluorides, and frequent dental recall visits (9). Part of the pre-radiation evaluation is an estimate of the patient's desire and ability to comply with the need for improved oral hygiene. In those patients who are not expected to be compliant, the extraction of many or all the remaining teeth is recommended to avoid extracting them after radiation therapy, thus decreasing the risk for the development of osteoradionecrosis. In patients who retain their dentition, custom-made mouth trays should be constructed to be used by the patient in applying the topical fluoride. During radiation therapy, a 1% neutral sodium fluoride such as Thera-Flur-N can be used for 5 minutes each day, usually at bedtime. The patient should be advised not to eat or drink for 30 minutes after the application. When the patient's oral mucosa has returned to normal, the fluoride can be changed to an acidulated form such as Gel-Kam (0.4% stannous fluoride gel). This treatment should be continued indefinitely. Dental evaluations should occur weekly during therapy and at least every 3 months upon completion of therapy. These recalls not only help to detect disease earlier but also reinforce the importance of oral hygiene maintenance to the patient.

Treatment of radiation caries can be problematic. In the early stages, routine restorative therapy and increased use of topical fluorides can be effective. Later stages often result in irreversible pulpal pathology. Endodontic therapy is the treatment of choice because the extraction of such teeth should be avoided if possible to prevent osteoradionecrosis. When extractions must be performed, they must be done as atraumatically as possible.

D. Osteoradionecrosis

Osteoradionecrosis is the most severe complication of radiation therapy in the head and neck region. Radiation, trauma, and infection are the three major factors involved in this pathologic process (10). Bone that has received heavy doses of radiation becomes hypovascular, hypocellular, and hypoxic. This results in permanent cellular and vascular damage. Trauma-induced spontaneous tissue breakdown occurs, which leads to a nonhealing wound. Teeth, gingiva, and damaged mucosa all can act as portals of entry for infectious agents. The resultant radionecrosis will, if untreated, ultimately involve all dysplastic bone. The spread of this process is usually accompanied by intense pain, production of bony sequestra, purulence, and a marked fetor oris. In one series, 5% of the patients died of this complication with no evidence of their original neoplastic disease (11). The incidence of this lesion ranges from 4% to 35% and the risk increases with increasing doses of radiation. Use of megavoltage instead of orthovoltage therapy has also decreased the risk of radionecrosis. With the advances in radiotherapy and proper dental management, the incidence should be in the 5% to 10% range.

1. Preradiation

The prevention of osteoradionecrosis begins during the admission process by obtaining a dental consult. If the maxillary or mandibular arches will be exposed to significant amounts of radiation, consideration is given to several preventive measures. First, all compromised teeth should be extracted 21 days before radiation therapy begins to allow for maximal healing. Alveolectomies and primary closure should be used to increase healing and decrease sharp bony spicules that might later damage the overlying soft tissues. Second, treatment of remaining dentition should be accomplished to prevent the need for later extractions in areas to be irradiated. Third, the importance of preventive oral hygiene must be emphasized to the patient. Fourth, shielding of nontumor areas should be accomplished when possible. At one time, it was recommended that all teeth in the path of the radiation be extracted before radiation therapy. However, a number of factors are taken into consideration when planning whether to retain or remove such teeth. Severe periodontal disease, irreversible pulpal pathology, and high caries index are indications for the extraction of the involved teeth. Patients who are thought to be motivated to maintain a high level of oral hygiene postoperatively would need fewer extractions. Because osteoradionecrosis more often occurs in the mandible, extractions of mandibular teeth are more frequently required. When the irradiation of the major salivary glands cannot be avoided, indications for the removal of teeth increase. Decreased dosage of radiation and poor prognosis for tumor controls are factors that decrease the necessity for dental extractions.

After the dental extractions but before radiation therapy, it is most important that the remaining teeth and periodontium be brought to a maximal state of health. Routine dental care should be provided to prevent acute periodontal and pulpal exacerbation from occurring in the postradiation phase. Emphasis must be placed on the maintenance of a high level of oral hygiene as well as the use of daily applications of topical fluoride.

A number of prosthodontic stents can be constructed. Indications for stents include shielding structures from the radiation, fixing movable structures (e.g., tongue), or assisting in the positioning of external beam source. If possible, dental extractions should not be performed during radiation therapy. The trauma from the extraction and radiation is additive and produces the highest risk for the development of osteoradionecrosis (10). When radiation therapy has begun, it is recommended that palliative measures be used until the mucositis/dermatitis signs and symptoms have subsided.

2. Postirradiation

The prevention of osteoradionecrosis after radiation therapy is accomplished by decreasing trauma to the bone. Therefore, both mechanical trauma (surgery) and microbiological trauma (periodontal disease, pulpal pathology, and surgery) need to be minimized. Maintenance of the optimal level of oral health established in the preradiation phase is the most effective way of preventing the development of osteoradionecrosis. During and immediately following radiation therapy, the patient should be evaluated weekly by the dental team. This allows detection of developing pathology and emphasizes the importance of good oral hygiene. Afterward, the patient may be placed on a 2- to 3-month recall interval. Topical fluorides and a reemphasis of the importance of proper oral hygiene are used to reduce the incidence of periodontal disease and dental caries. Reducing the risk of caries also decreases the likelihood of subsequent pulpal pathology.

If the patient is edentulous, the prostheses must be evaluated routinely to ensure that they fit properly, thus decreasing the chance for soft tissue ulceration and secondary infectious involvement of underlying irradiated bone.

When possible, the use of endodontic therapy in teeth with irreversible pulpal pathology is preferred over dental extractions. When dental extractions or other surgery must be performed on the postradiation patient, the development of osteoradionecrosis is a distinct possibility. Hyberbaric oxygen treatment should be used both before and after surgical treatment. Hyperbaric oxygen is more effective than prophylactic antibiotics in preventing osteoradionecrosis (12).

3. Therapy

In the past, treatment of osteoradionecrosis has been conservative. Topical application of zinc peroxide, antibiotics, and gentle wound irrigation were used. Systemic antibiotic therapy was administered when gross infection is found. Currently, hyperbaric oxygen therapy has become a mainstay of treatment (13–15). Loose, necrotic bone spicules should be judiciously removed. Surgical interventions such as partial or complete mandibulectomy are indicated when conservative measures fail to control infections. It has been recommended by some clinicians that hyperbaric oxygen be combined with aggressive surgical techniques to reduce morbidity in severe cases of osteoradionecrosis (16).

E. Altered Nutrition

Several radiation-induced problems may compromise the nutritional status of these patients. If the muscles of mastication, especially the masseters, lie in the path of radiation, trismus may result. This form of trismus is thought to result from muscle fibrosis, producing a severely limited mandibular function. The diminished opening interferes with the patient's ability to masticate food and perform oral hygiene procedures. It is thought that trismus can be prevented by the use of a set of 20 maximal opening exercises three times daily during and following radiation therapy. These exercises are also used to treat postirradiation trismus, but appear to be less successful when begun after therapy.

Dysgeusia is another side effect of therapy that may affect the nutritional status of the patient. The severity of these abnormal taste sensations ranges from loss of taste to altered perception of distinct flavors. Most patients are affected to some degree, and although apparently not preventable, taste sensations are reported to gradually return to near normal levels in the post-therapy period. Dysgeusia appears to contribute to the decrease in appetite that many patients experience.

III. CHEMOTHERAPY

Chemotherapy for neoplasia frequently results in oral complications. These may develop in more than 30% of patients undergoing treatment for malignancies other than of the head and neck (17). Infections and mucositis are the most common serious complications seen in patients receiving chemotherapy. By using proper management, major hemorrhagic episodes are seldom encountered. Also occurring frequently are pain, altered nutrition, and xerostomia, which significantly affect the quality of life of the patient. With proper precautions, routine dental treatment including periodontal therapy and the extraction of teeth can be performed immediately preceding chemotherapy for leukemia with minimal risk for significant infectious or hemorrhagic complications. Neutropenic patients with neutrophil counts less than 2,000/mm^3 should receive prophylactic antibiotics before procedures that produce bacteremia. Likewise, patients with platelet counts less than 50,000/mm^3 should receive platelet transfusions before surgical procedures.

A major responsibility in oncology is the prevention and treatment of infectious complications. The prevention of these complications is summarized in Table 3. Infection is a leading cause of morbidity and mortality in patients with cancer. The patient's malignant disease or its treatment alter the host defenses and diminish the patient's ability to inhibit infectious agents. Two normally chronic oral infections, periodontal disease and pulpal pathosis, may become acute during periods of granulocytopenia, leading to systemic sequelae. Viral and fungal infections are often seen in these patients. Their clinical presentations may be somewhat similar and resemble mucositis. A high index of suspicion and

Table 3 Prevention Protocol for Patients Receiving Myelosuppressive Chemotherapy

Protocol	Timing
A. Prior to chemotherapy	3–7 d before chemotherapy
1. Dental consultation	
Examination, radiographs, treatment plan	
2. Oral surgery	3 d before chemotherapy Platelet transfusion if platelets <50,000/mm^3 Prophylactic antibiotics if neutrophils <2,000/mm^3
3. Dental care	Prior to chemotherapy
Oral hygiene instruction	Prior to myelosuppression
Periodontics	Prior to chemotherapy
Endodontics	Prior to myelosuppression
Restorative	
B. During myelosuppression	
1. Oral hygiene care	Twice weekly
2. Peridex if indicated	Daily
C. After chemotherapy	
1. Routine care may be provided	

proper culturing techniques are important in the diagnosis and management of these entities.

A. Mucositis/Ulceration

Mucositis is a frequent oral complication of cancer chemotherapy. The oral mucosa is susceptible to the toxic effects of these agents because of its high mitotic index. Certain chemotherapeutic agents, such as 5-fluorouracil, methotrexate, and doxorubicin, are more commonly associated with the development of oral mucositis. It is postulated that the basal cell activity of the mucosa is impaired, reducing the ability of the epithelium to regenerate. The mucosa is also probably less resistant to the trauma these tissues receive. The mucosal integrity is broken and then is secondarily infected by the normal oral flora. The resultant ulcerations can also act as a portal of entry for pathogenic organisms into the patient's bloodstream and may lead to systemic infections. Additionally, these oral ulcerations can lead to severe pain. This pain can lead to a decrease in nutritional intake and a reduction in chemotherapy dose, which could alter the patient's prognosis. These lesions appear as oral ulcerations approximately 7 to 10 days after the initiation of chemotherapy and may be limited in range or they may involve more than 50% of the mucosa of the oral cavity. The severity and extent of oral mucositis vary with the patient, the drugs used, and the severity of myelosuppression that is induced.

1. Prevention

It has been suggested that improved oral hygiene results in a decreased incidence of oral mucositis. However, conclusive evidence is not available. It seems reasonable that improved oral hygiene would at least result in the diminished severity of the secondary infections associated with these toxic reactions. As is discussed later, reactivation of herpes simplex often cannot be clinically distinguished from mucositis. Prophylactic acyclovir effectively prevents much of the incidence of this form of mucositis. A number of agents have been used to reduce the incidence, severity, duration of chemotherapy-induced mucositis. Benzydamine hydrochloride, beta-carotene, cryotherapy, oral sucralfate, and diphenhydramine syrup plus kaolin-pectin (3,4) have all shown some degree of efficacy in the management of mucositis. Table 2 lists many of the drugs used to diminish the effects of mucositis. None of these have effectively prevented mucositis or the acute infections arising from mucositis. Further study in this area is needed.

2. Management

Treatment of oral mucositis is mainly palliative, but steps should be taken to minimize secondary pathogenic infections. Culture and sensitivity data should be obtained to select the appropriate therapy for the bacterial, viral, or fungal organisms found. Whereas numerous bacterial pathogens may be found, the most common fungi isolated are *Candida* sp., *Mucormycosis*, and *Aspergillus*. Herpes simplex and cytomegalovirus are the most frequent viral pathogens found in the oral cavity. They should be included in the differential diagnosis of any ulcerative lesions of the oral cavity.

A number of palliative treatments for mucositis are available. When the involved area is limited, topical application of Orabase with Benzocaine (Hoyt Laboratories, Norwood, MA) may be applied as necessary. The Orabase is a solubilized adherent ointment base that confines the anesthetic to the appropriate area as well as lengthens the period of anesthesia. When the mucosal involvement is widespread, a variety of topical rinses may be used. Such agents include lidocaine liquid, kaolin-pectin mixed equally with diphenhydramine elixir, dyclonine hydrochloride, and Tessalon Perles (R.P. Scherer Laboratories, Detroit, MI), which provide varying degrees of symptomatic relief. All should be expectorated and not swallowed. If these are ineffective or cannot be tolerated by the patient, systemic analgesics may be necessary.

B. Infections

1. *Periodontal Disease*

It has been estimated that more than 80% of patients age 15 to 19 years old and more than 90% of patients older than age 35 years are affected by periodontal disease. This disease represents the most common reason for the extraction of teeth in patients 35 years old or older. The periodontium is composed of four structures that maintain the teeth in the mouth. These are the gingiva, cementum, periodontal ligament, and the alveolar bone. Periodontal disease includes gingivitis and periodontitis, and is most commonly caused by poor oral hygiene, which allows for the accumulation of dental plaque and calculus. The microorganisms of the dental plaque that colonize the surface of the tooth adjacent to the gingiva induce a gingival inflammatory response. These microorganisms, chiefly bacteria, metabolize local nutrients and produce toxins, which eventually lead to the ulceration of the epithelium of the gingival sulcus. This process creates a gingival pocket or deepened gingival sulcus. The pockets next to the teeth further deepen and additional accumulation of plaque is promoted. The patient's ability to perform proper oral hygiene (remove all dental plaque) is then impaired. The earliest clinical signs of gingivitis are inflammation and gingival bleeding resulting from minimal trauma. The gingival bleeding arises from the ulcerated sulcular epithelium. The pockets in gingivitis are generally less than 3 mm in depth when measured with a small calibrated probe.

Histologically, periodontitis begins with the loss of the connective tissue attachment that connects the gingiva to the crown of the tooth. The pocket epithelium is then able to migrate further along the root surface toward the apex of the tooth, creating a periodontal pocket. The inflammatory process then involves the underlying alveolar bone. This bone is resorbed in response to the inflammation, producing a net loss of bony support. Clinically, this is characterized by mobility of the involved teeth and, unless treated, ultimately causes the loss of these teeth. As the ulcerated epithelium lining the periodontal pockets can cover several square centimeters in advanced periodontal disease, it is easily understood why this can lead to infectious complications in myelosuppressed patients.

The dental staff using clinical and radiographical examinations can best determine the extent of periodontal disease present in a cancer patient. Pocket measurements in periodontitis can range from 4 to 10 or more millimeters. The deeper pockets are associated with more advanced disease. Many patients are unaware of the presence of the disease because it is usually asymptomatic. The incidence and severity of periodontal disease in cancer patients are comparable to those found in the general population. The ulcerative nature of the disease enables these tissues to act as a portal of entry for infectious agents into the systemic circulation. In one study, up to 28% of all microbiologically or clinically documented infections in acute nonlymphocytic leukemia patients undergoing remission induction chemotherapy were periodontal in origin (18). These exacerbations are characterized by localized tenderness in the gingival area and a temperature in excess of 38.3°C. These acute exacerbations of a normally chronic disease usually occurred during periods of profound granulocytopenia. Untreated periodontal disease, therefore, exposes a patient about to undergo myelosuppression to an increased risk for infectious complications.

Hospital-acquired organisms have been reported to cause 47% of all acute infections in myelosuppressed leukemia patients (19). In addition, it has been shown that the oral cavity acquires an enteric gram-negative flora in such patients. However, the surveillance cultures used to produce these data sample the flora of the gingiva and oral mucosa and not that of the ulcerated periodontal pocket. Because periodontal disease is an infectious process, the oncologist must be aware of potential shifts in the oral flora during hospitalization, producing systemic infectious episodes requiring longer hospitalization or increased use of antibiotic therapy. *Staphylococcus epidermidis, Staphylococcus aureus*, and *Pseudomonas aeruginosa* have been found in the subgingival flora and are associated with acute periodontal infections in these patients.

(a) Prevention

When it was learned that the oral cavity could be a significant source of infection in chemotherapy-induced myelosuppressed patients, several recommendations were considered. Some centers recommend that manipulation of the oral hard and soft tissues while patients are myelosuppressed be avoided. Included in this recommendation was the elimination of oral hygiene aids such as brushing and flossing. This topic has been debated because oral hygiene measures, as well as the simple mastication of food, have been shown to produce transient bacteremias in noncancer patients with periodontal disease. However, it has been shown that oral hygiene measures do not result in an increase in systemic complications including infections of the respiratory and upper alimentary tracts (20). Moreover, improved oral hygiene and other preventive measures have reduced the number of acute periodontal exacerbations that occur in acute nonlymphocytic leukemia patients who undergo remission induction chemotherapy.

To prevent many of the oral complications, the dental evaluation must occur early in the admission work-up for any patient anticipated to receive myelosuppressive chemotherapy. Initial periodontal therapy, and scaling and polishing the teeth, in combination with proper oral hygiene, effectively prevent most acute exacerbations of mild to moderate periodontal disease during periods of profound granulocytopenia. A major goal in periodontal therapy is to reduce pocket depths to the point that the patient can effectively perform oral hygiene measures on a daily basis. This objective is also sought for patients about to receive myelosuppressive chemotherapy to reduce plaque accumulation and prevent this chronic infectious disease from becoming an acute infectious episode.

In patients with more severe periodontal disease, it has not been established whether initial periodontal therapy is the most efficacious method of preventing acute periodontal infections during periods of myelosuppression. Therefore, the extraction of such teeth is an alternative method of preventing acute infectious episodes (21). If extractions are contemplated, several objective should be met (see Table 3). First, the surgery must be accomplished quickly to allow for approximately 10 to 14 days of healing before the onset of severe bone marrow suppression. Second, if the patient is already thrombocytopenic ($<50{,}000/mm^3$), platelet transfusion should be given in order to reach that level. Third, the surgeon should use alveolectomies to obtain primary closure with nonresorbable sutures. No packing materials should be placed in the extraction site to prevent secondary infection. Some patients, especially those with leukemia, may be admitted with bone marrow suppression and thus not be candidates for dental extractions. They should, therefore, be managed more conservatively.

Emphasis on good oral hygiene (brushing and flossing) technique must be continually reinforced to prevent the accumulation of dental plaque. Some patients are physically unable to accomplish this, and it may be necessary for the dental or nursing staff to provide this care for the patient. The only mouth rinse that has been shown to be effective as a chemical plaque-inhibiting agent in these patients is chlorhexidene (22). It can be most beneficial for patients who are unable to properly remove plaque by mechanical means and for reducing the overall oral microbial flora.

Powered water irrigation devices should not be used for these patients. In addition to producing bacteremias in patients with healthy periodontium, they have been shown to be ineffective in removing dental plaque. These devices do not seem indicated in patients receiving chemotherapy.

(b) Treatment

When periodontal exacerbations do occur, they should be treated conservatively. These usually occur during periods of profound granulocytopenia and therefore the involved teeth should not be extracted. Acute periodontal infections are normally associated with mild gingival bleeding and some pain. The pain further diminishes the patient's ability to maintain proper oral hygiene. The staff can assist in the improvement of plaque removal. If the patient is not already using chlorhexidene rinses, they should be instituted at this time. Topical anesthetics such as dyclonine hydrochloride or lidocaine can be used to decrease the pain and allow the patient or staff to perform the oral hygiene procedures. All local irritants should be removed by gentle debridement.

Warm saline rinses and 3% hydrogen peroxide can be used as adjuncts to the regular brushing and flossing. If gingival bleeding occurs, topical thrombin (1000–2000 U/mL) can be applied. Generally, no treatment is needed because the gingival bleeding is usually self-limiting. Appropriate systemic antibiotics should be administered for febrile patients.

2. *Pulp and Periapical*

Within the pulp chamber of each tooth is the dental pulp or dental nerve. It is connective tissue that has vascular, lymphatic, neural, and undifferentiated connective tissue cell components. Its chief function is to form dentin, which it does at varying rates throughout life. It responds to minor injuries such as early caries by mounting an inflammatory response and forming increased amounts of dentin as a protective measure. This often causes the tooth to be more sensitive to thermal stimuli. These teeth can be treated conservatively. If the injury, most commonly caries or physical trauma, is too great, the inflammatory response becomes irreversible. Irreversible pulpal pathosis, including pulpitis and necrosis, cannot be treated conservatively and the tooth must be extracted or treated endodontically. Even though these pulpal pathoses are invariably infectious in nature, they are not necessarily painful. The lack of discomfort in up to half of teeth with irreversible pulpal pathosis can mislead the clinician when the patient is facing significant myelosuppression. A thorough dental evaluation should identify most of these asymptomatic processes.

An established pulpal infection spreads toward the apex of the tooth. Ultimately, the periapical region of alveolar bone can become involved and form a cyst, granuloma, or abscess. An abscess is usually painful but the former two are often asymptomatic. These entities may lie dormant at the end of the tooth root for months or years before evolving further into an acute abscess or osteomyelitis. The reason that acute pathology develops in a previously quiescent lesion is not known. Changes in the microflora may produce many of these exacerbations. The diminished host resistance of the myelosuppressed patient could conceivably contribute to this development. Pulpal pathosis accounts for up to 5% to 10% of all oral complications of chemotherapy. Periapical infections in myelosuppressed patients are serious infections that are difficult to manage when the patient is granulocytopenic (23).

(a) Prevention

During the admission work-up, the dental consultant evaluates clinical and radiographical evidence of pulpal or periapical pathology. When reversible pulpal pathology is found, conservative dental restorative treatment is appropriate. If a deep caries is found in a tooth but has not yet produced signs of irreversible pulpal pathosis, the dentist can remove it and place a treatment restoration of zinc oxide and eugenol. These restorations stop the progress of the caries and have a palliative effect on the pulp. Any tooth that has turned dark, is crowned, has a history of acute trauma, has deep caries, or a deep restoration is a possible candidate for irreversible pulpal pathosis. If the evaluation indicates such pathology, endodontic therapy or extraction of the tooth is indicated before initiation of chemotherapy (Table 4). If the infection is confined to within the pulp chamber, a one-appointment endodontic procedure appears to adequately protect the patient during subsequent chemotherapy. However, if radiographical or clinical evidence of asymptomatic periapical pathology exists, endodontic therapy or extraction is recommended. If symptomatic periapical pathology is found, extraction of the tooth is recommended when possible.

(b) Management

Successful treatment of pulpal pathology found during or immediately after chemotherapy diminishes with increasing severity of the pulpal involvement (Table 5). Shallow caries and reversible pulpal pathology confined to the pulp chamber can usually be managed with conservative restorative treatment. Infection that has spread beyond the pulp into the surrounding alveolar bone presents a more difficult situation to manage. Routine endodontic therapy is less predictable for these infections when found in patients with normal host defenses. Leaving the tooth open for drainage exposes the patient to the risk of acquiring a nosocomial infection. Closing the tooth may lead to the formation of a sinus tract and again risk acquiring a hospital organism. Extraction of the tooth creates an even larger wound. Management with broad-spectrum antibiotics is successful until resistant organisms are encountered. Prevention of these adverse sequelae is therefore preferable to treatment during periods of myelosuppression.

3. Fungal

Fungal infections of the oral cavity are seldom primary events. They are seen in infants or are secondary to either a systemic disease or systemic antibiotic ther-

Table 4 Guidelines for Dental Extractions in Patients Scheduled to Receive Myelosuppressive Cancer Therapy

Ten days between extraction date and granulocyte count of <500 mm^2
Platelet transfusion if platelet count is $<40{,}000$ mm^3
Prophylactic antibiotics if granulocyte count is <2000 mm^3
Avoidance of intra-alveolar hemostasis packing agents
Primary wound closure with multiple interrupted black silk sutures

Source: Ref. 21.

Table 5 Guidelines for Management of Patients with Pulpal Pathology Receiving Chemotherapy

Diagnosis	Prechemotherapy management	Postchemotherapy management
Reversible pulpitis	Caries control	Caries control
Irreversible pulpitis	Endodontics or extraction	Endodontics or extraction
Necrotic pulp with asymptomatic periapical pathology	Endodontics or extraction	Antibiotics if symptomatic
Necrotic pulp with acute periapical pathology	Extraction (endodontics only if extraction is not possible)	Antibiotics

apy. It is not unusual for oral fungal infections to develop in the patient receiving chemotherapy. The most common fungal infection seen is produced by *C. albicans*, a normal inhabitant of the oral cavity (24). Infections caused by *Aspergillus*. sp. and *Torulopsis glabrata* have also been reported with some frequency in recent years. Oral candidiasis may present as erythematous (diffuse mucosal erythema), pseudomembranous (white, creamy thrush with underlying ulceration), hyperplastic (leukoplakia-like), or angular cheilitis. The erythematous and pseudomembranous types are usually accompanied by complaints of generalized oral pain. Smears or cultures can be used to confirm the diagnosis.

(a) Prevention

Because oncologists already limit the use of systemic antibiotics when possible, little can be done to prevent fungal infections secondary to antibiotic therapy. Although many clinicians believe that improved oral hygiene will lead to decreased fungal infections, no clinical trial has confirmed this hypothesis.

(b) Management

Superficial candidiasis can be treated with either topical nystatin or clotrimazole troches. Patients place them four times a day in the mouth and leave them until they completely dissolve. This increases the contact time necessary to control the organism. For deeper infections, ketoconazole or amphotericin B can be used systemically. *C. albicans* can also complicate angular cheilitis. This usually can be controlled with Mycolog (Squibb and Sons, Inc., Princeton, NJ) cream.

Fungal infections often occur in patients who wear removable dental prostheses. In addition to instituting a patient regimen, the prosthesis must also be treated because the plastic used can act as a reservoir to reinfect the treated mucosa.

Prostheses may be placed in a denture cup with 100 mL of nystatin suspension overnight for 6 to 8 hours per day. Fungal infections caused by organisms other than *Candida* should be treated by the appropriate antifungal agent.

4. Viral

Viral infections in myelosuppressed patients can cause significant pain, interfere with function and nutrition, and be fatal under certain circumstances. Reactivation of latent herpes simplex virus infection is the most frequent viral complication, but primary herpes, varicella zoster, and cytomegalovirus infections are also seen in these patients. Such reactivation appears more commonly during therapy that produces intense and prolonged myelosuppression.

The clinical appearance of both recurrent herpes labialis and recurrent intraoral herpes in these patients presents in a much more severe form than in noncancer patients and may be overlooked in the differential diagnosis. Intraoral herpes simplex virus infection may present as a very difficult diagnostic challenge. Both forms of recurrent herpes labialis and intraoral herpes may begin as small vesicles. These vesicles quickly rupture, leaving small shallow punctate ulcers. Usually these ulcers quickly coalesce to form larger ragged-shaped ulcerations that are quite painful. Apparently, both forms of the infection are often not seen clinically until the latter stages. The lesions are then easily confused with chemotherapy-induced mucositis. The atypical presentations may account for the few descriptions of these lesions in the literature.

(a) Prevention

Because almost all herpes infections in these patients are reactivation of the latent virus, identification of those patients at risk for reactivation during intensive myelosuppressive therapy is the best method of prevention. Identification of seropositive patients during the admission work-up enables the clinician to administer prophylactic acyclovir or have a high index of suspicion when unidentified mucocutaneous lesions occur. Early diagnosis of these lesions is important institute effective therapy with acyclovir (25).

(b) Treatment

Intravenous or oral acyclovir is effective in treating herpes simplex infections. Use of oral acyclovir in these patients is often limited because of the presence of nausea, vomiting, oral ulcerations, and other gastroenterologic problems. Acyclovir therapy improves the quality of life, helps maintain nutrition, and helps prevent secondary bacterial and fungal infections in the ulcerated lesions.

5. Removable Dental Prosthesis

Approximately 20% of the population wears some type of removable dental prostheses, which serve functional and aesthetic purposes. However, prosthetic devices can lead to complications during the treatment of patients receiving chemotherapy. Dentures that are worn constantly or fit improperly can produce mucosal ulcerations that readily become contaminated by the oral flora. The prostheses, their cleaners, and the containers in which they are soaked can be a source of reinfection for the patient, as well as cross-contamination among patients and staff. *C. albicans* is a common contaminate of dentures in the noncancer patient population. High concentrations of *P. aeruginosa, Klebsiella* sp., *Enterobacter* species, *Escherichia coli*, other gram-negative bacilla, *S. aureus*, and *T. glabrata* are frequently found on the denture and denture-soaking containers of cancer patients. The potential for infection from such organisms in the myelosuppressed patient is readily apparent.

(a) Prevention

To lessen the risk for oral infections during chemotherapy, patients with removable dental prosthetic devices should receive a dental evaluation preoperatively. These prostheses assist in mastication and therefore are important in the maintenance of proper nutrition. In addition, these devices often promote the patient's self-image and loss of the prostheses can cause significant embarrassment. Therefore, the decision to remove the prosthesis during chemotherapy should not be made lightly. If time permits, improperly fitting prostheses should be modified to fit. However, the patient should not be allowed to use them if proper adaptation to the tissues cannot be established. Patients allowed to retain their dentures should not wear them more than 12 hours per each 24-hour period. When the prostheses are removed from the mouth, they should be scrubbed clean with a denture brush, rinsed, and placed in an appropriate denture antiseptic solution. Denture soaking agents with antiseptic properties include Efferdent (Warner-Lambert Co., Morris Plains, NJ), Polident (Block Drug Co., Jersey City, NJ), and Kleenite (Vicks Toiletry Products, Wilton, CT). These solutions must be changed daily. This prevents gross contamination, which may then allow growth of the pathogens described previously. As mentioned, these containers and solutions represent not only a source of patient reinfection but also a mechanism of cross-contamination via hospital staff members (26).

It must be kept in mind that the tissues beneath these prostheses continue to slowly change. Upon completion of chemotherapy, the adaptation of the dentures to the tissues must be periodically reevaluated by the dental staff to prevent subsequent complications.

(b) Management

Appropriate antibiotic therapy should be instituted for infections arising from prosthetic contamination. It must be remembered that, in the management of fungal infections, especially *C. albicans*, treatment of the prosthesis itself with the appropriate antifungal agent is important to prevent reinfection from the prosthesis. Additionally, the denture hygiene protocol and compliance should be reviewed to determine whether the infection was due to ill-fitting prosthesis, poor hygiene, or cross-contamination.

C. Hemorrhage

Bleeding complications occur commonly in patients receiving chemotherapy for cancer and are usually due to the associated thrombocytopenia. Most bleeding problems encountered are not seriously debilitating. Surgery, such as dental extractions, poses the greatest risk for bleeding diathesis. With proper evaluation and treatment before chemotherapy, there should seldom be a need for surgical procedures. Petechial hemorrhages are often seen in the gingiva, buccal mucosa, tongue, floor of the mouth, and the hard and soft palate. Ecchymosis is more likely found in the tongue and floor of the mouth. Because gingival bleeding is one of the earliest clinical signs of gingivitis, this also commonly occurs in the thrombocytopenic patient. As in patients not receiving chemotherapy, gingivitis and gingival bleeding are a response to dental plaque. Effective oral hygiene usually prevents most such hemorrhages.

Physical trauma is a frequent cause of oral hemorrhagic events. Physical trauma includes improper oral hygiene technique (especially floss), mastication of soft tissues, and periodontal therapy. Traumatic episodes are often followed by local tissue necrosis. Such lesions often become secondarily infected.

1. Prevention

Dental evaluation of patients at admission should obviate the need for most surgical procedures during times of thrombocytopenia. The most common exception is the patient with granulocytopenia or thrombocytopenia at admission. Hematoma formation in the floor of the mouth may slowly enlarge but seldom causes respiratory embarrassment. Serious hemorrhage is likely if surgery is performed in the presence of disseminated intravascular coagulation.

2. Treatment

Minor oral bleeding, commonly gingival in origin, can usually be controlled by pressure. Application of topical thrombin (1000–2000 U/mL) can be helpful if pressure is unsuccessful. Gingival bleeding is usually associated with the inflammation produced by dental plaque, and therefore improvement in the oral hygiene should be a primary goal. When estimating the amount of blood lost, the clinician and patient must be cognizant of presence of saliva, which dilutes the blood. This dilution significantly increases the apparent amount of bleeding that is observed.

Major oral bleeding most likely occurs when surgery is performed when platelet counts are below 50,000/mm^3. Ideally, procedures such as the extraction of teeth and periodontal surgery should have been accomplished before chemotherapy or should be delayed until the patient's platelet counts begin to return to normal. However, if necessary, teeth can be removed when appropriate platelet transfusions are given. Infection rather than hemorrhage is usually the greatest risk with surgery in the myelosuppressed patient. Platelet transfusions and primary closure of the surgical site can control bleeding from such wounds. No packing materials such as oxidized cellulose or bone wax should be placed in the extraction site (21).

D. Xerostomia

Xerostomia occasionally is a complication of chemotherapy, which can interfere with nutrition, taste, and speech. Normal salivary output also provides some protection against shifts in the oropharyngeal microbial flora (27), which may help protect against mucosal infection. Although xerostomia resulting from chemotherapy cannot be prevented, it usually can be managed.

1. Treatment

The primary goals in the management of xerostomia are restoration of moisture and alleviation of pain. Often, frequent rinses with sterile ice water or saline provide sufficient relief to the patient. Some patients prefer saliva substitutes, which replace many of the missing constituents of normal saliva. Chewing sugarless gum can be helpful in patients without oral mucositis. The patient must be advised to be careful not to damage the mucosa.

E. Graft-Versus-Host Disease

Except for graft-versus-host disease (GVHD), most oral complications in bone marrow transplant patients are similar to those found in patients receiving radiation or myelosuppressive chemotherapy (28–30). Acute GVHD (day 0–100 after transplantation) and chronic GVHD (day 100–400 after transplantation) are significant complications of allogeneic bone marrow transplantation. They result when immunologically active T cells are transplanted into a recipient who is genetically different than the donor.

1. Acute Graft-Versus-Host Disease

In the oral cavity, it is difficult to distinguish the oral complications of GVHD from those toxic and infectious side effects of the chemoradiotherapy. The lesions typically seen in acute GVHD are ulcers that are usually painful. Biopsies that could differentiate GVHD from side effects of the conditioning regimen are usually contraindicated during this time period. Because viral and bacterial infections are often included in the differential diagnosis, appropriate culture and sensitivity tests should be performed. Prevention and treatment of oral GVHD is accomplished through the systemic management of GVHD. A number of drugs have been found to be useful in ameliorating the symptoms of the disease; they include steroids cyclosporine, and antithymocyte globulin. The response to these has been mixed.

2. *Chronic Graft-Versus-Host Disease*

A number of oral manifestations of chronic GVHD have been described. These include mucosal erythema and atrophy, lichenoid reactions, pain, and xerostomia. In some cases, the mucosal atrophy becomes frankly ulcerative and is often consistent with erosive lichen planus. As with acute GVHD, prevention and treatment are mainly accomplished through the systemic management of the disease. Topical steroids, appropriate antimicrobial agents, topical anesthetics, and systemic analgesics may be needed to treat the painful oral lesions. Management of the xerostomia is similar to that for the patient who has received radiation therapy and includes salivary stimulants, saliva substitutes, and fluoride treatments.

REFERENCES

1. Wright W. Pretreatment and oral care intervention for radiation patients. Natl Cancer Inst Monogr 1990; 9:57–59.
2. Miaskowski C. Oral complications of cancer therapies. Management of mucositis during therapy. Natl Cancer Inst Monogr 1990; 9:95–98.
3. Barker G, Loftus L, Cuddy P, Barker B. The effects of sucralfate suspension and diphenhydramine syrup plus kaolin-pectin on radiotherapy-induced mucositis. Oral Surg Oral Med Oral Pathol 1991; 71:288–293.
4. Carl W, Emrich L. Management of oral mucositis during local radiation and systemic chemotherapy: a study of 98 patients. J Prosthet Dent 1991; 66(3):361–369.
5. Liu R, Fleming T, Toth B. Salivary flow rates in patients with head and neck cancer 0.5 to 25 years after radiotherapy. Oral Surg Oral Med Oral Pathol 1990; 70:724–729.
6. Valdez I, Wolff A, Atkinson J, Macynski A, Fox P. Use of pilocarpine during head and neck radiation therapy to reduce xerostomia and salivary dysfunction. Cancer 1993; 71:1848–1851.
7. Johnson JT, Ferretti GA, Nethery WJ, Valdez IH, Fox PC, Ng D, Muscoplat CC, Gallagher SC. Oral pilocarpine for post-irradiation xerostomia in patients with head and neck cancer. N Engl J Med 1993; 329:390–395.
8. LeVeque PG, Montgomery M, Potter D, Zimmer MB, Rieke JW, Steiger BW, Gallager SC, Muscoplat CC. A multicenter, randomized, double-blind, placebo-

controlled, dose-titration study of oral pilocarpine for treatment of radiation-induced xerostomia in head and neck cancer patients. J Clin Oncol 1993; 11:1124–1131.
9. Epstein J, McBride B, Stevenson-Moore P, Merilees H, Spinelli J. The efficacy of chlorhexidine gel in reduction of *Streptococcus mutans* and *Lactobacillus* species in patients treated with radiation therapy. Oral Surg Oral Med Oral Pathol 1991; 71:172–178.
10. Marx R, RP J. Studies in the radiobiology of osteoradionecrosis and their clinical significance. Oral Surg Oral Med Oral Pathol 1987; 64(4):379–390.
11. Watson WL, Scarborough JE. Osteoradionecrosis in intraoral cancer. Am J Roentgenol Radium Therapy 1938; 40:524.
12. Marx R, Johnson R, Kline S. Prevention of osteoradionecrosis: a randomized prospective clinical trial of hyperbaric oxygen versus penicillin. J Am Dent Assoc 1985; 111:49–54.
13. Mainous E, Boyne P. Hyperbaric oxygen in total rehabilitation of patients with mandibular osteoradionecrosis. Int J Oral Surg 1974; 3(5):297–301.
14. Friedman R. Osteoradionecrosis: causes and prevention. Natl Cancer Inst Monogr 1990; 9:145–149.
15. Myers R, Marx R. Use of hyperbaric oxygen in postradiation head and neck surgery. Natl Cancer Inst Monogr 1990; 9:151.
16. Marx RE. Osteoradionecrosis: a new concept of its pathophysiology. J Oral Maxillofacial Surg 1983; 41:283–288.
17. Sonis ST, Sonis AL, Lieberman A. Oral complications in patients receiving treatment for malignancies other than of the head and neck. J Am Dent Assoc 1978; 97: 468–472.
18. Overholser CD, Peterson DE, Williams LT, Schimpff SC. Periodontal infection in patients with acute nonlymphocytic leukemia. Arch Intern Med 1982; 142:551–554.
19. Schimpff SC, Young VM, Greene WH, Vermeulen GD, Moody MR, Wiernik PH. Origin of infection in acute nonlymphocytic leukemia: significance of hospital acquisition of potential pathogens. Ann Intern Med 1972; 77:707–714.
20. Weikel DS, Peterson DE, Rubinstein LE, Samuels CM, Overholser CD. Incidence of fever following invasive oral interventions in the myelosuppressed cancer patient. Cancer Nurs 1989; 12:265–270.
21. Overholser CD, Bergman SA, Peterson DE. Dental extractions in acute and chronic myelogenous leukemia patients. Oral Surg 1982; 40:296–298.
22. Ferretti GA, Ash RC, Brown AT, Largent BM, Kaplan A, Lillich TT. Chlorexidine for prophylaxis against oral infections and associated complications in patients receiving bone marrow transplants. J Am Dent Assoc 1987; 114:461–467.
23. Peterson DE. Oral complications associated with hematologic neoplasms and their treatment. In: Peterson DE, Elias EG, Sonis ST, eds. Head and Neck Management of the Cancer Patient. Boston: Martinus Nihjoff 1986:351–361.
24. Dreizen S, Brown LR. Oral microbial changes and infections during cancer chemotherapy. In: Peterson DE, Sonis ST, eds. Oral Complications of Cancer Chemotherapy. The Hague: Martinus Nijhoff, 1983:41–77.
25. Bustamante CI, Wade JC. Herpes simplex virus infection in the immunocompromised cancer patient. 1991; 9(10):1903–1915.

26. DePaola LG, Minah GE. Isolation of pathogenic microorganisms from dentures and denture soaking containers of myelosuppressed cancer patients. J Prosthet Dent 1983; 49:20–24.
27. Laforce FM, Hopkins J, Trow R, Wang WL. Human oral defenses against gram-negative rods. Am Rev Respir Dis 1976; 114:929–935.
28. Schubert MM, Sullivan KM, Truelove EL. Head and neck complications of bone marrow transplantation. In: Peterson DE, Elias EG, Sonis St, eds. Head and Neck Management of the Cancer Patient. Boston: Martinus Nijhoff, 1986; 401–427.
29. Maxymiw WG, Wood RE. The role of dentistry in patients undergoing bone marrow transplantation. Br Dent J 1989; 167:229.
30. Brown AT, Shupe JA, Sims RE, Matheny JL, Lillich TT, Douglas JB, Henslee PJ, Raybould TP, Ferretti GA. In vitro effect of chlorhexidine and amikacin on oral gram-negative bacilli from bone marrow transplant recipients. Oral Surg Oral Med Oral Pathol 1990; 70:715–719.

10

Mucositis

James G. Gallagher
Penn State–Geisinger Health System, Danville, Pennsylvania

I. INTRODUCTION

Toxicity to gastrointestinal mucous membranes is a frequent side effect of treatment for malignancy. Probably no other side effects so interfere with quality of life than mucositis and diarrhea. Both cause pain and hemorrhage and interfere with adequate hydration and nutrition. In addition, interruption of alimentary tract membranes may allow local invasion by bacteria, fungi, or viruses, singly or in combination. Some of these localized ulcerations may lead to systemic infections (bacteremia and fungemia). All such mucous membrane injuries require time to heal, during which intense supportive care must be given, frequently in the hospital, and at great expense.

As newer chemotherapy and radiation therapy strategies are introduced, some of them result in unexpectedly severe mucositis or diarrhea. Each of these gastrointestinal toxicities can be fatal if not promptly recognized and treated. As long as aggressive treatment is done, mucositis and diarrhea will remain serious problems for oncologists. Recently, more attention has been paid to prevention and supportive care in this area. A number of international conferences on supportive care in cancer have been held in Europe and the United States. The practical applications of new knowledge in this area are presented in this volume and also in the new journal *Supportive Care in Cancer*.

II. DEFINITION AND MAGNITUDE OF THE PROBLEM

Inflammation of the oral mucous membranes is a common toxicity of chemotherapy or irradiation, with a wide spectrum of severity, from a few small patches of inflammation to widespread involvement causing severe pain and cessation of all oral intake. This process may extend down the esophagus, causing further dysphagia, odynophagia, and interrupted alimentation. Because this phenomenon is rarely seen outside cancer therapy or other acquired immunodeficiency states (e.g., acquired immunodeficiency syndrome and severe combined immunodeficiency), most general medicine and gastroenterology textbooks ignore mucositis. Because it is largely an iatrogenic phenomenon, stomatitis should be aggressively studied to minimize the suffering of those who must undergo systemic drug or oral irradiation treatment. Because mucous membranes are only one part of total oral care, dental prophylaxis (fluoride regimens for teeth before radiation therapy), endodontics, periodontics, and care of dental prostheses or intraoral or maxillofacial prostheses should also be considered at the outset of a treatment plan.

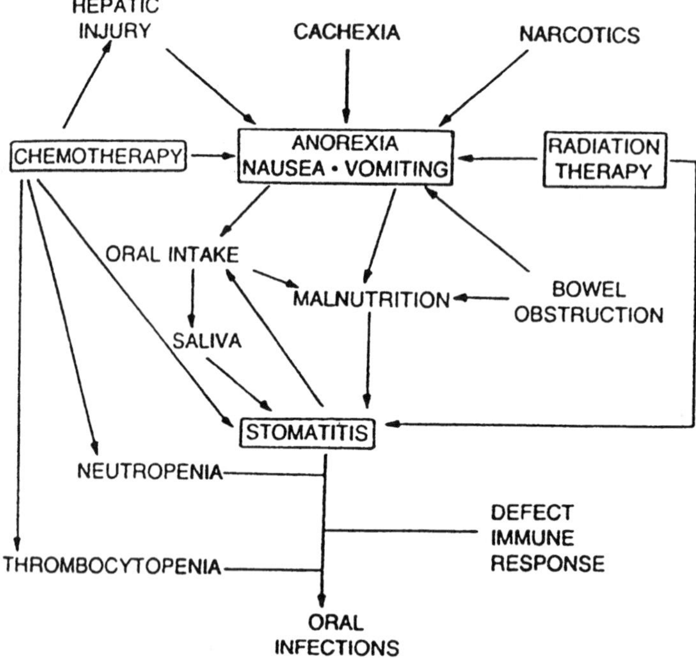

Figure 1 Interrelationships of common causal factors. (From Ref. 3a.)

These subjects are covered elsewhere (1–3). With increasing numbers of protocols delivering drugs on a ''dose intensity'' schedule, it should be expected that toxicity intensity will also result. Thus, the need for better supportive care to rescue surviving normal cells and ensure the survival of the individual should be apparent. Dose intensity makes sense only if it is both effective and results in less than fatal toxicity. Figure 1 shows the complex set of interactions that result in mucositis.

III. ETIOLOGY

Both irradiation and chemotherapy produce mucositis, and when both modalities and multiple agents are used to treat head and neck cancer, the toxicities are at least additive and result in a further cascade of morbidities: malnutrition, dehydration, bleeding, and infection. Many drugs have been observed to produce mucositis: 5-fluorouracil (5-FU), azathioprine, bleomycin, cyclophosphamide, dactinomycin, daunorubicin, doxorubicin, nitrogen mustard, melphalan, 6-mercaptopurine, methotrexate, mitomycin C, mitoxantrone (Novantrone), plicamycin (mithramycin), procarbazine, streptozotocin, 6-thioguanine, and vinblastine (Velban). Thus, about one-half of the most commonly used chemotherapy drugs have been reported to cause mucositis (4). Five drugs commonly cause severe mucositis: methotrexate, 5-FU, dactinomycin, doxorubicin, and daunorubicin. Combination chemotherapy with two or more of these drugs can be at least additive in toxicity to the mucous membranes. Other drugs that can occasionally produce clinically significant mucositis include nitrogen mustard, cyclophosphamide, ifosfamide, 6-thioguanine, idarubicin, mitoxantrone, vinblastine, bleomycin, mitomycin C, procarbazine, and malphalan. Methotrexate can be particularly toxic when given to those with pleural effusions or ascites. The drug enters the effusion and then slowly reenters the circulation, causing severe mucositis and bone marrow suppression. Radiation therapy to head and neck sites produces inflammation acutely and decreased salivary function on a subacute and chronic basis. Concomitant chemotherapy and irradiation can produce severe mucositis, and these treatments are often done sequentially to avoid the toxicity of simultaneous treatment. The most severe radiation mucositis occurs when 5-FU or methotrexate is given during a course of radiation to the head and neck region (5).

Besides direct toxicity to mucosal cells, immunosuppression and myelosuppression play a role in oral toxicity. Once the direct toxicity has occurred and is followed by immunosuppression or myelosuppression, infection is facilitated. This may be bacterial, fungal, or viral. In herpes simplex virus-seropositive bone marrow transplant (BMT) patients, the majority of cases reactivate within the first 5 weeks after transplant and manifest with severe, deep, painful ulcers. Herpes simplex virus (HSV) esophagitis occasionally follows the initial oral reactivation. None of these viral infections can be diagnosed on clinical grounds alone.

Candida albicans infection may present with any of several types of mucosal lesion: pseudomembranous candidiasis, chronic hyperplastic candidiasis, chronic erythematous candidiasis, and angular cheilitis (6).

Bacterial periodontal abscess, sialadenitis of major salivary glands, and gingivitis are seen and may be the portal of entry for bacteremia and sepsis (6). Empirical antibiotics are necessary while awaiting cultures and must include coverage for *Pseudomonas* species (6,7).

IV. PATHOPHYSIOLOGY

Cell death is the intended result of all cancer treatments. By whatever mechanism of injury to nucleic acid or protein synthesis, mitosis, or membrane integrity, it is hoped to kill more tumor than normal cells. This acknowledges the incidental killing of a fraction of normal cells, especially those with a rapid division rate and turnover time. Thus, mucosal and bone marrow cells sustain much of the incidental, unintended injury. This is particularly true when cell cycle–specific agents are used.

While sloughing of epithelial cells continues, replacement cells are slow to recover proliferative function. Histologically, dysplasia, hyperplasia, glandular degeneration, and collagen disruption are seen (8). Intact oral mucosa serves as a chemical and microbiological barrier by surface sloughing with regeneration time of 5 to 16 days, but this protective function is disrupted when turnover time is prolonged. Bacteria that adhere and are normally carried away by surface sloughing maintain their position on the mucosa long enough to proliferate and invade. Similarly, *C. albicans* may have more time to form germ tubes and penetrate mucosal epithelium, thus tipping the balance ordinarily present between mucosal clearance and pathogen (opportunist) virulence. Reduction in salivary gland and mucous gland function results in fewer humoral factors, such as antibody and antimicrobial proteins to degrade oral microorganisms.

Defenses against microorganisms are multifactorial. The importance of mucosal barrier and clearance mechanisms, as well as salivary flow, is most apparent when they are disrupted. Other host defenses are present in normal oral mucosa that are not as apparent but play an important role. Abundant lymphoid tissue is present in Waldeyer's ring and other oral mucosal sites. T cells, B cells, mast cells, and natural killer cells are all present. Secretory immunoglobulin (IgA) plays a role in preventing reinfection with previously recognized viruses and other microorganisms. Lymphoid tissue, with its important cellular and humoral defenses, is undoubtedly diminished by the same agents that injure mucosal epithelium directly. Thus, the final picture of inflamed, denuded epithelium, superficial or deep infection, and bleeding results from injury to all components of the oral defenses (6).

A. Bacterial Infections

Leukemic and other immunosuppressed cancer patients have a higher incidence of infection with gram-negative rods, such as *Escherichia coli*, *Klebsiella pneumoniae*, and *Pseudomonas aeruginosa*. Frequently, these occur as nosocomial infections when multiple-drug–resistant strains present in the hospital colonize the oropharynx and gastrointestinal tract or upper respiratory tract and then invade when mucosal barriers are disrupted. Because this usually coincides with a period of maximum neutropenia, systemic infections and endotoxic shock are likely events. Antibiotic prophylaxis for this is controversial. It may decrease gram-negative rod infections at the cost of increasing gram-positive coccal, fungal, and yeast infections. Empirical antibiotic therapy of the febrile neutropenic patient with many mucosal portals of entry is necessary and often lifesaving (9–11). Recently, gram-positive coccal organisms have become a more frequent cause of sepsis in granulocytopenic patients than gram-negative rods. These include *Staphylococcus epidermidis*, *Staphylococcus aureus, Streptococcus mitis*, and other strains. Multiple-drug–resistant *S. epidermidis* strains causing bacteremia in cancer patients have often been shown by DNA restriction endonuclease typing not to originate from contaminated intravenous catheters, as was thought, but to come from the gastrointestinal tract (12). These agents undoubtedly enter through disruptions of the mucosal barrier. Viridans streptococci from the mouth cause similar infections (4).

B. Fungal Infections

Candida, species are the most commonly isolated yeast from oral lesions. Increased adherence time to mucosal cells and decreased phagocytic activity allow invasion of mucosa. Declining phagocytic activity against *Candida* can be demonstrated starting 30 minutes after exposure to alkylating agents. *C. albicans* is most frequently encountered, but other species are seen in oral candidiasis: *Candida tropicalis*, *Candida krusei*, *Candida parapsilosis*, and *Candida glabrata*. The appearance of oral candidiasis ranges from discrete white ''curds'' to extensive white pseudomembranous lesions (4).

C. Viral Infections

Most oral viral lesions are caused by herpes simplex virus. In the normal host with reactivation of latent virus, the vesicles in the lips and oral mucosa have a characteristic appearance. In the compromised host, especially BMT patients, they are often far more extensive and their appearance is less characteristic or obscured altogether by concomitant mucosal inflammation and nonspecific ulceration, yeast infection (thrush), hemorrhage, and adherence of food particles and medicaments to the mucosa. Laboratory tests may be helpful in making a specific diagnosis.

In the compromised host with painful ulcerated lesions who is already receiving antibiotics and who does not have a fungal infection by clinical or laboratory criteria, the empirical use of acyclovir often produces clinical improvement. This may be the best test of whether HSV is part of a multiagent painful ulcerative process.

Graft-versus-host disease in BMT patients, either acute or chronic, affects both mucosal surfaces and salivary gland function.

V. CLINICAL PRESENTATION AND COURSE

Acute oral mucositis begins 7 to 10 days after cytoreductive therapy. Mucosal ''burning'' is often the first manifestation, accompanied by erythema. Erosion and ulceration next develop over a period of 3 to 5 days and then persist for days to weeks, depending on the dose and duration of the offending agents. This is accompanied by pain, bleeding, and infection. Brief pulses of chemotherapeutic drugs may produce short-duration patchy involvement of the mucosa, especially if the patient is practicing good oral hygiene. Continuous infusion of 5-FU or irradiation for head and neck tumors is often directly toxic to the entire mucosa, with extensive involvement, which may occur despite the best oral hygiene.

VI. DIAGNOSTIC TESTS

Although nonspecific ulcerations occur secondary to leukemia or profound neutropenia, infection must always be ruled out. In BMT patients, graft-versus-host disease may also be present and confuse the diagnostic picture (6). During acute oral mucositis, cultures and stains for bacteria and fungi can be helpful in assessing the etiological role of these agents in the current episode. Viral cultures of ulcers may yield HSV because this virus reactivates in many patients who are serologically positive. Swabs from ulcerated epithelium can be examined by immunofluorescence for HSV, but this is expensive and not always available. A new quantitative assay of chemotherapy-induced mucositis has been described (20).

There are tests for quantitating salivary flow and estimating the degree of xerostomia, but these are not of much benefit in managing acute toxicity. When esophagitis is also present, endoscopy may be most helpful in differentiating between lesions caused by *Candida* and those caused by HSV.

VII. TREATMENT

Many topical oral preparations have been used in the treatment of oral mucositis. A number were described as effective in the *National Cancer Institute Monograph* (6): benzylamine hydrochloride in head and neck cancer patients, β-carotene in oral squamous cell carcinomas, allopurinol in gastrointestinal cancers, and sucralfate in acute nonlymphocytic leukemia in adults but not in children. It is sometimes effective to use a combination of therapies given sequentially through the day. Sucralfate given as a slurry to ''swish and swallow'' may protect both oropharynx and esophagus. Viscous 2% lidocaine (Xylocaine), 15 mL diluted with a small amount of water in a swish and spit treatment, reduces pain if used before meals. It is important that the lidocaine be expectorated to avoid cardiac toxicity from systemic absorption. Newer preparations that combine a long-lasting (6 h) barrier for denuded epithelium with an analgesic seem to be a worthwhile addition for those with discrete ulcers. For oral candidiasis, nystatin, clotrimazole, or oral ketoconazole can be used. Low-dose (3–5 mg) intravenous amphotericin B has been used for lack of response to the other agents.

Acyclovir should be given either as prevention for HSV in high-risk patients, such as leukemic and BMT patients, or for lower risk patients therapeutically as needed.

Radiation-induced decreased salivary flow often results in rampant caries. Increased flow can be stimulated with sialogogues, such as pilocarpine, or, more inexpensively, with sugarless chewing gum.

Additional recommendations can be found in comprehensive monographs (4,6). The pain from mucositis can be severe and should not be underestimated. Appropriate analgesics must be given, and this frequently includes parenteral morphine for adequate relief.

Parenteral nutritional support either as peripheral protein-sparing solution or total parenteral nutrition must often be administered to those with severe mucositis to rest inflamed mucosa and to promote healing. For those with less severe mucositis, a full liquid diet (e.g., Ensure, Sustacal, or surgical liquid diet) may suffice. Consultation with the nutritional support service may be helpful for calculation of caloric requirements in a catabolic, malnourished patient and counting the actual number of calories delivered orally and intravenously, for example.

The Mayo Clinic North Central Cancer Treatment Group (NCCTG) has tried a number of palliative care strategies in controlled trials (14). Their placebo-controlled trial of sucralfate for radiation- or 5-FU–induced esophagitis was negative (15,16) but a nonabsorbable antibiotic lozenge did alleviate radiation-induced mucositis (17). A current trial compares sucralfate with vitamin E for mucositis.

Oral health care for cancer patients in general and hospice patients in particular has attracted considerable attention. Nurses and dental practitioners are frequent contributors to the palliative care literature on mucositis (18–21).

VIII. PREVENTION

Preexisting oral disease unrelated to the cancer or its therapy increases the complication rate after therapy. The mouth is a ''trauma-intense'' environment. Rough teeth, dental plates, bridges, and hard food particles frequently abrade the mucosa. If possible, a dental evaluation and corrective plan should be initiated before the onset of chemotherapy or radiation therapy. In this way, plaque can be removed and roughened or ill-fitting teeth and appliances can be repaired. Carious teeth should be repaired or removed. Gingivitis should be controlled before treatment because it can easily exacerbate and be a source for systemic infection.

While the patient is on therapy for cancer, consistent oral hygiene with a fluoride toothpaste and a soft toothbrush should be done after meals and at bedtime. For those in whom use of a toothbrush causes hemorrhage because of friability of thrombocytopenia, topical rinses, such as chlorhexidine, are available. Chlorhexidine with an aminoglycoside prevents the emergence of gram-negative rods. Oral nonabsorbable antibiotic mixtures, such as gentamicin, vancomycin, and nystatin, are falling from favor because their foul taste markedly reduces patient compliance. Less compromised hosts are often advised to rinse with normal saline solution, 3% hydrogen peroxide solution, or sodium bicarbonate solution. Other strategies include a soft diet to reduce mechanical trauma and avoidance of thermal trauma. A cooked food diet and avoidance of fresh fruit and vegetables reduce the acquisition of new gram-negative rods. For leukemic or BMT patients, antifungal prophylaxis and antiviral prophylaxis with acyclovir have been shown to be helpful (11). Not all preventive measures are effective. Citrovorum mouthwash during methotrexate infusion has failed to prevent mucositis. Recently, a controlled trial of oral cryotherapy for preventing stomatitis from 5-FU modulated with leucovorin was found to be effective (13). Patients used ice chips to cool the mouth for 30 minutes while a bolus of 5-FU was given. Because the drug has a half-life of 10 to 20 minutes, it was hoped that decreasing blood flow by cooling would limit exposure of mucosal cells. This is an inexpensive prophylactic against an expensive toxicity.

Synthetic saliva (Salivart) is often used to prevent dryness (xerostomia) when salivary flow is decreased. The duration of such an effect is usually brief. Longer acting saliva substitutes with mucopolysaccharides are becoming available (Mouth-Kote). Some add diphenhydramine or benzyl alcohol for anesthetic purposes.

Pilocarpine (Salagen) has been available for some time to stimulate salivary gland function after radiation-induced xerostomia. When pilocarpine is given after xerostomia is established, it may take considerable time to repair some measure of salivary gland output. More recent approaches have been to give pilocarpine concurrently with radiation to minimize gland injury while improving tumor kill (22,23). The result is more salivary flow and better mucosal integrity.

An interesting combination of pilocarpine, sucralfate, and diflucan was used in an uncontrolled study in similar patients with no interruption in treatment schedule owing to mucositis, a dramatic difference from previous experience (25). Even though pilocarpine probably does offer some preservation of salivary function, it is difficult to persuade patients to persist in taking it when they experience side effects and do not see immediate benefit similar to the benefit seen with antiemetics or analgesics.

Probably the most innovative recent approach to prevention and treatment of mucositis is the topical use of biological response modifiers (e.g., granulocyte colony-stimulating factor, granulocyte-macrophage colony-stimulating factor, and tumor growth factor beta) to prevent mucositis. Although these trials are few in number and mostly uncontrolled, it is striking how many different clinics seem to have noted similar activity (25–27). These growth factors may be a major, although expensive, advance in preventing therapy-related mucositis.

IX. FUTURE RESEARCH

Future cooperative group protocols should incorporate data collection on the incidence and prevalence of oral complications related to different types of anticancer therapies. These trials should also incorporate state-of-the-art treatment for oral toxicity. It would be useful to have radioprotective and chemoprotective agents. Further investigation of the role of biological response modifiers, such as the colony-stimulating factors, in the prevention of myelosuppression and mucositis is needed. Further definition of the patient populations that benefit from prophylactic antiviral therapy should be done. More information is needed about the optimal antifungal prophylaxis and therapy of overt infection. Controlled studies of chlorhexidine and other oral antimicrobials for the prevention of infection and control of mucositis are needed in defined patient populations. It will be useful to know the cost of oral toxicity to determine the cost-effectiveness of strategies for dealing with these toxicities.

Resource utilization, outcomes, and costs of complications are just beginning to be addressed and predictive models developed (28). It should not be surprising that, as treatments are intensified, more febrile days per cycle and more hospital days per cycle are recorded (28). If such research reveals disproportionate toxicity of a specific treatment in the aged or one gender rather than both, then strategies for relieving these toxicities must be sought (29).

It is expected that further studies with sucralfate, vitamin E, pilocarpine, and cryotherapy will advance current ability to prevent and treat mucositis. Working out the correct time sequence for these agents to be applied effectively will take time and carefully designed trials. Supportive care groups such as Multinational Association for Supportive Care in Cancer (MASCC) are conducting such trials and welcome new members to their cooperative group research efforts.

REFERENCES

1. McElroy TH. Oral care of the cancer patient. In: Schein PS, ed. Decision Making in Oncology. Philadelphia: BC Decker, 1989:230–231.
2. Toth BB, Frame RT. The management of disease and treatment-related oral dental complications associated with chemotherapy. Curr Probl Cancer 1983; 7:7–35.
3. McElroy TH. Infection in the patient receiving chemotherapy for cancer: oral considerations. J Am Dent Assoc 1984; 109:454–456.
3a. Daeffer R. Oral hygiene measures for patients with cancer, part I. Cancer Nurs 1980; 3:347–355.
4. Peterson DE. Oral toxicity of chemotherapeutic agents. Semin Oncol 1992; 19:478–491.
5. Perry MC. Toxicity: ten years later. Semin Oncol 1992; 19:453–457.
6. National Cancer Institute. Consensus Development Conference on Oral Complications of Cancer Therapies: Diagnosis, Prevention, and Treatment. NCI Monograph 1990; 9:95–98.
7. Gallagher JG. Empiric antimicrobial therapy in the community hospital setting for the cancer patient with fever and neutropenia: the need for vigilance and attention to detail. Rec Res Cancer Res 1993; 132:89–96.
8. Lockhart PD, Sonis ST. Alterations in the oral mucosa caused by chemotherapeutic agents. J Dermatol Surg Oncol 1981; 7:1019–1025.
9. Klastersky J, Zinner SH, Calandra T, et al. Empiric antimicrobial therapy for febrile granulocytopenic cancer patients: lessons from four EORTC trials. Eur J Cancer Clin Oncol 1988; 24(suppl 1):S35–S45.
10. Hughes WT, Armstrong D, Bodey GP, et al. Guidelines for the use of antimicrobial agents in neutropenic patients with unexplained fever. J Infect Dis 1990; 161:381–396.
11. Schimpff SC. Prevention of and therapy for infections in cancer patients. Curr Opin Oncol 1990; 2:919–923.
12. Wade J. Controversies in new anti-infectious therapies. Fourth International Symposium on Supportive Care in Cancer. St. Gall, Switzerland, February 24–27; 1993.
13. Mahood DJ, Dose AM, Loprinzi CL, et al. Inhibition of fluorouracil-induced stomatitis by oral cryotherapy. J Clin Oncol 1991; 9:449–452.
14. Loprinzi CL, Foote RL, Michalak J. Alleviation of cytotoxic-induced normal tissue damage. Semin Oncol 1995; 22(suppl 3)95–97.
15. McGinnis WI, Loprinzi CL, et al. Placebo-controlled trial of sucralfate for inhibiting radiation-induced esophagitis. J Clin Oncol 1997; 15:1239–1243.

16. Loprinzi CL, Ghosh C, et al. Phase III controlled evaluation of sucralfate to alleviate stomatitis in patients receiving fluorouracil-based chemotherapy. J Clin Oncol 1997; 15:1235–1238.
17. Okuno SH, Foote RL, Loprinzi CL, et al. A randomized trial of a nonabsorbable antibiotic lozenge given to alleviate radiation-induced mucositis. Cancer 1997; 79: 2193–2199.
18. Carl W. Oral complications of local and systemic cancer treatment. Curr Opin Oncol 1995; 7:320–324.
19. Sweeney MP, Bogg J. Oral care for hospice patients with advanced cancer. Dental Update 1995; 22:424–427.
20. Wymenga AN, van der Groff WT, et al. A new in vitro assay for quantitation of chemotherapy-induced mucositis. Br J Cancer 1997; 76:1062–1066.
21. Scully C, Epstein JB. Oral health care for the cancer patient. Eur J Cancer 1996; Part B, Oral Oncology 32B:281–292.
22. LeVeque F, Fontanesi J, et al. Salivary gland sheltering using concurrent pilocarpine (PC) in irradiated head and neck cancer patients (abstr. 1665). Proc Am Soc Clin Onc 1996; 15:516.
23. Zimmerman RP, Mark RJ, Jullard GF. Timing of pilocarpine treatment during head and neck radiotherapy: concomitant administration reduces xerostomia better than post-radiation pilocarpine (abstr). Int J Rad Onc 1996; 36(1):suppl.
24. Lozada-Nur F, Schoelch M, Fu K, et al. A pilot study to evaluate the effect of pilocarpine tablets on salivary flow and mucositis in head and neck cancer patients during radiotherapy (abstr 1541). Proc Am Soc Clin Oncol 1998; 17:399a.
25. Karthaus M, Rosenthal C, Paul H. Effect of topical oral G-CSF application on oral mucositis in high-grade lymphoma patients treated with HD-methotrexate—results of a randomized placebo-controlled trial (abstr 235). Proc Am Soc Clin Oncol 1998; 17:61a.
26. Ibrahim E, Al-Mulhim F. Use of granulocyte-macrophage colony stimulating factor in chemotherapy induced oral mucositis in non-neutropenic cancer patients (abstr 335). Proc Am Soc Clin Oncol 1998; 17:87a.
27. Wymenga ANM, van der Graaf WTA, Hofstra LA. Phase I Study of CGP-46614 (TGF-β3) mouthwash as prevention for chemotherapy induced mycositis (abstr 280). Proc Am Soc Clin Oncol 1998; 17:72a.
28. Manzullo E, Chambers B, Toth E. Outcomes and resource utilization in cancer patients with oral and gastrointestinal complications of chemotherapy (abstr 1605). Proc Am Soc Clin Oncol 1998; 17:416a.
29. Weinerman B, Rayner H, Venne A. Increased incidence and severity of stomatitis in women treated with 5-fluorouracil and leucovorin (abstr 1176). Proc Am Soc Clin Oncol 1998; 17:305a.

ANNOTATED BIBLIOGRAPHY

Fisher DS, Knobf MT. The Cancer Chemotherapy Handbook, 5th ed. St. Louis: Mosby-Year Book, 1997. The stomatitis section is a useful guide to management. The figure illustrating the multifactorial etiology of mucositis is helpful. The treatment of diarrhea is less adequate. Overall, this is an excellent example of the many such handbooks available.

National Cancer Institute. Consensus Development Conference on Oral Complications of Cancer Therapies: Diagnosis, Prevention, and Treatment. Natl Cancer Inst Monogr Vol. 9, 1990. This is the most extensive reference ever produced on oral toxicities and their management. A total of 30 presentations on pretreatment assessment, pretreatment strategies, management of acute problems, and management of chronic toxicities are followed by a consensus statement. There is more information about tooth and bone problems in irradiated and BMT patients than in most other reviews. The pediatric population is well covered.

National Institutes of Health. Oral Complications of Cancer Therapies: Diagnosis, Prevention and Treatment. NIH Consensus Development Conference Statement. 1989, Vol. 7, No. 7. This is the consensus statement alone and should not be confused with the much larger conference proceedings. This brief consensus statement, however, is a remarkable summary of current recommendations for the management of oral toxicities and directions for future research.

Peterson DE. Oral toxicity of chemotherapeutic agents. Semin Oncol 1992; 19: 478–491. This is a thorough treatment of oral toxicities emphasizing dental problems. Mucositis and salivary gland dysfunction are well covered, and the reference list is excellent: a recent and highly recommended reference.

Wilkes JD. Prevention and treatment of oral mucositis following cancer chemotherapy. Semin Oncol 1998; 25:538–551. Useful algorithm for nurses and physicians.

11

Diarrhea

James G. Gallagher
Penn State–Geisinger Health System, Danville, Pennsylvania

I. INTRODUCTION

Toxicity to gastrointestinal mucous membranes is a frequent side effect of treatment for malignancy. Probably no other side effects so interfere with quality of life as mucositis and diarrhea. Mucositis is covered in the previous chapter; diarrhea is the subject of this chapter. Both cause pain and hemorrhage and interfere with adequate hydration and nutrition. In addition, interruption of alimentary tract membranes may allow local invasion by bacteria, fungi, or viruses, singly or in combination. Some of these localized ulcerations may lead to systemic infections (bacteremia and fungemia). All such mucous membrane injuries require time to heal, during which intense supportive care must be given, frequently in the hospital and at great expense.

As newer chemotherapy and radiation therapy strategies are introduced, some of them result in unexpectedly severe mucositis or diarrhea. Each of these gastrointestinal toxicities can be fatal if not promptly recognized and treated. As long as aggressive treatment is done, mucositis and diarrhea will remain serious problems for oncologists. Recently, more attention has been paid to prevention and supportive care in this area. A number of international conferences on supportive care in cancer have been held in Europe and the United States. The practical applications of new knowledge in this area are presented in this volume and in the new journal *Supportive Care in Cancer*.

II. DEFINITION AND MAGNITUDE OF THE PROBLEM

Many cancer patients are troubled by diarrhea at some time during therapy for malignancy. Usually this is simply an excess number of loose stools for a limited time and is easily managed. Life-threatening diarrhea is seen infrequently and is observed mostly for those on continuous chemotherapy infusions, those receiving radiation to the abdomen or pelvis, and those with pseudomembranous enterocolitis or secretory diarrheas. The Cancer Clinical Trials common toxicity criteria for grading diarrhea are given in Table 1.

III. ETIOLOGY AND PATHOPHYSIOLOGY

A. Normal Bowel Function

Normal bowel function has considerable variation in the healthy adult human, but average values for frequency, weight, water content, and solids have been outlined (1). Normal frequency is defined as up to two stools per day. Diarrhea is defined by one or more of the following: (1) abnormal increase in stool frequency, (2) abnormal increase in stool liquidity, and (3) abnormal increase in stool weight (2,3). These are often accompanied by urgency, incontinence, and abdominal pain and cramps. In a normally nourished adult, approximately 9 L of fluid per day is delivered to the duodenum. Of this, the small bowel absorbs approximately 8 L, the colon absorbs approximately 0.9 L, and approximately 0.1 L is excreted as stool liquid. This is an enormous capacity for absorption of fluid while maintaining osmolality and ion concentrations, and there is little reserved capacity; therefore, normal bowel function is easily tipped toward constipation or diarrhea (2).

B. Physiology of Diarrhea

There are multiple causes of diarrhea: (1) unusual amounts of poorly absorbed osmotically active solutes, (2) intestinal ion secretion, (3) inhibition of normal ion absorption and stimulation of ion secretion (secretory diarrhea), (4) abnormal intestinal motility, and (5) inflammatory exudation of mucus, blood, and protein (1–3).

Osmotic diarrheas result from disaccharidase deficiency or mannitol, sorbitol, or lactulose ingestion or poorly absorbed salts and mineral ions in cathartics and antacids, such as magnesium citrate and magnesium hydroxide.

Secretory diarrhea results when enterotoxins or endocrine tumors elaborate secretagogues, such as vasoactive intestinal peptide (VIP) or serotonin, that cause net increases in luminal ions and water. This is often a combination of abnormal ion secretion and inhibition of normal ion absorption.

Table 1 Toxicity Criteria

Toxicity	Grade 0	1	2	3	4
Diarrhea	None	Increase of 2–3 stools/d over pretherapy	Increase of 4–6 stools/d, or nocturnal stools, or moderate cramping	Increase of 7–9 stools/d, or incontinence, or severe cramping	Increase of ≥10 stools/d or grossly bloody diarrhea, or need for parenteral support
Diarrhea + colostomy	None	Mild increase in loose watery colostomy output compared with pretreatment	Moderate increase in loose watery colostomy output compared with pretreatment	Severe increase in loose watery colostomy output compared with pretreatment	Grossly bloody diarrhea or loose water colostomy output requiring parenteral support

Deranged motility hurries fluid through the small intestine, with consequent reduced contact time between bowel mucosa and contents. The result is delivery of abnormally large and qualitatively abnormal boluses of fluid to the colon. Overwhelming of colonic absorption or reduced time in transit results in increased volume and liquidity of stools. A mild example is irritable bowel syndrome and a severe example is the diarrhea of carcinoid syndrome.

Exudation of fluid, mucus, and blood in variable quantities follows disruption of mucosal integrity by inflammation, infection, or cytotoxic drugs. Arrest of rapidly dividing mucosal cells in the crypts results in atrophy of villus formation and patches of inflamed and infected mucosa.

C. Etiologies of Diarrhea

Most diarrheas are not the result of a single operant mechanism. Most are a combination of mechanisms and may be further exacerbated by diabetic autonomic neuropathy, thyroid dysfunction, previous bowel surgery, radiation, or advanced age. See Table 2 for differential diagnostic information.

D. Chemotherapy-Associated Diarrhea

1. 5-FU +/− Leucovorin
2. CPT-11 (Irinotecan, Camptosar)

Clues to the etiology of an episode of diarrhea are provided in most patients with an established diagnosis of malignancy by their immediate previous therapies: 5-fluorouracil (5-FU) ± leucovorin, 5-FU by continuous infusion, abdominal or pelvic radiation, or antibiotic therapy predisposing to pseudomembranous enterocolitis. In a summary of the toxicity of the 33 most commonly used chemotherapy drugs, only 9 of 33 were noted occasionally to cause diarrhea (4). 5-Flourouracil was noted as a frequent cause of clinical diarrhea. When 5-FU is given over multiple days or as modulated by folinic acid (leucovorin), diarrhea is a major problem. In a study of 5-FU plus high-dose folinic acid for metastatic colon cancer, Asbury et al. Reported that 58% had enteritis severe enough for admission in 30% and fatal in 9% (5). Numerous other reports note that aggressive 5-FU therapy protocols, especially those with folate modulation, can result in death from either diarrhea and dehydration alone or combined with neutropenia and sepsis (6).

CPT-11 (Irinotecan, Camptosar) also can produce severe diarrhea. This late-onset diarrhea is particularly severe and has been fatal.

Table 2 Differential Diagnosis of Diarrhea in Cancer Patients

Excessive volume
- I. Impaired absorption
  - A. Malabsorption secondary to loss of normal mucosal integrity
    - 1. Inflammatory diseases
      - a. Radiation enteritis
      - b. Regional enteritis
      - c. Ischemic colitis
      - d. Ulcerative colitis
      - e. Stevens-Johnson syndrome
      - f. Celiac sprue
      - g. Pseudomembranous enterocolitis
    - 2. Invasive infectious diseases
      - a. Bacteria: *Shigella, Salmonella,* enteropathogenic *Escherichia coli*
      - b. Viruses
      - c. Protozoa: giardiasis, amebiasis
      - d. Helminths: *Ascaris lumbricoides, Necator americanus,* and *Strongyloides stercoralis*
    - *3. Infiltrative diseases*
      - a. Intestinal lymphoma
      - b. Intestinal amyloidosis
      - c. Intestinal scleroderma
    - 4. Miscellaneous
      - a. Massive small bowel resection
      - b. Postgastrectomy diarrhea
      - c. Bile salt diarrhea
      - d. Steatorrhea
  - B. Maldigestion
    - 1. Pancreatic insufficiency
    - 2. Lactase deficiency
    - 3. Disaccharidase deficiency
    - 4. Other enzyme deficiencies
- II. Increased secretion
  - A. Bacterial toxins
    - 1. *Clostridium difficile*
    - 2. Enterotoxigenic *E. coli*
    - 3. Food poisoning with *Staphylococcus, Bacillus,* or *Clostridium* species
  - B. Humoral factors
    - 1. Non-β islet cell tumors of the pancreas
      - a. Zollinger-Ellison syndrome (gastrin)
      - b. Vasoactive intestinal peptide (VIP-producing tumors)
      - c. Other vasoactive substances

Table 2 Continued

2. Medullary carcinoma of the thyroid
C. Miscellaneous: villous adenoma
Abnormal gastrointestinal motility
I. Hypermotility with decreased transit time
   A. Gastrointestinal hemorrhage
   B. Postgastrectomy with "dumping syndrome"
   C. Cathartics
   D. Carcinoid tumors
II. Hypomotility with intestinal stasis, bacterial overgrowth, secondary malabsorption, and maldigestion
   A. Stricture
   B. Diverticula
   C. Blind loops
   D. Neuromuscular disease
III. Miscellaneous
   A. Diabetic diarrhea
   B. Postvagotomy
   C. Irritable bowel syndrome

Diarrhea is categorized according to pathophysiological mechanisms as described in the text. Any one episode may be mediated by several mechanisms. All patients are presumed to have received chemotherapy drugs and/or radiation therapy.
Source: Adapted from Ref. 17.

E. Radiation-Induced Enteritis

Radiation-induced enteritis is most frequently observed after pelvic irradiation for prostate, bladder, or gynecological malignancies (3). Total dose, fractionation, vascular disease, and previous surgery that may have fixed bowel in the pelvis are important variables in the origin of enteritis. Most patients undergong pelvic irradiation have signs or symptoms of proctitis. Those with a history of ulcerative colitis or diverticular disease have less tolerance to radiation therapy. As with chemotherapy toxicity to the mucosa, there are acute reversible mucosal changes: reduction in the mitotic figures and progressive flattening of columnar cells. This results in villus flattening after 1 week. Late effects include ulceration, stricture, and even perforation. Connective tissue shows amorphous hyaline change and atypical fibroblasts. Smooth muscle atrophy is often present. Radiation vasculitis results in ischemic lesions (3). The bowel may ultimately become narrow, straight, and tubular and lose its haustra; it may resemble ulcerative colitis in gross appearance. The small bowel may histologically resemble Crohn's disease (3). Acutely, there is diarrhea with or without tenesmus and rectal bleeding. Malabsorption of Vitamin B_{12}, bile salts, lactose, and water are noted (7,8). Excess bile acids induce water and electrolyte secretion, increase motility, and decrease transit time (9–11).

F. Endocrine Functional Neoplasms

The diarrheas caused by endocrine neoplasms are secondary to the circulating hormones produced by these tumors. Their characteristics, diagnoses, and treatment are reviewed in standard texts (2,12,13).

G. Infectious Diarrheas and Pseudomembranous Enterocolitis

The infectious diarrheas are discussed in Chapter 1 and are not discussed here, except for pseudomembranous enterocolitis caused by *Clostridium difficile* toxin. This is an often serious and sometimes lethal diarrhea that follows antibiotic therapy, especially with clindamycin, ampicillin, and cephalosporines (2). In some patients, pseudomembranous enterocolitis seems to develop after combination chemotherapy, without recent exposure to antibiotics or gastrointestinal surgery. Pseudomembranes composed of fibrin, mucin, inflammatory cells, and sloughed mucosa are noted on examination of the colon. A more advanced stage shows gland disruption. The most advanced form shows necrosis down to the lamina propria, with a correspondingly thicker pseudomembrane (14). Infectious diarrheas have been reviewed in the literature (15).

IV. CLINICAL PRESENTATION AND COURSE

Many patients with mild to moderate diarrhea delay seeking help until they have tried an over-the-counter preparation that helped in the past. Because these have been intensely promoted in recent years, most patients have ready access to Kaopectate, antispasmodics, and anticholinergics.

Most diarrhea episodes are either self-limited or self-treated to resolution. Those that resist self-medication are accompanied by considerable spasm and pain, awaken the patient from sleep, or are accompanied by blood trigger medical consultation. Volume loss and dehydration do not, of themselves, seem to trigger appropriate concern in the sufferer. This is especially true in the elderly and very young. Fatalities have occurred in the elderly from excessive volume loss and failure of early recognition and correction of volume and electrolyte depletion (6). Most patients have some degree of crampy abdominal pain with the diarrhea. Varying amounts of mucus and blood may be present. Clinical symptoms at presentation may give some clues to the cause, as may the history of drug treatment, but diagnostic tests are necessary for definitive diagnosis because diverse etiologies may have similar clinical presentations.

V. DIAGNOSTIC TESTS

Diarrhea in a patient receiving chemotherapy or radiation therapy is usually attributed to the treatment modality involved. This is often the correct assessment, but it remains important to rule out other causes, such as infectious or toxin-mediated enterocolitis, because these may require specific therapies. A relatively simple and inexpensive diagnostic approach should narrow the differential diagnosis. White cells with or without blood in the stool denote inflammation and help to distinguish bacterial from nonbacterial causes of diarrhea. Blood without white cells indicates either tumor invasion of the bowel or recent bowel surgery. Cultures should be done to rule out *Salmonella*, *Shigella*, *Campylobacter*, and enterotoxigenic *Escherichia coli*. Smears for *Cryptosporidium* are occasionally indicated, especially in those with acquired immunodeficiency syndrome (AIDS). Toxin assay for *C. difficile* should not be overlooked. A problem-oriented approach to differential diagnosis is given in Table 2. This is intended as a first approach to diagnosis in an adult with an established diagnosis of malignancy undergoing treatment. For patients without a previous history of gastrointestinal illness and whose diagnosis does not appear in Table 2, consultation with a gastroenterologist or reference to a more comprehensive differential diagnosis is imperative (2,3,16–18).

Most acute diarrhea episodes resolve with a week or less of supportive care if the chemotherapy agents are discontinued and no other etiology is identified. Those that persist beyond this time must be evaluated for other etiologies besides chemotherapy association, for example, infectious agents, toxins, or ischemia. Most acute episodes of diarrhea following chemotherapy respond well to simple supportive measures, but those with grade III or IV toxicity (see Table 1) require considerably more attention and support to avoid catastrophic outcome.

VI. THERAPY FOR DIARRHEA

It is difficult to assess over the telephone the severity of diarrhea and the need for intervention. Many patients seem to underestimate the number of stools per day, duration of diarrhea, and extent of volume loss. Often when such patients are seen, they are significantly volume depleted, as manifested by postural hypotension, decreased skin turgor, and oliguria. Such acute fluid and electrolyte losses can be life threatening unless replaced in a timely fashion. Standard texts contain recommendations for estimating extracellular fluid and electrolyte deficits and acid-base imbalance (2,3,18). These recommendations should be followed to determine the volume and electrolyte composition of replacement fluids. Water deficit can be estimated by the following equation, in which body weight is estimated weight in kilograms when fully hydrated; Na^+ is serum or plasma sodium.

$$\text{Water deficit} = 0.6 \times \text{body weight} \times \left[1 - \left(\frac{140}{\text{Na}^+}\right)\right]$$

Corrected sodium is necessary if blood glucose is greater than 150, and for each kilogram of water deficit, 1 L of appropriate crystalloid is given as replacement (15,19).

Normal saline solutions can be given rapidly (300–500 mL/h) until 2 to 3 L is delivered, as long as the patient is closely observed for pulmonary edema and the solution does not result in the delivery of more than 10 mEq/h of potassium. Potassium deficit should be estimated based on the serum potassium concentration. A serum potassium of 3.0 to 3.5 corresponds to a 150 to 300-mEq deficit, a serum potassium of 2.5 to 3.0 is equivalent to a 300 to 500-mEq deficiency, and for each additional decrease in serum potassium by 1.0 mEq/L, there is approximately a 200 to 400-mEq additional deficit. Correction of hypokalemia is most important in patients with cardiac disease and those on digitalis to decrease conduction disturbances and dysrhythmias. For serum potassium levels greater than 2.5 mEq/L, potassium can be given at a rate of up to 10 mEq/H and in concentrations of up to 30 mEq/L. If estimated potassium deficit is large, a portion can be given orally to limit the intravenous (IV) amount so that rapid infusion rates and larger volumes can be delivered when necessary. It is inefficient to rehydrate at 100 to 200 mL/h when most adults without a history of congestive heart failure can tolerate 500 mL/h of crystalloid for long enough to replace a multiliter of volume deficit. This type of rehydration is best done in a hospital setting, especially if diarrhea remains an ongoing process. Strict measurements of input and output and electrolyte changes are required. A measure of successful hydration is a urine output $\geq$30 mL/h, urine specific gravity $\geq$1.010, and resolution of postural hypotension. For those with lesser volume deficits and some oral intake, daily IV hydration of 1 to 2 L may be sufficient. Some patients can use oral home hydration with isotonic fluids, such as Gatorade. Because chemotherapy-related acute diarrhea is often self-limited, rehydration and maintenance fluids for several days should be adequate therapy.

Patients often self-medicate or seek prescriptions for symptoms associated with diarrhea. Such adsorbents as Kaopectate do not affect the course of disease but, in milder cases, may help solidify stools and allow more voluntary control of defecation. They usually fail to help those diarrheas that need medical attention. Opiates diminish peristalsis and slow gut transit time but are contraindicated in toxin-mediated or infectious diarrheas because they allow the toxic gut contents to remain in mucosal contact in pooled secretions in hypoactive loops of bowel.

Anticholinergics, such as dicyclomine (Bentyl Hydrochloride), are not useful. Antisecretory agents, such as octreotide, may help in secretory diarrheas and are occasionally used empirically in other refractory diarrheas for which toxin and infectious etiologies have been excluded. For those who are febrile and neutropenic as well, empirical antibiotics are given. Specific antimicrobial therapies of infectious diarrheas are outlined in many references (e.g., Refs. 15 and 18).

An excellent guide to the assessment and treatment of diarrhea in children has been published recently (19). It contains useful information regarding at-home oral rehydration fluids as well as intravenous rehydration and nutritional support.

VII. PREVENTION OF DIARRHEA

There is no a priori method of determining who will have severe gastrointestinal toxicity from chemotherapy regimens. However, experience has identified those drugs and delivery strategies that place the patient at most risk. Thus, patients receiving 5-FU modulated with leucovorin, 5-FU by continuous infusion, or by multiple daily bolus doses to saturate degradation enzymes are at high risk. Those receiving CPT-11 (Irinotecan, Camptosar) are also at risk of grade 3 or 4 late-onset diarrhea (24). They should be cautioned that this treatment can induce life-threatening diarrhea so that early evaluation and therapy are possible. Most protocols require significant reductions in drug doses following an initial episode of severe diarrhea. The Cancer Clinical Trials common toxicity criteria for diarrhea are listed in Table 1. A grade II toxicity requires a 20% reduction in 5-FU in many colon cancer protocols, and grade III or IV toxicity requires a 30% reduction in drug dose. This strategy helps prevent subsequent episodes. For those patients for whom dose reduction does not prevent grade II or III recurrent episodes of diarrhea, daily outpatient hydration of 1 to 2 Liters of saline solution often reduces the worst of the volume, electrolyte, and acid-base disturbances so that the chemotherapy regimen need not be abandoned.

A. Sucralfate

Prevention of irradiation-induced bowel spasm and diarrhea has long been a desirable goal of research. Steroid enemas and bile acid sequestering resins have only provided brief palliation and may have a considerable number of side effects. A more effective therapy may be sucralfate, a sulfated sucrose compound used for healing gastric ulcers. In a prospective, randomized, double-blind placebo-controlled trial in pelvic malignancies treated with curative intent, to doses of 62 to 66 Gy, it was shown that sucralfate decreased stool frequency and increased stool consistency compared with placebo (20). Diminished bowel discomfort was also reported in the treated group. The authors speculate that sucralfate served as a protective barrier from acids, enzymes, and bacteria for denuded mucosa.

The increased concentrations of bile acids as a result of malabsorption are controlled by binding with sucralfate, reducing their activity on the mucosa. This study suggests real benefit from a simple oral therapy for the many patients who undergo definitive radiation therapy for bladder, prostate, and cervix cancers.

B. Nutritional Support

The role of nutritional support in limiting gastrointestinal toxicity and maintaining weight is an important area for research. It has been shown that maintaining normal protein intake during 5-FU chemotherapy of tumor-bearing animals resulted in decreased incidence and duration of diarrhea and increased body weight compared with similarly treated tumor-bearing animals fed a protein-depleted but isocaloric diet (21). Perhaps in humans, earlier therapy with intravenous protein-sparing solutions would similarly decrease the severity of mucositis and diarrhea compared with therapy when these toxicities are already well established. As with burns, mucosal injury is better prevented than treated.

VIII. FUTURE RESEARCH ON DIARRHEA

There is much research and progress on the roles of bile salts and disaccharides in chemotherapy-induced diarrhea. In addition, data are being gathered from cooperative group clinical trials on the grade and duration of diarrhea experienced, as well as the type and duration of supportive care required. Retrospective analysis of these data will better define risk of diarrhea by regimen, patient age, functional status at enrollment, and numerous other parameters. Thus, high-risk situations can be better defined, allowing the oncologist to closely watch the patients at highest risk.

A. Oral Rehydration Fluids

Further attention should be directed toward oral rehydration solutions for inexpensive therapy of less severe grades of diarrhea. Most patients can take oral fluid but often are not sure what to take. Cola or ginger ale (after decarbonation) is often recommended, but in my experience, Gatorade and similar dilute salt solutions with less carbohydrate are more tolerable and more effective as oral rehydration. A prospective randomized trial of Gatorade versus some more traditional rehydration fluid would be useful in advancing outpatient therapeutic options.

B. Octreotide

Some oncologists recommend empirical use of octreotide in secretory diarrheas for which toxins or infectious agents have been ruled out. Further definition of the role of octreotide in noncarcinoid diarrheal syndromes is needed. Further work on the role of cost-effective nutritional support in limiting gastrointestinal toxicity would be most helpful.

Recently, the Mayo Clinic oncology trials cooperative group (NCCTG) examined the differences in incidence and severity of acute diarrhea in patients receiving surgical adjuvant pelvic radiation alone or combined with 5-FU for rectal cancer (22). The combined modality patients had a higher rate of severe and life-threatening diarrhea. They next performed a multi-institutional trial of sucralfate during pelvic irradiation and concluded it did not prevent bowel toxicity (23). These conflicting results with sucralfate require further studies.

Following a number of reports on the efficacy of octreotide after chemotherapy (24,25), a U.S. intergroup trial (1,295) compares 5 days of high-dose octreotide (1500 mcg. t.i.d.) versus conventional dose octreotide (150 μg tid) versus loperamide (4 mg initially, followed by 2 mg after each unformed stool to a maximum of 16 mg per day for 5 days). Results of the trials should enhance treatment of diarrhea more effectively.

C. Glutamine

The NCCTG has begun a trial of oral glutamine versus placebo to reduce acute and chronic bowel enteropathy secondary to pelvic radiation.

REFERENCES

1. Davenport HW. Physiology of the Digestive Tract, 4th ed. Chicago: Year Book Medical, 1977.
2. Slesinger MH, Fordtran JS. Gastrointestinal Diseases, 4th ed. Philadelphia: WB Saunders, 1989.
3. Spiro HM. Gastroenterology, 3rd ed. New York: Macmillan, 1983.
4. Mitchell EP. GI toxicity of chemotherapeutic agents. Semin Oncol 1992; 19:572–579.
5. Asbury RF, Boros L, Brower M, et al. 5-FU and high dose folic acid treatment for metastatic colon cancer. Am J Clin Oncol 1987; 10:47–49.
6. Grem JL, Shoemaker DD, Petrelli NJ, Douglass HO Jr. Severe and fatal toxic effects observed in treatment with high- and low-dose leucovorin plus 5-fluorouracil for colorectal carcinoma. Cancer Treat Rep 1987; 71:1122.
7. Thomas PRM, Lindblad AS, Stablein DM. Toxicity associated with adjuvant

postoperative therapy for adenocarcinoma of the rectum. Cancer 1986; 57:1130–1134.

8. Kelvin FM, Gramm HF, Gluck WL, et al. Radiologic manifestations of small bowel toxicity due to floxuridine therapy. Am J Radiol 1986; 146:39–43.
9. Arlow FL, Dekovich AA, Priest RJ, et al. Bile acids in radiation-induced diarrhea. South Med J 1987; 80:1259–1261.
10. Yeoh EK, Lui D, Lee NY. The mechanism of diarrhea resulting from pelvic and abdominal radiotherapy; a prospective study using selenium-75 labeled conjugated bile acid and cobalt-58 labeled cyanocobalamin. Br J Radiol 1984; 57:1131–1136.
11. Fernandez-Banares F, Villa S, Esteve M, et al. Acute effects of abdominal pelvic irradiation on the orocecàl transit time: its relation to clinical symptoms, and bile salt and lactose malabsorption. J Gastroenterol 1991; 86:1771–1776.
12. Moossa AR, Schimpff SC, Robson MC. Comprehensive Textbook of Oncology. Baltimore: Williams & Wilkins, 1991.
13. Krejs GJ, ed. Diarrhea. Clin Gastroenterol 1986; 15:603–629.
14. Bartlett JG. The pseudomembranous enterocolitides. In: Slesinger MH, Fordtran JS, eds. Gastrointestinal Diseases, 4th ed. Philadelphia: W. B. Saunders, 1989.
15. Woodley M, Whelan A, eds. Manual of Medical Therapeutic. Boston: Little, Brown, 1992:261–264.
16. Friedman HH, ed. Problem-Oriented Medical Diagnosis, 5th ed. Boston: Little, Brown, 1991.
17. Gottlieb AJ, Zamkoff KW, Jastremski MS, Scalzo A, Imboden KJ. The Whole Internist Catalog. Philadelphia: WB Saunders, 1980.
18. Eastwood GL, Avunduk C, eds. Manual of Gastroenterology, Diagnosis, and Therapy. Boston: Little, Brown, 1988.
19. U.S. Public Health Service. The management of acute diarrhea in children. MMWR Morbid Mortal Wkly Rep 1992; 41:RR–16.
20. Henriksson R, Franzen L, Littbrand B. Prevention of irradiation-induced bowel discomfort by sucralfate: a double-blind placebo-controlled study when treating localized pelvic cancer. Am J Med 1991; 91(suppl 2A):151S–156S.
21. Torosian MH, Jaloli S, Nguyaen HQ. Protein intake and 5-fluorouracil toxicity in tumor bearing animals. J Surg Res 1990; 49:298–301.
22. Miller RC, Martenson JA, et al. Acute diarrhea during rectal surgical adjuvant postoperative pelvic radiation therapy (RT) with or without 5-fluorouracil: a detailed analysis of toxicity from a randomized North Central Cancer Treatment Group study. Proc Am Soc Clin Oncol 1998; 17:279a.
23. Martenson JA, Bollinger JW, Sloan JA, Urias RE, Dick SJ, Gagnon JD, Longo JM, Moore RL: Sucralfate does not prevent bowel toxicity during pelvic radiation therapy: results of a randomized North Central Cancer Treatment Group Study, Proc Am Soc Clin Oncol 1998; 17:64a.
24. Characterisation and clinical management of CPT-11 (Irinotecan)-induced adverse events: the European perspective. Eur J Cancer 1996:32A (suppl 3):S18–23.
25. Geller RB, Gilmore CE, Dix SP, Lin LS, Topping DL, Davidson TG, Holland HK, Wingard JR. Randomized trial of loperamide versus dose escalation of octreotide acetate for chemotherapy-induced diarrhea in bone marrow transplant and leukemia patients. Am J Hematol 1995; 50(3):167–172.

ANNOTATED BIBLIOGRAPHY

Davenport HW. Physiology of the Digestive Tract, 4th ed. Chicago: Yearbook Medical, 1977. An excellent compendium of human gastrointestinal motility secretion, digestion, and absorption.

Mitchell EP. GI toxicity of chemotherapeutic agents. Semin Oncol 1992; 19: 572–579. This is the most recent and comprehensive review of the subject. The table on pages 454–455 summarizes a great deal of reference material in a concise manner. Highly recommended reading.

U.S. Public Health Service. The management of acute diarrhea in children: oral rehydration, maintenance, and nutritional therapy. 1992; MMWR 41:RR-16. This ''recommendation and report'' discusses home as well as hospital rehydration solutions. It is an excellent guide to assessment and treatment.

Slesinger MH, Fordtran JS. Gastrointestinal Diseases, 6th ed. Philadelphia: WB Saunders, 1998. A comprehensive two-volume work. Of interest are chapters on neoplasms causing secretory diarrhea, lymphoma of the gastrointestinal tract, and AIDS enteropathy.

Spiro HM. Gastroenterology, 4th ed. New York: McGraw-Hill, 1993. A classic reference, slightly dated. Radiation enteritis is well considered here.

Taplin C, Blanke CD, Baughman C. Nursing care strategies for the management of side effects in patients treated for colorectal cancer. Semin Oncol 1997; 24(suppl 18):S18-64–S18-70. Deals with diarrhea from newer drugs.

12

Chemotherapy Side Effects and Their Management

Pavel Klener
Charles University Hospital, Prague, Czech Republic

I. INTRODUCTION

The management of undesirable side effects of chemotherapy is an important part of supportive care in cancer. Although side effects may occur following the administration of any drug, after cytotoxic chemotherapy they are almost inevitable. This results from the nonspecic effect of cytotoxic drugs, which inhibits proliferation not only in tumor cells but also in normal cells. Consequently, the most frequent side effects can be seen in tissues with high proliferative activity (e.g., bone marrow, the epithelium of the gastrointestinal tract, hair follicles). The incidence of other less frequent side effects are connected with the chemical structure of particular drugs or with the mechanism of their action, distribution, metabolism, or excretion.

The classification of side effects can be viewed from various standpoints. For convenience, we have classified the side effects of cytotoxic drugs as immediate, early, delayed, and late (Table 1). Immediate side effects are those that occur within 24 hours (nausea and vomiting). Early side effects have their onset within days to weeks (leukopenia, stomatitis). Delayed effects are those occurring within weeks to months after administration (cardiomyopathy, peripheral neuropathy). Late effects are those that become evident months to years later (secondary malignancies).

The intensity of toxic effects depends not only on the characteristics of the

Table 1 Side Effects of Antineoplastic Agents

	Common for different agents	Special for particular agents
Immediate (hours, days)	Nausea, vomiting, phlebitis, hyperuricemia, anaphylaxis, skin rash	Hemorrhagic cystitis (cyclophosphamide, Ifosfamide) Fever (bleomycin) Hypocalcemia (mithramycin) "Recall reaction" (actinomycin D) Hypersensitivity (paclitaxel)
Early (days, weeks)	Leukopenia Thrombocytopenia Alopecia, stomatitis, diarrhea	Paralytic ileus (vincristine) Retention of fluids (estrogens) Pancreatitis (L-asparaginase) Lung infiltrates (methotrexate) Ototoxicity (cisplatin) Flu-like syndrom (DTIC, interferons)
Delayed (weeks, months)	Anemia, azoospermia, hyperpigmentation, lung fibrosis	Peripheral neurophathy (vincristine) Cardiotoxicity (anthracyclines) SIADH (cytarabine, vincristine) Cholestasis (mercaptopurin) Addison-like syndrome (busulfan)
Late (months, years)	Sterility, hypogonadism Secondary malignacies	Cataracts (busulfan) Bladder carcinoma (cyclophosphamide) Osteoporosis (glucocorticoids) Encephalopathy (methotrexate)

Table 2 Estimated Cumulative Doses for Different Intercalating Agents

Drug	mg/m^2
Daunorubicin	400–450
Doxorubicin	500–550
Epirubicin	800–1000
Pirarubicin	500–870
Idarubicin	100–150[a]
Mitoxantrone	120–160[b]
Amsacrine	350–400

[a] Oral idarubicin is less cardiotoxic.
[b] In patients previously treated with anthracyclines, the cumulative dose should be only 120 mg/m^2.

drug but also on the dose used, single or cumulative (Table 2). However, even the dose used currently can cause damage under certain circumstances, for example, if the elimination of the drug is impaired (e.g., in liver or kidney disease), or if its metabolic inactivation is inhibited (e.g., with simultaneous administration of 6-mercaptopurine and allopurinol). Furthermore, there are striking individual interpatient differences; consequently, the symptoms of toxicity can be different even after the same dose.

The management of some toxicities is described in detail elsewhere in this book. This chapter focuses on toxicity to apparently nonproliferating cell populations in specific parenchymal organs such as the heart, lungs, kidney and bladder, peripheral nerves, and central nervous system.

II. CARDIOTOXICITY

Some cytotoxic drugs can affect the heart, causing dose-limiting myocardial damage. Occasional reports of cardiotoxicity have been published in association with the administration of alkylating agents (cyclophosphamide or ifosfamide at very high doses), some antimetabolites (5-fluorouracil), and miscellaneous agents (vincristine, taxanes) (1). However, the most prominent cardiotoxicity is caused by anthracycline antibiotics or some other intercalators (mitoxantrone, amsacrine).

A. Pathogenesis of Cardiotoxicity

Pathogenesis of cardiac damage is complicated and is not fully elucidated. Anthracyclines are capable of undergoing single electron reduction in the hydroxyquinone moiety of chromophore rinstructure. The free radical species generated in this process may react with membrane lipids, causing oxidative damage to myocardial cells. Such damage has been observed in the cell membrane, the mitochondrial membrane, and the sarcoplasmic reticulum. Although free radical formation can occur in other tissues, the heart has low levels of catalase, the enzyme that detoxifies free radicals, and is therefore particularly susceptible to free radical–induced damage. In addition, anthracyclines chelate iron, with an affinity similar to that of desferrioxamine. The doxorubicin–iron complex catalyzes the formation of extremely reactive hydroxyl radicals at the site of binding of the complex to membrane, implicating the complex in the development of cardiotoxicity (1).

Cardiotoxicity is primarily related to the cumulative dose of the drug administered. Although anthracycline-related congestive heart failure may occur after a cumulative dose as low as 100 mg/m^2, the incidence of drug-induced cardiomyopathy increases steeply starting at a total dose of 500 to 550 mg/m^2. For this reason, many current treatment regimens include a predetermined limit to the total planned anthracycline dose, as well as serial measurements of cardiac function.

Estimated cumulative dose for different anthracycline derivatives and other intercalators is summarized in Table 2.

B. Clinical Presentation

Myocardial toxicity can present in three ways:

1. *Acute toxicity* occurs within hours after bolus administration and consists primarily of supraventricular tachyarrhythmias. Electrocardiographic changes occurring most commonly include decrease in voltage, ST-T segment changes, and T-wave flattening. The changes are transient and do not appear to be dose dependent.

2. *Subacute toxicity* noted within days of administration is rare and consists of toxic myocarditis.

3. *Chronic toxicity* occurs weeks or months after administration and consists of cumulative dose–related myocardial cell damage (cardiomyopathy that may ultimately culminate in congestive heart failure).

Late sequelae occurring more than 5 years after exposure to anthracyclines manifests like chronic heart failure, or life-threatening arrhythmias.

Factors other than cumulative dose that can increase the risk of anthracycline cardiotoxicity are preexisting cardiac disease and hypertension, irradiation of mediastinum, malnutrition, concomitant adminsitration of some other cardiotoxic agents, and administration of anthracycline as a bolus (1).

C. Prevention and Management

Cardioprotection using free radical scavengers has received the most clinical attention. In animal models, administration of alpha-tocopherol and *N*-acetylcysteine has cardioprotective effect. However, no study has demonstrated protection from anthracycline-induced cardiac damage in clinical trials (2).
Subsequently, the ability of iron chelation to protect against anthracycline cardiac toxicity was investigated. ICRF-159 (razoxane) and its soluble enantiomer ICRF-187 (dexrazoxane) are chelating agents originally developed as antitumor compounds (3). Dexrazoxane would chelate the intracellularly available iron, leaving doxorubicin unable to form drug–iron complexes and less able to generate cardiotoxic activity, without affecting the antitumor action of doxorubicin. Recommended dose of dexrazoxane is 1000 mg/m^2 in short intravenous infusion of Ringer's solution, administered 30 minutes before anthracyclines.

Several studies have shown that anthracycline cardiotoxicity can be diminished by administration of vasoactive amine blockade consisting of various combinations of alpha- and beta-blockers (4).

Other drugs under clinical or experimental investigation can be useful in prophylaxis and therapy of cardiotoxicity. The imbalance of antioxidant systems is associated with selenium deficiency. Therefore, selenium can play a role in preventing cardiac functional disorder attributable to oxygen free radical formation induced by anthracycline (5). Decreased glutathion peroxidase activity, which contributes to the development of free radicals, was shown to recover by the combined flavonoids such as alpha-G-rutin and luteolin (6). In several experimental models, nitroxides have been shown to exert antioxidant effects. Piperidine nitroxide (tempol) has been found particularly effective (7). Also, a new antithrombotic agent aspalatone (acetylsalicylic acid maltol ester) was suggested to possess an antioxidant effect (8). Prolonged treatment with aspalatone significantly reduced toxicity and ablated histopathological evidence of cardiomyopathy after administration of anthracyclines in animals.

III. PULMONARY TOXICITY

Pneumotoxicity following cytotoxic therapy was first reported in 1961 following busulfan therapy. In the following years, observation of pulmonary toxicity has grown, and there are currently at least 40 such agents that may produce adverse pulmonary effect.

A. Pathogenesis of Pneumotoxicity

Pulmonary toxicity may produce a wide variety of clinicopathological syndromes, depending on their pathogenesis. Drug-related pulmonary disease may be a result of toxicity, hypersensitivity, or idiosyncrasy. A rare manifestation of cytotoxic drug injury is pulmonary veno-occlusive disease with vasculitis and intimal fibrosis, resulting in pulmonary hypertension (9).

The injury the most commonly seen is interstitial pulmonary fibrosis. The prototype of such damage is pulmonary fibrosis associated with bleomycin treatment (10).

Bleomycin has a direct action on capillary endothelium and type I pneumocytes. The biochemical basis of its toxicity is oxidant injury, with subsequent destruction of type I pneumocytes, followed by fibrinous exudation into alveoli. Then there is an influx of granulocytes with release of chemotactic factors, elastase, collagenase, and myeloperoxidase (9). Growth factors released from pulmonary macrophages and lymphocytes are responsible for attracting and stimulating fibroblasts with subsequent collagen deposition and fibrosis. Mitomycin C produces lung injury by means of similar mechanism. Nitrosoureas additionally inhibit glutathion reductase in alveolar macrophages (11). Other agents that possibly affect the lung are summarized in Table 3.

B. Clinical Presentation

The clinical features of pulmonary fibrosis are usually dyspnea, and crackles are present on physical examination. However, routine pulmonary function tests are not very sensitive to early changes (12). Therefore, in some patients, deterioration of pulmonary function may be sudden and may occur many months after completing therapy.

Pulmonary infiltrates may occur after the administration of methotrexate. The pulmonary infiltrates may occur as peripheral consolidations similar to those described in chronic eosinophilic pneumonia and may be accompanied by transient hilar and paratracheal adenopathy. A diffuse nodular pattern may also be present radiographically. The usual presentation is a subacute illness characterized by malaise, myalgias, fever, chills, headache, dyspnea, and cough developing within several hours or days after initiation of therapy. Skin rash and peripheral eosinophilia are frequent.

Pulmonary edema, induced by capillary leak with features of adult respiratory distress syndrome (ARDS), has been described after high-dose ara-C (13) and after administration of some cytokines (interleukin-2, interferon [IFN]-gamma). Pleural effusion has been reported after fludarabine phosphate therapy.

Pulmonary veno-occlusive disease is a rare cause of pulmonary hypertension,

Table 3 Cytotoxic Drugs Producing Different Manifestations of Pulmonary Toxicity

Lung fibrosis	Lung infiltrate	Pulmonary edema	Pleural effusion	Veno-occlusive disease
Bleomycin	Methotrexate	High-dose cytarabine	Fludarabine	Bleomycin
Busulfan	Cyclophosphamide	Aldesleukin		Mitomycin C
Carmustine	Chlorambucil	Interferon gamma		Carmustine
Mitomycin C	Melphalan			

which can occasionally occur after chemotherapy. Several cases have been described after bleomycin, mitomycin C, and BCNU therapy.

C. Prevention and Management

The best prophylaxis is to keep a watchful eye on the total dose of bleomycin administered. Cumulative dose should never be greater than 350 mg/m^2. When concurrent risk factors are present, the minimal cumulative dose should be lower. Risk factors include being older than age 70 years, previous radiotherapy to chest, oxygen therapy, and bolus intravenous administration of the drug.

Once bleomycin toxicity is diagnosed, morbidity and mortality risks are considerable and no treatment is fully effective. Administration of glucocorticoids does not stop the fibrotic process and the disease most often progresses despite institution of this therapy (9).

Some degree of protection against subclinical BCNU pulmonary toxicity was described after therapy with ambroxol (12). This drug enhances alveolar surfactant synthesis and decreases influx of neutrophils, macrophages, and lymphocytes into the lung. On the other hand, corticosteroids may be effective in resolution of infiltrates after methotrexate or cyclophosphamide treatment. Even bilateral infiltrates may resolve within a week. Supportive care with bronchodilators, expectorants, and antibiotics can be beneficial for symptom relief.

Pulmonary edema and ARDS after high-dose ara-C therapy may be helped by the administration of high-dose methylprednisolone (9). In general, there is no adequate therapy for pulmonary veno-occlusive disease. Heparin and pentoxyfylline can be beneficial.

Understanding new molecular mechanisms, involving immediate cytokine release in the initiation of the fibrosis process, opens the door for intervention and protection using some cytokines. Experimentally, the administration of exogenous keratinocyte growth factor (KGF)—a member of the fibroblast growth factor family (FGF-7)—prevents or attenuates several forms of oxidant-mediated lung injury (14).

Alveolar type II cell proliferation is thought to minimize the fibrotic response after lung injury. Because KGF stimulates type II cell proliferation in the rat, intratracheal KGF was proved to prevent lung injury after intratracheal bleomycin (15,16). It was also demonstrated that interferon-gamma has antifibrotic effect in the mouse model of bleomycin-lung fibrosis. It is believed that IFN-gamma down-regulates the bleomycin-induced overexpression of TGF-beta mRNA, and subsequently procollagen mRNAs, leading to decreased collagen content (17).

Experimentally, vitamin E considerably reduces the fibrotic effect of bleomycin on lung tissue in mice, probably as a result of its antioxidant role (18). Another potent inhibitor of bleomycin-induced pulmonary fibrosis, studied in rats, is halofuginone, a novel inhibitor of collagen I synthesis (19).

IV. NEPHROTOXICITY AND UROTOXICITY

A. Pathogenesis of Nephrotoxicity

Damage to kidney caused by anticancer chemotherapy can be caused by indirect effect, resulting from hyperuricemia induced by cytotoxic therapy or by drug-induced renal lesions.

In patients with tumors highly sensitive to chemotherapy, uric acid nephropathy may develop. Hyperuricemia results from rapid release and catabolism of intracellular nucleic acids. Purine nucleic acids are catabolized to hypoxanthine, then to xanthine, and finally to uric acid by xanthine oxidase. Uric acid is filtered by the glomeruli and is reabsorbed and secreted by the tubules. Urates have a decreased solubility in acid urine and thus precipitation may occur, particularly in distal tubules and renal collecting ducts, resulting in anuria. Hyperuricemia may be a part of so-called ''tumor lysis syndrome'' manifested not only by hyperuricemia but also by severe life-threatening metabolic abnormalities, including hyperkalemia, hyperphosphatemia, and hypocalcemia.

Direct damage either is the consequence of mechanic blockade of nephron or is the direct toxic effect of cytotoxic drug or its metabolite on kidney tissue. The former can be seen after methotrexate treatment. Methotrexate and its metabolite 7-OH methotrexate has a tendency to precipitate in renal tubules and collecting ducts at high concentration or in low urinary pH. Oliguria or anuria can develop, particularly after high doses of methotrexate (20).

Toxic effects to the kidneys were observed following administration of many cytotoxic drugs. However, some of them are almost regularly nephrotoxic, These are particularly cisplatinum and nitrosoureas (Table 4).

The types of injury observed after cisplatinum therapy include proximal and distal tubule damage. Cisplatin decreases metabolic activity of tubular mitochon-

Table 4 Anticancer Agents Causing Kidney Toxicity and Urotoxicity

Drug	Toxic dose range
Nephrotoxicity	
Cisplatin	50–200 mg/m^2
Carmustine	1200 mg/m^2
Streptozotocin	Conventional dose
Pentostatin	>5 mg/m^2/d
Mitomycin C	25–30 mg/m^2
Urotoxicity	
Cyclophosphamide	50 mg/kg
Fosfamide	1.2 g/m^2

dria, inhibits glutathion peroxidase, and stimulates lipoperoxidases. This results in cell membrane damage and necrosis of tubular cells (21). Cisplatin has also been implicated in several electrolyte abnormalities. The most frequent is hypomagnesemia and hypocalcemia resulting from urinary wasting.

Streptozotocin damages the renal tubular functions with consequent proteinuria, aminoaciduria, and hypokalemia. Lomustine and carmustine can cause similar renal injuries. Mitomycin C has been associated with a syndrome of renal failure and microangiopathic hemolytic anemia. Distal tubules can be damaged by ifosfamide or cyclophosphamide. They may also induce hyponatremia and decrease urine production by inducing an antidiuretic hormone-like excess syndrome called SIADH.

B. Pathogenesis of Urotoxicity

Toxicities to the genitourinary tract may occur in patients administered cyclophosphamide or ifosfamide. Cyclophosphamide undergoes a multistep activation in vivo, resulting in a range of biologically reactive products, including phosphoramide mustard and acrolein (22). Whereas phosphoramide mustard provides the major antitumor effects of the drug, acrolein has negligible antitumor activity but contributes significantly to the toxic effect of both cyclophosphamide and ifosfamide to bladder epithelium. After administration of these drugs, hemorrhagic cystitis develops in approximately 10% of patients being administered standard therapy and in up to 40% of patients given high-dose therapy.

C. Prevention and Management of Nephrotoxicity and Urotoxicity

1. Hyperuricemia

Prevention and best management of hyperuricemia is maintaining an adequate urinary output, alkalinizing the urine, and using allopurinol before initiation of chemotherapy. Intravenous hydration, preferably with isotonic saline at 2,500 to 3,000 mL/m^2/24 hours, should begin 24 hours before initiation of chemotherapy. For alkalinization, 50 to 100 mEq of sodium bicarbonate may be added to each liter of intravenous fluids to obtain an isotonic solution. Acetazolamide, a carbonic anhydrase inhibitor, may also be used for urinary alkalinization. (150–500 mg/m^2/d). Standard prophylaxis and treatment of chemotherapy-associated hyperuricemia is allopurinol.

Allopurinol is a potent inhibitor of xanthine oxidase and blocks the conversion of hypoxanthine and xanthine to uric acid. It is generally given at a dose of 300 to 400 mg/m^2/d. Recently, an alternative therapy has been under clinical investigation. Urate oxidase (Uricozyme), the enzyme that converts uric acid to allantoin (a readily excreted metabolite that is 5- to 10-fold higher solubility than uric acid) is a more effective uricolytic agent than allopurinol (23). Patients given urate oxidase had rapid and significantly greater decrease in their blood uric acid level than did the historical controls. Urate oxidase treatment can be associated with acute hypersensitivity reaction, even in patients without a history of allergy.

If urate nephropathy unexpectedly develops and the aforementioned measures are ineffective, hemodialysis should be initiated.

Patients must be carefully followed up, because prophylactic measures may cause fluid overload and metabolic alkalosis with associated hypokalemia.

2. *Cisplatin Nephrotoxicity*

Cisplatin nephrotoxicity can be prevented by the induction of a brisk diuresis during drug administration. There is convincing experimental evidence that hydration should always be given using chloride-containing solution, such as normal saline or glucose 5% in saline solution. As a general rule, cisplatin should only be given to patients with a urinary output of at least 100 mL/h during and immediately after drug administration. Vigorous hydration and osmotic diuresis significantly diminished the risk of acute renal toxicity (22). However, cumulative renal toxicity still occurs. Because of this cumulative toxicity, initial therapy is commonly limited, even though a patient might benefit from additional treatment with cisplatin. The most promising protective agent in this situation seems to be amifostine (Ethyol). Amifostine, an organic thiophosphate, is dephosphorylated at the tissue site by alkaline phosphatase to form the active metabolite or free thiol (24). Once inside the cell, the free thiol can bind with and neutralize the reactive species of cisplatin. Thus, the free thiol can detoxify cisplatin before it damages DNA and RNA. Additionally, the free thiol is a potent scavenger of oxygen-free radicals. It has been demonstrated that amifostine has no detectable effect on the antitumor efficacy of cisplatin-based chemotherapy in advanced ovarian cancer (25). Amifostine should be administered as an intravenous infusion over a period of 15 minutes, begining 30 minutes before cisplatin chemotherapy. Because amifostine may cause severe nausea and vomiting, patients should receive antiemetic therapy that includes intravenous dexamethasone (20 mg) and serotonin receptor antagonist before amifostine is administered (26). Another side effect of amifostine is temporary hypotension. Therefore patients should remain in the supine position and should be adequately hydrated. Usual dosage for adults is 740 to 910 mg/m^2/d (27).

Sodium thiosulphate can react covalently with cisplatin, reducing its cytotoxicity. However, it may also protect tumor cells from drug effects (28). Sodium thiosulphate is highly concentrated in the renal tubules and may be particularly useful if administered intravenously while cisplatin is given intraperitoneally as, for instance, in the case of ovarian cancer. Under the latter conditions, it may allow the administration of significantly higher doses of cisplatin (up to 270 mg/m^2) without significant renal toxicity.

Diethyldithiocarbamate is a strong SH group chelator, which has also been shown to protect cisplatin nephrotoxicity in animal models (29). This effect probably depends on the competition with cisplatin for protein-bound SH groups in the renal tubules.

The angiotensin inhibitor captopril and the calcium channel blocker verapamil have also been shown to reduce cisplatin toxicity. This effect may be related to an inhibitory effect on plasma-related reduction of renal plasma flow.

3. *Protection Against Urotoxic Effects*

Urotoxic effects are seen after administration of oxazaphosphorines (cyclophosphamide and ifosfamide). The protection is offered by sodium-2 mercapto-ethane sulphonate-mesna (Uromitexan), administered either concomitantly or shortly before administration of oxazaphosphorines. Mesna reduces the speed of degradation of the 4-hydroxymetabolite in the urine.

A bladder-untoxic condensation product from 4-hydroxy cyclophosphamide or 4-hydroxy ifosfamide and mesna is formed. By such stabilization, mesna inhibits the further degradation of previously mentioned metabolites and hence the formation of acrolein. In addition, mesna causes direct detoxification of acrolein, forming a stable thio ether as an additional compound. Mesna should be administered intravenously, usually at doses of 20% of the respective cyclophosphamide or ifosamide dose at time 0 (administration of oxazaphosphorine), 4 hours, and 8 hours. In case of a continuous infusion (24 h) of oxazaphosphorines, the mesna regimen has to be modified. Mesna should be administered as a bolus injection at time 0. Furthermore, mesna is added to oxazaphosphorine continuous infusion (up to 100% of oxazaphosphorine dose) and given simultaneously with the cytostatic agent. It is advisable to continue the uroprotection (up to 50% of oxazaphosphorine dose) for about 6 to 12 hours after oxazaphosphorine administration is finished.

Once hemorrhagic cystitis develops, the drug must be discontinued and vigorous hydration initiated. If gross hematuria is present, a large catheter must be placed and hydration or irrigation continued.

V. NEUROTOXICITY

Chemotherapy-induced neurotoxicity has become a frequent side effect of anticancer treatment. Increasing incidence of neurotoxic effects is a consequence of advances in supportive care, which permit the use of higher doses of drugs and prolong patient survival, allowing some treatment-related neurotoxicity with a long latency to become evident.

A. Clinical Presentation

Clinical presentations of neurotoxicity are dependent on the specific agent, route of administration, and the dose used. The most common neurological syndromes are peripheral neuropathy, encephalopathy, and cerebellar dysfunction. Other possible presentations are summarized in Table 5.

B. Peripheral Neuropathy

Peripheral neuropathy is the most frequent toxicity associated with tubulin-binding agents, particularly with vincristine (30). The toxicity is usually dose dependent. Tubulin binding of these substances may cause disruption of the axonal tubular system, thereby impairing the axonal transport. Paresthesias in the hands or feet is the most common complaint. With continued drug administration (usually for cumulative dose more than 15 mg), distal and symmetrical weakness starting at the lower limbs occurs gradually.

Paresthesias usually disappear in a few weeks if vincristine is discontinued at onset. Resolution of motor weakness may take months and may be incomplete. Cranial nerves may also be affected. In addition to peripheral neuropathy, autonomic neuropathy presents with obstipation, or paralytic ileus can develop. Atonic bladder and urinary retention are less frequently seen. Neuropathy after taxol to promote stabilization of microtubules is predominantly sensory, particularly affecting small sensory fibers. Neuropathy generally occurs at doses greater than 200 mg/m^2. Peripheral neuropathy is also the most common neurotoxicity associated with cisplatin (31). The neuropathy predominantly involves the large sensory fibers, which mediate vibration and proprioceptive function (32). The development of neuropathy is dose related (when cumulative dose exceeds 300 mg/m^2).

Peripheral neuropathy has been reported also in patients after administration of procarbazine, hexamethylmelamine, or high-dose cytarabine.

C. Acute Encephalopathy

Encephalopathic syndromes are related most often to administration of high-dose intravenous methotrexate (more than 3 g/m^2) or to its intrathecal administration. Less frequently it has been observed after cytarabine therapy. In most cases, the somnolence and lethargy completely resolved soon after completion of chemotherapy. Severe encephalopathy has been reported in patients receiving ifosfam-

Table 5 Cytotoxic Drugs that Cause Different Manifestations of Neurotoxicity

Peripheral neuropathy	Acute encephalopathy	Chronic leukoencephalopathy	Seizures	Cerebellar toxicity
Vincristine	High-dose cytarabine	Intrathecal MTX	Cisplatin	High-dose methotrexate
Cisplatin	Ifosfamide	Intrathecal ara-C	Ifosfamide	High-dose cytarabine
Taxol	Nitrosoureas	Intrathecal thiotepa	High-dose methotrexate	Procarbazine
Procarbazine	Interferons		High-dose cytarabine	Hexamethylmelamine
Cytarabine	Vincristine		Busulfan (bone marrow transplant preparative regimens)	
Interferons	Aldesleukin		L-asparaginase	
Hexamethylmelamine				

ide. Within hours of receiving the drug, confusion, hallucinations, and aphasia are the most common initial signs (33). Nitrosoureas, most commonly carmustine, can cause encephalopathy characterized by a progressive decline of cognitive function, with subsequent development of seizures, coma, and death. Confusion, lethargy, and loss of cognitive function are the most common central nervous system (CNS) effects associated with the use of interferons. Drug-related encephalopathy was described also after the therapy with ifosfamide, probably caused by mitochondrial toxicity of ifosfamide metabolites. Another mechanism of ifosfamide encephalopathy may be excessive quantity of NADH formed during ifosfamide metabolism.

D. Cerebellar Toxicity

5-fluorouracil causes acute cerebellar dysfunction. Patients show the development of moderate to severe gait ataxia, scanning speach, and often nystagmus. Global cerebellar dysfunction is manifested in about 20% of patients receiving high-dose cytarabine. Reported risk factors include cumulative dose, age, and renal dysfunction with impaired drug clearence.

E. Prevention and Management

No specific measures exist to prevent or reverse most chemotherapy-related neurotoxicity. That is why the focus should be on monitoring of toxicity so that treatment can be modified before the development of severe CNS dysfunction. Many treatments have been tried to relieve neurotoxic symptoms. Encouraging results have been reported with gangliosides or glutamic acid in the treatment of vincristine neuropathy. An ACTH analog, ORG 2766, has been reported to protect against cisplatin neuropathy. This drug was tested in a double-blind placebo-controlled trial in patients with ovarian cancer undergoing intensive cisplatin treatment. It is suggested that Org 2766 works synergistically with trophic factors such as nerve growth factor and promotes nerve regeneration (34). Another protective agent against cisplatin-induced neurotoxicity is amifostine (Ethyol). This drug is particularly useful in patients with ovarian cancer receiving the combination cisplatin-taxol. Leucovorine may be helpful in reversing methotrexate-induced encephalopathy. Dose-limiting neurotoxicity of alkylating chemotherapy with ifosfamide can be overcome by the administration of methylene blue. The prophylactic administration of methylene blue is equally effective. It has been suggested that methylene blue exhibits several modes of action (35). It prevents formation of the neurotoxic chloroacetaldehyde from ifosfamide-derived chloroethyl amine, and its electron-accepting property can substitute for the demonstrated flavoprotein deficiency. Thus, its administration leads to resolution of the encephalopathy (36).

All cancer chemotherapeutic agents have produced at least an isolated instance of some untoward side effect. The majority may be reversible spontaneously if they are recognized early and if administration of the appropriate drug is discontinued. On the other hand, some side effects may be life threatening. Therefore, the appropriate diagnosis is critical and clinicans should be vigilant about the possibilty of serious toxic effect associated with any chemotherapeutic regimen.

REFERENCES

1. Allen A. The cardiotoxicity of chemotherapeutic drugs. Semin Oncol 1992; 19:529–542.
2. Carlson RW. Reducing the cardiotoxicity of anthracyclines. Oncology 1992; 6:95–100.
3. Hochter H, Wasserheit C, Speyer J. Cardiotoxicity and cardioprotection during chemotherapy. Curr Opin Oncol 1995; 7:304–309.
4. Legha SS, Benjamin RS, Mackay B, et al. Reduction of doxorubicin cardiotoxicity by prolonged continuous intravenous infusion. Ann Intern Med 1982; 96:133–139.
5. Matsuda A, Kimura M, Itokawa Y. Influence of selenium deficiency on the acute cardiotoxicity of adriamycin in rats. Biol Trace Elem Res 1997; 57:157–167.
6. Sadzuka Y, Sugiyama T, Shimoi K, et al. Protective effect of flavonoids on doxorubicin-induced cardiotoxicity. Toxicol Lett 1997; 92:1–7.
7. Monti E, Cova D, Guido E, et al. Protective effect of the nitroxide tempol against the cardiotoxicity of adriamycin. Free Radic Biol Med 1996; 21:463–470.
8. Kim C, Nam SW, Choi DY, et al. A new antithrombotic agent, aspalatone, attenuated cardiotoxicity induced by doxorubicin in the mouse. Life Sci 1997; 60:75–82.
9. Kreisman H, Wolkove N. Pulmonary toxicity of antineoplastic therapy. Semin Oncol 1992; 19:506–520.
10. Budd GT, Ganapathi R, Adelstein DJ, et al. Randomized trial of carboplatin plus amifostine versus carboplatin alone in patients with advanced solid tumors. Cancer 1997; 80:1134–1140.
11. Weinstein AS, Diener-West M, Nelson DF, et al. Pulmonary toxicity of carmustine in patients treated for malignant glioma. Cancer Treat Rep 1986; 70:943–946.
12. Lehne G, Lote K. Pulmonary toxicity of cytotoxic and immunosuppressive agents. A review. Acta Oncol 1990; 29:113–124.
13. Anderson BS, Cogan BM, Keating MJ, et al. Subacute pulmonary failure complicating therapy with high-dose ara-C in acute leukemia. Cancer 1985; 56:2181–2184.
14. Deterding RR, Havill AM, Yano T, et al. Prevention of bleomycin-induced lung injury in rats by keratinocyte growth factor. Proc Assoc Am Phys 1997; 109:254–268.
15. Takeoka M, Ward WF, Pollack H, et al. KGF facilitated repair of radiation-induced DNA damage in alveolar epithelial cells. Am J Physiol 1997; 272:1174–1180.
16. Yi ES, Williams ST, Lee H, et al. Keratinocyte growth factor ameliorates radiation-

and bleomycin-induced lung injury and mortality. Am J Pathol 1996; 149:1963–1970.
17. Gurujeyalaksmi G, Giri SN. Molecular mechanisms of antifibrotic effect of interferon gamma in bleomycin-mouse model of lung fibrosis. Exp Lung Res 1995; 21: 791–808.
18. Kilinic C, Ozcan O, Karaoz E, et al. Vitamin E reduces bleomycin-induced lung fibrosis in mice. J Basic Clin Physiol Pharmacol 1993; 4:249–269.
19. Nagler A, Firman N, Feferman R, et al. Reduction in pulmonary fibrosis in vivo by halofuginone. Am J Respir Crit Care Med 1996; 154:1082–1086.
20. Kintzel PE, Dorr RT. Anticancer drug renal toxicity and elimination: dosing guidelines for altered renal function. Cancer Treat Rev 1995; 21:33–64.
21. Patterson WP, Reams GP. Renal toxicities of chemotherapy. Semin Oncol 1992; 19:521–528.
22. Perry MC, ed. Toxicity of chemotherapy. Baltimore, Williams & Wilkins, 1992.
23. Pui CH, Relling MV, Lascombes F, et al. Urate oxidase in prevention and treatment of hyperuricemia associated with lymphoid malignancies. Leukemia 1997; 11:1813–1816.
24. McCauley DL. Amifostine. A novel cytoprotective agent. Cancer Pract 1997; 5: 189–191.
25. Kemp G, Rose P, Lurain J, et al. Amifostine pretreatment for protection against cyclophosphamide-induced and cisplatin-induced toxicities. J Clin Oncol 1996; 14: 2101–2112.
26. Schiller JH, Storer B, Berlin J, et al. Amifostine, cisplatin, and vinblastine in metastatic non-small-cell lung cancer. J Clin Oncol 1996; 14:1913–1921.
27. Spencer CM, Goa KL. Amifostine. Drugs 1995; 50:1001–1031.
28. Vogelzang NJ. Nephrotoxicity from chemotherapy. Prevention and management. Oncology 1991; 5:97–105.
29. Derry JM, Jacobs C, Sikio B, et al. Modification of cisplatin toxicity with diethyldithiocarbamate. J Clin Oncol 1990; 8:1585–1590.
30. Kaplan RS, Wiernik P. Neurotoxicity of antineoplastic drugs. Semin Oncol 1982; 9:103–130.
31. Roberts JA, Jenison EL, Kim K, et al. A randomized, multicenter, double-blind, placebo-controlled, dose-finding study of ORG 2766 in the prevention or delay of cisplatin-induced neuropathies in women with ovarian cancer. Gynecol. Oncol. 67, 1977, p. 172–177.
32. Mollman JE. Cisplatin neurotoxicity. N Engl J Med 1990; 322:126.
33. Curtin JP, Koonigs PP, Guttirez M, et al. Ifosfamide-induced neurotoxicity. Gynecol Oncol 1991; 42:193–197.
34. Apfel SC, Lipton RB, Arezzo JC, et al. Nerve growth factor prevents toxic neuropathy in mice. Ann Neurol 1991; 29:87–91.
35. Kupfer A, Aeschlimann C, Cerny T. Methylene blue and the neurotoxic mechanisms of ifosfamide. Eur J Clin Pharmacol 1996; 50:249–252.
36. Alonso JL, Nieto Y, Lopez JA, et al: Ifosfamide encephalopathy and methylene-blue: a case report Ann Oncol 1996; 7:643–44.

13

Management of Cancer Anorexia and Cachexia

Prema P. Peethambaram and Charles L. Loprinzi
Mayo Clinic, Rochester, Minnesota

I. INTRODUCTION

Cancer cachexia is a wasting syndrome associated with the presence of uncontrolled malignancy and usually characterized by loss of appetite (anorexia), weight loss, and weakness. Cancer anorexia/cachexia is commonly seen in advanced malignancy, involving up to 85% of patients with cancer (1). This syndrome can occur early in the course of cancer in a minority of patients (2). Cancer anorexia/cachexia leads to inanition and may be the most direct cause of death in some patients. In addition, anorexia/cachexia can cause major physical and psychological morbidity, and usually signifies a poor prognosis (3).

II. MECHANISM OF CANCER ANOREXIA AND CACHEXIA

There is still no clear explanation for the majority of weight loss caused by malignancy. It is partly a result of a reduced caloric intake and partly related to alterations in energy expenditure. Poor oral intake of food can occur from disorders of the alimentary tract, such as dysphagia, gastrointestinal obstruction, xerostomia, malabsorption from pancreatic insufficiency or short bowel syndrome after surgical resection of a cancer. Chemotherapy or radiation therapy can cause nausea, vomiting, or inflammation of the gastrointestinal tract and can lead to poor oral intake. More commonly, poor oral intake is a result of anorexia. Anorexia can be attributed to cytokines released from the tumors, such as interleukin-1 (IL-1) or tumor necrosis factor; a result of mental depression from cancer diagnosis (4); associated with raised intracranial pressure; or a result of cancer therapy.

A possible association between increased concentration of brain tryptophan and serotonin and the presence of anorexia represents one potential mechanism for cancer anorexia/cachexia. Krause et al. inoculated rats with an experimental tumor and demonstrated that these rats progressively had reduced food intake (5). The brain concentrations of tryptophan, serotonin, and 5-hydroxyindoleacetic acid in these anorexic rats were increased significantly compared to control rats. Laviano and colleagues infused IL-1 in normal rats and induced anorexia similar to that seen in cancer anorexia (6). Interestingly, they found that brain tryptophan and serotonin levels increased in these animals. In addition, 45 patients with cancer-associated anorexia had measurements of plasma free tryptophan and large neutral amino acids. An increased ratio of free tryptophan to other competing acids was reported, denoting an increased availability of brain tryptophan (7). In 1990, Cangiano et al. reported increased tryptophan concentrations in the cerebrospinal fluid of anorectic cancer patients, which correlated positively to the ratio of plasma tryptophan to large neutral amino acids (8). Muscaritoli et al., in 1996, published results showing that anorexia developed in tumor-bearing rats coincident with increased plasma free tryptophan to large neutral amino acid ratios and there was an increase in brain serotonin levels, as measured by using whole brain tissue (9). Cangiano et al., in 1994, studied anorexic and non-anorexic cancer patients both before and after surgical removal of their tumors. They found that the ratio of free tryptophan to large neutral amino acid levels was increased in anorexic patients only and that this ratio decreased when the cancer was removed and the anorexia resolved (10). In patients with chronic liver or renal failure and anorexia, a similar increase in brain availability of tryptophan has been found (11,12). To further validate the hypothesis that increased brain serotonin concentration leads to tumor-induced anorexia, rats with tumors and anorexia as well as non-anorexic control rats were randomly injected with mianserin, a serotonin antagonist, in the venteromedial hypothalamus (which is a predominantly serotoninergic nucleus and is known to be involved in the development of reduced food intake) or with isotonic saline (13). They reported that this serotoninergic block of the hypothalamus increased appetite and food intake in tumor-bearing rats, whereas anorexic tumor-bearing rats with the isotonic saline injection continued to have a decreased food intake.

Derangements in carbohydrate, glucose, protein, and fat metabolism have been reported in a large number of studies performed in patients with cancer anorexia/cachexia. These patients appear to have relative insulin resistance and diminished insulin levels and tend to overproduce glucose (14,15). Patients with cancer cachexia also have higher lactate levels than do control subjects during starvation becasue of utilization of the anaerobic gluconeogenesis pathway (16). Thus, in cancer anorexia/cachexia, protein stores form skeletal muscle are commonly mobilized before fat and carbohydrate stores are depleted (17). In association, there is increased protein turnover and decreased skeletal muscle protein synthesis (18–20). The abnormal protein metabolism seen in cancer cachectic patients may be causative of skin atrophy, disminished wound healing, and an increased risk of infection.

Several humoral factors have been postulated as mediators of the process of cancer cachexia. Tumor necrosis factor alpha (TNF-α), initially termed cachectin, is thought to suppress lipoprotein lipase (21), an enzyme that prevents adipocytes from extracting fatty acids from plasma lipoproteins for storage. When TNF-α is given to animals, weight loss results (22). When Chinese hamster ovarian cells were transfected with a gene for producing TNF-α, a syndrome resembling cancer cachexia was seen (23). However, when TNF-α antibodies were given to rats with sarcoma, anorexia was delayed but not prevented and no overall effect on weight loss was noted (24); multiple other studies also failed to note reversal of anorexia and cachexia by these antibodies (25,26). The TNF-α was not elevated in the serum of human cancer patients in some studies (25,26), but in a study of children with cancer, TNF-α was elevated but did not correlate with weight loss (27). In total, despite some suggestive evidence that TNF-α causes cancer anorexia/cachexia, its exact role in humans still needs to be delineated.

Interleukin 6 (IL-6) is another cytokine that can be seen in elevated levels in patients with cancer anorexia/cachexia (28). Monoclonal antibodies to IL-6 have been reported to partially reverse the weight loss (29). It has been postulated that IL-6, like TNF-α, decreases adipose tissue liposomal protein lipase activity (30). Further studies are needed at this point to evaluate the exact role of IL-6 in cancer cachexia. Similarly, preliminary information in animals report that gamma interferon may play a role in the pathogenesis of cachexia and that blocking its activity may be able to reduce weight loss and increase food intake (31,32). Lastly, several studies have reported, in patients with cancer anorexia/cachexia, the presence of substances called lipid-mobilizing factors (LMF) (33–35), which cause the breakdown of triglycerides with the release of fatty acids and glycerol. The role of this in cancer anorexia/cachexia remains to be determined.

III. TREATMENTS EVALUATED FOR CANCER ANOREXIA/CACHEXIA

Many trials have evaluated several potential agents that might be able to reverse cancer anorexia/cachexia. Before reviewing these, the methods of evaluating patient appetites in such trials should be discussed. Although the instruments used in such trials are varied and have not generally undergone formal validity testing, these tools appear to be reliable measures of appetite as evidence by the following: (1) several trials evaluating a single agent have all reported benefit over a placebo (36–38); (2) different but similar appetite questions all provide similar information in a single trial (36,39,40); and (3) appetite improvement, as measured by such a questionnaire instrument, positively correlated with the amount of nonfluid weight gain (40).

A. Parenteral Nutrition

Treatment of cancer anorexia/cachexia would be beneficial if it could reverse the prominent symptoms associated with this syndrome and be well tolerated. Total parenteral nutrition had been studied for patients with cancer anorexia/cachexia but has not been demonstrated to be beneficial in this situation. Therefore, it is not generally recommended, with few exceptions (41).

B. Anabolic Steroids

There has been interest in evaluating anabolic steroids as a means of increasing appetite and providing increased muscle mass, given the information that these drugs do appear to increase muscle bulk in athletes. A pilot study suggested that there might be some benefit to this approach (42). Pursuant to this information, the North Central Cancer Treatment Group did conduct a randomized controlled trial to compare megestrol acetate (800 mg/d) to fluoxymesterone (10 mg po b.i.d.). In this trial, the anabolic steroid, fluoxymesterone, performed much less well than did megestrol acetate (43). Thus, at this time, anabolic steroids are not recommended as a therapy for cancer anorexia/cachexia.

C. Pentoxifylline

Preliminary reports suggested that pentoxifylline was able to inhibit tumor necrosis factor (44). In response, a placebo-controlled trial was conducted to look at this drug. This trial did not suggest any benefit for pentoxifylline as a means for alleviating cancer anorexia/cachexia (45).

D. Cyproheptadine

Cyproheptadine, a serotonin antagonist, has been shown to increase weight in children with asthma and pulmonary tuberculosis, children who are small for their age, and adults who are thin but otherwise healthy (46–48). At the Mayo Clinic, 16 patients with metastatic carcinoid were entered into a study and received cyproheptadine to evaluate whether it had any antitumor activity in this disease (49). No evidence of cytotoxic activity was seen, but 12 of the patients who received the drug for at least 2 months gained a median of 9 lb (5–30 lb). Based on these observations, 295 patients with advanced malignant disease were randomized to receive cyproheptadine or a placebo; the patients receiving cyproheptadine had a very mild enhancement in their appetite but this did not translate into weight gain (39). It was thought that the mild appetite enhancement from cyproheptadine was "a little too little, too late."

E. Hydrazine Sulfate

Hydrazine sulfate is a substance that inhibits the enzyme, phosphoenolpyruvate kinase. Following the reports of several small clinical trials (50–54), three large placebo-controlled studies were conducted (55–57). None of these three trials reported any suggestion of benefit for this drug.

F. Branched Chain Amino Acids

Branched chain amino acids are thought to decrease tryptophan transport to the brain by competitive inhibition and, in turn, lead to decreased brain serotonin. In animals, lower levels of brain serotonin can lead to an improved appetite. Preliminary data suggest that branched chain amino acids given orally can alleviate cancer-associated anorexia (58). In a prospective study by Hunter et al., cachectic cancer patients were given either branched chain amino acid enhanced or standard total parenteral nutrition. There was increased protein and albumin synthesis and a decrease in tyrosine oxidation (indicating improved protein utilization), supporting a positive benefit from branched chain amino acid enhanced nutrition in cancer cachexia (59). At this time, however, it is premature to recommend branched chain amino acids as a therapy for cancer anorexia/cachexia. Further work is planned to evaluate branched chain amino acids for cachectic patients.

G. Dronabinol

Tetrahydro-cannabinol (dronabinol) has been studied in acquired immunodeficiency syndrome (AIDS)-associated anorexia/cachexia. A randomized trial reported that dronabinol increased appetite in AIDS patients, resulting in Food and Drug Administration (FDA) approval of this drug for treatment of anorexia in this population (60). A few pilot studies have suggested that dronabinol also increases appetite in patients with advanced cancer (61,62). The precise mechanism of action of this in alleviating anorexia is not known. Further work is ongoing to prospectively evaluate the use of dronabinol as a drug to treat cancer anorexia/cachexia.

H. Corticosteroids

The first drugs to be studied for cancer anorexia/cachexia were corticosteroids. The first such trial was a double-blind clinical trial conducted at the Mayo Clinic in the 1970s (63). This trial evaluated dexamethasone in 116 patients with far advanced colon cancer. These patients were randomized to receive dexamethasone at 0.75 mg four times a day versus 1.5 mg four times a day versus a placebo. This trial reported a transient but statistically significant improvement in patient appetites for those randomized to receive dexamethasone. Two other randomized, double-blind, placebo-controlled studies evaluated (1) oral prednisolone (5 mg three times a day) (64) or (2) methylprednisolone (15 mg b.i.d.) (65) in patients with advanced cancer given for a short period of time (5–14 days). In these two studies, a significant improvement in anorexia was reported with the use of steroids. In another trial, methylprednisolone (125 mg/d) (66) was given intravenously for 8 weeks to female patients with advanced cancer. Again, this corticosteroid considerably improved appetites in the studied women.

I. Progestational Agents

The most extensively studied agent for cancer anorexia/cachexia is megestrol acetate. Less well studied is another progestational agent, medroxyprogesterone acetate, a drug that appears to have similar effects on appetite as does megestrol acetate (67). Megestrol acetate is a progestational agent, which, when used in patients with breast cancer or prostate cancer, was noted to be associated with weight gain (68,69). This observation led to several placebo-controlled randomized trials investigating its use in cancer cachexia (with doses ranging from 240 to 1,600 mg/d). Each of these trials demonstrated that this drug significantly improved appetites (36,70,71). In addition to showing that megestrol acetate improves appetites, several trials have also demonstrated that megestrol acetate leads to nonfluid weight gain (37,38,70,71). Furthermore, three placebo-controlled trials have reported statistically significant antiemetic properties of megestrol acetate (36,72). A dose-response trial, evaluating drug doses of 160, 480, 800, and 1,280 mg/d, demonstrated a positive dose-response as megestrol acetate increased from 160 mg/d up to 800 mg/d (40). A trial in AIDS patients also reported a similar dose-response effect (73).

Megestrol acetate is well tolerated overall. Withdrawal menstrual bleeding occurs within 1 to 4 weeks after discontinuing megestrol acetate and other irregularities of menses may occur (74). Impotence, which is reversible, occurs in a minority of men (73). Patients may experience minimal peripheral edema, which can be managed easily with a low dose of a diuretic. Megestrol acetate may slightly increase the risk of thromboembolic phenomenon, especially when used with chemotherapy (40,75). Patients receiving high doses of megestrol acetate can have suppression of adrenal-pituitary axis and can have an addisonian crisis upon abrupt withdrawl of the drug (76,77). Therefore, stress doses of corticosteroids are recommended if patients on megestrol acetate, or those who recently stopped it, experience either addisonian symptoms or the stress of surgery, trauma, or sepsis.

IV. TREATMENT RECOMMENDATIONS

Who should be teated for cancer anorexia/cachexia? When should they be teated and for how long? What should be used?

Because prophylactic use of megestrol acetate was unable to improve survival rate or quality of life when administered to newly diagnosed patients with extensive stage small cell lung cancer (75), the treatment of cancer anorexia/cachexia should be used only when anorexia and cachexia starts to be a bothersome clinical problem in an individual patient. For such a patient, megestrol acetate appears to be the most reasonable agent to use. It is rational to initially use a dose of 800 mg/d, given the results from the dose-response studies (40,73). However, it is also reasonable to start at lower doses (240–400 mg/d), given the placebo-controlled trials demonstrating benefit at these dose levels and the expense of high drug doses (37,38). In the United States, a liquid megestrol acetate formulation is considerably less expensive than a tablet formulation; although, even with the liquid preparation, the drug can cost several dollars per day. The effect of megestrol acetate on appetite stimulation is usually evident within several days. If the drug is ineffective after a week, then changes in approach are reasonable (going up to a higher dose, or stopping the drug if high doses are not helping). For patients who are gaining too much weight at higher doses of megestrol acetate, lower doses can be used, or the drug can be stopped and then restarted if appetite loss again becomes problematic.

As an alternative to using megestrol acetate, a corticosteroid (e.g., dexamethasone 0.75 mg po q.i.d.) can be used for treating cancer anorexia/cachexia. A potential advantage of this approach is that drug costs are considerably less than with megestrol acetate, but there is concern that corticosteroids might be more toxic. A randomized trial by the North Central Cancer Treatment Group (NCCTG) has been conducted to compare megestrol acetate to dexamethasone, the final results of which are pending.

V. CONCLUSION

Cancer-induced anorexia/cachexia is a significant and common problem. The exact mechanisms of pathogenesis of anorexia and cachexia are not well understood. Abnormalities in carbohydrate, fat, and protein metabolism have been described. Several humoral factors such as TNF-α, IL1, IL-6 and LMF have been implicated as mediators of this syndrome. Increased brain serotonin concentration resulting from increased availability of its precursor, tryptophan, in the brain may be a common final pathway in the pathogenesis of anorexia/cachexia. Megestrol acetate and corticosteroids represent proven means for abrogating cancer anorexia/cachexia, although only to a limited degree.

REFERENCES

1. Warren S. The immediate cause of death in cancer. Am J Med Sci 1932; 184:610–614.
2. Shils M. Nutritional problems induced by cancer. Med Clin North Am 1979; 63: 1009–1025.
3. Dewys W, Begg C, Lavin P, et al. Prognostic effect of weight loss prior to chemotherapy in cancer patients. Am J Med 1980; 69:491–497.
4. Bernstein I. Etiology of anorexia in cancer. Cancer 1986; 58:1881–1886.
5. Krause R, Humphrey C, von Meyenfeldt M, et al. A central mechanism for anorexia in cancer. Cancer Treat Rep 1981; 65:15.
6. Laviano A, Renvyle T, Meguid MM, et al. Relationship between interleukin-1 and cancer anorexia. Nutrition 1995; 11:680–683.
7. Rossi-Fanelli F, Cangiano C, Ceci F, et al. Plasma tryptophan and anorexia in human cancer. Eur J Cancer Clin Oncol 1986; 22:89.
8. Cangiano C, Cascino A, Ceci F, et al. Plasma and CSF tryptophan in cancer anorexia. J Neural Transm 1990; 81:225–233.
9. Muscaritoli M, Meguid M, Beverly L, et al. Mechanism of early tumor anorexia. J Surg Res 1996; 60:389–397.
10. Cangiano C, Testa U, Muscaritoli M, et al. Cytokines, tryptophan and anorexia in cancer patients before and after surgical tumor ablation. Anticancer Res 1994; 14: 1454.
11. Cangiano C, Alegiani F, Bartoli R, et al. Effetti clinici e nutrizionali della somministrazione di una nuova miscela di amino acidi essenziali in pazienti in trattamento dialitico continuato. Riv It Nutr Clin 1987; 5:27.
12. Kopple J, Jones M, Fukuda S, et al. Amino acid and protein metabolism in renal failure. Am J Clin Nutr 1978; 31:1532.
13. Laviano A, Cangiano C, Preziosa I, et al. Serotoninergic block in the venteromedial nucleus of hypothalamus improves food intake in anorectic tumor bearing rats. In Gea, F., ed. Recent Advances in Tryptophan Research. New York: Plenum Press, 1996.
14. Bennegard K, Lundgren F, Lundholm K. Mechanisms of insulin resistance in cancer associated malnutrition. Clin Physiol 1986; 6:539–547.
15. Rofe A, Bourgeois C, Coyle P, et al. Altered insulin response to glucose in weight-losing cancer patients. Anticancer Res 1994; 114:647–650.

16. Lundholm K, Byland A, Schersten T. Glucose tolerance in relation to skeletal muscle enzyme activities in cancer patients. Scand J Clin Invest 1977; 37:2670–2672.
17. Norton J, Stein T, Brennan M. Whole body protein turnover studies in normal humans and malnourished patients with and without cancer. Ann Surg 1980; 31:94–96.
18. Carmichael M, Clague M, Kier M, et al. Whole body protein turnover, synthesis, and breakdown in patients with colorectal carcinoma. Br J Surg 1980; 67:736–769.
19. Shaw J, Humberstone D, Wolfe R. Energy and protein metabolism in sarcoma patients. Ann Surg 1988; 207:283–289.
20. Shaw J, Humberstone D, Douglas R, et al. Leucine kinetics in patients with benign disease, non-weight losing cancer, and cancer cachexia: studies at the whole-body and tissue level and the response to nutritional support. Surgery 1991; 109:37–50.
21. Beutler B, Cerami A. Cachectin and tumor necrosis factor as two sides of the same biological coin. Nature 1986; 320:584–588.
22. Mahony S, Beck S, Tisdale M. Comparison of weight loss induced by recombinant tumor necrosis factor with that produced by a cachexia-inducing tumor. Br J Cancer 1988; 57:385–389.
23. Oliff A, Defeo-Jones D, Boyer M, et al. Tumors secreting human TNF/cachectin induce cachexia in mice. Cell 1987; 50:555–563.
24. Sherry B, Gelin G, Fong Y, et al. Anticachectin/tumor necrosis factor-α antibodies attenuate development of cachexia in tumor models. FASEB J 1989; 3:1956–1962.
25. Yoneda T, Alsina M, Chavez J, et al. Evidence that tumor necrosis factor plays a pathogenetic role in paraneoplastic syndromes of cachexia, hypercalcemia and leukocytosis in a human tumor in nude mice. J Clin Invest 1991; 87:977–985.
26. Mulligan H, Mahony S, Ross J, et al. Weight loss in a murine cachexia model is not associated with the cytokines tumor-necrosis factor α or interleukin-6. Cancer Lett 1992; 65:239–243.
27. Saarinen U, Koskelo E-K, Teppo A, et al. Tumor necrosis factor in children with malignancies. Cancer Res 1990; 50:592–595.
28. Jablons D, McIntosh J, Mule JJ, et al. Induction of interferon β2/interleukin-6 (IL-6) by cytokine administration and detection of circulating IL-6 in the tumor bearing state. Ann N Y Acad Sci 1989; 577:157–160.
29. Strassman G, Fong M, Kenney J, et al. Evidence for the involvement in interleukin-6 in experimental cancer cachexia. J Clin Invest 1992; 89:1681–1684.
30. Greenberg A, Nordan R, McIntosh J, et al. Interleukin 6 reduces lipoprotein lipase activity in adipose tissue of mice in vivo and in 3T3-L1 adipoyctes: a possible role for interleukin 6 in cancer cachexia. Cancer Res 1992; 52:4113–4116.
31. Langstein H, Doherty G, Fraker D, et al. The roles of γ interferon and tumor necrosis factor α in an experimental rat model of cancer cachexia. Cancer Res 1991; 51: 2302–2306.
32. Matthys P, Hermnas H, Opdenakker G, et al. Anti-interferon γ antibody treatment, growth of Lewis lung tumors in mice and tumor associated cancer cachexia. Eur J Cancer 1991; 27:182–187.
33. Masuno H, Yamasaki N, Okuda H. Purification of and characterization of a lipolytic factor (toxohormone-L) from cell free fluid of ascites sarcoma 180. Cancer Res 1981; 41:284–288.

34. Masuno H, Yoshimura H, Ogawa N, et al. Isolation of a lipolytic factor (toxohormone-L) from ascites fluid of patients with hepatoma and its effect on feeding behavior. Eur J Cancer Clin Oncol 1984; 20:1177–1185.
35. Kitada S, Hays E, Mead J. A lipid mobilizing factor in serum of tumor-bearing mice. Lipids 1980; 15:168–174.
36. Loprinzi C, Ellison N, Dose A, et al. Controlled trial of megestrol acetate for the treatment of cancer anorexia and cachexia. J Natl Cancer Inst 1990; 82:1127–1132.
37. Feliu J, Gonzalez-Baron M, Berrocal A, et al. Treatment of cancer anorexia with megestrol acetate: which is the optimal dose? J Nat Cancer Inst 1991; 83:449.
38. Bruera E, Macmillan K, Kuehn N, et al. A controlled trial of megestrol acetate on appetite, caloric intake, nutritional status, and other symptoms in patients with advanced cancer. Cancer 1990; 66:1279–1282.
39. Kardinal C, Loprinzi C, Scaid D, et al. A controlled trial of cyproheptadine in cancer patients with anorexia and/or cachexia. Cancer 1990; 65:2657–2662.
40. Loprinzi C, Michalak J, Schaid D, et al. Phase III evaluation of four doses of megestrol acetate as therapy for patients with cancer anorexia and/or cachexia. J Clin Oncol 1993; 11:762–767.
41. Loprinzi CL. Should cancer patients with incurable disease receive parenteral or enteral nutritional support-bridging (editorial). Eur J Cancer 1998; 34:284–285.
42. Chlebowski R, Herrold J, Ali I, et al. Influence of nandrolone decanoate on weight loss in advanced non-small cell lung cancer. Cancer 1986; 58:183–186.
43. Loprinzi CL, Kugler J, Sloan J, Mailliard J, Krook J, Wilwerding M, Rowland K, Camoriano J. Phase III randomized comparison of megestrol acetate, dexamethasone, and fluoxymesterone for the treatment of cancer anorexia cachexia. Proc Am Soc Clin Oncol 1997; 48:167.
44. Dezube B, Fridovbich-Keil J, Bouvard I, et al. Pentoxifylline and wellbeing in patients with cancer. Lancet 1990; 335:662.
45. Goldberg R, Loprinzi C, Mailliard J, et al. Pentoxyfylline for the treatment of cancer anorexia/cachexia? A randomized, double-blinded, placebo controlled trial. J Clin Oncol 1995; 13:2856–2859.
46. Antoon A, Bode H, Crawford J. Effect of cyproheptadine on growth in short underweight children. Pediatr Res 1973; 7:310–382.
47. Lavenstein A, Dacaney E, Lasagna L, et al. Effect of cyproheptadine on asthmatic children: study of appetite, weight gain, and linear growth. JAMA 1962; 180:912–916.
48. Shah N. A double-blind study on appetite stimulation and weight gain with cyproheptadine as adjunct to specific therapy in pulmonary tuberculosis. Curr Med Pract 1968; 12:861–864.
49. Moertel C, Kvols L, Rubin J. A study of cyproheptadine in the treatment of metastatic carcinoid tumor and the maliganant carcinoid syndrome. Cancer 1991; 67:33–36.
50. Lerner H, Regelson W. Clinical trial of hydrazine sulphate in solid tumors. Cancer Treat Rep 1976; 60:959–960.
51. Spermulli E, Wampler G, Regelson W. Clinical study of hydrazine sulphate in advancd cancer patients. Cancer Chemother Pharmacol 1979; 3:121–124.
52. Gold J. Use of hydrazine sulphate in terminal and preterminal cancer patients: results

of a new investigational drug (IND) study in 84 evaluable patients. Oncology 1975; 32:1–10.
53. Chlebowski R, Heber D, Richardson B, et al. Influence of hydrazine sulphate on abnormal carbohydrate metabolism in cancer patients with weight loss. Cancer Res 1984; 44:857–867.
54. Ochua MJ, Wittes R, Krakoff L. Trial of hydrazine sulphate (NSC 150014) in patients with cancer. Cancer Chemother Rep 1975; 59:1151–1153.
55. Loprinzi C, Kuross S, O'Fallon J, et al. Randomized placebo-controlled evaluation of hydrazine sulphate in patients with advanced colorectal cancer. J Clin Oncol 1994; 12:1121–1125.
56. Loprinzi C, Goldberg R, Su J, et al. Placebo-controlled trial of hydrazine sulphate in patients with newly diagnosed non-small cell lung cancer. J Clin Oncol 1994; 12:1126–1129.
57. Kosty M, Fleishman S, Herndon J, et al. Cispaltin, vinblastine and hydrazine sulphate (NSC # 150014) in advanced non-small cell lung cancer (NSCLC): a randomized, palcebo-controlled, double-blind phase III study. Proc Am Soc Clin Oncol 1992; 11:294.
58. Cangiano C, Laviano A, Meguid MM, et al. Effects of administration of oral branched-chain amino acids on anorexia and caloric intake in cancer patients. J Nat Cancer Inst 1996; 88:550–552.
59. Hunter DC, Weintraub M, Blackburn GL, et al. Branched chain amino acids as the protein component of parenteral nutrition in cancer cachexia. Br J Surg 1989; 76: 149–153.
60. Beal J, Olson R, Laubenstein L, et al: Dronabinol as a treatment for anorexia associated with weight loss in patients with AIDS. J Pain Sympt Manag 1995; 10:89.
61. Nelson K, Walsh D, Deeter P, et al. A phase II study of delta-9-tetrahydrocannabinol for appetite stimulation in cancer-associated anorexia. J Palliat Care 1994; 10:14–18.
62. Plasse T, Gorter R, Krasnow S, et al. Recent clinical experience with dronabinol. Pharm Biochem Behav 1991; 40:695–700.
63. Moertel C, Schutt A, Reitmeier R, et al. Corticosteroid therapy of preterminal gastrointestinal cancer. Cancer 1974; 33:1607–1609.
64. Willox JC, Corr J, Shaw J, et al. Prednisolone as an appetite stimulant in patients with cancer. BMJ 1984; 288:27.
65. Bruera E, Roca E, Cedaro L, et al. Action of oral methylprednisolone in terminal cancer patients: a prospective randomized double-blind study. Cancer Treat Rep 1985; 69:751–754.
66. Popiela T, Lucchi R, Giongo F. Methylprednisolone as palliative therapy for female terminal cancer patients. Eur J Cancer Clin Oncol 1989; 25:1823–1829.
67. Simons JP, Aaronson NK, Vansteenkiste JF, et al. Effects of medroxyprogestrone acetate on appetite, weight, and quality of life in advanced-stage non-hormone sensitive cancer: a placebo-controlled study. J Clin Oncol 1996; 14:1077–1084.
68. Gregory E, Cohen S, Oines D, et al. Megestrol acetate therapy for advanced breast cancer. J Clin Oncol 1985; 3:155–160.
69. Bonomi P, Pessis D, Bunting N, et al. Megestrol acetate used as primary hormonal therapy in stage D prostate cancer. Semin Oncol 1985; 12:36–39.

70. Tchekmediyan N, Hickman M, Siau J, et al. Megestrol acetate in cancer anorexia and weight loss. Cancer 1992; 69:1268–1274.
71. Tchekmediyan N, Tait N, Moody M, et al. Appetite stimulation with megestrol acetate in cachectic cancer patients. Semin Oncol 1986; 13:37–43.
72. Tchekmedyian N, Hickman M, Siau J, et al. Treatment of cancer anorexia with megestrol acetate: impact on quality of life. Oncology 1991; 5:119–126.
73. Von Roenn J, Armstrong D, Kotler D, et al. Megestrol acetate in patients with AIDS-related cachexia. Ann Intern Med 1994; 121:393–399.
74. Loprinzi C, Michalak J, Quella S, et al. Megestrol acetate for the prevention of hot flashes. N Engl J Med 1994; 33:347–352.
75. Rowland KJ, Loprinzi C, Shaw E, et al. Randomized double blind placebo controlled trial of cisplatin and etoposide plus megestrol acetate/placebo in extensive stage small cell lung cancer: a North Central Cancer Treatment Group study. J Clin Oncol 1996; 14:135–141.
76. Loprinzi CL, Jensen M, Jiang N, et al. The effect of megestrol acetate on the human pituitary-adrenal axis. Mayo Clin Proc 1992; 12:1160–1162.
77. Leinung M, Liporace R, Miller C. Induction of adrenal suppression by megestrol acetate in patients with AIDS. Ann Intern Med 1995; 122:843–845.

14

Sexual Health and Functioning After Cancer

Patricia A. Ganz
University of California, Los Angeles, and Jonsson Comprehensive Cancer Center, Los Angeles, California

Beth E. Meyerowitz and Martin A. Perez
University of Southern California, Los Angeles, California

I. INTRODUCTION

Among the many aspects of health and well-being, sexual health is seldom discussed by the patient and physician unless there are medically related symptoms (e.g., sexually transmitted diseases) or there is severe disruption of sexual functioning related to physical or psychological illness. Humans are sexual beings, yet sexual health is often taken for granted. Sexuality is considered a private matter and not usually the domain of the physician's office. Thus, most physicians have little experience discussing sexual health with their patients and are poorly prepared to address their sexual concerns.

Sexual health and functioning can be important to the cancer patient. Lifesaving cancer treatments often affect physical and psychological well-being, and pose a serious threat to body image. Many surgical procedures have direct physical effects on the organs of sexual functioning. While struggling to overcome their cancer, many patients forego normal sexual relations because of the severe fatigue and symptoms that decrease their sexual interest; however, during recovery from treatment, resumption of normal sexual relations is often a signal of return to health. At any point during the cancer experience, patients can benefit from the advice and counsel of their physicians on issues related to sexual health and functioning.

This chapter reviews normal sexual health including the human sexual response cycle, age-related changes in sexual health and functioning, and common sexual problems and syndromes. This review is followed by a discussion of some of the effects of cancer therapies on sexual functioning. Finally, a brief assessment of sexual problems in the cancer patient is described and simple recommendations are made on how to intervene effectively on these issues. This chapter gives the reader the basic knowledge and skills to address these issues with patients, knowing that the oncologist is the central professional providing support to patients during their experience with cancer.

II. SEXUAL HEALTH

To understand the impact of cancer and its treatments on sexuality, patients must place these changes in the context of healthy sexual functioning. However, despite the importance of sexuality in people's lives, very few individuals are knowledgeable about sexual anatomy, physiology, or functioning. These aspects of sexuality are rarely taught or discussed. Thus, when cancer is diagnosed and treated, both the patient and his or her partner are likely to lack information and to hold misperceptions about sexuality and sexual functioning. Moreover, many patients are already dealing with the changes in sexuality associated with aging. In this section, basic sexual functioning is described with an emphasis on common misperceptions and on changes that occur with aging, in order to provide a context in which to understand sexual functioning after cancer. This information can alert clinicians to areas in which patients may frequently need education.

A. Human Sexual Response Cycle

Approximately 40 years ago, Masters and Johnson (1) began laboratory studies of sexual functioning. Their goal was to describe the physiological changes that women and men undergo when they are aroused sexually. On the basis of observing and measuring thousands of orgasmic cycles, they concluded that there is a four-phase human sexual response cycle. Their research indicated that, with adequate arousal, the physiological responses in each of the four phases are similar in healthy individuals regardless of the source of arousal (e.g., vaginal or penile intercourse, clitoral stimulation through masturbation, oral sex), the sexual orientation of the individual, or the feelings or thoughts involved in the arousal. The physiological changes that occur at each phase for women and men are listed in Tables 1 and 2. Most patients are likely to be unfamiliar with this basic information about sexual functioning. Rather, they are likely to hold some of the misperceptions described in the following paragraphs.

Table 1 Human Sexual Response Cycle in Women

Excitement
Vaginal lubrication begins
Heart rate and muscle tension increase
Breasts swell and nipples become erect
Uterus enlarges from vascular engorgement
Uterus begins to elevate
Labia majora separate and elevate
Vaginal canal lengthens
Plateau
Vasocongestive response of the primary sex organs reaches its peak
Labia minora swell and become darker in color
Uterus completes ascent from the pelvic floor
Outer two-thirds of vagina swells to form the "orgasmic platform"
Clitoris retracts under clitoral hood
Inner third of vagina widens to create tenting effect
Orgasm
Contractions of the circumvaginal and perineal muscles
Resolution
Thin film of perspiration covers body
Body returns to its basal state

1. Excitement Phase

Shortly after the start of sexual stimulation, a vasocongestive response begins that is marked by blood flowing into the gentials and breast tissue. This vasocongestion, which is responsible for erection in men and vaginal lubrication and nipple erection in women, continues throughout the excitement and plateau phases. This phase is also marked by increased muscle tension, heart rate, blood pressure, and respiratory rate. As excitement continues, the testes and uterus enlarge and elevate. The vaginal canal, which is usually a potential space, begins to lengthen.

Some patients may be unaware that vasocongestion is responsible for erection and vaginal lubrication. A more common, and potentially problematic misconception, is that the start of vaginal lubrication is a sign that the woman is physically ready for vaginal penetration. If penetration occurs before the uterus elevates and the vagina lengthens, however, pain can result from thrusting that hits the cervix. Many couples also may be unaware that, because nerve endings in the clitoris are very sensitive, direct stimulation can be painful for many women. For most women, however, indirect stimulation of the clitoris, through movement of the labia minora and clitoral hood or through stimulation above or to the side of the clitoris, is likely to be more arousing than vaginal stimulation

Table 2 Human Sexual Response Cycle in Men

Excitement
Penile erection begins
Heart and muscle tension increase
Scrotum thickness
Testes elevate
Plateau
Testes enlarge to 150% their basal size
Testes elevate close to perineum
Vasocongestive response of the primary sex organs reaches its peak
Urethra increases in diameter
Drops of clear mucoid fluid from the Cowper's gland appear on the tip of the penis
Point of "ejaculatory inevitability" is reached
Orgasm
Emission
Ejaculation
Contractions of the penile urethra and perineal and bulbocavernosus muscles
Resolution
Thin film of perspiration covers body
Body gradually returns to its basal state
Refractory period temporarily prevents sexual arousal

alone. With very few nerve endings, especially in the upper two-thirds of the vaginal canal, the vagina is not a particularly sensitive organ for most women, and vaginal stimulation alone is not sufficient for orgasm for many women.

2. *Plateau Phase*

The plateau phase involves a continuation of the processes begun in the excitement phase—vasocongestion of pelvic area and breasts, myotonia, quickened breathing, and increased heart rate and blood pressure. In women, although nipple erection continues, swelling of the areola makes it appear that the nipple has withdrawn. The clitoris pulls up under the clitoral hood.

Some partners think that the apparent withdrawal of the clitoris and nipples means that the woman is not enjoying stimulation of these areas, when actually the withdrawal is a sign of increasing arousal. There are also several internal changes, as noted in Tables 1 and 2. By the end of the plateau phase in women, the outer portion of the vagina has swollen to the extent that the vaginal walls will almost touch if nothing is inserted or will expand to accommodate and to grip what has been inserted, such as a penis or fingers. Near the end of the plateau phase in men, the Cowper's gland secretes a few drops of fluid. Many individuals are unaware of the fact that Cowper's secretions can contain live sperm.

3. Orgasm Phase

Orgasm is the contractions of the genitals and pelvic floor muscles. Many couples do not know that for most women to experience a complete orgasm, or multiple orgasms in some cases, stimulation is necessary throughout the orgasm phase. Several different types of orgasms have been described for women, ranging from strong and intense contractions to mild and wavelike contractions. Women who experience milder orgasms are not always certain that orgasm has occurred.

The orgasm phase for men differs from that of women in several ways. According to Masters and Johnson, men do not report the same variety of orgasmic experiences that women do. Rather, men typically experience a fairly strong series of several muscle contractions, except for some older men for whom the intensity of contractions decreases. For men, the orgasm occurs in two stages—(1) emission, the contraction of internal and external reproductive organs, and (2) ejaculation, the expulsion of seminal fluid and sperm through the urethra. Emission and ejaculation usually occur almost simultaneously, although certain physical problems can disrupt one or the other process. In contrast to women, men reach a "point of ejaculatory inevitability" immediately before orgasm. At that point, even if stimulation ceases entirely, men will experience orgasm, although perhaps with less intensity than if stimulation had continued. Some men may attempt to distract themselves at this point in hopes of delaying the onset of orgasm. This approach results only in decreasing the enjoyment of the orgasm, but it is not successful in delaying it. Finally, Masters and Johnson reported that men, unlike women, are incapable of having multiple orgasms, although more recently there has been some controversy on this point.

4. Resolution Phase

Immediately following orgasm, a thin film of perspiration forms over the body and nipple erection becomes obvious once again. Most individuals experience a sense of relaxation and calm as the body returns to the prearousal state. The orgasm causes the blood in the pelvic region to return to the rest of the body, and the uterus, vagina, and testes return to their usual positions. If orgasm does not occur following the plateau phase, both men and women can experience an uncomfortable pelvic heaviness for some time until pelvic vasocongestion decreases. For men, the resolution phase occurs in two stages. The first stage takes place immediately following orgasm and involves a partial reduction in erection. The second stage takes place more gradually, as the remaining penile vasocongestion decreases and the erection disappears. Men also experience a refractory period, ranging from minutes in young men to a day or more in older men, during which they are physically unable to become aroused. It is important for partners to know that penile stimulation can be unpleasant during the refractory period; some partners can feel hurt if the man rejects stimulation even though he appears to have a partial erection.

B. Changes in Sexuality with Aging

Even without the effects of illness and medication, older patients may have a decline in sexual capacity that is normal to the aging process. Some of these patients may misinterpret these natural changes as sexual dysfunction related to the cancer experience, unless they receive accurate information about changes in sexuality related to aging. The oncology team can play an important role in providing this basic information.

The most common changes in sexual functioning associated with age are listed in Table 3. For most older men and women, the vasocongestion process is slowed, the duration of some phases of the sexual response cycle is increased, and the intensity of orgasm is decreased. More tactile stimulation is usually required for arousal and orgasm than is needed in younger men or women. In addition to these physical changes, many older men and women report declines in sexual desire and the frequency of sexual thoughts (2,3).

Age-related declines in sexual capacity do not imply an absence of sexual interest, however. Many healthy older adults remain interested in sex and continue to report sexual satisfaction throughout their lives. Frequency of sexual activity in older adults appears to be related primarily to level of sexual activity during younger years, with those who were active when younger showing less

Table 3 Age-Related Changes in Sexual Response

Older men
Sexual desire declines
Erections are less rigid
Erections take longer to achieve
Erections require more direct tactile stimulation
Ejaculation is less forceful
Refractory period is longer
Older women
Vaginal lubrication decreases
Vaginal lubrication takes longer to achieve
Vaginal walls thin
Vaginal barrel shrinks and loses elasticity

of a decline with aging (2). However, an absence of sexual activity should not be taken to mean an absence of sexual desire or interest. Many older adults who would like to be sexually active may lack a willing and able partner, and they may have moral constraints against engaging in self-pleasuring activities. Also, individuals who react negatively to normal changes in sexuality may become anxious regarding their sexual capacity and sexual difficulties may develop; others may be aware that the changes are normal and adapt their sexual behavior accordingly.

C. Menopause and Sexual Functioning

In addition to these general changes in sexuality that both men and women experience, many women also experience physical changes with menopause. A woman is not considered ''menopausal'' until she has gone without a menstrual period for 1 full year. Women between the ages of 40 and 50 are considered ''perimenopausal,'' and this is often described as the transition phase from premenopausal to postmenopausal status. During this time, ovarian function begins to diminish (irregular menses, anovulatory cycles), and women may experience a variety of menopausal symptoms including hot flashes, vaginal discomfort, changes in bladder function, and beginning of acceleration in bone loss (osteoporosis). Women also often experience mood changes and changes in sexual desire during this time. These symptoms frequently develop during the perimenopausal phase and may continue into the postmenopausal years.

For women without other significant illness, the menopause is often a gradual process. For women who have had cancer, however, it may be more abrupt, caused by a surgical procedure that removes the ovaries, or by chemotherapy or hormone therapy, which may damage or diminish ovarian function. Menopause may occur after certain chemotherapy (e.g., alkylating agents) at any age; however, the closer a women is to the age of normal menopause, the more likely she is to lose her ovarian function as a result of chemotherapy. Younger women who stop ovulating for a period of time sometimes later regain ovarian function. There is a general belief that a more abrupt menopause is more difficult to cope with and that the consequences may be more severe, both symptomatically and sexually.

Coping with the effects of estrogen loss can be a daunting experience for some women. Each person is different, and the combination of symptoms and experiences often varies significantly from one woman to the next. Hot flashes and vaginal dryness are two problems that appear to be the most disturbing. The former can indirectly have an impact on sexuality through its effect on fatigue and energy level, whereas the latter may contribute directly to poor vaginal lubrication and sexual dysfunction.

D. Triphasic Model of Sexual Functioning

Subsequent to the publication of Masters and Johnson's findings, other sexologists, most notably Kaplan (4), argued that a complete description of the human sexual response cycle required inclusion of a desire phase prior to the start of arousal. Desire is a multidimensional construct including emotional, cognitive, hormonal, physical, interpersonal, and motivational components. With the addition of a desire phase, researchers suggested a model of sexual functioning to include desire, arousal (subsuming the excitement and plateau phases of the sexual response cycle identified by Masters and Johnson), and orgasm phases. This triphasic model has served as the basis for diagnostic categorization of sexual dysfunctions.

III. COMMON SEXUAL DYSFUNCTIONS AND PROBLEMS

The sexual response requires a complex interplay of biological/physical, psychological, interpersonal, and cultural variables. Cancer and its treatments can disrupt one or all of these variables. The following is an overview of the most common sexual dysfunctions and problems, so that changes resulting from cancer can be placed in this broader context. It can be important for patients and their partners to realize that almost all couples, even happily married ones, experience sexual difficulties at some point in their lives.

A. Diagnosable Sexual Dysfunctions

A deficiency in any of the phases of the triphasic sexual response cycle is a diagnosable sexual dysfunction. Table 4 provides a description for each of the sexual dysfunctions that appear in the *Diagnostic and Statistical Manual of Mental Disorders* (5). In addition to meeting criteria for the essential feature of the disorder, a patient must report that the problem is recurrent or persistent and that he or she experiences individual or relationship distress because of the sexual problem.

For all diagnoses of sexual dysfunction, the clinician must use his or her judgment to determine what factors may be contributing to the problem. Not surprisingly, rates of all of the dysfunctions listed herein tend to be higher in individuals in poor health (6). With cancer patients, a sexual problem may or may not be a direct result of the cancer treatment. A sexual problem may be better accounted for by another psychological disorder such as depression, or it may be related to an individual's age, sexual experience, or duration and type of sexual stimulation. Furthermore, it is important to consider the nature of patients' relationships with their sexual partners as a possible contributor to the dysfunc-

Table 4 Sexual Dysfunctions

The sexual dysfunctions are disturbances that cause marked distress or interpersonal difficulty as a result of persistent or recurrent problems in the following areas:

Sexual desire disorders

Hypoactive sexual desire disorder—Deficiency or absence of sexual fantasies and desire for sexual activity

Sexual aversion disorder—Aversion to and active avoidance of genital sexual contact with a sexual partner

Sexual arousal disorders

Female sexual arousal disorder—Persistent or recurrent inability to attain or to maintain until completion of the sexual activity an adequate lubrication-swelling response of sexual excitement

Male erectile disorder—Persistent or recurrent inability to attain or to maintain until completion of the sexual activity an adequate erection

Orgasmic disorders

Female orgasmic disorder—Persistent or recurrent delay in, or absence of, orgasm following a normal sexual excitement phase

Orgasmic disorders in males:

Male orgasmic disorder—Persistent or recurrent delay in, or absence of, orgasm following a normal sexual excitement phase

Premature eiaculation—Persistent or recurrent onset of orgasm and ejaculation with minimal sexual stimulation before, on, or shortly after penetration and before the person wishes it

Sexual pain disorders

Dyspareunia—Genital pain that is associated with sexual intercourse; most commonly experienced during coitus but may also occur before or after intercourse

Sexual pain disorder in females (vaginismus)—Recurrent or persistent involuntary contraction of the perineal muscles surrounding the outer third of the vagina when vagina penetration with penis, finger, tampon, or speculum is attempted

Source: Ref. 5.

tion. A sexual dysfunction may be generalized, occurring in all instances, or situational, specific to certain situations or sex partners.

1. Sexual Desire Disorders

Hypoactive sexual desire is by far the more common of the desire disorders (see Table 4), and its prevalence appears to have increased markedly over the past 2 decades. The prevalence of hypoactive sexual desire in the general population is approximately 16% for men and 33% for women according to a recent national survey of adults younger than 60 years old (6). However, up to 55% of clinical samples have the disorder, with some studies indicating higher rates in men and others indicating higher rates in women (7). It can be difficult to make a differential diagnosis because hypoactive sexual desire usually presents with other sexual disorders, such as arousal disorders, making the primary cause of the problem difficult to isolate. Additionally, psychogenic desire disorders need to be distinguished from deficiencies in desire caused by medication, drug or alcohol abuse, depression, or serious relationship problems.

Sexual aversion disorder, an active avoidance of genital sexual contact with a sexual partner, can be associated with the experience of disgust, fear, or anxiety when the patient is confronted with a sexual opportunity with a partner. The prevalence rate for this disorder is not well documented, perhaps because of the difficulty of differentiating it from hypoactive sexual desire.

2. *Arousal Disorders*

Female sexual arousal disorder is the most common sexual problem reported by women seeking both sex therapy and marital therapy. In community studies, rates range from as low as 11% to as high as 48% (6,7). In making the diagnosis, it is especially important to distinguish age or medically related decreases in lubrication from overall failure to experience the excitement and plateau phases of the response cycle.

In men, erectile disorders may involve the inability to attain any kind of erection during sexual activity or the loss of erection prior to, attempting, or during sexual intercourse. Men with psychogenic origin of their erectile dysfunction usually experience nocturnal erections and may be able to attain erections during masturbation. As many as 50% of men report experiencing erectile difficulties at some point in their lives (7). The prevalence of diagnosable erectile disorder in the general population of men younger than 60 is approximately 10% (6), whereas rates for men by age 75 are close to 25% or more. In a clinical setting, erectile disorder is one of the most commonly diagnosed sexual problems in men, with close to half of men who seek treatment listing erectile disorder as a primary complaint. Rates of erectile disorder are especially high in clinical settings, such as those in urology departments, that have a medical, versus a psychological, focus.

3. *Orgasmic Disorders*

Female orgasmic disorder is reported by close to one fourth of women in community samples (6), with rates in clinical settings being substantially higher. Rates of primary anorgasmia, never having had an orgasm, are typically less than 10%, whereas some studies find a majority of women experience lack of orgasm through coitus alone (7). As noted earlier, many women require some degree of clitoral stimulation to reach orgasm, and the need for this stimulation should not be considered evidence of orgasmic disorders. The clinician must draw on his or her expertise to determine whether the level of stimulation the woman is receiving should be considered adequate for orgasm.

Orgasmic disorders in men can be indicated by either delayed or absent orgasm or by very rapid orgasms. In both cases, it requires considerable clinical experience to determine whether these problems are within normal limits or are indicative of sexual dysfunction. Male orgasmic disorder is relatively rare in clinical settings and has approximately an 8% prevalence rate in the general population (6). In contrast, premature ejaculation is commonly diagnosed in clinical settings and has a prevalence of approximately 30% in the general population (6). Many men experience rapid ejaculation at some points in their lives or in some sexual interactions (8). The clinician must make a judgment about the extent to which ejaculation is ''too rapid'' and about how often the rapid ejaculation has to occur in order for the man to have a diagnosable disorder. Rates of rapid ejaculation appear to decrease with age.

4. *Sexual Pain Disorders*

Although not specific to any one stage of the sexual response cycle, sexual pain disorders are diagnosable as sexual dysfunctions. Dyspareunia, genital pain associated with intercourse, is rarely diagnosed in men, occurring in only 3% of the general population (6). Pain in men is often associated with urinary tract infection or other medical causes. In contrast, dyspareunia is one of the more common complaints reported by women in clinical settings and in approximately 14% of the general population. The diagnosis of vaginismus is more difficult to make. The diagnosis should not be made on the basis of self-report alone, but requires pelvic examination. Reported rates of vaginismus in clinic populations vary widely across studies, with some studies indicating that it is a fairly common complaint (7). In diagnosing pain disorders, it is important to consider the possibility that the patient has experienced sexual abuse or trauma.

B. Other Sexual Problems

In addition to diagnosable disruption in physiological sexual functioning, other aspects of sexuality—sexual behaviors, sexual satisfaction, dyadic adjustment, and body image—need to be considered to provide a comprehensive assessment. The frequency and type of sexual behavior may change regardless of whether a patient meets criteria for a sexual dysfunction. For example, inability to engage in penile-vaginal intercourse may cause considerable distress for couples whose primary way of interacting sexually is through intercourse. This view may exacerbate or contribute to the onset of a diagnosable sexual dysfunction, unless alternative forms of sexual interaction can be integrated into the relationship. Many men are able to achieve orgasm regardless of erectile functioning and many couples may already include noncoital sexual activity in their sexual repertoire. Some data indicate that men who had experienced noncoital orgasms with their partner before cancer treatment had sexual activity more frequently following treatment than men who did not experience noncoital orgasm before treatment. Couples who are comfortable and knowledgeable regarding noncoital sexual activity are able to compensate for disruption in sexuality that renders the patient incapable of engaging in sexual intercourse or other previously enjoyable activities.

Another distinct component of sexuality is level of sexual satisfaction. Sexual satisfaction is an individual's subjective feeling of sexuality regardless of ability to progress through the human sexual response cycle. When sexual dysfunction has a primarily organic origin, a focus on sexual performance with the goal of restoring a patient's physical ability to engage in sexual activity may need to be replaced with a focus on improving subjective feelings regarding sexuality and sexual satisfaction.

For most people, a satisfying sexual relationship requires a healthy partner relationship in other areas, as well. Communication difficulties and lack of intimacy or trust are frequent contributors to sexual dysfunction (8). The relation between sexual dysfunctions or problems and relationship problems is typically bidirectional, with each exacerbating the other. Clinicians need to be aware that changes in relationships can be at the core of sexual problems.

Finally, body image can also be associated with problems in sexuality. Patients who experience difficulties in body image caused by disfiguring treatments or disruptions in bodily functioning may have an added barrier to overcome in restoring satisfying sexual relations. Additionally, some patients who do not experience any extreme physical alteration as a result of treatment, nonetheless can hold negative and deprecating images of their physical bodies that require assessment for a comprehensive analysis of sexual functioning.

IV. EFFECTS OF CANCER THERAPIES

An understanding of normal human sexual response helps explain why cancer and its treatments can be so disruptive, often bringing about physiological, psychological, personal, and interpersonal changes that affect sexual behavior. The following are some of the most common problems:

1. Chemotherapy can cause vaginal irritation and discharge, and sometimes ovarian failure that leads to menopause. Menopause can decrease the amount of vaginal lubrication, which is important for comfortable sexual intercourse.
2. All treatments can cause fatigue. Nausea and moderate to severe fatigue

are reported by 90% of patients on chemotherapy. When "not feeling well," most people lose interest in sex.

3. Radiation to the pelvic region can cause shrinkage, irritation and drying of the vagina, pain, nausea, gastric distress, and serious fatigue. Many of these conditions, however, can be treated. In men, pelvic irradiation can cause vascular damage that may lead to erectile dysfunction.

4. Surgery can change body appearance and can create issues between patients and partners about touching the areas where surgery has recently occurred. It is not uncommon for problems to arise after surgery. The partner may not want to hurt the patient and backs off from lovemaking or any physical contact. The patient then may think that the partner is not interested or is put off by the physical changes and thus feels rejected. This dynamic often can be stopped if the partner and the patient talk about what each is feeling and perceiving. Surgery can also involve dissection of nerves crucial to sexual arousal in men.

5. A mastectomy, surgery scars, a stoma, weight loss or gain, and hair loss are among the common changes to a person's body that can decrease body image and feelings of sexual attractiveness. In turn, this can affect sexual functioning.

6. Cancer treatments may cause changes in the sensitivity of sexual organs. If the sensitivity is increased and the patient experiences pain, the ability to become aroused may change, which affects the sexual relationship.

7. The effects of hormone therapy as a cancer treatment may vary, depending on the specific treatments used. Tamoxifen, for example, often does not have a negative effect on sexual function because, for some women, it works like an estrogen on the vaginal tissues. On the other hand, androgen deprivation (e.g., orchiectomy, gonadotropin-releasing hormone analogues) used in prostate cancer treatment, has a profound effect on a man's libido.

8. The sexuality of men and women with cancer who are in their childbearing years can be affected by the possible loss of fertility or concerns about whether to conceive a child.

V. THE EFFECT OF DIFFERENT TYPES OF CANCER ON SEXUAL FUNCTION

The impact of cancer and its treatment on sexual functioning varies by cancer site. This section describes common sequelae for several major cancers.

A. Breast Cancer

Treatment for breast cancer often produces the side effects of fatigue, diminished lubrication, nausea, and significant body changes, including the loss of a breast from mastectomy. Early menopause is common. The use of hormone replacement therapy is controversial in this population because of the concern that it will stimulate tumor growth. Tamoxifen, which is often used, can create vaginal dryness and vaginal discharge in some women. In a large cross-sectional survey of North American women, sexual functioning was similar to a group of age-matched menopausal women who had not had breast cancer (9). Breast cancer survivors who received adjuvant chemotherapy reported poorer sexual functioning than those who had not (9).

B. Testicular Cancer

Findings from studies that assess sexuality in testicular cancer patients are mixed, possibly because samples have been made up of patients with different tumor types who received different treatments. Rates of decreased sexual desire are moderately low for all treatment modalities and may improve with time. Occasional erectile problems are more common than permanent dysfunction, particularly in patients who received adjuvant radiation treatments. Problems with orgasm, particularly intensity of orgasm and ejaculatory function, are the most common type of dysfunction documented. Problems in sexuality appear to be largely explained by ejaculatory dysfunction, which occurs more often in patients who received radiation therapy or retroperitoneal lymph node dissection in addition to orchiectomy. Despite disruption to physiological sexual functioning, most men are sexually satisfied and only some report decreases in sexual activity.

C. Prostate Cancer

With the exception of advanced prostate cancer patients who undergo surgical or hormonal castration, global sexual desire is not disrupted drastically for most patients following radiation or radical prostatectomy, regardless of erectile ability. Erectile function is the area of sexuality that is most disrupted following radiation or prostatectomy, with most patients reporting some decrease in erectile ability (10–12). Moderate to high levels of disruption in orgasm and sexual activity also are common. Although more data are needed, body image appears to be disrupted in a minority of prostatectomy patients. This may be a more common problem in patients receiving hormonal or surgical castration.

D. Bladder Cancer

Most patients with cystectomy experience some problems with sexuality following treatment. A minority of men experience some disruption in sexual desire, but the most drastic impact is in erectile function, with most men reporting severe dysfunction. The proportion of erectile dysfunction has been reported to be lower in nerve-sparing procedures. The frequency of sexual intercourse is decreased with greater levels of posttreatment sexual activity reported by men who engaged in noncoital sex before treatment. It appears that sexuality also is significantly influenced by treatment choice, with bladder-sparing procedures and the absence of a stoma being related to greater levels of sexual desire and activity. Body image is often disrupted in stoma patients. In addition to disruption in sexuality, urinary leakage (resulting from the presence of a urostomy) during sexual activity may occur in some patients and may interfere with sexual functioning.

E. Lung Cancer

Most patients with lung cancer are given the diagnosis of advanced disease and thus often have severe physical symptoms. Shortness of breath, fatigue, and pain are important problems that can limit sexual activity in this group of patients.

F. Colorectal Cancer

Treatment of colorectal cancer initially may increase fatigue, and many patients may find that their bowel habits change. If they have surgery that leads to an ostomy, their feelings about their body image may become negative. In addition, some surgical procedures for colorectal cancer have the potential to damage the pelvic nerves leading to erectile dysfunction in men. Overall, patients who undergo abdominoperineal resection report worse sexual outcomes than patients who undergo low anterior resection. Poor sexual outcomes in the former may be related to erectile dysfunction, bowel dysfunction, or the presence of a stoma.

G. Gynecological Cancers

With gynecological cancers, surgery and radiation can cause changes to the pelvis and sexual organs. The vagina frequently becomes less elastic and shorter. Changes in vaginal sensation, shape, and lubrication also are common. Chemotherapy or surgery may throw a woman into early menopause, and some patients may not be able to have hormone replacement therapy because of its potential to stimulate cancer growth (e.g., uterine adenocarcinoma).

H. Hematological Cancers—Leukemias and Lymphomas

The treatments for hematological diseases are often toxic and can produce considerable fatigue and other side effects. Even though many of these diseases are curable, the chemotherapy and radiation may lead to toxicity in other organs that can increase fatigue. The treatments often induce early menopause and lead to a need for hormone replacement therapy.

VI. ASSESSMENT AND INTERVENTION

A. Assessment

The comprehensive assessment of sexual dysfunctions is complex, requiring consideration of medical, psychological, interpersonal, and cultural components of sexuality. It is often impossible to distinguish a precise etiological factor because many sexual problems are multidetermined by interacting causes. The assessment of a couple's problems in a standard course of sex therapy typically requires three to four 1-hour sessions. This assessment can include reports of physiological evaluation, comprehensive interviews, and administration of self-report questionnaires. Although a comprehensive assessment is necessary before the start of intensive therapy, it is not the role of the oncology team to conduct such an assessment. Rather, the oncology clinician's goal should be limited to obtaining enough information to determine whether and what type of a referral is needed. This effort depends primarily on discussions with the patient and his or her partner.

In many cases, the medical team can handle the concerns of patients and partners effectively without the need for more intensive therapy. For example, clinicians can introduce the subject of sexual health as follows: ''Sexuality is an important part of people's lives, but one that many patients and partners may feel uncomfortable discussing. Therefore, I like to ask all of my patients about this aspect of their lives directly, in case there are some problems we might be able to address.'' Such an approach allows the patient to share concerns that he or she might have been reluctant to volunteer or discuss. This should be followed by specific questions about desire (''Are you interested in having sex with your partner?''), arousal (''Do you have trouble becoming lubricated?'' or ''Do you have trouble getting an erection?'') and orgasm (''Do you have trouble reaching orgasm?''). Finally, one can assess overall satisfaction (''Are you satisfied with your sexual relationship?). This brief interview is within the practical realm of the oncologist and can serve to identify patients who are having significant problems.

In the following sections, we suggest a graduated approach to interventions for sexual problems that can be used in oncology practices.

B. Interventions for Sexual Problems: The P-LI-SS-IT Model

In addressing sexual problems in cancer patients and their partners, the level of intervention should be matched to the intensity of the problems. There are four general levels of strategies that Annon has summarized using the acronym P-LI-SS-IT (13). According to the P-LI-SS-IT model, the range of interventions includes *giving* ***permission***, *providing* ***limited information***, *offering* ***specific suggestions***, and *conducting* ***intensive therapy***. Table 5 lists specific steps that the

Table 5 P-LI-SS-IT Model

Permission
Invite patient and partner to raise concerns and ask questions about sexuality
Encourage patient to communicate with partner about cancer and sexuality
Normalize broad definition of sexuality
Limited information
Provide information about sexual functioning, aging, and sexual problems related to the cancer experience
Offer relevant written materials about cancer, sexuality, and community resources
Describe options for psychosocial and medical interventions for enhancing sexual functioning
Specific suggestions (targeted to individual patient concerns)
Discuss possibilities for increasing vaginal lubrication
Offer recommendations for use of erectile aids
Suggest positions for sexual activity to reduce discomfort
Intensive therapy
Provide referral for individual, couples, or sex therapy, as indicated

oncology team could take at each level of intervention to help patients and their partners deal with sexual concerns and problems.

1. *Permission*

Perhaps the most important intervention that oncologists and oncology nurses can make is to raise the issue of sexuality with patients and give them permission to discuss their concerns. Research documents that physicians rarely raise these issues with patients, but may be more likely to draw assumptions about patients' concerns that are often inaccurate. When patients are encouraged to ask questions, they report greater satisfaction with medical care. Patients, especially older patients, may be highly reluctant to bring up sexuality without receiving explicit permission from the medical team to do so. Clinicians should be careful in these conversations to use a broad, inclusive, culturally sensitive definition of sexuality that is not limited to penile/vaginal intercourse. They also should be careful not to make assumptions about patients' sex lives (e.g., assuming heterosexuality or assuming that a patient has a partner). In addition to broaching discussion of sexuality with the patient, the oncology team can help the patient by encouraging communication between the patient and his or her partner or partners about cancer and sexuality.

2. Limited Information

The medical team is in the ideal position to offer patients and partners basic information about sexual functioning in the context of the cancer experience. Throughout this chapter we have suggested areas where patients may have a lack of knowledge or may hold specific misperceptions. In addition to discussing this information, patients may find it useful to receive written information, such as the pamphlets on sexualtiy published by the National Cancer Institute and the American Cancer Society or a recently published book by Schover (14).

3. Specific Suggestions

For many sexual problems facing cancer patients, fairly simple suggestions are effective. For example, all oncologists should ask about problems with vaginal lubrication in female patients who have had chemotherapy or may be menopausal. This can be followed by suggestions for treating inadequate lubrication. Hormone therapy with vaginal or systemic estrogen should be prescribed if not contraindicated. Androgen supplementation may help some women who have diminished desire or sexual interest. Similarly, men whose erectile functioning has been disrupted through surgery, chemotherapy, or hormonal therapy might benefit from suggestions about erectile aids (such as vacuum constriction devices, penile injections, penile implants, and oral medication) and referral to a urologist. The specific suggestions need to be targeted to the patients' presenting problems and should be offered only after providing permission and limited information. Without the assessment gained through these earlier stages, the oncologist may risk making inappropriate suggestions based on an incorrect or incomplete understanding of the problem.

4. Intensive Therapy

When information and relatively straightforward suggestions are insufficient, clinicians should make referrals for more intensive therapy. It is helpful to have available referrals for male and female therapists who have training in sex therapy and psychosocial oncology. Mental health professionals with special training can conduct a comprehensive assessment and determine whether sex therapy, couples therapy, or individual therapy is called for. Although the oncologist is not in a position to offer intensive sex therapy, she or he plays a pivotal role in ensuring the success of the treatment. By making appropriate referrals that normalize the need for intervention and describe treatment in a positive tone, patients are far more willing to enter treatment with an optimistic outlook. For more information about the specific methods of assessment or sex therapy, there are several good books and articles available on the topic (e.g., Refs. 7, 8, 15, and 16).

C. Integrating Psychological and Medical Approaches

Although physicians typically are not expected to conduct sex therapy per se, they are responsible for medical interventions. Sex therapy often involves integrating hormonal or surgical approaches with the more traditional psychosocial therapies. Recently, there have been major improvements in medical interventions aimed at correcting sexual problems, especially in men. Unlike current psychological interventions that aim to treat multiple components of sexuality, these medical approaches primarily treat erectile dysfunction without necessarily addressing psychological and relationship issues. However, it is important to consider that a patient's emotional well-being and relationship status or quality may play a role in the success of the medical treatment aimed at sexual rehabilitation. In addition to providing information on medical treatments for sexual dysfunction, physicians should attempt to identify whether patients receiving medical treatment for their sexual dysfunctions would also benefit from psychological interventions. Patients often consider their problems to be strictly of a medical nature and may feel uncomfortable with the idea of receiving psychological support. Support from the physician is required so that patients understand that the role of the mental health professional is optimizing treatment success by integrating medical and psychosocial treatments.

VII. CONCLUSIONS

Sexual functioning is often taken for granted and it is only when it is lost, or when there is temporary dysfunction, that the individual appreciates its complexity. As has been described, the normal human sexual response cycle is triphasic and can be disrupted at various places by cancer and its treatment. It is essential that oncology specialists have an understanding of normal sexual health and functioning in order to understand the disorders associated with cancer. Even without specialized sex therapy training, the attentive clinician can identify patients who are having difficulties, provide them with basic information and assistance, and refer them for more intensive therapy when appropriate. The clinician who begins the dialogue on this topic is appreciated by his or her patients. Early intervention with cancer patients in whom sexual dysfunction has developed may prevent long-term and permanent difficulties.

REFERENCES

1. Masters WH, Johnson VE. Human Sexual Response Cycle. Boston: Little, Brown, 1966.

2. Bancroft J. Human Sexuality and Its Problems. Edinburgh: Churchill Livingstone, 1989.
3. Schiavi RC, Schreiner-Engel P, Mandeli J, Schanzer H, Cohen E. Healthy aging and male sexual function. Am J Psychiatr 1990; 147:766–771.
4. Kaplan HS. Disorders of Sexual Desire. New York: Brunner/Mazel, 1979.
5. American Psychiatric Association. Diagnostic and Statistical Manual of Mental Disorders. 4th ed. Washington, DC: American Psychiatric Association, 1994.
6. Laumann EO, Gagnon JH, Michael RT, Michaels S. The social organization of sexuality: Sexual practices in the United States. Chicago: The University of Chicago Press, 1994.
7. Wincze JP, Carey MP. Sexual dysfunction: A guide for assessment and treatment. New York: Guilford Press, 1991.
8. Rosen RC, Leiblum SR. Treatment of sexual disorders in the 1990s: an integrated approach. J Consult Clin Psychol 1995; 63:877–890.
9. Ganz PA, Rowland JH, Desmond K, Meyerowitz BE, Wyatt GE. Life after breast cancer: understanding women's health-related quality of life and sexual functioning. J Clin Oncol 1998; 16:501–514.
10. Talcott JA, Rieker P, Propert KJ, Clark JA, Wishnow KI, Loughlin KR, Richie JP, Kantoff PW. Patient-reported impotence and incontinence after nerve-sparing radical prostatectomy. J Nat Cancer Inst 1997; 89:1117–1123.
11. Litwin MS, Hays RD, Fink A, Ganz PA, Leake B, Leach GE, Brook RH. Quality-of-life outcomes in men treated for localized prostate cancer. JAMA 1995; 273:129–135.
12. Perez MA, Meyerowitz BE, Liesovsky G, Skinner DG, Reynolds B, Skinner EC. Quality of life and sexuality following radical prostatectomy in patients with prostate cancer who use or do not use erectile aids. Urology 1997; 50:740–746.
13. Annon J. Behavioral Treatment of Sexual Problems. Honolulu: Enabling Systems, 1974.
14. Schover L. Sexuality and Fertility After Cancer. New York: John Wiley & Sons, 1997.
15. Leiblum SR, Rosen RC, eds. Principles and Practice of Sex Therapy: Update for the 1990's. New York: Guilford Press, 1989.
16. Schover LR, Jensen SB. Sexuality and Chronic Illness: A Comprehensive Approach. New York: Guilford Press, 1988.

15

Pain Control in Patients with Cancer

Stuart A. Grossman
The Johns Hopkins Oncology Center, Baltimore, Maryland

I. IMPORTANCE OF CANCER PAIN

Pain is one of the most common and feared symptoms associated with cancer. Approximately 20% to 50% of patients with cancer are first seen with pain, 33% have pain during the treatment of their disease, and 75% to 90% in the advanced stages of their disease experience moderate to severe pain requiring treatment with opioids (1–5). Unrelieved pain has a substantial effect on patients' activities, affect, motivation, interactions with family and friends, and overall quality of life.

The importance of this symptom and the excellent therapies available make it imperative that physicians and nurses caring for cancer patients be adept at the assessment and treatment of cancer pain. This requires familiarity with the pathogenesis of cancer pain, pain assessment techniques, the common barriers to the delivery of appropriate analgesia, and the pertinent pharmacological anesthetic, neurosurgical, and behavioral approaches to the treatment of cancer pain.

II. ETIOLOGY OF CANCER PAIN AND IMPLICATIONS FOR THERAPY

Approximately 70% of all pain in cancer patients results from tumor invading or compressing soft tissue, bone, or neural structures (3,5). Common cancer pain

Table 1 Etiology of Pain in Cancer Patients

A. Direct tumor involvement (70%)
   1. Invasion of bone
   2. Invasion or compression of neural structures
   3. Obstruction of hollow viscus or ductal system of solid viscus
   4. Vascular obstruction or invasion
   5. Mucuous membrane ulceration or involvement

B. Associated with antineoplastic therapy (20%)
   1. Diagnostic and staging procedures
   2. Postoperative (acute postoperative pain or postsurgical syndromes, i.e., postmastectomy, postthoracotomy, postamputation)
   3. Postradiation (injury to plexus or spinal cord, mucositis, enteritis)
   4. Postchemotherapy (mucositis, peripheral neuropathy, aseptic necrosis)

C. Cancer-induced syndromes (<10%)
   1. Paraneoplastic syndromes
   2. Pain associated with debility (bed sores, constipation, rectal or bladder spasm)
   3. Other (post-herpetic neuralgia)

D. Pain unrelated to the malignancy or its treatment (<10%)

syndromes are listed in Table 1. Failure to define the origin of pain is a common reason for inadequate pain relief and for poor patient outcomes. This is exemplified by the following case history.

> A 65-year-old woman with lung cancer had a 3-week history of worsening pain in the midthoracic region. She had no other symptoms on a complete review of systems and a careful neurological examination was normal. Her chest roentgenograph revealed a posterior mediastinal mass, which had not changed since her last evaluation. Oral opioids were initiated and the doses were rapidly increased in an unsuccessful attempt to control her pain. Two weeks later, bilateral lower extremity weakness with loss of bowel and bladder continence developed suddenly. She had a T6 sensory level and myelography, which revealed a T6–9 epidural cord compression. Despite aggressive treatment with surgery, radiation therapy, and glucocorticoids, she failed to regain strength in her lower extremities or sphincter function.

Impending epidural cord compressions are an important cause of unrelieved pain in patients with cancer (6,7). These patients usually have weeks to months of back pain, which may have a radicular component. Tumor can reach the epidural space from a metastatic site in the vertebrae or from a posterior mediastinal or retroperitoneal mass that extends through the intervertebral foramina. More than 70% of patients with cancer, back pain, a normal neurological examination, and an abnormal roentgenogram of the spine have epidural tumor evident on myelography or magnetic resonance imaging (MRI) (7,8). These patients often remain in substantial pain on opioids before an acute and usually irreversible loss of neurological function develops. A high index of suspicion and early evaluation allows the diagnosis to be made before neurological function is compromised. Pain relief with the administration of glucocorticoids can be dramatic and radiation usually provides excellent local control. Thus, the patient presented in the case study could have received excellent pain relief and preservation of neurological function with a prompt evaluation and appropriate therapy.

Other common clinical scenarios also highlight the need for a proper pain diagnosis rather than the ''empirical'' use of opioids in this patient population. Headaches in cancer patients may result from many causes, and opioid analgesics are often not the treatment of choice. Herniation and death may result from untreated brain metastases. Progressive pain and irreversible cranial nerve palsies occur when metastases to the base of the skull are not suspected and treated with radiation therapy. Multifocal neurological signs and symptoms and a rapid demise are likely in patients with untreated leptomeningeal metastases. Likewise, pain in the hip can result from extensive bone metastases and an impending pathological fracture or from referred pain secondary to a spinal lesion. Proper treatment of the pain, in these and other situations, requires an accurate diagnosis.

Pain also occurs from causes other than the cancer itself. Nearly 20% of all cancer pain results from diagnostic tests, staging procedures, or antineoplastic therapy (3). Surgery can result in significant pain. In 10% of women who undergo a mastectomy for breast cancer, a tight, burning pain in the posterior arm, axilla, or anterior chest develops following surgery. This postmastectomy syndrome must be differentiated from brachial plexus involvement by tumor, a transient inflammatory plexopathy, radiation fibrosis, or an injury related to surgical positioning. Post-thoracotomy syndromes are also common. Radiation and chemotherapy can also cause significant discomfort. Severe oral mucositis is common with these treatment modalities. Cisplatin, vincristine, and taxol can produce painful peripheral neuropathies and other agents, such as cyclophosphamide, can cause a painful hemorrhagic cystitis. In addition, many patients have pain from illness unrelated to their neoplasm. Migraine headaches, osteoarthritis, gout, and degenerative disc disease are examples of painful illnesses that are frequently seen in patients with cancer.

Pain is often classified as nociceptive, neuropathic, or sympathetically maintained to guide the evaluation and therapy in cancer patients. Nociceptive pain occurs with the activation of somatic or visceral nociceptors. Painful bone metastases are a common example of somatic nociceptive pain whereas visceral nociceptive pain occurs with organ distention. The referral of visceral pain to cutaneous sites can be confusing to the examiner. Neuropathic pain results from direct injury to peripheral or central nervous system structures. It is typified by the burning discomfort or shocklike paroxysms seen in brachial plexopathies. This pain may not respond to opioids, but sometimes improves with agents that affect spontaneous discharges in nerves, such as anticonvulsants or antidepressants. Sympathetically maintained pain is much less prevalent than nociceptive or neuropathic pain in cancer patients. It is characterized by a burning discomfort, allodynia, hyperpathia, brawny edema, and osteoporosis. Prompt sympathetic blockade and physical therapy are important in the management of this type of cancer pain.

III. THE ASSESSMENT OF CANCER PAIN

The goals of a comprehensive cancer pain assessment are to estimate the severity of pain, formulate a differential diagnosis for the etiology of the pain, determine the need for further diagnostic studies, and to plan therapy that considers the patient's overall medical and psychosocial status (5). The assessment of cancer pain, not unlike the assessment of any other serious medical problem, is comprised of a detailed history, physical examination, and review of available records, laboratory data, and imaging studies. Aggressive treatment with analgesics should be initiated while the etiology of the pain is being evaluated. This facilitates the evaluation and reassures patients that their discomfort is being taken seriously. The entirely subjective nature of pain, the complex multisystem involvement in patients with advanced malignancies, and the ever-changing clinical situation in this patient population pose special challenges in the assessment of cancer pain.

A detailed pain history is the cornerstone of the assessment. This may be complex in that most patients with advanced cancer have several painful sites and almost one-third have four or more separate pains (1). Each pain must be identified and characterized as to its intensity, location, and radiation; how and when it began; how it has changed over time; and what makes it better or worse. The quality of each pain (e.g., burning, stabbing), its temporal pattern (e.g., constant, intermittent), whether it is associated with neurological or vasomotor abnormalities, how it interferes with the patient's life, and an account of the successes and failures of current and prior therapies can provide valuable insight.

Patients with severe, chronic pain often do not ''appear'' to be in pain (9). Thus, it is imperative that health care providers believe the patient's report of their pain and use their pain intensity ratings to assess the efficacy of therapeutic interventions. The most useful measure of a patient's pain is his or her subjective pain rating. A formal assessment of pain intensity should be performed using a validated pain intensity scale such as the visual analogue or visual descriptor scale. Many instruments have been developed to aid in pain assessment (Table 2)

Table 2 Valid and Practical Cancer Pain Assessment/Staging Tools

Wisconsin Brief Pain Inventory
Memorial Pain Assessment Card
Hopkins Pain Rating Instrument
Edmonton Staging System

(10,11). These attempts to characterize and quantify the quality or intensity of a patient's pain represent the best available means to document the discomfort and to serially follow up the results of therapy.

Several of these instruments have been validated in patients with cancer pain and can be practically incorporated into clinical practice. Most contain a variant of the unidimensional visual analogue scale (VAS) and a schematic representation of the body for the patient to indicate where their pain is located. The Wisconsin Brief Pain Inventory provides information on the characteristics, severity, and location of the pain, its interference with normal life functions, and the efficacy of prior therapy (12). The Memorial Pain Assessment Card is a simple instrument that can be completed in less than 1 minute and features scales for the measurement of pain intensity and pain relief (13). It is also designed to provide some insight into global suffering or psychological distress. The Hopkins Pain Rating Instrument is a validated plastic version of the VAS, which obviates the need for the paper, pencil, ruler, and measurements associated with the standard VAS (14). This simplifies repeated pain intensity measurements, making it easier to reassess the efficacy of therapeutic endeavors frequently. The Edmonton Staging System for Cancer Pain provides information on how likely a specific patient is to respond to therapy (15). This staging system relies on the underlying reason for the pain, prior treatment with opioids, and presence of incident pain, impaired cognitive function, psychological distress, tolerance to opioids, and history of alcoholism or drug abuse.

A complete oncological history is essential because 70% of the pain in cancer patients results from tumor invading or compressing normal tissues and 20% stems from surgery, radiation, chemotherapy, or diagnostic studies performed to evaluate the extent of the tumor. As a result, information about the histology, presentation, stage, sites of involvement, and natural history of the tumor is indispensable. All surgery, radiation, chemotherapy, and hormonal treatments should be noted as should as should the dates, doses, toxicities, and responses to each. In addition, it is important to determine whether the malignancy is responding to therapy, is stable, or is progressing.

Pain treatments can affect coexisting medical problems, exacerbate constitutional symptoms, or interact with other medications. As a result, a general medical

Table 3 Important Definitions in the Treatment of Cancer Pain

Physical dependence
- A normal physiological response to chronic opioid administration characterized by development of the abstinence syndrome on abrupt withdrawal of opioids
- A potential problem in virtually all patients receiving moderate to high doses of opiates

Tolerance
- A normal pharmacological response to chronic opioid therapy characterized by the development of a relative resistance to analgesic and other effects of the drug
- Overcome by increasing the dose administered

Psychological dependence (addiction)
- Abnormal behavior pattern characterized by an all-consuming desire to obtain opioids for reasons other than pain relief. This often occurs at the expense of the patient's physical, social, and environmental well-being
- Extraordinarily rare in patients with cancer pain
- Not to be confused with "pseudoaddiction," which is behavior commonly seen in patients who are undertreated and in pain attempting to obtain appropriate analgesia

history is critical. A history of severe peptic ulcer disease, benign prostatic hypertrophy, or obstructive pulmonary disease with CO_2 retention is significant in decisions to prescribe potent anti-inflammatory drugs or opioids. The route of drug administration is influenced by a patient's ability to take food or fluids by mouth, the presence of an indwelling venous access device, or a history of substance abuse. The patient's age, functional status, social support, education, residence, health insurance, finances, and religious and cultural background may also figure prominently in planning therapy.

A through physical examination with emphasis on the neurological system can also provide important clues as to the origin of the pain. Added insight may come form a review of available laboratory and imaging data, medical records, and from discussions with family members and physicians familiar with the patient and his or her illness. Appropriate diagnostic studies may include blood tests, bone scans, plain roentgenograms, myelography, lumbar puncture, electromyelogram (EMG), nerve conduction studies, or computed tomography (CT) or MRI scans of the head, brachial plexus, chest, abdomen, pelvis, or spine.

The history, physical examination, laboratory, and other data should provide the clinician with sufficient information to formulate a differential diagnosis for each of the patient's distinct pains and to make recommendations regarding the work-up and therapy. However, frequent reassessment of cancer pain relief is key to providing optimal care. Excellent pain relief suggests an accurate initial diagnosis and appropriate therapy, whereas suboptimal control or new symptoms may prompt a new treatment approach or a search for a different origin of the pain. The toxicities of the analgesic therapies must also be periodically reevaluated. Many of the agents used to treat cancer pain can substantially affect quality of life and can be replaced by alternate approaches if they are associated with excessive toxicity. One of the most difficult aspects of cancer pain management is that the patient's clinical situation is rarely static. His or her underlying malignancy, antineoplastic therapy, tolerance to opioids, and psychosocial status change continually during the course of the illness. As a result, the origin and intensity of each new or worsening pain must be reassessed.

IV. TREATMENT OF CANCER PAIN

More than 80% of patients with cancer pain can receive excellent analgesia with conventional oral medications (16). More aggressive or invasive therapies should provide pain relief in an additional 10% of patients, leaving only a small portion of cancer patients with inadequate pain relief. However, current data suggest that a minority of patients with cancer pain receive adequate analgesia (4,5,17–19). Many reasons have been proposed to explain these therapeutic inadequacies. Some of these have to do directly with patient concerns or misconceptions. Many patients are reluctant to take opioids fearing addiction, tolerance, and the potential side effects of these agents. Others fail to communicate the intensity of their discomfort to their health care provider. Some patients elect not to discuss pain with their caregivers, believing that cancer pain is unavoidable or fearing that it signifies progressive cancer or that they may divert physician attention from treating the tumor.

Health care providers also contribute to inadequate pain treatment for these patients. Physicians and nurses receive little formal cancer pain instruction during their training. As a result, studies demonstrate that physicians and nurses neglect pain control issues, fail to evaluate the underlying origin of cancer pain, are overly concerned about addiction, tolerance, and opioid toxicities, lack essential opioid prescribing skills (20), and have little understanding of the intensity of cancer pain in patients (21). In addition, they are frequently confused by the differences between opioid tolerance, dependence, and addiction (Table 3), and are intimidated by young patients and those with cognitive or communication handicaps or a history of substance abuse. Regulatory efforts to control opioid diversion also result in physicians being overly cautious in prescribing these important drugs (22–24).

Pharmacological approaches are the most commonly used treatments for cancer pain because they are effective, safe, and inexpensive (25–27). Aspirin, acetaminophen, or nonsteroidal anti-inflammatory agents (NSAIDs) are preferred for mild to moderate pain. If these do not provide adequate analgesia, codeine, oxycodone, or hydrocodone frequently provide excellent relief. For persistent or severe pain, codeine (or its congener) can be replaced by a potent opioid such as morphine. Drug substitution should be considered before an entire class of agents is abandoned, because patients frequently tolerate one NSAID or opioid better than another.

Most cases can be managed with oral opioids (Tables 4, 5, and 6). These are best given "around the clock" to keep pain under control. Although tolerance to these agents occurs, tumor progression is the most common reason for increasing opioid requirements. Tolerance can be easily overcome by increasing opioid doses. Addiction is rare in cancer patients taking opiates for pain relief. Constipation can be anticipated and should be treated prophylactically. Other opioid side effects can be managed without excessive difficulty.

"Adjuvant" drugs can be beneficial in specific circumstances. Glucocorticoids are effective anti-inflammatory agents and reduce the edema associated with brain and epidural metastases. Antidepressants may elevate mood, help with insomnia, and alleviate neuropathic pain (28). Anxiolytic agents are indicated in selected patients and may potentiate the effect of the opioids. Anticonvulsants, such as carbamazepine, phenytoin, or gabapentin, may be effective in neuropathic pain and amphetamines can decrease opioid-induced sedation. Caution must be exercised in the use of adjuvant drugs with sedative properties, because the dose of opioids should not be compromised by the toxicities of these secondary agents. Bisphosphonates increase osteoclastic activation and reduce bone resorption and appear to have an important role in the treatment of osteolytic bone metastases (29,30). Besides reducing hypercalcemic episodes, they can diminish pain, reduce the incidence of pathological fractures, and promote healing.

Patients with severe pain should receive aggressive treatment. Opioids with short half-lives permit rapid oral or intravenous dose escalations. Patient-controlled analgesia is an effective means to titrate opioid doses and toxicities in patients with normal mentation. Once pain is well controlled, opioid requirements frequently diminish without other interventions. A narcotic equivalency table should be used to convert the doses taken parenterally or the short-acting oral agents to an approximately equianalgesic dose of standard or controlled-release oral preparations. Patients with substantial pain who are unable to take oral medications may benefit from parenteral infusions or transdermal opioids. The chronic use of rectal suppositories or injections are usually unnecessary and unacceptable to patients.

Antineoplastic therapy can provide significant analgesia if it reduces the size of lesions invading or compressing normal tissues (17). Radiation therapy is the

Table 4 Weak Opioids for Moderate Pain

Drug	Route	Equianalgesic dose (mg)[a]	Peak effect (h)	Duration of effect (h)	Comments
Codeine	PO	200	0.5	3–6	Ceiling for analgesia reached at doses >240 mg/d orally
	IV/IM	130	0.5	3–6	
Oxycodone	PO	30	0.5	3–6	Parenteral formulation not available
Hydrocodone	PO	NA	0.5	4–6	Only available as fixed combination with acetaminophen or aspirin
Propoxyphene	PO	NA	1.0	4–6	100 mg napsylate = 65 mg hydrochloride salt
Pentazocine	PO	NA	2.0	3	Oral form also available in combination with naloxone
	IV		0.25	1	Not recommended for treatment of cancer pain

[a] Approximate potency relative to 10mg of parenteral morphine
Abbreviations: PO, oral; IV, intravenous; NA, not available.
Source: Modified from Grossman SA, Gregory E. Management of Cancer Pain in Cancer. Current Therapeutics, 1994.

Table 5 Strong Opiates for Severe Cancer Pain

Drug	Route	Equianalgesic dose (mg)[a]	Peak effect (h)	Duration of effect (h)	Comments
Morphine	PO	30–60	1.5–2.0	4–6	Preferred opiate for management of cancer pain
	PO (SR)		2.0–3.0	8–12	
	IV/IM	30–60	0.5–1.0	3–6	
		10			
Hydromorphone	PO/PR	7.5	1.0–2.0	3–4	Good choice for SQ because of its potency
	IV/IM	1.5	0.5–1.0	3–4	
Meperidine	PO	300	1.0–2.0	3–6	Not preferred because CNS toxic metabolites accumulate in renal failure
	IV/IM	75	0.5–1.0	2–3	
Levorphanol	PO	4.0	1.0–2.0	6–8	Long half-life (11 h) necessitates slow dose titration; drug accumulation may occur
	IV/IM	2.0	1.0–1.5	6–8	
Fentanyl	TD	0.1 (?)	72	12 or >	Short half-life (<1 h). TD dose titration difficult with depot in SQ adipose tissue.
	IV/IM	0.1	<1.0	0.5–1.0	
Methadone	PO	20	?	4–6	Despite long half-life (15–150+ h), duration of analgesia is not prolonged; however, drug accumulation can result in toxicities
	IV/IM	10	0.5–1.5	4–6	
Butorphanol	IN	2	1.0	3–4	Mixed agonist-antagonist may precipitate withdrawal in patient previously receiving a pure agonist, thus not generally recommended for cancer pain
	IV/IM	2	0.5–1.0	3–4	

[a] Approximate potency relative to 10 mg of parenteral morphine

Abbreviations: PO, oral; SR, sustained release; IV, intravenous; PR, per rectum; SQ, subcutaneous; IN, intranasal; TD, transdermal; CNS, central nervous system

Source: Modified from Grossman SA, Gregory E. Management of Cancer Pain in Cancer. Current Therapeutics, 1994.

Table 6 Opioid Analgesics: Routes of Administration

Route of administration	Comments	Cost considerations[a]
Oral	Preferred route for cancer pain management	$: D
Buccal/Sublingual	Avoids first pass through the liver. Otherwise no advantage over oral and unavailable in United States.	$: D
Rectal	Available for morphine, oxymorphone, and hydromorphone. Dosing is considered equivalent to oral, but absorption may be erratic and incomplete.	$: D
Transdermal	Available for fentanyl. Absorption rates may be affected by subcutaneous fat stores, hypothermia or hyperthermia, placement in a radiation port, and ambient temperature. Controversial conversion recommendations.	$: D
Intranasal	Available for buprenorphine, but not evaluated for management of chronic pain.	$: D
Subcutaneous	Bioavailability similar to that for IV. Infection, bleeding, and irritation at injection site may occur.	$$$: D,(P),S,Ph,RN,C
Intramuscular	Contraindicated for management of chronic pain.	$$: D,S,RN
Intravenous	Indicated only when other routes have failed.	$$$: D,P,S,Ph,RN,(SF),C
Epidural/Intrathecal	May be useful for avoiding systemic side effects of opiates. Usually not effective if systemic treatment has failed.	$$$$: D,P,S,Ph,RN,SF,C

[a] $ = overall costs ($ = least expensive, $$$$ = most expensive). Specific costs for each therapy include D, drug; P, pump rental; S, supplies (tubing, filters, batteries, tape, heparin); Ph, pharmacy services; RN, nursing services; SF, surgical fee, C, risk of costly complications; ( ), may or may not be necessary for this route of delivery.

Source: Modified from Grossman SA, Gregory E. Management of Cancer Pain in Cancer. Current Therapeutics, 1994.

treatment of choice for most patients with local pain from tumor invasion. It is frequently administered to patients with symptomatic bone, brain, epidural, and plexus metastases. Systemic radiotherapy, using isotopes such as strontium^{89}, which are concentrated in areas of new bone formation, provide local radiation at the site of metasases. These may provide considerable pain relief months after administration but can be associated with myelosuppression in patients with limited bone marrow reserve. Surgery is effective in relieving pain from intestinal obstruction, pathological fractures, and obstructive hydrocephalus. Chemotherapy can provide substantial pain relief in chemotherapy-sensitive tumors.

Nonpharmacological approaches such as progressive muscle relaxation, massage, guided imagery, biofeedback, and hypnosis are useful adjuncts to pain management. Although psychotherapy is indicated for an associated depression, unrelieved pain often results in depression and is best treated with appropriate pain management techniques.

Neurostimulatory techniques such as transcutaneous electrical nerve stimulation (TENS), peripheral nerve stimulation, dorsal column stimulation, and deep brain stimulation have been used to treat cancer pain (15). The TENS is safe, noninvasive, relatively inexpensive, and easily added to other analgesic approaches. It can provide short-term benefits in cancer patients and a 2 to 4 week trial often determines its clinical utility. Peripheral nerve stimulation is invasive, feasible only in the extremities, and of limited benefit in cancer pain. Dorsal column stimulation is usually performed with an epidural electrode that is introduced with a Tuohy needle. It may be helpful in mild to moderate neuropathic pain. Deep brain stimulation is rarely used because it requires placement of stimulating electrodes into the internal capsule, thalamus, or hypothalamus. It is ineffective in deafferentation pain.

Regional analgesia can be achieved with long-acting local anesthetics (such as bupivacaine), which provide pain relief for 3 to 12 hours; neurolytic agents (alcohol or phenol), which produce analgesia that can last for weeks to months; or opioids injected into the epidural or subarachnoid space (17). Anesthetic blocks can be used diagnostically or to predict the efficacy and side effects of neurolytic blocks or neurosurgical operations. They can also be useful at ''trigger points'' in myofascial pain syndromes. Local administration of anesthetic agents are occasionally complicated by hypotension, toxic reactions from accidental intravenous or subarachnoid administration, or pneumothorax following needle placement.

Neurolytic blocks are primarily indicated in patients with localized or regional pain. Subarachnoid and extradural phenol or alcohol destroys nociceptive fibers in the dorsal rootlets, simulating a surgical rhizotomy. This can be useful in thoracic pain in which few motor effects are noted. However, in cervical and lumbar regions, motor or sphincter dysfunction develops in nearly 20% of patients and may be permanent. Celiac plexus blocks relieve pain originating in the pancreas, stomach, gallbladder, or other upper abdominal viscera in most patients. Intercostal blocks are helpful in chest or abdominal wall pain. Less commonly used blocks include gasserian ganglion neurolysis (pain in the anterior two-thirds of the head) and brachial plexus blocks (for patients with preexisting limb paralysis). Because neurolytic blocks will eventually produce a painful chemical neuropathy, they are limited to patients with advanced disease and a limited life expectancy.

Intraspinal opioids produce analgesia without blocking other sensory, motor, or sympathetic functions. The total daily dose of opioid required with intraspinal administration is one-tenth to one-hundredth of an equianalgesic dose of oral or parenteral opioid and is thus associated with fewer systemic toxicities. Chronic epidural or intrathecal opioids are invasive, expensive, and usually ineffective in patients requiring high doses of systemic opioids. Tolerance, pruritus, urinary retention, and nausea and vomiting occur in up to 20% of patients receiving spinal opiates. Respiratory depression is unusual. The addition of low doses of anesthetic agents to intrathecal and epidural opioids may add considerably to pain relief.

Neuroablative procedures are infrequently performed on cancer patients because of the success of more conservative therapies. The open unilateral anterolateral cordotomy, percutaneous cordotomy, and commissural myelotomy are the most commonly performed procedures (17). An open cordotomy is performed through a T2 or T3 laminectomy and produces excellent pain relief in the lower part of the body in 80% of patients. A 5% to 10% mortality rate and significant morbidity in an additional 15% of patients is reported with this procedure. Hemiparesis, urinary retention, sexual impotence, unmasking pain on the opposite side of the body, and late sensory abnormalities are seen. Bilateral cordotomies are associated with higher complication rates. Percutaneous cordotomy is safer and provides excellent pain relief. However, the pain recurs in about 50% of patients within 3 months. A commissural myelotomy can be considered in selected patients with bilateral pelvic and perineal pain. This involves a laminectomy and surgical division of the crossing fibers of the spinal cord. Although it may result in pain relief with sphincter sparing, there are few neurosurgeons with extensive expertise in this procedure.

V. SUMMARY

Pain occurs in more than 70% of patients with cancer and, in the vast majority, can be well controlled with the currently available treatmetns. Providing optimal pain relief to cancer patients should be a priority for health care providers, especially in view of mounting data that confirm the undertreatment of cancer pain. A careful and formal pain assessment is required to determine pain intensity, the origin of the pain, the need for furhter evaluation, and an appropriate therapeutic plan. Frequent reassessment is required because the underlying malignancy, the antineoplastic therapy, tolerance to opioids, and the patient's psychosocial status change continually during the course of the illness.

SELECTED READINGS

Bonica JJ. The Management of Pain. 2nd ed., Philadelphia: Lea & Febiger, 1990. This exhaustive reference text contains extensive chapters on cancer pain and the use of anesthetic and neurosurgical procedures.

Cleeland CS, Gonin R, Hatfield AK, et al. Pain and its treatment in outpatients with metastatic cancer. N Engl J Med 1994; 330:592–596. This study documents the difficulties patients with cancer have receiving adequate pain control.

Grossman SA. Undertreatment of cancer pain: barriers and remedies. Support Care Cancer 1993; 1:74–78. This paper explores the reasons for the continued undertreatment of cancer pain and suggests practical approaches to correct these therapeutic inadequacies.

Jacox A, Carr DB, Payne R, et al. *Management of Cancer Pain: Clinical Practice Guideline No. 9*. AHCPR Publication No. 94-0592. Rockville, MD: Agency for Health Care Policy and Research, US Dept of Health and Human Services, Public Health Service, 1994. This publication describes in detail the results of a comprehensive US government sponsored review of the management of cancer pain. It provides a carefully considered summary of the state-of-the-art on the assessment and treatment of cancer pain.

Levy MH. Pharmacologic treatment of cancer pain. N Engl J Med 1996; 335:1124–1132. This manuscript provides an excellent discussion of pharmacologic therapy of cancer pain.

Marks RM, Sachar EJ. Undertreatment of medical inpatients with narcotic analgesics. Ann Intern Med 1973; 78:173–181. This classic paper is credited with raising the consciousness of clinicians to the undertreatment of pain. It continues to be cited as evidence continues to mount that too little has changed in the treatment of cancer pain in the past 2 decades.

Martin LA, Hagen NA. Neuropathic pain in cancer patients: mechanisms, syndromes, and clinical controversies. J Pain Symptom Manage 1997; 14:99–117. This review addresses the treatment of neuropathic pain which is one of the most difficult types of pain to treat in patients with cancer.

Mercadante S. Malignant bone pain: pathophysiology and treatment. Pain 1997; 69:1–18. This recent review summarizes the management of the most common source of pain in patients with cancer.

REFERENCES

1. Twycross RG. Incidence of pain. Clin Oncol 1984; 3:5–15.
2. Daut RL, Cleeland CS. The prevalence and severity of pain in cancer. Cancer 1982; 50:191–198.
3. Portenoy RK. Cancer pain: epidemiology and syndromes. Cancer 1989; 63:2298–2307.
4. Cleeland CS, Gonin R, Hatfield AK, et al. Pain and its treatment in outpatients with metastatic cancer. N Engl J Med 1994; 330:592–596.
5. Jacox A, Carr DB, Payne R, et al. Management of Cancer Pain: Clinical Practice Guideline No. 9. AHCPR Publication No. 94-0592. Rockville, MD: Agency for Health Care Policy and Research, US Dept of Health and Human Services, Public Health Service, 1994.
6. Rodichok LD, Harper GR, Ruckdeschel JC, et al. Early diagnosis of spinal epidural metastases. Am J Med 1981; 70:1187–1188.
7. Byrne TN. Spinal cord compression from epidural metastases. N Engl J Med 1992; 327:614–619.
8. Grossman SA, Weissman DE, Wang H, et al. Early diagnosis of spinal epidural metastases using out-patient computed tomographic myelography. Eur J Cancer Clin Oncol 1990; 26:495–499.
9. Foley KM. The treatment of cancer pain. N Engl J Med 1985; 313:84–95.
10. Chapman CR, Casey KL, Dubner R, et al. Pain measurement: an overview. Pain 1985; 22:31.
11. Williams CR. Toward a set of reliable and valid measures for chronic pain assessment and outcome research. Pain 1988; 35:239–251.
12. Cleeland CS. Assessment of pain in cancer. In: Foley KM, Bonica JJ, Ventafridda V, eds. Advances in Pain Research and Therapy. Vol. 16. New York: Raven Press, 1990:47–55.
13. Fishman B, Pasternak S, Wallenstein S, et al. The Memorial Pain Assessment Card: a valid instrument for the evaluation of cancer pain. Cancer 1987; 60:1151–1158.
14. Grossman SA, Sheidler VR, McGuire DB, et al. A comparison of the Hopkins Pain Rating Instrument with standard visual analogue and verbal descriptor scales in patients with cancer pain. J Pain Symptom Manage 1992; 7:196–203.
15. Bruera E, MacMillan K, Hanson I, et al. The Edmonton staging system for cancer pain: Preliminary report. Pain 1989; 37:203–209.
16. Stjernsward J, Teoh N. The scope of the cancer pain problem. Adv Pain Res Ther 1990; 16:7–12.
17. Bonica JJ. The Management of Pain. 2nd ed. Philadelphia: Lea & Febiger, 1990.
18. Grossman SA. Undertreatment of cancer pain: barriers and remedies. Support Care Cancer 1993; 1:74–78.
19. Koshy RC, Rhodes D, Devi S, Grossman SA. Cancer pain management in developing countries: a mosaic of complex issues resulting in inadequate analgesia. Support Care Cancer. In press.
20. Grossman SA, Sheidler VR. Skills of medical students and house officers in prescribing narcotic medications. J Med Educ 1985; 60:552–557.

21. Grossman SA, Sheidler VR, Swedeen K, et al. Correlations of patient and caregiver ratings of cancer pain. J Pain Symptom Manage 1991; 6:53–57.
22. Angarola RT. National and international regulation of opioid drugs: purpose, structures, benefits and risks. J Pain Symptom Manage 1990; 5:S6–S11.
23. Joranson DE. Federal and state regulation of opioids. J Pain Symptom Manage 1990; 5:S12–S23.
24. Joranson DE. Availability of opioids for cancer pain: recent trends, assessment of system barriers, new World Health Organization guidelines, and the risk of diversion. J Pain Symptom Manage 1993; 8:353–360.
25. Inturrisi CE. Opiate analgesic therapy in cancer pain. Adv Pain Res Ther 1990; 16: 133–154.
26. Levy MH. Pharmacologic treatment of cancer pain. N Engl J Med 1996; 335:1124–1132.
27. Cherny NI, Foley KM. Nonopioid and opioid analgesic pharmacotherapy of cancer pain. Hematol Oncol Clin North Am 1996; 10:79–102.
28. Martin LA, Hagen NA. Neuropathic pain in cancer patients: mechanisms, syndromes, and clinical controversies. J Pain Symptom Manage 1997; 14:99–117.
29. Body JJ, Piccart M, Coleman RE. Use of bisphosphonates in cancer patients. Cancer Treat Rev 1996; 22:265–287.
30. Berenson JR, Lichtenstein A, Porter L, et al. Efficacy of pamidronate in reducing skeletal events in patients with advanced multiple myeloma. N Engl J Med 1996; 333:488–493.

16

Psychiatric Disorders in Cancer Patients

Darius Razavi
Centre Hospitalier Universitaire Saint-Pierre, Brussels, Belgium

Friedrich Stiefel
University Hospital, Lausanne, Switzerland

I. INTRODUCTION

An important prevalence of psychiatric disturbances in cancer patients has been reported in many studies. In 1983, the Psychosocial Collaborative Oncology Group observed a prevalence rate of 47% for *Diagnosic and Statistical Manual of Mental Disorders-III*-defined psychiatric disorders in a cohort of cancer patients (inpatient and outpatient populations of three cancer centers). Most importantly, this rate was approximately twice that reported for psychiatric disorders in medical patients, and three times the modal estimate appearing in the literature for the general population. As a diagnostic category, adjustment disorders (ADs) accounted for 68% of all diagnoses. Other diagnoses were major affective disorders (13%), organic mental disorders (8%), personality disorders (7%), and anxiety disorders (4%). Nearly 85% of patients with a positive psychiatric condition indicated that depression or anxiety was the principal symptom.

Most of these conditions were judged by the authors to be highly treatable disorders (1). In a 1987 study, approximately one in three oncology outpatients, assessed with the Brief Symptom Inventory, reported moderate to high levels of depression and anxiety (2). A 1989 Swedish study (in Sweden all cases of cancer have been, by law, notified and recorded since 1958) reported that cancer patients seem to have an increased suicide rate compared with that of the general population, particularly during the first year after diagnosis, when the rate is multiplied by 15 (3). Finally, the high risk of medium- and long-term sequelae of cancer and its treatments has come to light, even if the exact prevalence of these problems remains to be assessed in future prospective research (4).

Therefore, the assumption that emotional distress was just a foreseeable and ordinary reaction to cancer had to be reviewed and the need for comprehensive therapeutic models to care for patients in whom psychological disorders develop was recognized.

Before reviewing recent advances in treating the psychologic conditions related to cancer, three concepts that have a major influence on the current literature must be considered: stress, rehabilitation, and quality of life.

First, physicians have come to accept the view that cancer and its treatments constitute a stress imposed on a previously healthy individual, involving adjustment efforts (or coping) and possibly adjustment disorders. This stress concept treats psychological disturbances as the consequence of a sustained stressful situation. Several recent articles evaluated the psychosocial disorders associated with cancers in terms of adaptation (5) or adjustment (6).

Second, improvement in cancer treatments and prognosis means that a diagnosis of cancer can no longer be equated with a death sentence. Survivorship, especially in patients with cured hematological malignancies (7), has increased, and with it the need for achieving and maintaining optimal quality of life has become apparent for these patients. Consequently, oncologists are increasingly aware of the patient's needs regarding the return to a normal and useful life, and they therefore feel more concerned not only about the short-term psychological effects of their treatments (8) but also about their long-term outcomes in terms of a patient's quality of life (9) and rehabilitation (10). In particular, the psychological distress after surgical treatment of breast cancer is still the center of a controversial debate on partial versus total mastectomy (11,12). At the same time, surgical and medical treatment decision makers increasingly consider the psychosocial factors predictive of a treatment's success or failure (13).

Rehabilitation of the cancer patient, which seems to be the current leading concept, includes specific support by a multidisciplinary team. From this perspective, psychosocial and psychopharmacological interventions will become a part of large programs oriented toward the rehabilitation and quality of life of cancer patients.

Although most recent articles are related to these promising topics, only a minority investigated the ways to make them operational (i.e., the two types of interventions known to be effective for common psychiatric or psychological disorders), which are psychological support and psychotropic medications. The literature of the past years had to be reviewed to provide a valid picture of the current situation in this new area.

II. ADJUSTMENT DISORDERS

A. Definition and Clinical Presentation

Cancer and its treatments are stressful life events producing an acute stress reaction or a significant life change leading to continued unpleasant circumstances that may result in an adjustment disorder. Adjustment disorders are thought to arise as a direct consequence of stress or trauma. It is assumed that AD would not have occurred without the impact of cancer stress or trauma.

As discussed in the International Classification of Diseases by the World Health Organization (WHO), AD should be differentiated from acute stress reactions, which are transient disorders of significant severity. This disorder usually subsides within hours or days. Symptoms of acute stress reactions usually appear within minutes of the impact of the stressful event (e.g., cancer diagnosis) and disappear within 2 or 3 days: inattention, daze, numbness, and inability to comprehend stimuli in a first phase, followed by withdrawal, agitation, or anxiety.

Adjustment disorders are states of subjective distress and emotional disturbance interfering with social functioning and performance. The onset of AD is usually within 1 month of the occurrence of a stressful event and the duration does not usually exceed 6 month. The manifestations include depressed mood, anxiety, feeling of inability to cope, loss of control, and low self-esteem.

Adjustment disorders should also be differentiated from posttraumatic stress disorder, which occurs as a delayed or protracted response to a stressful event or situation. Typical symptoms include episodes of repeated reliving of the trauma in intrusive memories, dreams, and nightmares, and avoidance of activities and situations reminiscent of the trauma or its causes. Thus, there is commonly fear and avoidance of what is reminiscent of the original trauma. Moreover, patients may avoid situations to which they attribute the stressful event. There may be acute outbursts of fear, panic, or aggression. Anxiety and depression are also common. There is support for conceptualizing events in the life of the cancer patients as analogous to suffering physical traumas such as natural disaster or any victimization. Cancer-related events are often of sudden onset and frequently unexpected. They are also associated with physical discomfort and feelings of helplessness (14).

Postchemotherapy nausea and vomiting, often associated with helplessness, may lead to the development of anticipatory nausea and vomiting. During the course of chemotherapy, an important percentage of patients become sensitized to treatment, reporting anxiety, depression, and nausea in anticipation of chemotherapy (conditioned symptoms). For these reasons, chemotherapy may be considered as a severe stressor and it could be useful to assess psychological and pharmacological interventions designed to reduce, retard, or prevent these consequences.

B. Etiology

Cancer patients experience periods of extreme stress. Hospitalization, illness, surgery, and nonoperative procedures are stressful to all patients and may produce AD, because coping with pain, disability, or death challenges human adaptation. Stressors not related to medical problems such as marital problems, job difficulties, or financial problems can also contribute to the development of AD.

The number and significance of psychosocial stressors, whether they are related to cancer or not in a patient's life, are important factors in determining the degree of disability. The more stressors the patients experiences at one time and the more disturbing the stressors are to the patient, the greater is the effect on the patient's ability to adjust.

Vulnerability factors are not available to help predict in which patients AD will develop. Even if it has not been clearly demonstrated, patients with a previous history of AD or complicated prolonged psychological reaction to stressors may be at increased risk for development of these disorders.

C. Major Diagnostic Procedures

The medical interview is the major mean of establishing a diagnosis of AD and a therapeutic relationship with the patient. The interview allows the clinician to define past and present problems.

A diagnosis of AD should be considered in patients who have symptoms of anxiety or depression, who are experiencing a major psychosocial stressor, and who do not meet the criteria for an anxiety disorder, a depressive disorder, or a posttraumatic stress disorder.

It could be argued that the training of health care professionals may be a way to improve early detection and recognition of psychological problems or psychiatric disorders. This is probably true, but considering that traditional standardized interviews leading to early detection are time-consuming (15,16), it would not be reasonable to assign all specialized staff to this procedure. A balance should be found between time allocated on the one hand and to treatment or support on the other. The type of health care available and the skills of the health care provider are important factors affecting health policy in this area.

The fact that effective methods of treatment are available for several psychological problems and psychiatric disorders associated with cancer is another argument that justifies the cost of the development and implementation of a screening procedure.

The question as to whether screening for the need of psychosocial interventions may be harmful to an individual should also be considered (17). Screening for the need of psychosocial interventions in a cancer population is difficult compared to other psychiatric screening.

In traditional psychiatric screening, it has been argued that the stigma of a psychiatric label may have negative consequences for the patient in terms of income (18), friendships, and social interaction (19). Moreover, referral to mental health specialists is poorly accepted by some patients (20).

For cancer patients, the same arguments fall short. First, one study showed that 85% of cancer patients who reported significant emotional problems said they definitely or probably would go to a mental health professional if they were referred by a medical staff member. Second, 72% responded positively to meeting a mental health professional together with their families (21). These results confirm results of previous studies (22).

Moreover, for cancer patients, it could not be argued that the stigma of a psychiatric label might have a harmful effect on a condition in which the stigma of being a cancer patient is already distressing and replete with psychosocial consequences. It seems also that psychosocial studies are viewed by most patients as a helpful extension to their treatment (23).

Are specific and sensitive screening methods available at a reasonable cost? Screening methods are beginning to be studied in psychosocial oncology. Most of the methods tested have been self-administered questionnaires because standardized research interviews require time and training.

Beck's Depression Inventory (24), Zung's Self-Rating Depression Scale (25), the General Health Questionnaire (26), Hopkins Symptom Checklist (27), the Rotterdam Symptom Checklist (28), and the Hospital Anxiety and Depression Scale (29) are the most frequently used screening methods in psychiatry for depression or for general psychopathology.

These screening instruments generally take less than 15 minutes to complete and have proven to be acceptable to most patients. Most of these questionnaires have been tested in oncology and in primary care settings. The validity of the oral administration of some of these scales for inpatients has also been studied (30).

The verbally administered questionnaire allows participation by patients who have difficulties in writing or who have organic mental disorders. The determination of optimal cut-off points is a major issue for screening instruments. The optimal cut-off point curve is generally determined by a cost-benefit analysis.

Cost and benefit should be objective. One must take into account the medical costs implicated in the decision to screen for a given condition and the benefits in terms of quality of life. The medical costs include the expenses related to the screening method and the optimal treatment of the disorders screened for. The benefits derive from the improvement of quality of life for patients and their families. This issue is closely related to the effectiveness of the interventions designed for the treatment of the disorders.

At this point, most of the research efforts have been focused on the screening of anxiety and depression, which are the most frequent symptoms of ADs and anxiety and ADs associated with the diagnosis of cancer and its treatment and evolution. For these conditions, self-administered anxiety and depression questionnaires are methods with sufficient sensitivity and specificity that can be used for screening. The few studies that assess the performance of the screening methods report a sensitivity and specificity of approximately 75% (31,32).

D. Therapy

In this article, the term "psychological support" includes all the psychosocial interventions relevant to oncology. Psychological support may thus range from the information provided by the general practioner who suspects a diagnosis of cancer to the use of sophisticated techniques performed by well-trained oncologists and psychiatrists. Evidence has been found that cancer psychologically affects not only the patients but also their relatives and the health professionals dealing with them (33). Family interventions and psychological training or support for health professionals should thus also be included in psychological support programs (34).

Not surprisingly, therefore, the literature includes various techniques, more or less explicitly described, dealing with this question: What can we do, without medications, to help the cancer patient cope? Despite the multiplicity of approaches and the objectives they openly declare, (i.e., to reduce psychological morbidity, enhance quality of life, improve communication, provide information, and teach skills), their purpose can be summarized as optimization of the patient's adaptation to the consequences of the disease. Although techniques constantly overlap in clinical practice, they can be divided schematically according to (1) their degree of directivity, for example, nondirective versus directive and (2) their form, for example, individual, family, or group (Table 1).

1. Directive Psychological Support Techniques

Behavioral therapies are based on conditioning theories. They involve precise observation of behavior and use directive methods to achieve determined goals. Their results can be directly observed by the disappearance or persistence of the symptom. The positive effects of the behavioral techniques in treating adverse reactions are well documented by controlled studies. These techniques are especially effective for anticipatory nausea and vomiting related to cancer chemotherapy (35). They are also proposed for controlling and treating psychological reac-

Table 1 Common Psychological Support Techniques in Oncology

Type of interventions	Nondirective techniques	Directive techniques
Individual	Information	Behavior therapy
		Hypnosis
	Counseling	Relaxation
		Progressive muscle relaxation training
Family	Psychotherapy	Electromyographic biofeedback
	Supportive	Guide imagery
	Psychodynamic	Systematic desensitization
Group		Distraction
		Cognitive therapy

tions secondary to painful procedures and acute pain, and adverse reactions to surgery, radiotherapy, and hyperthermia treatment. Recently, they have been proposed for treating postprostatectomy urinary incontinence (36) and for treating anxiety and depression in patients with early breast cancer (37). These uses would represent a considerable and promising increase in indications for the use of behavioral techniques.

Cognitive therapy deals with present problems and tries to identify maladaptive thoughts, irrational beliefs, and inner factors that are responsible for psychological or somatic symptoms. Once identified, these thoughts are confronted with reason and reality. Self-monitoring automatic thoughts, restructuring, and learning coping strategies are commonly used with cancer patients.

2. Nondirective Psychological Support Techniques

Providing information is the first step in helping patients cope with cancer. Information on diagnosis, prognosis, treatments, and long-term sequelae is given by oncologists and general practitioners, but they can be further delivered by other medical staff members and members of self-help groups, either alone or in groups. Information can be provided to the patient alone, to the patient in the presence of family members, or to family members apart from the patient. Perception of information by the patient or the patient's family may be distorted by intellectual and psychological factors, especially in the case of negative information (38). Another bias can be the patient's inability or unwillingness to attend to all presented information.

Counseling is a special form of help performed by persons whose purpose is to listen to the patients, help them express and understand their feelings about cancer, and encourage them to cope with their current situation. Counselors can be specialized nurses, veteran patients, or even volunteers (39). Counseling is a ubiquitous term, but the technique is used to provide cancer patients with first-line support and continuity when no other more specialized help is available.

Psychotherapy is the development of a trusting relationship that allows free communication between patient and specialized therapist. Two models of psychotherapy are used with the cancer patient: supportive and dynamic. Supportive psychotherapy is based on a short-term, crisis-intervention model. This technique is useful in restoring or maintaining the status quo in a crisis. Individuals, families, or groups can be treated. One article concluded that, although group support was effective in providing information and new friends, it did not help patients cope better with cancer (40). Dynamic psychotherapy, based on the psychoanalytical model, is useful when patients desire to explore further their reactions and feelings to promote personality changes and when unconscious or preconscious conflicts are responsible for a large part of the psychic symptoms. Because its duration can be long, psychotherapy is indicated for cancer patients with good prognosis.

Nondirective therapies achieve their supposed wide field of action at great cost: no definite conclusion can be drawn on their efficiency because there are methodological deficiencies. For example, terms are too broad and include different techniques, there is a lack of fully completed interventional descriptions, there is vague determination of which patients could benefit from these interventions, there is nonhomogeneous constitution of the patient groups studied, and there is absence of control groups or randomization in most studies. A recent comprehensive review about the effectiveness of psychological intervention has been recently published (41). The assessment of nondirective therapies have failed to provide unequivocally positive results in oncology. Even so, general agreement exists, supported by clinical experience, that nondirective therapies are effective and feasible in a cancer setting.

3. Psychotropic Medications

Clinical experience supports the need and usefulness of psychotropic medications in oncologic settings. However, because psychotropic medications have been too rarely tested rigorously in oncology, any advances in the treatment of psychological disturbances remains dependent on progress in the clinical psychiatric research. With the exception of treatment for pain, which is discussed elsewhere, very few psychotropic medications have been tested in oncology: mianserin (42) and methylphenidate (43) have been tested for treating depression, and alprazolam (44,45) and lorazepam (46) have been tested for treating phobic nausea and vomiting related to chemotherapy.

It may be useful to recall that alprazolam has been already tested to treat aversion to chemotherapy and adjustment disorders. Greenberg et al. demonstrated in a double blind crossover design study that alprazolam significantly reduced nausea before and vomiting during and after chemotherapy in patients in whom an aversive syndrome developed (44). Patients receiving the active agent typically took 0.25 mg at dinner, 0.5 mg at bedtime, 0.5 mg on morning awakening, and 1.0 mg at noon before chemotherapy. Following chemotherapy, they continued 0.5 mg four times daily as tolerated for an additional 2 days.

Both alprazolam and relaxation reduce cancer-related anxiety and depression (mostly adjustment disorders) (45). Although both treatment arms were effective, patients receiving alprazolam (0.5 mg three times a day) showed a slightly more rapid decrease in anxiety and greater reduction of depressive symptoms.

A recent double blind, placebo controlled study has shown that patients receiving fluoxetine reported at the end of the study statistically significantly less psychological distress than patients receiving placebo (47). Concepts and research about anxiety and depression treatment or control for cancer patients are in their infancy. Goals of anxiety and depression treatment or control may be therefore different for cancer patients who experience numerous daily stressors related to oncological treatments, fear of relapse, or difficulties of coping with sequelae. Therefore, it is not surprising that a complete remission of an anxiety and depressive episode is infrequent. At the end of this study, only 7% in the placebo arm (PA) and 11% in the fluoxetine arm (FA) had a score lower than 8 on the Hospital Anxiety and Depression Scale. The infrequent rate of complete response seems to support the idea of the need to introduce—especially because cancer diseases are generating chronic stress—the concept of controlling anxiety and depression rather than treating AD and major depressive disorder (MDD).

Studies comparing the efficacy and safety of second generation antidepressants versus benzodiazepines in the treatment of adjustment disorders are also needed. A randomized pilot unpublished study comparing trazodone to chlorazepate showed that patients receiving trazodone reported less psychological distress (not statistically significant because of the small sample size) than patients receiving chlorazepate. Number of subjects reporting at least one adverse effect is moreover similar in the chlorazepate arm (37%) and in the trazodone arm (39%). This pilot study indicates the need to further compare antidepressants and benzodiazepines with regard to their impact on psychological distress control and side effect profile.

There is a high prevalence of psychiatric disorders in oncology, and there is an undoubtful interest in preventing these conditions from occurring. A study designed for this purpose failed to show that the adjunct of low doses of alprazolam to a psychological support program may prevent adjustment disorders. However, this study showed that the adjunct of alprazolam to a psychological support program delays the occurrence of anticipatory nausea to cancer chemotherapy. This result indicates the need to further improve the effectiveness shown in this study by finding more effective drug dosages and combinations and to design more appropriate psychological support programs for a preventive aim (48).

One of the reasons for underusing antidepressants is the importance given to interference with cytotoxic drugs, morphinics, steroids, and anticoagulants (49). The limited use of antidepressants is also due to some badly tolerated side effects, particularly in elderly patients. There are some cardiovascular risks (conduction disorders and low blood pressure), neurological risks (sedation, confusion, seizure), and risks of developing visual disorders, constipation, and urinary retention. In elderly patients having cardiac disorders, an electrocardiogram, a monitoring of arterial pressure, and a plasmatic dosage of antidepressants are usually required (50). Trials assessing this issue of potential interference are needed. Moreover, the assumption that trials are difficult to conduct because of possible drug interactions and altered pharmacokinetics caused by medications prescribed for the malignancy is irrelevant, especially in the case of psychotropic drugs, which are generally well tolerated.

Over the past several years, news that antidepressant drugs accelerated tumor growth in rodent studies created a stir among researchers and clinicians (51). Several mechanisms have been suggested. Because tricyclics, phenothiazines, benzodiazepines, and barbiturates are hepatic microsomal enzyme inducers, they are capable of enhancing estrogen metabolism (52). This induction may increase cancer risk by elevating gonadotropin levels. In this hypothesis, estrogen passing through the portal circulation is degraded and does not reach the pituitary to exert its feedback control (53).

Another mechanism suggested is a direct stimulation of malignant growth by antidepressants. Rodent and cell culture studies have shown that certain arylalkylamine (antidepressants, H_1-antihistamines, and benzodiazepines) may stimulate malignant tumors. Dose-response for tumor growth stimulation appears to be bell shaped or biphasic rather than linear: growth enhancement has been found to occur at low or average doses and reversion occurs at higher doses. It is hypothesized that drugs compete for histamine binding on cytochrome P-450 enzymes; in this hypothesis, histamine is considered as being able to modulate the activity of various P-450 enzymes involved in proliferation (51,54,55).

There are contradictory results about the possible role of antidepressants on carcinogenesis and tumor growth promotion (56). The conclusion of a Food and Drug Administration (FDA) study report was that there was no evidence that these drugs increased tumor growth in test tubes or laboratory rodents (57). These controversies indicate the need to study more carefully antidepressant use in a cancer patient population.

III. ANXIETY DISORDERS

A. Definition and Magnitude of the Problem

Anxiety can be classified according to the *Diagnostic and Statistical Manual of Mental Disorders* (DSM-IVH) (58). These definitions are of help for research purposes but not for daily clinical work, because anxiety may be caused by different events in cancer patients than in the psychiatric setting. In a recent study of more than 700 cancer patients (59), clinically relevant anxiety—assessed with a psychometric instrument—was diagnosed in 13% of the patients. Not all anxious states, however, are pathological or clinically relevant. Anxiety serves as a physiological reaction to signal danger to human beings and is, in a way, part of the somatic disease. Anxiety is known by every human being, and the clinical presentation of anxious mood, increased attention, fearfulness, inability to concentrate, and restlessness is easy to diagnose. However, the associated somatic symptoms such as dyspnea, tremor, palpitations, or sweating can also be due to the cancer or its treatment and are therefore less reliable in the diagnosis of anxiety.

B. Etiology

Anxiety can be reactive to a stressor and may be a consequence of an underlying somatic process or a symptom of a psychiatric disturbance. The following arbitrary classification should help to conceptualize states of anxiety in cancer patients and serve for differential diagnostic considerations.

Anxiety as a reaction to a stress is the most common form of anxiety in oncology. In the DSM-IVH classification, this is called an adjustment disorder with anxious mood, alone or in combination with depressed mood (58). Stressors include the diagnosis of cancer, uncontrolled symptoms, or treatment side effects, as well as any other stressor (e.g., conflictual relationships with significant others) that may be perceived as more harmful under the circumstances of a serious disease.

Anxiety may arise in adjustment disorders and less often in phobias activated by some aspects of medical care, panic, and generalized anxiety disorders. Phobias (e.g., claustrophobia) may complicate medical procedures and result in the refusal of a necessary medical intervention. Patients have insight that their fears are unrealistic and are compliant with psychopharmacological or behavioral interventions to help them to overcome their difficulties. Panic disorders, sudden attacks of intense discomfort and fear with physical symptoms such as shortness of breath and palpitations, may be difficult to differentiate from somatic disorders. Generalized anxiety disorders can arise in patients who have had this problem before or as a consequence of repressed fears surrounding the diagnosis of cancer.

Anxiety is also a prominent symptom of delirium (acute confusional states): up to 50% of delirious patients express anxiety as one of the main symptoms (60). Withdrawal from alcohol and benzodiazepines is also often associated with mild to severe anxiety and other psychiatric disorders—such as depressive disorders.

Different somatic processes can cause anxiety in cancer patients. Acute pain is one of the most common causes of anxiety, but hypoxia or metabolic disorders (e.g., hypercalcemia) can also be associated with anxiety. A variety of drugs provoke anxiety as known side effects: corticosteroids (and corticosteroid withdrawal) and morphine, by inducing hallucinatory states (61). Akathisia, a side effect of neuroleptics, is commonly misdiagnosed as anxiety and can be discomforting for the patient.

There are many other forms of anxiety in cancer patients, and some of them have a spiritual and existential dimension, illustrating that not all anxious states are the domain of the medical doctor or the psychiatrist.

C. Major Diagnostic Procedures

To assess anxiety, the main diagnostic tool remains the dialogue with the cancer patient and his or her family. Possible misconceptions, unrealistic fears, psychiatric disorders, and somatic complaints can be questioned, and if an organic cause is suspected to provoke anxiety, additional medical examinations and laboratory work-up, as well as a chart review for side effects of administered drugs, are required. Repeated examinations of cognitive functions are also useful because delirium in cancer patients is often not diagnosed. To assume that an anxious patient has ''the right to be anxious since he has cancer'' is probably the most common obstacle to diagnosis and appropriate treatment.

D. Therapy

Any therapeutic approach requires a discussion with the patient about how he or she copes with the illness and the patient's future to understand possible reasons of the patient's anxiety. A discussion on what the patient thinks of the situation and what the physical symptoms are is necessary for proper treatment and is, in itself, therapeutic. Often, the dialogue with the treating physician, in which a patient is allowed to express his or her feelings and possible misconceptions and fears, is the best therapeutic procedure. If organic causes or psychiatric disturbances as source of anxiety are ruled out, and psychotherapeutic and spiritual support are not successful, then symptomatic treatment with psychotropic medication is indicated.

Benzodiazepines and sometimes low doses of neuroleptics are frequently successfully used for symptomatic treatment of anxious states in cancer patients. Benzodiazepines (e.g., diazepam) with long half-lives and active metabolites can cause profound and prolonged sedation, and should therefore be used with caution (62); newer benzodiazepines with short half-lives, such as lorazepam, are more suited to treat anxiety in cancer patients. In the elderly patient, benzodiazepines can sometimes induce paradoxical excitement and low-dose neuroleptics may be the better choice (63).

IV. DEPRESSIVE DISORDERS

A. Definition and Clinical Presentation

The frequency of depression in cancer patients ranges from 4.5% to 58% in the different studies. One study (1), using DSM-III criteria, has reported a rate of 13% of cancer patients with a major affective disorder (unipolar and bipolar depression, atypical depression, and dysthymic depression) among patients who met criteria for psychiatric disorder.

The clinical presentation includes psychological and somatic symptoms: dysphoric and diurnal mood changes, feelings of hopelessness and helplessness, suicidal ideation, guilt, poor concentration, and rarely delusional thoughts; somatic symptoms such as constipation, insomnia, pain, fatigue, anorexia, and psychomotor retardation or agitation are not reliable signs in cancer patients, because they can be caused by the tumor or its treatment (61).

B. Etiology

Patients with a family or a personal history of depression are at greater risk of development of a depression during the course of cancer. As in the general population, alcohol abuse is also a risk factor for depression, a fact that is also illustrated by the higher incidence of depression in patients with head and neck cancer (64). Patients with pancreatic cancer also have a higher risk for depression (65); the causes for this phenomenon is still unknown, but a paraneoplastic syndrome is suspected (66). Other common causes for depression in cancer patients include chronic, unrelieved pain, medications (e.g., corticosteroids, vincristine, interferon, cimetidine), metabolic alterations (e.g., hypercalcemia), or damage to the central nervous system by the tumor or its treatment (62).

C. Major Diagnostic Procedures

Clinical evaluation includes a careful assessment of the aforementioned symptoms; the fact that depression in cancer patients remains undiagnosed is often related to the fear of the treating physicians to ask direct questions about the feelings of their patients. However, the daily clinical experience with cancer patients demonstrates that patients do not feel such questions to be stressful as long as they are posed in an empathetic way. In contrary, most of the cancer patients feel relief when talking about their feelings.

The differential diagnosis of depression includes sadness, adjustment disorders with depressed mood, grief, and delirious states with depressed affect. If the aforementioned psychological symptoms are present and the cognitive state of the patient is not altered, then the diagnosis of depression is likely and a treatment should be considered. It may sometimes be difficult to diagnose depression in cachectic cancer patients with advanced disease, and confirmation of the diagnosis by a consultation-liaison psychiatrist may be necessary.

Criteria have been suggested to be used in diagnosing major depressive syndromes in medical patients (67). Somatic items of DSM-III criteria such as problems with appetite and sleep, fatigue, and complaints about lessened concentration could be replaced by psychological items such as fearfulness or depressed appearance, social withdrawal or decreased talkativeness, brooding self pity, and pessimism.

D. Therapy

Once the cause of depression has been established and a causal therapeutic approach (e.g., treatment of hypercalcemia) is not possible, short-term psychotherapy supporting past strengths and successful coping strategies becomes necessary. If possible and helpful, the inclusion of family members in the therapy may be beneficial. Severe depressive states usually also require treatment with psychotropic drugs. Antidepressants used in cancer patients include the tricyclic and second generation antidepressants started in low doses, monoamine oxidase inhibitors, benzodiazepines, and stimulants (like dextroamphetamine). Cancer patients respond to lower doses of psychotropic medications because of their altered metabolism and they may be more sensitive to side effects (62). Second generation antidepressants may be more appropriate for cancer patients because they have less anticholinergic side effects thant tricyclic antidepressant.

The effectiveness of mianserine versus placebo has been tested in a double blind design. The doses used were 3 × 10 mg/d in the first week and 3 × 20 mg/d in the following weeks. Twenty-eight patients in the mianserine groups and 18 in the placebo groups benefited from the treatment (42).

In 1988, an uncontrolled pilot study in which imipramine ''or its equivalent'' was used suggested the efficacy of antidepressants in treating major depression in cancer patients (68). One recent controlled, double blind study confirmed the usefulness of mianserine (69).

The lack of controlled studies on psychotropic compounds in oncology is explained in part by the lack of recognition for psychiatric disturbances in oncology. Another factor is the relatively small number of psychiatrists specializing in this field. Moreover, the assumption that trials are difficult to conduct because of possible drug interactions and altered pharmacokinetics caused by medications prescribed for the malignancy is irrelevant, especially in the case of psychotropic drugs, which are generally well tolerated. Table 2 reviews the principal psychotropic drugs currently admitted to be effective in oncology.

One of the reasons for underusing antidepressants is the importance given to interference with cytotoxic drugs, morphinics, steroids, and anticoagulants. The limited use of antidepressant is also due to some badly tolerated side effects,

Table 2 Commonly Prescribed Psychotropic Medications in Oncology

Psychotropic agent	Dosage	
	Initial[a]	Range[b]
Antidepressants		
Tricyclics		
Amitryptiline[c]	25 mg/d	50–150 mg/d
Imipramine	25 mg/d	50–150 mg/d
Nortyptiline	10 mg/d	25–75 mg/d
Desipramine	25 mg/d	50–150 mg/d
Doxepin[c]	25 mg/d	50–150 mg/d
Second generation antidepressants		
Maprotiline	25 mg/d	50–150 mg/d
Mianserin	10 mg/d	10–30 mg/d
Trazodone	50 mg 3 × daily	150–300 mg/d
Fluoxetine	20 mg/d	20–60 mg/d
Venlaflaxine	80 mg/d	80–300 mg/d
Monoamine oxidase inhibitors		
Isocarboxazid	10 mg 2 × daily	20–40 mg/d
Phenelzine	15 mg 2 × daily	30–60 mg/d
Tranylcypromine	10 mg 2 × daily	20–40 mg/d
Moclobemide	150 mg 2 × daily	300–450 mg/d
Triazolobenzodiazepine		
Alprazolam	0.25 mg 3 × daily	0.75–6 mg/d
Stimulants		
Dextroamphetamine	2.5 mg/d in the AM	5–10 mg/d
Methylphenidate	5 mg/d in the AM	10–20 mg/d
Lithium		
Lithium carbonate	250 mg 3 × daily	750–1250 mg/d
Anxiolitics		
Long half-life benzodiazepines		
Diazepam[c]	5 mg 3 × daily	15–30 mg/d
Clorazepate[c]	5 mg 3 × daily	15–30 mg/d
Short half-life benzodiazepines		
Lorazepam[c]	1 mg 3 × daily	3–7.5 mg/d
Oxazepam	15 mg 3 × daily	45–90 mg/d
Alprazolam	0.25 mg 3 × daily	0.75–6 mg/d
Antipsychotics		
Phenothiazine		
Thioridazine	25 mg 3 × daily	75–300 mg/d
Butyrophenone		
Haloperidol[c]	1 mg 3 × daily	3–30 mg/d

[a] Suggested oral dosage, administered once daily at bedtime unless otherwise noted.
[b] Suggested oral dosage.
[c] Available for parenteral use.

particularly in elderly patients. There are some cardiovascular risks (conduction disorders and low blood pressure), neurological risks (sedation, confusion, seizure), and risks of the development of visual disorders, constipation, and urinary retention. In elderly patients having cardiac disorders, an electrocardiogram, a monitoring of arterial pressure, and a plasmatic dosage of antidepressants are usually required (50).

Like with the anxiety disorders, a major setback to effective treatment is that depression often remains unrecognized and, if it is recognized, it remains untreated (62). The knowledge about psychiatric complication in medically ill patients is not extensive among nonpsychiatrists, and future medical education should include these subjects during training.

V. DELIRIUM IN CANCER PATIENTS

A. Definition and Clinical Presentation

Delirium (acute confusional states) is a common psychiatric complication of patients with cancer (70). It is the most common neglected psychiatric syndrome, partly because it is a psychiatric syndrome mainly seen by nonpsychiatric physicians (71). Since Engel and Romano's classic studies (72) investigating delirium, there is a lack of research into classification, epidemiology, pathophysiology, etiology, clinical presentation, diagnostic procedure, treatment, and prevention of delirium (60). With these facts in mind, this section presents a brief overview on the current literature of delirium in cancer patients.

Early symptoms of delirium are often unrecognized or misdiagnosed as depression or dementia (73). Delirium has usually an acute onset and is of brief duration; three clinically distinctive types can be distinguished: the hyperactive-hyperalert, mixed, and hypoactive-hypoalert type (74). In a retrospective study with referred delirious cancer patients (75), the hyperalert subtype was found to be most common with the shortest duration and the best outcome. However, these results may be biased by the fact that this subtype is most often recognized and referred, whereas hypoalert and mixed delirious states remain undetected.

Delirium is often reversible; the clinical course and consequences of delirium (mortality, cognitive impairment, and length of hospitalization) are not well elucidated. However, the onset of delirium is always a serious sign of a dangerous underlying somatic process and can serve as a predictor of shortened survival (76).

Lipowski, who is devoted to the elucidation of this syndrome and has edited one of the most comprehensive books on this subject (77), described the core features as "disorders of cognition, attention, sleep-wake cycle, and psychomotor behavior" (78). According to DSM-IV criteria (58), delirium is characterized by impairment in responsiveness and alertness as manifested by fluctuating inability to maintain and shift attention, by cognitive dysfunction of recent onset (development over a period usually hours or days), and by the evidence from history, physical examination, or laboratory findings of organic factors judged to be etiologically related to the disturbance (such an etiological agent may not always be found in a patient population in which investigations are limited).

The magnitude of the problem can be concluded from different studies on the prevalence of delirium in cancer patients, which has ranged from 5% to 25% (73). These differences are based on variations in population samples and are largely dependent on age, preexistent brain damage (especially dementia), level of physical disability, and stage of disease, which are all risk factors of delirium in cancer patients (79).

B. Etiology

Different hypotheses on the etiology of delirium exist in the literaute, and it may be that different mechanisms are contributing simultaneously to a delirious state of a cancer patient, or that the pathophysiology may differ according to the underlying etiology.

The following hypotheses have been posited to explain the onset of delirium (70,60): (1) Any factor that reduces cerebral oxidative metabolism can lead to changes in the functional metabolism of cerebral neurons; (2) an imbalance of neurotransmitters (imbalance between acetylcholine and dopamine by anticholinergic drugs or other reasons); (3) hypercortisolism caused by stress or external agents; (4) neuroanatomical models (brain metastases); (5) changes in endorphine levels, and (6) other hypotheses.

A range of factors causes delirium in cancer patients. They can be classified as direct and indirect effects on the central nervous system (Table 3) (80). Direct effects are those that are related to primary brain tumor or metastatic spread; indirect effects are more frequent and are due to infections, vascular complications, metabolic abnormalities, hematological complications, nutritional deficiencies, treatment side effects, and paraneoplastic syndromes.

The following causes of delirium in cancer patients are most important (79): metabolic abnormalities (organ failure, electrolyte imbalance), infections (pneumonia, sepsis), vascular complications (thromboembolic cerebral infarction), metastatic brain disease, and treatment effects including withdrawal. Among treatment side effects, corticosteroids, narcotic analgesics, psychotropics, and other drugs with anticholinergic properties and chemotherapeutic agents are the most common causes of delirium in cancer patients (73,79,81).

Patients with cancer who are seriously ill often have multiple causes for delirium. In a study of patients with advanced and terminal disease, in only 1 of 11 patients with delirium was a single cause established. The remaining patients' delirium was attributed to multiple factors. In a retrospective study (70) on cogni-

Table 3 Causes of Delirium in Cancer Patients

1. Direct effects
   a. Primary tumor
   b. Metastatic lesions by local extension, hematogenous, or lymphatic routes
2. Indirect effects
   a. Metabolic problems (organ failure and electrolyte imbalance)
   b. Treatment effects (chemotherapeutic agents, radiation, medications)
   c. Infections (pneumonia) and systemic infections
   d. Vascular complications (thromboembolic cerebral infarction, intracranial hemorrhage)
   e. Hematologic abnormalities (anemias, coagulopathies)
   f. Nutritional deficits (general malnutrition and vitamin deficits)
   g. Paraneoplastic syndromes

Source: Ref. 80.

tive failure in cancer patients with advanced disease, the causal agent remained unknown in 75%. This may be due to the fact that an extensive work-up in terminally ill patients is rarely appropriate.

C. Major Diagnostic Procedures

The diagnosis of delirium relies heavily on the history and the presence of an abruptly altered mental state, with identification of an inability to maintain or shift attention and cognitive impairment. Clinical examination, laboratory data, assessment instruments, and other investigations assist in establishing etiology and diagnosis (79). Unlike other medical patients, many cancer patients are faced with dealing with a fatal disease, and normal stress reactions, depression, and other psychiatric disturbances may be difficult to differentiate. Subtle changes in mental status and behavior are therefore apt to go unnoticed or to be attributed to the stress of cancer diagnosis. A close watch of mental functions and comparison with its prior level (history by family members, chart review) help to differentiate delirium from normal stress reactions, adjustment disorders, or early dementia.

D. Therapy

Management of delirium is first directed toward determining the underlying cause and toward treatment, when possible, of the etiological agent to reverse the condition. However, because this is rarely possible, symptomatic treatment becomes necessary. General supportive and nonspecific treatments may help in milder forms of delirium: environmental manipulation with a clock at bedside to help the patients orientation, avoidance of hypostimulation or hyperstimulation, and staff instructions to minimize the number of different members involved in the care of the patient (79).

More often, acute confusion with hallucinations, delusions, anxiety, agitation, and disruptive behavior requires symptomatic treatment with psychotropic drugs. The cornerstone of symptomatic psychotropic therapy is neuroleptic and benzodiazepine drugs.

Haloperidol is a commonly prescribed antipsychotic drug in the cancer setting because of its low incidence of cardiovascular and anticholinergic effects (62). Hospitalized cancer patients usually respond to low doses of psychotropic medication, such as 0.5 mg of haloperidol given two or three times daily; acute extrapyramidal side effects, although not common at these dose levels, are usually controlled by diphenhydramine or benztropin twice a day (79). The addition of lorazepam for sedation or a continuous subcutaneous infusion of midazolam in severe cases is being increasingly used (77).

Despite these clinical observations, benzodiazepine may have limited benefit in delirium. In a double blind, randomized trial in patients with acquired immunodeficiency syndrome, Breitbart and colleagues (82) demonstrated that lorazepam alone was ineffective in the treatment of delirium and contributed to worsening delirium and cognitive impairment. On the other hand, both neuroleptic drugs used in this study—haloperidol and chlorpromazine—were effective in low doses to control the symptoms of delirium and to improve cognitive function. Suggestions from the literature remain on empirical grounds.

VI. CONCLUSIONS

First, a precise and comprehensive assessment of the patient's psychological and psychiatric problems and a good understanding of the patient's social situation are of the utmost importance for any reasonable therapeutic intervention. Developing specific assessment methods is still necessary, as are simple, reliable, and valid tools for the early screening of psychological disturbances in an oncology population. Early detection of mild psychological distress may identify patients who could be helped with psychosocial interventions. Moreover, even if no data are available stating that early treatment could have therapeutic results superior to those of delayed treatment, early treatment has a positive effect on quality of life. Along the same line, early recognition of distress among family members and caretakers is another promising subject of research to improve the quality of support.

Second, the diversity of, and lack of precise description for, most psychological interventions remains an obstacle to any progress in this field. Especially for nondirective techniques, the indications for and purposes of psychological support remain unclear. The type of cancer and treatment; the time in the illness course; the patient's personality, gender, and age; and the quality of social support are all factors that should be taken into account to increase the relevance and validity of research in this area. The question of whether appropriate psychological support has a positive influence on cancer patient survival has recently come to the fore. This topic requires careful examination and further controlled studies (83). Studies have been undertaken in the United States and in Canada for that purpose.

Third, it is unfortunate that the qualifications of the person performing the therapy are hardly defined. Should a general practitioner, an oncologist, a nursing staff member, a mental health professional (e.g., psychiatrist, psychologist, or trained therapist), or a nonprofessional (e.g., veteran patient or voluntary organization member) intervene? Specific training should be designed and organized for each of these categories (34,84,85). More research comparing the efficacy of the same treatments performed by differently trained persons must be done, not only to provide patients with the most effective therapy but also to take into account its cost and feasibility in a cancer setting. In conclusion, without rigorous research and controlled studies, psychological support will continue to be suspected of empiricism, although its efficacy as adjuvant therapy in oncology can no longer be questioned (86).

Despite recognition of the high prevalence of psychiatric and psychosocial disturbances associated with cancer and its treatments, and inclusion of the psychosocial factors in quality of life assessments and rehabilitation programs, very few articles rigorously investigate what can actually be done to prevent and alleviate these disturbances. In particular, research should be encouraged in the newly identified class of adjustment disorders that occur so frequently in oncology; new concepts to understand and treat them are dramatically needed. The respective indications of psychological support, psychotropic medications, or both are based on clinical experience and rarely on large, controlled, prospective studies. A first step should be to recognize the respective usefulness of single psychological interventions and single medical agents in specific situations. A second step should be to compare different techniques for their efficacy, cost, and feasibility in a cancer setting. A third step should be to test for the possible superior effectiveness of combinations, such as nondirective technique with directive technique, individual psychological support with family support, psychological support with psychotropic medication, and antidepressant with benzodiazepine.

First, because the psychiatric conditions found in cancer patients are reported to be quite different from those encountered in the general population and in other medically ill patients, further development of specific tools is needed to assess psychiatric morbidity in oncology. Second, controlled studies have to test the usefulness of psychotropic agents for major depressive disorders, delirium, and insomnia. The complete lack of controlled studies in the field of adjustment disorders must be addressed without delay. Third, the feasibility and effectiveness of using specific classes of psychotropic medications for preventing psychological and psychiatric disorders in cancer patients should be evaluated in prospective studies at each phase of the illness course. For example, concepts and research about preventive use of psychopharmacotherapy for patients undergoing stressful medical procedures or treatment (e.g., chemotherapy) is in its infancy so that, at present, only tentative guidelines can be offered to oncologists. Goals of a preventive treatment should be the reduction of psychological and psychiatric morbidities and the reduction in the delay of symptom control when some symptoms may be frequent and expected (e.g., sleeping problems, conditioned symptoms, adjustment disorders). More studies are needed to find the most effective drug combinations, optimal drug dosage, and treatment duration. The ideal evaluation of the efficacy of prevention programs requires randomized controlled trials that compare not only prevention to normal clinical follow-up but also to early detection and early treatment. Finally, more research on the development of the most frequent psychological or psychiatric conditions encountered in oncology will allow selections of which drugs should be combined for a preventive use on a less empirically basis.

The important prevalence of psychosocial problems and psychiatric disturbances that have been reported in oncology underlines the need for a comprehensive psychosocial support of cancer patients and their families. Psychosocial support is designed to preserve, restore or enhance quality of life. Quality of life refers not only to psychosocial distress and adjustment related problems but also to the management of cancer symptoms and treatment side effects. Psychosocial interventions designed for this purpose should be divided in five categories: prevention, early detection, restoration, support, and palliation. First, preventive interventions are designed to avoid the development of predictable morbidity secondary to treatment or disease. Second, early detection of patient's needs or problems refers to the assumption that early interventions could have therapeutic results superior to those of delayed support, both for quality of life and survival. Third, restorative interventions refer to actions used when a cure is likely, the aim being the control or elimination of residual cancer disability. Fourth, supportive rehabilitation is planned to lessen disability related to chronic disease characterized by numerous cancer illness remissions and progressions, and to active treatment. Fifth, palliation is required when curative treatment is likely to be no more effective and when maintaining or improving comfort becomes the main goal. Psychosocial interventions are often multidisciplinary with a variety of content. The content of psychological interventions ranges from information and education to more sophisticated support programs including directive (behavioral or cognitive) therapies, or nondirective (dynamic or supportive) therapies. Social interventions usually include financial, household, equipment, and transport assistance depending on individual and family needs and resources. These interventions may be combined with the prescription of pharmacological (psychotropic, analgesic), physical, speech, or occupational therapy, especially in rehabilitation programs. Health care services devoted to delivering these interventions are hospital, hospice, or home based and are organized very differently depending on already available community resources.

REFERENCES

1. Derogatis LR, Morrow G, Fetting J, Penman D, Piatesky S, Schmale AM, Hendricks M, Carnicke C. The prevalence and severity of psychiatric disorders among cancer patients. JAMA 1983; 249(6):751–757.
2. Stephanek ME, Derogatis LP, Shaw A. Psychological distress among oncology outpatients. Psychosomatics 1987; 28:530–539.
3. Allebeck P, Bolund C, Ringbäck G. Increased suicide rate in cancer patients: a cohort study based on the Swedish Cancer-Environment Register. J Clin Epidemiol 1989; 42:611–616.
4. Loescher L, Welch-McCaffrey D, Leigh S, Hoffman B, Meyskens F. Surviving adult cancers: part 2: psychosocial implications. Ann Intern Med 1989; 111:517–524.
5. Eil K, Nishimoto R, Morvay T, Mantell J, Hamovitch M. A longitudinal analysis of psychological adaptation among survivors of cancer. Cancer 1989; 63:406–413.
6. Vinokur A, Threatt B, Caplan R, Zimmerman B. Physical and psychosocial functioning and adjustment to breast cancer: long-term follow-up of a screening population. Cancer 1989; 66:394–405.
7. Lesko L, Holland J. Psychological issues in patients with hematological malignancies. Rec Res Cancer Res 1988; 108:243–270.
8. Love R, Leventhal H, Easterling D, Nerenz D. Side effects and emotional distress during cancer chemotherapy. Cancer 1989; 66:604–612.
9. Ochs J, Mulheim R, Kun L. Quality-of-life assessment in cancer patients. Am J Clin Oncol 1988; 11:415–421.
10. Kurtzman S, Gardner B, Kellner W. Rehabilitation of the cancer patient. Am J Surg 1988; 155:791–801.
11. Kemeny M, Wellisch D, Schain W. Psychosocial outcome in a randomized surgical trial for treatment of primary breast cancer. Cancer 1988; 62:1231–1237.
12. Wolberg W, Romsaas E, Tanner M, Malec J. Psychosexual adaptation to breast cancer surgery. Cancer 1989; 66:1645–1655.
13. Salmon S. Factors predictive of success or failure in acquisition of esophageal speech. Head Neck Surg 1988; 10:5105–5109.
14. Cella D, Mahon S, Donovan M. Cancer recurrence as a traumatic event. Behav Med 1990; spring:15–21.

15. Hamilton M. The assessment of anxiety states by rating. Br J Med Psychol 1959; 32:50–58.
16. Wing JK, Cooper JE, Sartorius N. The Measurement and Classification of Psychiatric Symptoms. London: Cambridge University Press, 1974.
17. Ford DE. Principles of screening applied to psychiatric disorders. Gen Hosp Psychiatry 1988; 10:177–188.
18. Link B. Mental patient status, work and income: an examination of the effects of a psychiatric label. Am Sociol Rev 1982; 47:202–215.
19. Phillips D. Public identification and acceptance of the mentally ill. Am J Pub Health 1966; 56:755–763.
20. Bursztajn H, Barsky AJ. Facilitating patient acceptance of a psychiatric referral. Arch Intern Med 1985; 145:73–75.
21. Houts P, Lipton A, Harvey H, Simmonds M, Cadieux R, Bartholomew M. Willingness to use mental health services by cancer patients with emotional problems. International Conference on Supportive Care in Oncology. Abstracts. Princeton: Symedco, 1988:182.
22. Worden JW, Weisman AD. Do cancer patients really want counseling? Gen Hosp Psychiatry 1980; 2:100–103.
23. Fallowfield L. Do psychological studies upset patients? In: Holland JC, Massie MJ, Lesko LM, eds. Current Concepts in Psycho-Oncology and AIDS. Syllabus of the Postgraduate Course/Memorial Sloan-Kettering Cancer Center, New York, 1987:335.
24. Beck AT, Beck RW. Screening depressed patients in family practice. Postgrad Med J 1972; 52:81–85.
25. Zung WWK. A self-rating depression scale. Arch Gen Psychiatry 1965; 12:63–70.
26. Goldberg DP. A Technique for the Identification and Assessment of Nonpsychotic Psychiatric Illness. London: Oxford University Press, 1972.
27. Derogatis DL. The SCL-90 Administration, Scoring and Procedures Manual I. Baltimore: Clinical Psychometric Research, 1977.
28. de Haes JCJM, Pruyn JJA, Knipperberg FCG. Klachtenlijst voor kankerpatienten, eerste ervaringen. Ned Tijdschr Psych 1983; 38:403–422.
29. Zigmond AS, Snaith RP. The Hospital Anxiety and Depression Scale. Acta Psychiatr Scand 1983; 67:361–370.
30. Griffin Pht, Kogut D. Validity of orally administered Beck and Zung depression scales in a state hospital setting. J Clin Psychol 1988; 44:756–759.
31. Razavi D, Delvaux N, Farvacques C, Robaye E. Screening for adjustment disorders and major depressive disorders in cancer in-patients. Br J Psychiatry 1990; 156:79–83.
32. Razavi D, Delvaux N, Brédart A, Paesmans M, Debusscher L, Bron D, Stryckmans P. Screening for psychiatric disorders in a lymphoma out-patient population. Eur J Cancer 1992; 28A(11):1869–1872.
33. Delvaux N, Razavi D, Farvacques C. Cancer care—a stress for health professionals. Soc Sci Med 1988; 27:159–166.
34. Razavi D, Delvaux N, Farvacques C, Robaye E. Immediate effectiveness of brief psychological training for health professionals dealing with terminally ill cancer patients: a controlled study. Soc Sci Med 1988; 27:369–375.

35. Morrow GR, Morrel C. Behavioral treatment for the anticipatory nausea and vomiting induced by cancer chemotherapy. N Engl J Med 1982; 307:1476–1480.
36. Burgio K, Stutzman R, Engel B. Behavioral training for post-prostatectomy urinary incontinence. J Urol 1989; 141:303–306.
37. Bridge L, Benson P, Pietroni P, Prest R. Relaxation and imagery in the treatment of breast cancer. BMJ 1988; 297:1169–1172.
38. Mackillop W, Stewart W, Ginsburg A, Stewart S. Cancer patient's perceptions of their disease and its treatment. Br J Cancer 1988; 58:355–358.
39. Fallowfield L. Counseling for patients with cancer. BMJ 1988; 297:727–728.
40. Deans G, Bennett-Emslie J, Weir J, Smith D, Kaye S. Cancer support groups—who joins and why? Br J Cancer 1988; 58:670–674.
41. Fawzy FI, Fawzy NW. Psychoeducational Interventions. In: Holland JC, ed. Psycho-Oncology. New York: Oxford University Press, 1998:548–563.
42. Costa D, Mogos I, Toma T. Efficacy and safety of mianserin in the treatment of depression of women with cancer. Acta Psychiatr Scand 1985; 72:85–92.
43. Fernandez F, Adams F, Holmes VF. Methylphenidate for depressive disorders in cancer patients. Psychosomatics 1987; 28:455–461.
44. Greenberg DB, Surman OS, Clarke J, Baer L. Alprazolam for phobic nausea and vomiting related to cancer chemotherapy. Cancer Treatment Reports 1987; 71(5): 549–550.
45. Holland JC, Morrow GR, Schmale A, Derogatis L, Stefanek M, Berenson S, Carpenter PJ, Breitbart W, Feldstein M. A randomized clinical trial of alprazolam versus progressive muscle relaxation in cancer patients with anxiety and depressive symptoms. J Clin Oncol 1991; 9(6):1004–1011.
46. Greenspoon J, Leuchter RS, Semrad N. Lorazepam for chemotherapy-induced emesis. Arch Intern Med 1984; 144:2432–2433.
47. Razavi D, Allilaire JF, Smith M, Salimpour A, Verra M, Desclaux B, Saltel P, Piollet I, Gauvain-Piquard A, Trichard C, Cordier B, Fresco R, Guillibert-E, Sechter D, Orth JP, Bouhassira M, Mesters P, Blin P. The effect of fluoxetine on anxiety and depression symptoms in cancer patients. Acta Psychiatr Scand 1996; 94:205–210.
48. Razavi D, Delvaux N, Farvacques Ch, De Brier F, Van Heer C, Kaufman L, Derde M-P, Beauduin M, Piccart M. Prevention of adjustment disorders and anticipatory nausea secondary to adjuvant chemotherapy: a double-blind placebo controlled study assessing the usefulness of alprazolam. J Clin Oncol 1993; 11:1384–1390.
49. Stoudemire A. Expanding psychopharmacologic treatment options for the depressed medical patient. Psychosomatics 1995; 2(1):19–26.
50. Razavi D, Mendlewicz J. Tricyclics antidepressant plasma levels: the state of the art and clinical prospect. Neuropsychobiology 1982; 8:73–95.
51. Brandes LJ, Arron RJ, Bogdanovic RP, Tong J, Zaborniak CLF, Hogg GR, Warrington RC, Fang W, LaBella FS. Stimulation of malignant growth in rodents by antidepressant drugs at clinically relevant doses. Cancer Res 1992; 52:3796–3800.
52. Cramer DW, Welch WR. Determinants of ovarian cancer risk II. Inferences regarding pathogenesis. J Natl Cancer Inst 1983; 71:717–721.
53. Harlow BL, Cramer DW. Self-reported use of antidepressants or benzodiazepine tranquilizers and risk of epithelial ovarian cancer: evidence from two combined case-

control studies (Massachusetts, United States). Cancer Causes and Control 1995; 6: 130–134.

54. Lishi H, Tatsuta M, Baba M, Taniguchi H. Enhancement by the tricyclic antidepressant, desipramine, of experimental carcinogenesis in rat colon induced by azoxymethane. Carcinogenesis 1993; 14:1837–1840.
55. Brandes LJ, Friesen LA. Can the clinical course of cancer be influenced by non-antineoplastic drugs? Can Med Assoc J 1995; 153(5):561–566.
56. Bendele RA, Adams ER, Hoffman WP, Gries CL, Morton DM. Carcinogenicity studies of fluoxetine hydrochloride in rats and mice. Cancer Res 1992; 52:6931–6935.
57. News: Concern over prozac-induced tumor growth may dwindle following FDA study. J Natl Cancer Inst 1995; 87(17):1285–1287.
58. American Psychiatric Association. DSM-IV. Diagnostic and Statistical Manual of Mental Disorders. 4th ed. Washington DC: American Psychiatric Association, 1994.
59. Aass N, Fossa SD, Dahl A, More TJI. Prevalence of anxiety and depression in cancer patients seen at the Norwegian Radium Hospital. Eur J Cancer 1997; 33(10):1597–1604.
60. Stiefel F. Age and the Syndrome of Delirium-Ein Workshop des National Institut of Mental Health, Washington, DC, June 1989. Schweiz Rundschau Med (PRAXIS) 1989; 78:1329.
61. Massie MJ, Popkin MK. Depressive Disorders. In: Holland JC, ed. Psycho-Oncology. New York: Oxford University Press, 1998:518–540.
62. Stiefel F, Kornblith A, Holland J. Changes in the prescription patterns of psychotropic drugs for cancer patients during a 10-year period. Cancer 1990; 65:1048–1053.
63. Noyes R, Craig SH, Massie MJ. Anxiety Disorders. In: Holland JC, ed. Psycho-Oncology. New York: Oxford University Press, 1998:548–563.
64. Baile WF, Gibertini M, Scott L, Endicott J. Depression and tumor stage in cancer of the head and neck. Psycho-Oncology 1992; 1:15–24.
65. Holland JC, Hughes AH, Tross S, Silberfarb P, Perry M, Comis R, Oster M. Comparative disturbance in patients with pancreatic and gastric cancer. Am J Psychiatry 1986; 143:982–986.
66. Pomara NP, Gershon S. Treatment-resistant depression in an elderly patient with pancreatic carcinoma. J Clin Psychiatry 1984; 45:439–440.
67. Endicott J. Measurement of depression in patients with cancer. Cancer 1984; 53(10): 2243–2248.
68. Evans DL, McCartney CF, Haggerty JJ, Nemeroff CB, Golden RN, Simon JB, Quade D, Holmes V, Droba M, Mason GA, Fowler WC, Raft D. Treatment of depression in cancer patients is associated with better life adaptation: a pilot study. Psychosom Med 1988; 50:72–76.
69. Van Heeringen K, Zivkov M. Pharmacological treatment of depression in cancer patient. A placebo-controlled study of mianserin. Br J Psychiatry 1996; 169:440–443.
70. Stiefel F, Fainsinger R, Bruera E. Acute confusional states in patients with advanced cancer. J Pain Symptom Manage 1992; 7:25–29.
71. Levine PM, Silberfarb PM, Lipowski ZJ. Mental disorders in cancer patients. A study of 100 psychiatric referrals. Cancer 1978; 42:1385–1391.

72. Engel GL, Romano G. Delirium, a syndrome of cerebral insufficiency. J Chron Dis 1959; 9:260–277.
73. Lesko LM, Massie MJ, Holland JC. Oncology. In: Principles of Medical Psychiatry. Grune Stratton, 1987:501–503.
74. Stiefel F, Bruera E. Psychostiumulants for hypoactive-hypoalert delirium? J Palliat Care 1991(b); 7(3):25–26.
75. Oolfsson SM, Weitzner MA, Valentine AD, Baile WF, Meyers CA. A retrospective study of the psychiatric management and outcome of delirium in the cancer patient. Support Care Cancer 1996; 4:351–357.
76. Bruera E, Miller MJ, Kuehn N, MacEachern T, Hanson J. Estimate of survival of patients admitted to a palliative care unit: a prospective study. J Pain Symptom Manage 1992; 7:82–86.
77. Lipowski ZJ. Delirium: Acute Confusional States. New York: Oxford University Press, 1990.
78. Lipowski ZJ. Transient cognitive disorders (delirium, acute confusional states) in the elderly. Am J Psychiatry 1983; 140:1426–1436.
79. De Stoutz ND, Stiefel F. Assessment and management of reversible delirium. In: Portenoy RK, Bruera E, eds. Topics in Palliative Care. New York: Oxford University Press, 1997:21–43.
80. Posner JB. Neurologic complications of systemic cancer. Dis Month 1978; 25:1–60.
81. Breitbart W, Stiefel F, Kornblith AB, Panullo S. Neuropsychiatric disturbance in cancer patients with epidural spinal cord compression receiving high dose corticosteroids; a prospective comparison study. Psycho-Oncology 1993; 2:233–245.
82. Breitbart W, Marotta R, Platt MM, et al. A double-blind trial of haloperidol, cholorpromazine and lorazepam in the treatment of delirium in hospitalized AIDS patients. Am J Psychiatry 1996; 153:231–237.
83. Spiegel D, Kraemer H, Bloom J, Gottheil E. Effects of psychosocial treatment on survival of patients with metastatic breast cancer. Lancet 1989; 2:888–891.
84. Razavi D, Delvaux N, Farvacques C, Robaye E. Brief psychological training for health care professionals dealing with cancer patients: a one-year assessment. Gen Hosp Psychiatry 1991; 13:253–260.
85. Razavi D, Delvaux N. Communication skills and psychological training in oncology. Eur J Cancer 1997; 33:15–21.
86. Moorey S, Greer S. Psychological Therapy for Patients with Cancer: A New Approach. Oxford: Heinemann Medical Books, 1989.

17

Obstructive Syndromes

Anne O'Donnell
Royal Prince Alfred Hospital, Camperdown, New South Wales, Australia

Martin H. N. Tattersall
University of Sydney, Sydney, New South Wales, Australia

I. INTRODUCTION

Early identification of symptoms and signs attributable to organ obstruction by malignancy and effective treatment thereof can make a significant contribution to patient care. Where early treatment may avert major morbidity, obstructive syndromes in cancer patients must be regarded as medical emergencies. In other contexts, prompt identification of the symptoms of an obstructive syndrome and successful management may lead to improved symptom control even if the obstruction itself is not completely reversible.

An obstructive syndrome may be the primary presentation of a cancer or, more commonly, it may develop with progressive disease. In the assessment of these syndromes, it is important to establish clearly the major symptoms experienced by the patient and then to determine whether an obstructed organ is responsible. Useful features of the patient history are the pattern of the symptoms and their rate of evolution, which may reflect the biology of the obstruction. Equally important, however, is the background against which the problem has developed in the patient. For example, is it an isolated event in a patient with good performance status or is it the culmination of progressive disease in a patient with advanced malignancy? It is this context that should determine not only the investigations but also the treatment options that are realistic.

The importance of good communication between the patient, the patient's family, and the clinical team cannot be overemphasized. All need to understand not just the problem at hand but the overall situation, so that appropriate actions are undertaken. It may not always be appropriate to identify precisely the site and origin of the obstruction, but efforts should be directed at controlling the symptoms, which arise from it. All investigations have varying degrees of morbidity and inconvenience associated with them. There is a vast array of techniques to image organs and assess their function. It is rarely necessary to undertake them all, rather the skill lies in selecting those that will provide optimal information for a particular patient. It is important that persons recommending either investigations or treatments are aware of the effectiveness and morbidity of these interventions. In many situations, the patient and his or her unique history is unknown to the person undertaking the procedure and sometimes even to those providing treatment.

Evaluating the management options available, then selecting the appropriate intervention can be difficult, even for an experienced clinician. How much more difficult it must be then for the patient and the patient's family, who have only a limited and rapidly gained knowledge of medicine to grasp these issues, often in very emotional circumstances? They deserve full support from the management team, with careful and compassionate explanation.

All treatment must be continuously evaluated against the intended goal. If a treatment proves ineffective and additional intervention is justified, one must clarify again the objective and decide whether the intervention or even investigation is reasonable in the context of the patient's circumstances. It is important throughout that symptom control be the primary goal. Commonly, a palliative care physician can assist with management.

The patient must not be led to believe that nothing further can be done, rather the patient should know that treatment must be changed to achieve new goals. Arriving at understanding and acceptance of this is an index of successful communication between clinician and patient.

In general, management options for an obstructive syndrome may be thought of in two categories: (1) those techniques designed to shrink or eliminate the obstructing tumor itself (e.g., radiotherapy, chemotherapy, surgical excision) and (2) those designed to bypass the problem. (e.g., surgery or mechanical stenting). The background of the patient influences the choice of approach but several other issues are important:

- The probable chemosensitivity of the tumor or the need to treat several sites simultaneously
- The radiosensitivity of the tumor or the availability of radiotherapy
- The availability of suitable surgical or interventional radiological expertise and the acceptability of the patient as a surgical candidate.
- The rate of progression of the patient's symptoms or syndrome and tumor with the expected speed of a response to these differing modalities

II. ALIMENTARY TRACT OBSTRUCTION

The symptoms experienced by patients with alimentary tract obstruction vary with the site of the obstruction, as detailed in Table 1.

In patients with known malignant disease, obstruction of the digestive tract is most commonly directly related to the cancer; however, other possibilities should be kept in mind:

- Prior surgery may have led to the development of adhesions causing intestinal obstruction
- Prior abdominal radiotherapy may have led to stricture development causing esophageal or small bowel obstruction
- Drug therapy may be responsible (or at least contributory), as in the high prevalence of constipation with narcotic usage, vinca alkaloids, and serotonin antagonists

In some situations when the obstruction is due to cancer, antitumor treatment may relieve the obstruction and benefit the patient; for others, however, a conservative approach is more appropriate.

A. Conservative Measures

High-dose corticosteroids (e.g., dexamethasone $\geq$ 8 mg) may induce rapid functional improvement and symptom relief through reduction in edema. Drugs that may aggravate the obstruction (e.g., prokinetics) or its symptoms (e.g., tricyclic antidepressants) should be avoided.

Decisions about parenteral fluid support in patients with bowel obstruction can be difficult and need to be negotiated with patient, family, and nursing staff. Subcutaneous infusion is convenient and effective in hydrating patients. There may occasionally be a place for the temporary use of parenteral fluid, in the

Table 1 Alimentary Tract Obstruction

Site	Symptoms
Pharyngeal	Choking, dysphagia, pain
Esophageal	Dysphagia, weight loss, regurgitation, cough
Gastroduodenal	Nausea, early satiety, vomiting, dehydration
Biliary	Jaundice, pruritus, pain, diarrhea
Small bowel	Central colicky pain, distention, vomiting, transient diarrhea
Large bowel	Constipation, colicky lower abdominal pain, vomiting
Anorectal	Tenesmus, pain, constipation

context of realistic optimism regarding relief of the obstruction. However, in irreversible alimentary tract obstruction, infusions are not necessary to maintain patient comfort and may prolong the act of dying. Advances in therapeutics have led to the feasibility of obtaining and maintaining comfort and dignity for the patient, without these measures. Mouth care is crucial, usually including antifungal therapy. The focus of care is to alleviate the patient's symptoms rather than the academic exercise of maintaining fluid balance, which can be both invasive and problematic by exacerbating vomiting.

B. Esophageal Obstruction

The esophagus may be imaged directly by endoscopy or functionally with the use of barium. Plain x-ray and computed tomography (CT) scanning may better delineate the site of obstruction and the site of any associated mass. Tissue can be obtained at endoscopy or via fine needle aspiration biopsy.

Treatment options vary greatly in their morbidity, mortality, and cost-effectiveness. For some patients, the tumor may be treated with chemotherapy, radiotherapy, or a combination of the two in order to alleviate the occlusion. An example is the result achieved with chemoradiation for esophageal cancer. Randomized data suggest that combined modality therapy is comparable to surgery and outperforms radiotherapy alone. In RTOG 85-01 chemoradiation showed not only an overall survival advantage (30% at 5 y) but also improved local control when compared with radiotherapy alone (1).

Palliative surgical bypass has a mortality rate of up to 60% with significant morbidity in the recovery phase. Although it may palliate dysphagia in almost all patients, the associated complications commonly make it inappropriate (2). Laser therapy is expensive and must be repeated frequently (4–6 weekly) to manage recurrent tumor problems (3). Rigid endoprostheses are associated with major procedure-related morbidity and mortality rates (up to 36% in some series) (3). Self-expanding esophageal stents have gained popularity recently. Such stents may be metal or plastic, although the latter appear to have a higher rate of early complications (20%) and procedure-related mortality (3%–5%). Tumor ingrowth and stent migration are significant problems, which are only partially resolved by coating the metal stent. When occlusion occurs, it is usually feasible to revise such endoprostheses, at least initially (2–7).

Radiation alone palliates the dysphagia in less than 40% of patients depending somewhat on the site of obstruction and tumor histology. The relief may not be achieved for up to 2 months after radiation is initiated and treatment may be complicated by painful dysphagia requiring hospitalization and nutritional support (8).

When such maneuvers are unsuccessful and the condition of the patient warrants an aggressive approach, a feeding gastrostomy or fine bore nasogastric feeding tube can provide ongoing nutrition. Total parenteral nutrition is seldom justified in cancer patients, with an exception being the highly catabolic situation of high-dose chemotherapy or aggressive chemoradiation complicated by mucositis. Although such therapy may be technically feasible, the primary goal of treatment must be foremost in determining what is appropriate.

C. Intestinal Obstruction

Plain abdominal films (supine and erect or decubitus) retain their place in assessment of the patient because, despite their low specificity, they are inexpensive and noninvasive. Direct examination of the small bowel is difficult via endoscopy and barium studies are uncomfortable for the patient and may be difficult to interpret. Colonoscopy permits direct examination of the large bowel with potential for biopsy to establish etiology. It may be complemented by barium studies, but the use of barium may interfere with the accuracy of other investigations. Increasingly, CT scanning, with its relative noninvasiveness, is gaining in popularity to assess the level of intestinal obstruction and the extent of disease, as well as providing anatomical detail for consideration of surgery. Rarely, laparotomy may be not only diagnostic but also the means by which decompression or bypass is achieved. In patients with symptoms of a large or small bowel obstruction, an expert surgical opinion should be sought, even though a surgical approach may not be technically possible or appropriate when the situation is evaluated. Chemotherapy is rarely helpful unless the tumor is exquisitely chemosensitive and may lead to pancytopenia, rendering surgery hazardous.

The care of the patient with unrelieved intestinal obstruction requires skill and experience, which is most commonly concentrated in palliative care units. Patients are welcome to drink (and eat a little if they wish). Ice, offered to suck occasionally, may be useful to relieve distress. Glycerine can keep the lips moist. In most cases, such measures are highly successful but require care and experience. In a small minority of patients with gastroduodenal obstruction, a nasogastric tube is necessary, and occasionally stenting gastrostomy may be of benefit. Neither of these measures should be considered before an adequate trial of conservative management has been competently undertaken.

Specific measures for particular symptoms may include

1. Relief of colic
   Stopping gastrokinetics (e.g. cisapride/metaclopramide in high obstruction) or stimulatory laxative drugs (e.g., senna).
   Instituting regular subcutaneous morphine in small doses
   Using antispasmodics by subcutaneous bolus or infusion (e.g., hyoscine)
2. Control of nausea
   Centrally acting antiemetics such as haloperidol or cyclizine
   Rectal prochlorperazine

Hyoscine, which may reduce gastric secretions and thereby alleviate vomiting

Octreotide has gained favor in the palliative management of intestinal obstruction in reducing both gastric and intestinal secretions and motility. Subcutaneous delivery makes it attractive but the short half-life of the current preparation and its considerable expense precludes widespread use.

D. Biliary Obstruction

The pruritus that occurs with cholestasis is commonly very uncomfortable. Symptomatic measures such as cholestyramine may be helpful but it is unpleasant to take and can cause significant diarrhea.

Identification of the level of the obstruction is crucial in planning management, because endoscopic biliary drainage procedures are largely successful only for occlusion of the extrahepatic ducts. Abdominal ultrasound is the simplest procedure to determine the level of the obstruction. A CT scan may add further information but either percutaneous transhepatic cholangiography (PTC) or endoscopic retrograde choleopancreatography (ERCP) provide the most detailed images of the biliary system. Dilatation of the biliary tree may not develop for several days after the onset of symptoms.

Occasionally, a surgical resection to overcome the obstruction is both technically possible and appropriate (9). However, biliary tract obstruction often occurs when the patient is not imminently terminal. Surgical resection is often not possible and obstruction may be overcome by passage of a stent either endoscopically or percutaneously. Several randomized trials have demonstrated that stent insertion by either technique is not only as successful as a surgical approach but also is associated with a shorter duration of stay in hospital and fewer complications (10–13). The advent of self-expandable metal stents has reduced complications resulting from sludging and tumor ingrowth. Episodic cholangitis may relate to siting of the stent at the ampulla. It responds to the use of antibiotics, which may be required long term as prophylaxis (10,14–16). In the event of blockage, stent replacement is usually a safe and straightforward procedure. Intraluminal brachytherapy with iridium wires has been shown to be successful at maintaining patency of stents in sensitive tumors (15). External beam radiotherapy may be an alternative approach but requires careful planning because of the intricate anatomical relationships in this area. Liver irradiation commonly causes anorexia and nausea during the treatment course (17).

III. RESPIRATORY OBSTRUCTION

Major airway obstruction, whether it occurs at the time of a patient's initial presentation or with tumor recurrent after therapy, is a distressing problem that engenders much fear. Obstruction may occur at any level in the airway, from the larynx through to the bronchi. It may result from extrinsic compression, intraluminal disease, or difficulty clearing secretions. Occasionally, obstruction may be the result of a distant effect such as in bilateral recurrent laryngeal palsy or a consequence of treatment such as in a radiotherapy induced stricture.

Patients with major airway occlusion require urgent care because they are at high risk for respiratory failure or postobstructive pneumonia. Sometimes, conventional treatment, although ultimately effective, does not bring relief fast enough and supportive measures are required.

Symptomatic treatment can include oxygen, mucolytics, humidification of inhaled air, active physiotherapy, and inhaled bronchodilators. Other correctable causes of dyspnea should be addressed (e.g., pleural effusions, pneumonia), but as patients approach the terminal phase of their illness, many are too ill to tolerate aggressive treatment. Breathlessness and cough may respond to pharmacological maneuvers such as glucocorticoids, sodium chromoglycate, and opioids, which may be delivered successfully by mouth, by nebulizer (18), or subcutaneously. Acupuncture has also been of assistance in introductory trials, with 70% of patients reporting marked benefit, which was maximal at 90 minutes (19).

A. Laryngeal Obstruction

Emergency tracheostomy may sometimes be necessary although, in patients with laryngeal tumors, this is frequently performed as an elective procedure before local treatment.

B. Endobronchial Disease

It is important to consider the possibility of endobronchial obstruction in patients with dyspnea, wheeze, or hemoptysis with no apparent radiographic cause.

In one prospective series, radiographic signs of obstruction were seen in 44% of patients who had completely obstructive endobronchial lesions at bronchoscopy. There was a greater tendency for radiographically undetectable lesions to be located in segmental rather than mainstem bronchi, but in 16% of the patients with endobronchial disease in this series, the chest radiograph was reported as normal (20).

Palliation of symptoms attributable to endobronchial tumor can be achieved in a variety of ways:

External beam radio therapy with or without steroids
Endobronchial stents (21–24)
Nd- YAG laser resection (21,23,25)
Endobronchial brachytherapy (21,23,26)
Direct resection or intralesional chemotherapy (17,23,27)

External beam radiotherapy treats a relatively large tumor mass but its palliative value is limited by the cumulative toxicity to surrounding lung, mediastinal structures, and the spinal cord. Steroids may reduce edema associated with the tumor mass and allow temporary respite while definitive treatment is completed.

Brachytherapy with afterloading machines is ideal because there is only brief patient exposure (15 to 20 minutes), but the equipment is expensive.

Endobronchial stents have been used successfully for both extrinsic occlusion and intraluminal tumor invasion. Bare and covered metal stents can be inserted under local anesthesia but those of covered metal are preferred. They seem to be associated with a reduced rate of restenosis by tumor ingrowth.

Endoscopic resection of the malignant occlusion has been attempted by direct laser excision, by photodynamic therapy (which has been complicated by a photosensitive skin reaction), and by direct excision. Laser treatment has the advantage of immediate effect but it appears that brachytherapy usually maintains a longer response.

Cytotoxic drugs have been injected directly into endobronchial tumors with success, with subsequent bronchoscopic removal.

Randomized controlled trials comparing these treatment options are not reported and the selection of treatment therefore depends on local equipment and expertise.

IV. URINARY TRACT OBSTRUCTION

The clinical presentation of urinary tract obstruction is variable. It may be characterized by subtle changes in mentation and progressive lethargy or by anorexia with associated nausea. Some patients are seen with abrupt anuria or life-threatening sepsis. Changes in micturition patterns and urine quality may have been observed. Pain is not a constant feature, and when it occurs, it can range from minor discomfort in the back to the acute severe pain of urinary retention.

The patient's history and examination findings often allow the clinician to determine the level of the obstruction with confidence and thus consider appropriate investigations. As with obstruction in other systems, it is important to consider both benign and malignant causes, and screening for other sites of metastasis may contribute.

The diagnosis of uremia is readily established with routine biochemistry. Abdominal and pelvic ultrasound can demonstrate hydronephrosis, and the depth of the renal cortex provides an indication of renal reserve. Ultrasonography may also demonstrate the location of the obstruction without the need to resort to more invasive investigations such as retrograde pyelography. Intravenous contrast must be used with caution in the face of renal impairment.

Management of obstructive renal failure depends very much on the long-term goal of therapy. If the patient is faced with an irreversible condition and the condition is clearly terminal, it may be most appropriate to refrain from any attempt to correct the obstruction and to allow the patient to die of biochemical derangement. Death arising in this clinical context is usually peaceful but it may not be rapid. Twitching can be controlled with benzodiazepines, such as clonazepam. Rarely, anticonvulsant therapy may be required for seizures.

On occasion, the management team may have anticipated such a crisis and the approach to be taken may have been discussed with the patient and family. However urinary obstruction with secondary renal failure may develop suddenly and such discussions may not have occurred or be precluded by the changes in mentation, which accompany the metabolic disturbance. If the patient's condition is otherwise reasonable, urgent measures to correct metabolic abnormalities (elevated potassium) are appropriate. Dialysis may be essential in the first instance, but other pharmacological maneuvers can be used, including insulin and glucose, calcium gluconate, or the use of resonium.

In some patients, the degree of ureteric obstruction can be improved by moderate doses of corticosteroids (e.g., dexamethasone, 8 mg daily, intravenously, subcutaneously, or orally). The benefit is usually temporary and these agents should not be continued long term.

Ureteric obstruction may be overcome by percutaneous nephrostomy or by a stenting procedure, but the renal function does not always recover. An internalized system that is preferable for the patient usually requires general anesthesia. These systems are not without complications such as infection and may need to be regularly revised.

Percutaneous nephrostomy can commonly be associated with leaking, infection, and local discomfort. Such devices are prone to dislodge and overall can significantly increase the complexity of patient care and reduce quality of life. Detailed assessments of quality of life in patients who undergo percutaneous nephrostomy are lacking in the literature.

It has been argued that relieving urinary obstruction arising from malignancy prevents a humane death from progressive renal failure and provides a short period of life of poor quality ending in eventual death from symptomatic cancer. In early surgical series of stenting and nephrostomy, 40% of patients died without being discharged from the hospital. Recent prospective data are more encouraging (21% surviving to return to the community), but one recent report calculated that 24% of the patient's remaining life was spent in the hospital. Clearly, the patients who are likely to benefit from nephrostomy or stenting are those for whom there are options available (such as chemotherapy or radiotherapy) to alleviate the source of the obstruction (28,29).

When ureteric obstruction is unilateral, stenting may still be appropriate, although in the absence of symptoms, the morbidity of the procedure must be acknowledged. On occasion, such a procedure may facilitate definitive treatment of the underlying malignancy.

In patients with urethral, bladder neck, or prostatic obstruction, urological advice should be sought. It is important to consider the contribution that other factors such as concomitant drugs or constipation may be making. Again, the clinical background of the patient should be assessed before embarking upon invasive procedures such as permanent catheterization, urethral stents, or suprapubic cystostomy.

V. VASCULAR OBSTRUCTION

A. Superior Vena Caval Obstruction

The development of superior vena caval obstruction may be insidious and lead to considerable delay in diagnosis. The initial changes of suffusion, sometimes improved by sitting erect, facial plethora, and periorbital edema may be subtle. With time, the full symptom complex includes

Distention of internal and external jugular veins
Development of visible collateral veins of the chest wall
Upper limb and facial edema

Superior vena caval obstruction without airway compression is not a medical emergency but it demands prompt consideration of the cause and effective treatment options. Superior vena caval obstruction with a mediastinal mass may be the presenting sign of a malignancy. To a large extent, management is contingent upon the underlying histological diagnosis: thymoma may be excised; lymphoma and germ cell and small cell carcinoma of the lung are usually exquisitely chemosensitive, at least de novo; and tumors such as non-small cell lung cancer are best addressed by external beam radiotherapy. Tissue diagnosis must therefore be pursued if possible. Biopsy of the mediastinal mass itself may be associated with significant risk to the patient because there may be airway compression distal to that able to be maintained by intubation and because bleeding may cause increased mediastinal compression after biopsy. Careful examination for other disease in sites amenable to biopsy and assessment of markers (e.g., BHCG, alphafetoprotein) may be valuable. In some cases, a bone marrow aspiration can establish the diagnosis.

In addition to cytotoxic treatments, supportive measures can assist the patient. High-dose corticosteroids may temporarily reduce the compression. Anticoagulation is advocated by some. More recently, particularly when the patient has had a long disease-free interval and the disease is controlled at other sites, self-expanding stents are effective and should be considered (30,31). As yet, the effectiveness of these devices in comparison to standard treatment (chemotherapy, radiotherapy with or without anticoagulation) has not been tested in randomized trial.

Indwelling central vascular catheters for chemotherapy delivery have gained popularity but are clearly associated with a risk of thrombosis (3%–16%). The catheter type, side of insertion (right or left) and catheter tip position are all risk factors for occlusion. Thrombosis in this context can be treated successfully by thrombolysis (up to 90% success in one series), in this way salvaging the catheter for further use. Anticoagulation is useful to prevent propagation of the thrombus and, in some situations, the catheter requires removal, but not without careful thought (32–34).

B. Peripheral Venous Occlusion

The risk of deep venous thrombosis is increased in patients with malignancy. The mechanism of the hypercoagulable state is multifactorial:

- Tumor release of procoagulants (such as tissue factor and cancer procoagulant)
- Patient factors such as immobility and lymphadenopathy in pelvis or axilla, causing local compression
- Concomitant drug therapy such as hormones

Anticoagulation practices differ worldwide depending on the availability of pharmaceuticals and the feasibility of local monitoring. The duration of anticoagulant therapy in a patient with malignancy is also debated (35).

C. Lymphatic Obstruction

Lymphatic obstruction may be (but is not always) accompanied by venous obstruction, and evaluation by Doppler ultrasound is efficient and noninvasive. Massive lymph edema can be a source of major patient inconvenience and distress. Effective massage and compression bandages or stockings to minimize the reaccumulation of fluid can reduce symptoms and swelling.

D. Arterial Obstruction or Embolization

Arterial occlusion complicating malignancy is rare. The majority are associated with either an atrial mass or a lung malignancy invading the pulmonary vein. Arterial embolism may also occur in the context of the tumor lysis syndrome.

Effective treatment of the underlying disease forms the basis of management and, at times, surgical removal of the clot is indicated. Anticoagulation alone may be the only treatment option, but it can also assist the efficacy of these other maneuvers.

VI. NEUROLOGICAL OBSTRUCTION

Spinal cord compression is a common complication of malignant disease and, when it occurs, can be a source of much distress to patients and their caregivers because of a severe impact on quality of life. This is often intensified as spinal cord compression develops, most commonly in the context of widely disseminated cancer. If treatment is unsuccessful, the development of paralysis, sensory loss, and sphincter incontinence are lifelong sequelae.

Metastases to the spine are far more common than primary spinal neoplasms and may be epidural (most common), leptomeningeal, or intramedullary in location. Approximately 50% of the cases of metastatic epidural compression in adults arise from breast, lung, or prostate cancer. In children, the most common tumors are sarcoma, neuroblastoma, and lymphoma. In about 70% of the cases, the compression occurs at the thoracic level, with lumbar (20%) and cervical (10%) lesions occurring much less frequently. The tumor deposits usually occupy the anterior or anterolateral portion of the spinal cord.

The most important factor determining outcome is the level of neurological function of the patient at the commencement of therapy. The clinical challenge is therefore to diagnose imminent spinal cord compression and begin treatment before major (and pehaps permanent) neurological injury occurs. This is one of the true oncological emergencies.

The initial symptom of metastatic epidural compression is usually pain, which may be felt in the back but is often referred or radicular in distribution. The pain is generally aggravated by movement, particularly activities such as straight leg raising and neck flexion. Weakness, sensory deficits, and incontinence typically develop after the pain, which may have been present for several weeks. Once neurological dysfunction has appeared, paraplegia may develop over only a few hours. The clinical history may arouse considerable suspicion, but the examination findings such as an equivocal plantar response can appear unsupportive in a patient with significant spinal cord compression. To wait for ''hard'' neurological signs in a patient with back pain may be to wait too long. Of patients who underwent radiotherapy for spinal cord compression, more than 80% of those who were ambulatory before commencing therapy retained the ability to walk, compared to less than 10% of those who were paraplegic (36).

Controversy exists regarding the diagnostic steps with which to assess such patients. Plain radiographs identify vertebral metastases in about 85% of adults with metastatic epidural compression. Their sensitivity is influenced by the underlying tumor histology; less than 30% of patients with lymphoma have an abnormal x-ray.

In a patient with a strong clinical picture and an abnormal x-ray finding, the decision to proceed to further imaging is difficult and must be balanced against the expense of the imaging technique and any possible delay in commencing treatment. Several studies have shown that metastatic epidural compression occurs at multiple noncontiguous levels in up to one-third of patients. Definitive imaging has the advantage of identifying unexpected disease outside that which would otherwise be contained within the planned radiotherapy port. Magnetic resonance imaging (MRI) is the preferred noninvasive investigation, which usually provides exquisite neuroanatomical detail. Myelography should be considered when MRI is not available, but it is important to monitor the neurological signs after the lumbar puncture because there may be a rapid deterioration. Cerebrospinal fluid (CSF) findings are nonspecific in spinal cord compression: cell counts are usually normal, protein levels may be elevated, and the cytology may be negative because CSF flow is impeded.

As discussed in the previous sections, in common with other obstructive syndromes, the management of spinal cord compression is, to a large extent, dependent upon the underlying tumor histology and the concomitant medical problems facing the patient. Corticosteroids should be administered immediately to patients in whom compression is strongly suspected on clinical grounds as well as to those in whom cord compression is demonstrated by diagnostic imaging. Studies have demonstrated that steroids improve neurological function and alleviate pain in the short term, although their contribution to ultimate neurological function is unclear. The most commonly recommended dosage of dexamethasone is 4 mg given four times per day. Some authors have shown a dose-related benefit with dexamethasone that has led to clinical use of doses of up to 100 mg per day (37).

Anterior decompression should be considered if the compression appears largely mechanical (as in a pathological vertebral fracture), if a tissue diagnosis is required, or if the lesion has proven refractory to other treatment modalities. A surgical approach may not be possible in patients with poor performance status, or who have extensive vertebral disease. In highly chemosensitive tumors, such as lymphoma, chemotherapy may be effective. The mainstay of treatment, however, is radiotherapy. Several retrospective studies and a single prospective study have demonstrated no difference in overall neurological outcome between radiotherapy alone and laminectomy followed by radiotherapy (36).

Pain management in patients with spinal cord compression should include nonsteroidal anti-inflammatory drugs (NSAIDs) and opioids if necessary. The increased risk of gastrointestinal bleeding seen with the use of NSAIDs in the presence of steroids must be considered and agents such as misoprostol (a prostaglandin E_2 analogue) may reduce this risk. Paracetamol may also be helpful as an additional analgesic (36).

Neuropathic pain can prove resistant to these agents and, at times, is of excruciating intensity. Drugs relevant to neuropathic pain should be considered, for example, a tricyclic antidepressant if the pain is dysesthetic or burning in quality. Anticonvulsants such as sodium valproate, carbemazepine, or clonazepam may help if the pain is lancinating. Flecainide and mexilitine can also be useful. Careful review of potential contraindications should be made.

A similar analgesic pathway is appropriate for patients with nerve and nerve root compression. In some settings, local decompression or radiotherapy in sensitive tumors relieves symptoms and achieves return of function.

Obstructive hydrocephalus may require immediate treatment by steroid or osmotic diuretics if subsequent surgical or radiotherapeutic interventions are possible. The case for shunting depends very much on the patient's status, the location of the tumor, and whether antitumor treatment options are available. In many cases, if obstructive hydrocephalus develops late in the disease, symptomatic measures only may be preferred.

VII. CONCLUSION

There are many areas of controversy in the management of the various obstructive syndromes that occur in patients with malignant disease. In most situations, an appropriate management pathway can be devised by compassionate multidisciplinary consideration of the patient and the context of the problem. Well-designed randomized trials are still needed to compare outcomes in patients with obstructive syndromes.

REFERENCES

1. Herskovic A, Martz L, et al. Combined chemotherapy and radiotherapy compared with radiotherapy alone in patients with cancer of the esophagus. N Engl J Med 1992; 326:1593–1598.
2. Winkelbauer F, Schofi R, et al. Palliative treatment of obstructing esophageal cancer with nitinol stents. Am J Radiol 1996; 166:79–84.
3. Adam A, Ellul J, et al. Palliation of inoperable esophageal carcinoma: a prospective randomised trial of laser therapy and stent placement. Radiology 1997; 202:344–348.
4. de Palma G, Galloro G, et al. Self expanding metal stents for palliation of inoperable carcinoma of the esophagus and gastroesophageal junction. Am J Gastroenterol 1995; 90(12):2140–2143.

5. Ell C, Hochberger J, et al. Coated and uncoated self-expanding metal stents for malignant stenosis in the upper GI tract: preliminary clinical experiences with wallstents. Am J Gastroenterol 1994; 89(9):1496–1500.
6. Warren W, Smith C, et al. Clinical experience with montgomery salivary bypass stents in the esophagus. Ann Thorac Surg 1994; 57:1102–1107.
7. Watkinson A, Ellul J, et al. Esophageal carcinoma: initial results of palliative treatment with covered self-expanding endoprostheses. Radiology 1995; 195:821–827.
8. Saxon R, Morrison K, et al. Malignant esophageal obstruction and esophagorespiratory fistula: palliation with a polyethylene-covered Z-stent. Radiology 1997; 202: 349–354.
9. Nakeeb A, Lillemoe K, et al. The role of pancreaticoduodenectomy for locally recurrent or metastatic carcinoma to the peri-ampullary region. J Am Coll Surg 1995; 180:188–192.
10. Clements W, Diamond T, et al. Biliary jaundice in obstructive jaundice: experimental and clinical aspects. Br J Surg 1993; 80(7):834–842.
11. Lammer J, Hausegger K, et al. Common bile duct obstruction due to malignancy: treatment with plastic versus metal stents. Radiology 1996; 201:167–172.
12. Anderson JR, Sorenson SM, et al. Randomised trial of endoscopic endoprosthesis versus operative bypass in malignant obstructive jaundice. Gut 1989; 30:1132–1135.
13. Smith A, Dowsett J, et al. Randomised trial of endoscopic stenting versus surgical bypass in malignant low bile duct obstruction Lancet 1994; 344:1655–1660.
14. Vitale GC. Interventional ERCP. J Roy Coll Surg Edinburgh 1992; 37:291–297.
15. Kim G, Shin H, et al. The Role of Radiation Treatment in Management of Extrahepatic Biliary Tract Metastasis from Gastric Carcinoma. Int J Radiat Oncol Biol Phys 1994; 28(3):711–717.
16. Davids P, Groen A, et al. Randomised Trial of self-expanding metal stents versus polyethylene stents for distal malignant biliary obstruction. The Lancet 1992; 340: 1488–1492.
17. Celikoglu S, Karayel T, et al. Direct injection of anti-cancer drugs into endobronchial tumours for palliation of major airway obstruction. Postgrad Med 1997; 73:159–162.
18. Farncombe M, Chater S, et al. The use of nebulised opioids for breathlessness: a chart review. Palliative Medicine 1994; 8:306–312.
19. Filshie J, Penn K, et al. Acupuncture for the relief of cancer related breathlessness. Palliat Med 1996; 10:145–150.
20. Shure D. Radiographically occult endobronchial obstruction in bronchogenic carcinoma. Am J Med 1991; 91:19–22.
21. Bowman R. Endo-bronchial palliative therapy. Med J Aust 1997; 166(suppl):s17–s20.
22. De Souza A, Keal A, et al. Use of expandable wire stents for malignant airway obstruction. Ann Thorac Surg 1994; 57:1573–1578.
23. Hertzel M, Smith S. Endoscopic palliation of tracheobronchial malignancies. Thorax 1991; 46:325–353.
24. Tojo T, Iioka S, et al. Management of malignant tracheobronchial stenosis with metal stents and Dumon stents. Ann Thorac Surg 1996; 61:1074–1078.

25. Moghissi K, Dixon K, et al. Endoscopic laser therapy in malignant tracheobronchial obstruction using sequential Nd YAG laser and photodynamic therapy. Thorax 1997; 52:281–283.
26. Gustafson G, Vincini F, et al. High dose endobronchial brachytherapy in the management of primary and recurrent bronchogenic malignancies. Cancer 1995; 75:2345–2350.
27. Sutedja G, van Kralingan K, et al. Fibreoptic bronchoscopic electrosurgery under local anaesthesia for rapid palliation in patients with central airway malignancies: a preliminary report. Thorax 1994; 49:1243–1246.
28. Harrington K, Pandia H. Palliation of obstructive nephropathy due to malignancy. Br J Urol 1995; 76:101–107.
29. Jones S. Interventional radiology in a palliative care setting. Palliat Med 1995; 9: 319–326.
30. Nicholson A, Ettles DF, et al. Treatment of malignant superior vena cava obstruction: metal stents or radiation therapy. J Vasc Intervent Radiol 1997; 8(5):781–788.
31. Watkinson A, Hansell DM. Expandable wallstent for the treatment of obstruction of the superior vena cava. Thorax 1993; 48(9):915–920.
32. Koksoy C, Kuzu A, et al. The risk factors in central venous catheter related thrombosis. Austr N Z J Surg 1995; 65:796–798.
33. Mayo D, Pearson D, et al. Superior vena cava thrombosis associated with a central venous access device: a case report. Clin J Oncol Nurs 1997; 1(1):5–10.
34. Horatus MC, Wright DJ, et al. Changing concepts of deep venous thrombosis of the upper extremity—report of a series and review of the literature. Surgery 1988; 104:561–567.
35. Northsea C. Using urokinase to restore patency in double lumen catheters. ANNA J 1994; 21(5):261–264.
36. Byrne T. Spinal cord compression from epidural metastases. N Engl J Med 1992; 327(9):614–619.
37. Greenberg H, Kim JH, et al. Epidural spinal cord compression from metastatic tumour: results with a new treatment protocol. Ann Neurol 1980; 8:361–366.

18

Management of Malignant Effusion

Nobukazu Fujimoto
Okayama University Medical School, Okayama, Japan

Kenji Eguchi
National Shikoku Cancer Center Hospital, Matsuyama, Japan

I. MALIGNANT PLEURAL EFFUSION

A. Etiology

The pleural space consists of a continuous serosal lining. The side of the surface toward the lung is the visceral pleura and the other side, which covers the chest wall, is the parietal pleura. In the parietal pleura, a single sheet of the mesothelial cells lies on a connective tissue layer. The endothoracic fascia consists of the part of the parietal pleura adjacent to the muscle layer of the chest wall. The single layer of mesothelial cells, the thin layer of connective tissue, the chief layer of connective tissue rich in collagen and elastic fibers, and the vascular layer adjacent to the limiting membrane of the lung parenchyma constitute the structure of the visceral pleura. Unique to the parietal pleura are openings or stomata situated between mesothelial cells and centered over dilated lacunar portions of lymphatic channels (1). These stoma function as one-way valves for the removal of particulate matter. There is no communication between lymphatics of the visceral pleura and the pleural space.

It is generally accepted that the passage of protein-free fluid across the pleural space is dependent on the hydrostatic and colloid-osmotic pressures of the membranes and such passage obeys Starling's equation. About 5 to 10 L of fluid has been said to move through the pleural space per day. But these concepts of normal fluid formation and removal have been modified in view of new knowledge of the anatomy and histology of the pleural membranes. The parietal pleura is distinguished by the presence of stomata, 2- to 12-μm openings between mesothelial cells (2). These stomata are essential for the exit of pleural fluid, protein, and cells from the pleural space. From the pleural space, the stomata communicate directly with lymphatic channels and drain to mediastinal nodes. A low-protein filtrate from the systemic capillaries enters the parietal pleural interstitium, is concentrated to up to 1 to 1.5 g of protein/dL, and subsequently leaks through the mesothelium. Pleural fluid and protein then exit via parietal pleural stomata into the lymphatic channels. The visceral pleura contributes little to the formation or resorption of pleural fluid. Because the rate of entry into the pleural space is equal to the rate of exit of fluid, no net fluid accumulates. Contrary to prior views regarding pleural fluid formation, only 100 to 200 mL of pleural fluid is produced each day in humans (3).

The mechanisms of malignant pleural effusion are thought to be as follows: (1) increased capillary permeability as a result of inflammation or disruption of the capillary endothelium, (2) impaired lymphatic drainage or decreased drainage in the pulmonary vein secondary to obstruction by the tumor, (3) direct invasion of the pleural space by the tumor, (4) hypoalbuminemia caused by the malnourished state of cancer patients, and (5) chylous pleural effusion arising from obstruction of the thoracic duct.

The types of cancer causing malignant pleural effusions are lung, breast, lymphoma, gastrointestinal, and genitourinary malignancies. Lung cancer and breast cancer account for approximately 75% of malignant effusions. The prognosis of malignant pleural effusions depends on the type of tumor; gastric cancer has one of the worst prognoses and breast cancer the best. In patients with primary lung cancer, pleural effusion is sometimes revealed to be benign, especially in epidermoid histology, which is caused by atelectasis resulting from bronchial obstruction by tumor, mediastinal node involvement, superior vena cava obstruction, and so on. It is called ''paramalignant effusion.'' According to a large-scale study of prognostic factors in patients with small cell and non-small cell lung cancer by the Veterans Administration Lung Group and the Eastern Cooperative Oncology Group, pleural effusions were not the independent prognostic factors for survival.

B. Clinical Manifestation and Examination

Dyspnea, cough, and chest pain are three common symptoms in patients with pleural effusion. Dry cough when the patient changes position or progressive shortness of breath on exertion are the symptoms suggestive of pleural effusion. Patients with pleural effusion sometimes complain of chest oppression or dull back pain. Mechanical disturbance of lung expansion and compression atelectasis by the massive pleural effusion cause respiratory symptoms. Some patients are seen with severe progressive dyspnea because of malignant pleural effusion accompanied by disseminated carcinomatous lymphangitis of the lung.

The symptoms caused by the pleural effusion may sometimes be the initial manifestation of malignancy. Only one-fourth of patients with pleural effusion are asymptomatic at their initial visit. Decrease in breath sounds, increased dullness in percussion, and undetectable diaphragmatic excursion are the common physical findings.

The chest x-ray film is the most practical method for assessment of the pleural effusion. The ground-glass appearance of a fluid collection blurring the costophrenic angle and the diaphragm is the typical x-ray finding of pleural effusion. In massive effusion, one side of the lung shows complete opacity on a chest x-ray film. X-ray findings can differentiate massive pleural effusion, complete effusion, and complete atelectasis of the one-sided lung with the findings of reduction in the volume of the hemithorax. The shift of the mediastinal structure to the opposite side, expansion of the intercostal space, and downward shift of an intestinal or stomach air bubble are the x-ray findings for increased volume of the hemithorax with massive pleural effusion. The lateral decubitus view is useful for finding small amounts of free pleural fluid. These x-ray findings are easily observed using computed tomography (CT) of the thorax. Compared with conventional x-ray film, CT scan is a powerful tool to identify the solid mass or collapsed lung in massive pleural effusion. Ultrasonography (US) is also useful for differentiating free pleural effusion from organized thickening of the pleura and for detecting minimal free effusion. One can see the movement of reactive fibrous strings floating in the pleural effusion and surmise the content of the effusion.

Chest radiograph can fail to detect small effusions, even when decubitus views are included, until the amount of pleural fluid exceeds 500 mL. In contrast, US detects the presence of as little as 5 to 50 mL of pleural fluid and is 100% sensitive for effusions of $\geqq$100 mL. Computed tomography is superior to US for assessing disease status of the pleural space and other intrathoracic structures.

C. Diagnosis

If pleural effusion arises in a cancer patient, it is important to find the definitive cause. There are many causes of nonmalignant pleural effusion in patients who also have malignancies: cardiogenic, infection related, from pulmonary infarction, or a result of cirrhosis of the liver.

Thoracentesis is the first and most productive diagnostic procedure (Fig. 1). Chest x-ray films or ultrasonography is useful to determine the puncture site. The procedure should be performed with the patient sitting erect or lying on the bed. One should be careful to observe even minimal changes in the physical findings of the patient during the procedure, and vital signs should be monitored by nursing staff. All procedures should be done using sterilized techniques. Following

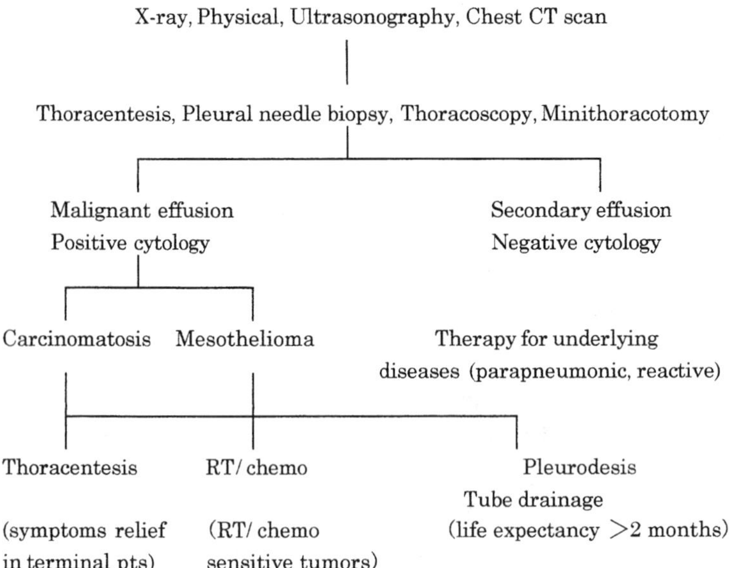

Figure 1 Diagram of the management for pleural effusion. RT, radiation therapy; pts, patients.

local anesthesia, a 14- to 18-gauge elastic needle attached to a syringe through a three-way stopcock is inserted into the desired puncture site. To avoid injury of the intercostal artery or nerve, one should choose the puncture site over the lower rib. When the tip of the needle reaches the parietal pleura and the pleural cavity, one can feel the subtle sense of resistance of the tissue through the needle. To avoid excessive pain in the patient, it is wise to give sufficient local anesthesia, especially in the area of the parietal pleura. ''Pleural shock,'' severe bradycardia, and hypotension may occur as irritable reactions of the vagal nerve in the parietal pleura. There are no absolute contraindications (4), and relative contraindications include a bleeding diathesis, systemic anticoagulation, a small volume of pleural fluid, mechanical ventilation, inability of the patient to cooperate, and cutaneous disease such as herpes zoster infection at the needle entry site (5). The complications of the thoracentesis are rare if the procedure is done carefully. In minimal effusion or compartmentalized effusion, ultrasonography is helpful for determining the puncture site.

Specimens from pleural fluid are routinely sent for various laboratory measurements, such as for protein, lactate dehydrogenase (LDH), and glucose levels. In addition, cell counts, cultures, and cytology are commonly undertaken. It is helpful to determine whether the pleural fluid is a transudate or exudate. Transudative effusion is caused primarily by an increased leakage of water. The abnormal accumulation of protein in the pleural space results in exudative effusion. Malignant pleural effusions are most commonly exudates with an LDH value greater than 200 U, fluid-to-serum LDH ratio greater than 0.6, and fluid-to-serum protein ratio greater than 0.5.

Transudates occur in approximately 10% of cases and are usually found early in the course of a malignant effusion when there is impaired lymphatic drainage secondary to involved mediastinal nodes and before protein has accumulated in the pleural space. The return of bloody fluid with a red blood cell count of greater than $100{,}000/mm^3$ in the absence of trauma suggests a malignant effusion. However, only 33% of patients with malignant effusions have bloody fluid (6).

There are many laboratory examinations for specimens of effusion to differentiate malignant effusion from others, such as LDH, adenosine deaminase, and glucose; however, none of them are definitive. Among the tumor markers, elevation in carcinoembryonic antigen (CEA) is indicative of malignant effusion. Values from 2.5 to 12.5 ng/mL have been used to separate benign from malignant cases, and the reported sensitivities in malignant pleural effusion range from 25% to 57% using these values as a cut-off level. The pleural fluid of chylothorax can be diagnosed by its milky appearance, positive fat staining, and elevated triglyceride level (>110 mg/dL).

Cytology is the best means for diagnosis of malignant effusion. Using thoracentesis, a cytological diagnosis of malignancy can be made, and more than 60% of patients are found to have malignant pleural effusion. The diagnostic efficacy also increases on repeated aspirations, from approximately 50% positivity on initial thoracentesis, to 65% on the second sample, to 70% on the third (7,8). Chromosomal analysis of cells found in the pleural space is reported to be useful in patients with lymphoma and leukemia. A chromosomal abnormality indicates a high probability that the effusion is malignant.

Pleural biopsy with Cope's or Abram's needle sometimes gives more information than the results of thoracentesis (Fig. 2). The combination of percutaneous pleural biopsy with cytological examinations correctly diagnoses about 80% of malignant pleural effusions. However, in a direct comparison of closed pleural biopsy with cytological examination, pleural biopsy was positive in only 45% of cases (versus 71% for cytology) and provided a diagnosis in only 3% of cases in which cytology was negative (9). The low yield of pleural biopsy is probably the result of the focal nature of the disease, and, hence random sampling and the inexperience of the operator.

The diagnostic role of thoracoscopy was recently reevaluated. Television-guided thoracoscopic surgery is applied for this purpose. Thoracoscopy is a high-yield procedure compared with thoracentesis or pleural biopsy, but the need for general anesthesia makes the procedure less indicative. Thoracoscopy is contraindicated for obliteration of the pleural space by adhesions. Thoracoscopy is gener-

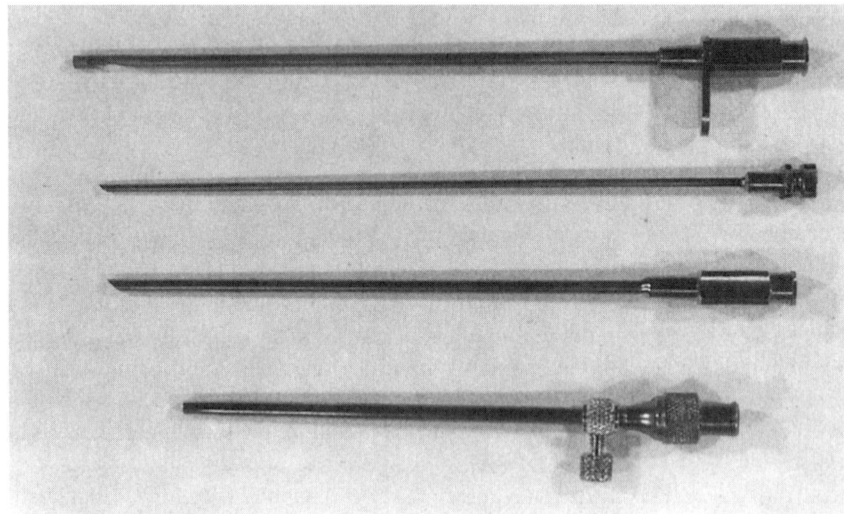

(A)

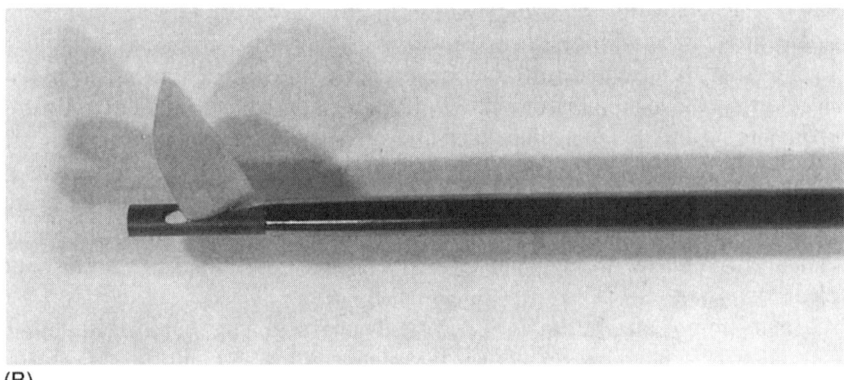

(B)

Figure 2 Needle biopsy of the pleura. (A) Cope pleural needle: hollow, blunt-tipped, hooked biopsy, trocar, obturator or stylet, hollow-beveled trocar, and outer cannula. (B) The parietal pleura is hooked with the hollow, blunt-tipped biopsy trocar. The biopsy specimen is obtained by advancing the outer cannula with a rotary motion to sever the engaged piece of pleura.

ally considered the final approach in patients whose diagnosis cannot be made with other methods. The sensitivity of thoracoscopy for the diagnosis of malignancy ranges from 80% to 100%.

There is no definitive diagnostic method to differentiate malignant effusion accompanied by primary malignant mesothelioma from that with metastatic tumors. Elevation in the concentration of hyaluronic acid in effusion and negative values of CEA tend to be higher in primary malignant mesothelioma than in other conditions. Using the immunohistochemistry, a negative stain reaction for epithelial mucin, that is, a negative diastase-periodic acid-Schiff stain, is suggestive of mesothelioma. In patients with both metastatic adenocarcinoma and mesothelioma, cytokeratin may be positive, and weak or absent CEA staining may be indicative of mesothelioma.

D. Treatment

1. Consideration of the Indication for Treatment Methods

For patients with chemoendocrine therapy or chemotherapy-sensitive tumors, such as breast cancer, small cell lung cancer, and lymphoma, systemic treatment is effective in relieving the symptoms of pleural effusion. If a patient who suffered from refractory pleural dissemination, such as postoperative relapse of non-small cell lung cancer, complains of severe chest wall pain caused by direct invasion of tumor to the chest wall, external irradiation may be a choice as palliative therapy to lessen severe pain. Another possible indication for external irradiation is in patients who suffer from lymphoma with mediastinal lymphadenopathy and pleural effusion.

There are potential advantages and disadvantages to each form of treatment. The relief of symptoms to maintain the quality of life is the goal of treatment for malignant effusion. Median survival after treatment for malignant pleural effusion has varied from 3 to more than 12 months. Some patients with breast cancer and well-differentiated adenocarcinoma of the lung survive more than 1 year after treatment for malignant effusion.

2. Thoracentesis

Thoracentesis is a tentative treatment to reduce malignant pleural effusion. In patients of poor performance status with refractory tumors or with bilateral malignant effusion, tube drainage is a good alternative. However, the effect of thoracentesis is temporary and it is often necessary to repeat it. The mean time for effusion to recur in one series was 4.2 days, with most recurring in 1 to 3 days (10). The efficiency in removing effusion is diminished after repeated thoracentesis. Pneumothorax, bleeding, and "pleural shock" are possible complications of thoracentesis. Repeated thoracentesis may increase the risks of pneumothorax, empyema, and pleural fluid loculation.

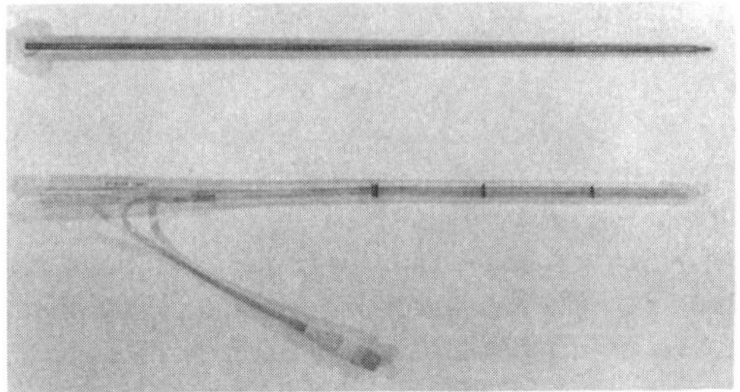

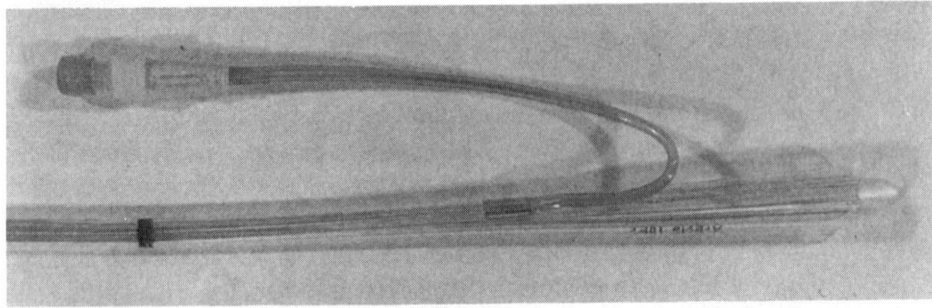

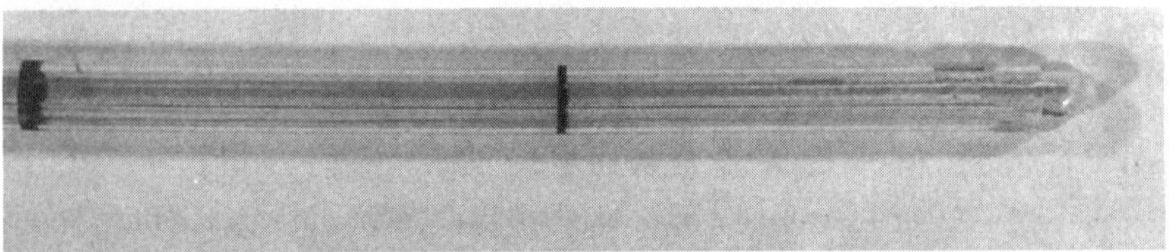

(A)

Figure 3 Pleural drainage systems: (A) double-lumen catheter; (B) suction and three-bottle collection system (Pleurievac). There are four kinds of available drainage systems, such as one-way valve (Heimlich valve, a one-way flutter valve assembly), one-bottle collection system, two-bottle collection system, and suction-control, water-seal collection system.

3. Tube Drainage

Tube drainage is a popular maneuver to relieve respiratory symptoms. The disadvantages of the procedure are similar to those of thoracentesis. Local anesthesia and disclosure of the insertion route using a hemostat through the chest wall before insertion of the tube make the procedure safe and easy without excessive trauma. Because significant force is required to insert the trocar, operative tube thoracostomy is probably safer than trocar tube thoracostomy. A 16- 20-F double-

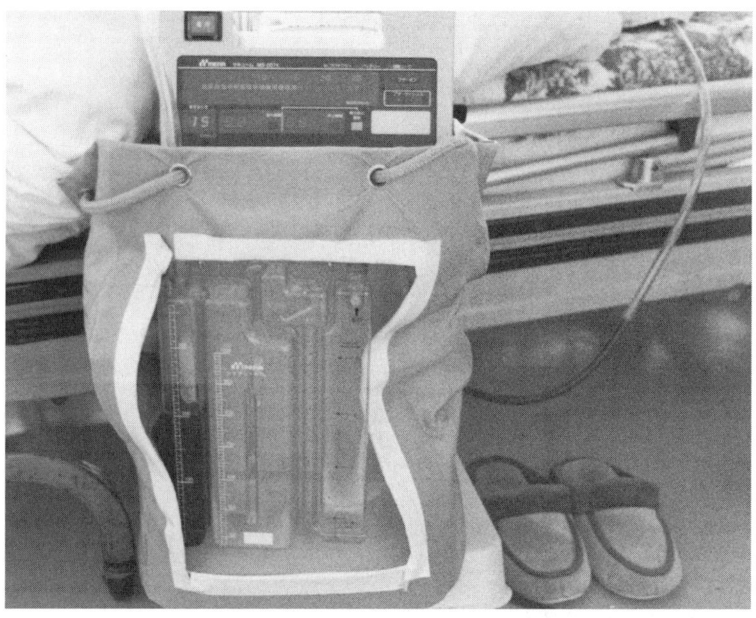

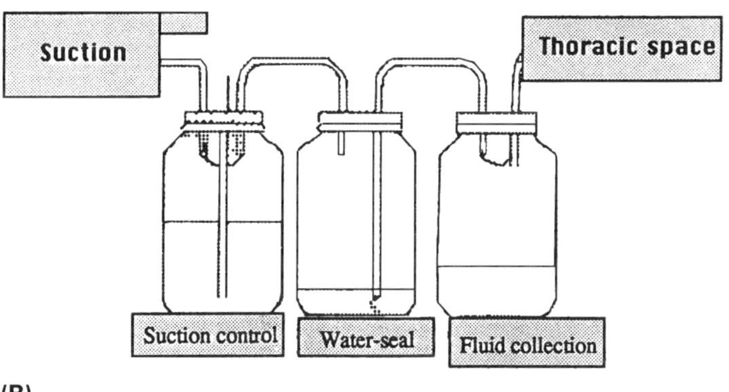

(B)

lumen catheter is used to remove effusion to avoid obstruction and to instill sclerosing agents (Fig. 3). Recently, a small-bore Silastic catheter has been used as a substitute for large catheters. Safe insertion of the drainage tube can be done using ultrasonography or x-ray fluoroscopy.

The following questions are asked in care of a chest tube to maintain efficient drainage: (1) Is there bubbling through the water-seal bottle or the water-seal

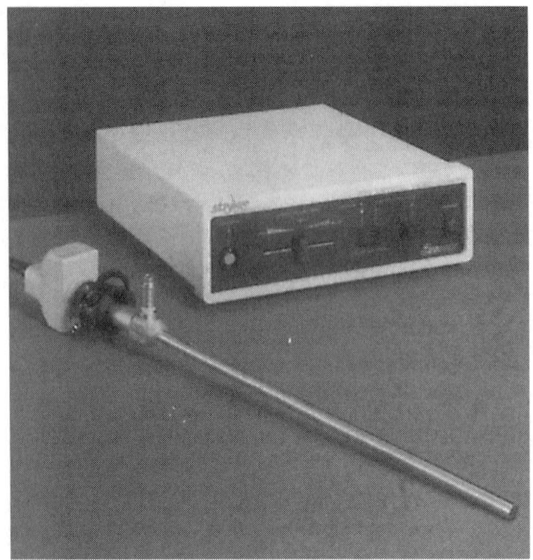

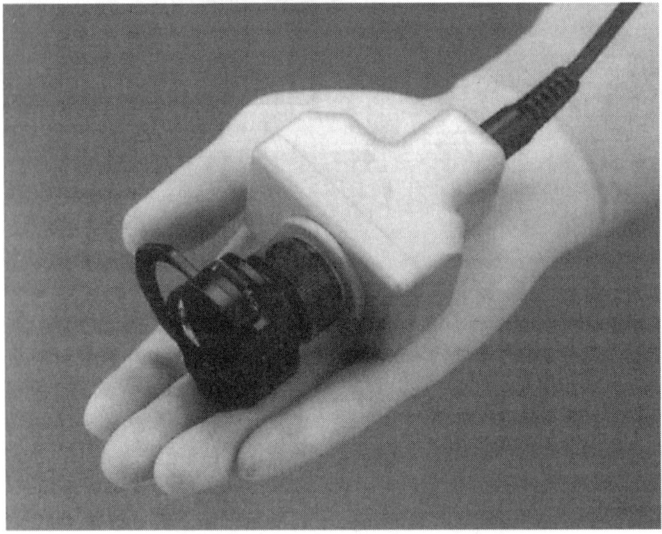

(A)

Figure 4 Video-assisted thoracoscopy: (A) thoracoscope and surgery; (B) under general anesthesia. (Courtesy of Dr. Tsuguo Naruke.)

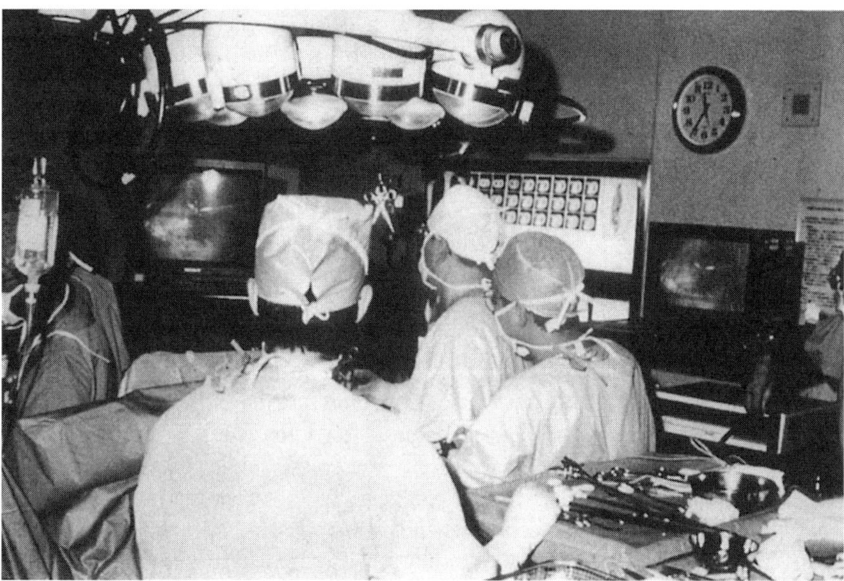

(B)

chamber on the disposable unit? (2) Is the tube functioning? (3) What are the amounts and type of drainage from the tube? These are important check points to find air leakage from the lung, disconnection of the tube, or decreased patency of the tube. The amount and character of the drainage fluid should be recorded for each 24-hour period. The tube can be removed when the drainage volume of effusion is reduced below 100 mL per day. Tube drainage alone is effective in reducing pleural effusion in a few cases.

The adverse complications of tube drainage are similar to those of thoracentesis. Circulatory disturbances, such as hypotension, after rapid reduction of massive pleural effusion and reexpansion pulmonary edema are rare complications of tube drainage. During prolonged tube drainage and repeated instillation of drugs, the chance of infection increases. The local implantation of tumors in the chest wall may occur along the tube, probably because of leakage of effusion.

4. Thoracoscopy

Video-assisted thoracoscopy has become popular in thoracic surgical oncology (Fig. 4). There have been some studies on the application of the thoracoscope as a useful tool for the instillation of a sclerosing agent, such as talc. Direct observation of the thoracic cavity and many techniques to obtain biopsy specimens and to instill agents are advantages of thoracoscopy. Although talc instillation via thoracoscopy seems to be the most effective management, general anesthesia and the cost of the maneuver are disadvantages compared with those of tube drainage.

5. *Instillation Therapy*

There have been many studies on the efficacy of sclerosing and nonsclerosing agents for controlling malignant effusion. The most common agents are tetracycline, bleomycin, and talc (Table 1) (11–32). Talc is usually poured via thoracoscopy, and the effectiveness of using a chest tube for talc instillation needs further confirmation. Tetracycline was the agent of choice for clinicians, but injectable tetracycline was discontinued in 1991 because the manufacturer did not meet U.S. Food and Drug Administration purity standards. So both minocycline and doxycycline have been used as replacements for tetracycline. Pleurodesis with doxycycline resulted in a 90% success rate and some studies have corroborated that the response rate of doxycycline compares favorably to that of tetracycline. Doxycycline is also cost-effective when compared to other agents. Bleomycin has been shown to be an effective although costly agent. A cumulative review reported a mean response rate of 84% (33). The usual dose of bleomycin is 60

Table 1 Overall Results of Controlled Trials of Intracavitary Therapy for Malignant Effusions

Number of patients	Treatment	Response (%)	Research group
67	Drainage	44	Izbicki et al. 1975 (Ref. 11)
	Drainage + ^{32}P	61	
38	Drainage	11	Mejer et al. 1977 (Ref. 12)
	Quinacrine	64	
	Thio-TEPA	27	
20	Tetracycline	80	Bayly et al. 1978 (Ref. 13)
	Quinacrine	60	
18	Mustine hydrochloride	45	Millar et al. 1979 (Ref. 14)
	Corynebacterium parvum	100	
29	Drainage	36	O'Neil et al. 1980 (Ref. 15)
	Tetracycline	72	
25	Bleomycin	54	Gupta et al. 1980 (Ref. 16)
	Tetracycline	58	
22	pH 2.8	11	Zaloznik et al. 1983 (Ref. 17)
	Tetracycline	69	

Table 1 Continued

Number of patients	Treatment	Response (%)	Research group
37	Mustine hydrochloride	53	Fentiman et al. 1983 (Ref. 18)
	Talc	90	
53	ADM[a]	48	Urata et al. 1983 (Ref. 19)
	ADM + OK 432	72	
62	Bleomycin	87	Johnson et al. 1984 (Ref. 20)
	Tetracycline	56	
21	Drainage	58	Sorenson et al. 1984 (Ref. 21)
	Talc	100	
32	Tetracycline[b]	56	Leahy et al. 1985 (Ref. 22)
	Tetracycline[c]	86	
	C. parvum	88	
30	Mustine hydrochloride	44	Kefford et al. 1986 (Ref. 23)
	Adriamycin	73	
	Tetracycline	70	
33	Tetracycline	48	Fentiman et al. 1986 (Ref. 24)
	Talc	92	
31	Tetracycline	65	Kessinger et al. 1987 (Ref. 25)
	Bleomycin	62	
50	Tetracycline, single	84[d]	Landvater et al. 1988 (Ref. 26)
	Repeated	84[d]	
44	Bleomycin	72	Ostrowski et al. 1989 (Ref. 27)
	C. parvum	47	
85	Bleomycin	70[d]	Ruckdeshel et al. 1991 (Ref. 28)
	Tetracycline	47[d]	
99	Bleomycin	64	Hartman et al. 1993 (Ref. 29)
	Tetracycline	33	
	Talc	97	
30	Mepacrine chloride	86	Bjermer et al. 1995 (Ref. 30)
	Mitoxantrone	93	
60	Tetracycline	95	Emad et al. 1996 (Ref. 31)
	Bleomycin	100	
	Tetracycline and bleomycin	100	
29	T Talc slurry	90	Zimmer et al. 1997 (Ref. 32)
	Bleomycin	79	

[a] ADM, Adriamycin (doxorubicin HCL); OK 432 is a streptococcal preparation.
[b] Through needle.
[c] Using tube drainage.
[d] Rate of no relapse (within 90 days).

Table 2 Results of Trials of Intracavitary Therapy for Pleural Effusions Secondary to Breast Cancer

Number of patients	Treatment	Response (%)	Research group
52	Drainage	50	Izbicki et al. 1975 (Ref. 11)
	Drainage + ^{32}P	54	
10	Drainage	33	Mejer et al. 1977 (Ref. 12)
	Quinacrine	75	
	Thio-TEPA	67	
10	Tetracycline	71	Bayly et al. 1978 (Ref. 13)
	Quinacrine	67	
37	Mustine hydrochloride	53	Fentiman et al. 1983 (Ref. 18)
	Talc	90	
12	pH 2.8	43	Zaloznik et al. 1983 (Ref. 17)
	Tetracycline	40	
33	Tetracycline	48	Fentiman et al. 1986 (Ref. 24)
	Talc	92	
22	Bleomycin	67[a]	Hamed et al. 1989 (Ref. 35)
	Talc	100[a]	
11	Mepacrine chloride	80	Bjermer et al. 1995 (Ref. 30)
	Mitoxantrone	100	

[a] Rate of no recurrence.

mg dissolved 10 to 100 mL of normal saline. Following administration of the agent, a drainage tube is usually clamped for a few hours and then suction is restarted. Pain and fever are common side effects of instillation therapy, especially for tetracycline or doxycycline, but they can be prevented with nonnarcotic analgesics, such as indmethacin, or more potent analgesics, such as pentazocine and morphine sulfate. Careful explanation of the pain associated with instillation therapy to the patient before administration of the agent and full premedication against pain may effectively relieve the patient's fear of severe pain. Like the systemic administration of antineoplastic agents, mild to moderate myelosupression, nausea, vomiting, and hair loss may occur after the instillation of anticancer agents.

The results of randomized control trials of sclerosing therapy are shown in Tables 2 and 3 (11–14,17,18,24,30,35–38). Although the criteria for response were different, most results showed a high response rate. However, there was no evidence of a survival advantage in choosing any of these agents. The superiority of anticancer agents (e.g., adriamycin, mitomycin, and cisplatin) to control malignant effusion, comparing with other sclerosing agents, has not yet been con-

Table 3 Results of Controlled Trials of Intracavitary Therapy for Pleural Effusions Secondary to Lung Cancer

Number of patients	Treatment	Response (%)	Research group
16	Drainage	0	Mejer et al. 1977
	Quinacrine	40	(Ref. 12)
	Thio-TEPA	29	
5	Tetracycline	75	Bayly et al. 1978
	Quinacrine	0	(Ref. 13)
16	Mustine hydrochloride	44	Millar et al. 1979
	Corynebacterium parvum	100	(Ref. 14)
11	pH 2.8	20	Zaloznik et al. 1983
	Tetracycline	67	(Ref. 17)
34	ADM or MMC[a]	62	Saijo et al. 1983 (Ref.
	ADM or MMC + N-CWS[b]	83	36)
68	ADM or MMC[a]	60	Yamamura et al.
	ADM or MMC + N-CWS[b]	86	1989 (Ref. 37)
53	OK432[c]	88	Luh et al. 1992 (Ref.
	MMC	67	38)
7	Mepacrine	100	Bjermer et al. 1995
	Mitoxantrone	100	(Ref. 30)

[a] ADM, Adriamycin (doxorubicin HCL); MMC, mitomycin.
[b] N-CWS, *Nocardia rubra* cell wall skeleton.
[c] OK 432, streptococcal preparation.

firmed. There have been several clinical trials on the efficacy of biological response modifiers, including recombinant cytokines (Table 4) (39–52). But, to date, no superiority in antitumor or sclerosing effect of these recombinant products has been clearly demonstrated compared with conventional treatment. Recently, elastance of pleural space was suggested to be a predictor for the outcome of pleurodesis in patients with malignant pleural effusion. The elastance of the pleural space was defined as the decline in pleural fluid pressure in cm H_2O after removal of 500 mL of effusion. Patients with an elastance of 19 cm H_2O or more had a significantly higher incidence of trapped lung than did those with an elastance less than 19 cm H_2O (34). One prospective randomized trial of talc slurry versus instillation of bleomycin had shown talc slurry via bedside thoracostomy was well tolerated without significant adverse effects. Talc is a much less costly agent than bleomycin and may be the agent of choice using pleurodesis for malignant pleural effusion (32).

Table 4 Recent Results of Nonrandomized Trials of Intracavitary Therapy for Malignant Pleural Effusions

Number of patients	Treatment	Response (%)	Research group
50	*Corynebacterium parvum*	100[a]	Casali et al. 1988 (Ref. 41)
50 Breast	*C. parvum*	100[a]	Contegiacomo et al. 1987 (Ref. 39)
25	Tetracycline	15[a]	Gravelyn et al. 1987 (Ref. 40)
37	Cisplatin + cytarabine	49	Rusch et al. 1991 (Ref. 42)
34	Iodized talc	100[a]	Webb et al. 1992 (Ref. 43)
29	Natural IFN-β ($5 \sim 20 \times 10^6$ U)	27	Rosso et al. 1988 (Ref. 44)
10	rhIL-2 (1×10^3 U/day)	30[a]	Suzuki et al. 1989 (Ref. 46)
4	rhIFN-β ($3 \times 10^6 \sim 1.8 \times 10^9$ U)	75	Tanaka 1988 (Ref. 45)
35 Lung	rhIL-2 (1×10^3 U/day)	37[a]	Yasumoto et al. 1991 (Ref. 47)
14 Lung	IFN-α (2×10^6 U)	79	Tercelj-Zorman et al. 1991 (Ref. 48)
22	rhIL-2 ($3 \sim 24 \times 10^6$ U)	45	Astoul et al. 1993 (Ref. 49)
38	Pirarubicin (20 ~ 80 mg/body)	74	Gotoh et al. 1996 (Ref. 50)
26	rHuTNF (0.10 ~ 0.50 mg/body)	87	Rauthe et al. 1997 (Ref. 51)
21	rhIFN-α2b	100	Wilkins et al. 1997 (Ref. 52)

[a] Complete response.

II. MALIGNANT PERICARDIAL EFFUSION

A. Etiology

The pericardial sac normally contains a small amount of fluid. The fluid is produced in the myocardium and diffuses through the mesothelial tissue of the visceral pericardium into the sac. Most of the fluid is reabsorbed by the parietal lymphatics at the base of the heart and drains into the thoracic duct. Some of the fluid may be reabsorbed by the visceral pericardial lymphatics and capillaries connected to the coronary sinus. Because of its anatomical characteristics, the lymphatic drainage of the heart and pericardium has a narrow zone. Metastatic tumors may block lymphatic drainage progressively without the development of collateral flow. Malignant pericardial effusion occurs by direct infiltration and hematogeneous and lymphatic spread of tumors. Bulky involvement of mediastinal lymph nodes may be a cause of retrograde lymphatic spread. Obstruction of lymphatic drainage and blood vessels of the heart disrupts the equilibrium between capillary filtration and osmotic pressure. As a result, the pericardial effusion appears in the pericardial sac. Disseminated tumors on the pericardial surface cause exudation. The consequences of the accumulation of pericardial effusion partly depend on the rate of exudation and the compliance of the pericardial cavity. A rapid accumulation of fluid and a thickened pericardium with tumor infiltration or fibrosis cause cardiac tamponade. The elevation of intrapericardial pressure interferes with ventricular movement, and the cardiac output decreases. The increased ventricular diastolic pressure results in right-sided cardiac failure. Tachycardia and increased peripheral vascular tone are signs of hemodynamic crisis caused by cardiac tamponade. Shock and cardiac arrest occur if these compensatory responses fail. A thickened pericardium with tumor infiltration causes constrictive pericarditis, and cardiac tamponade may occur without fluid accumulation.

Metastatic cancer to the heart or pericardium is surprisingly common at autopsy, with most investigators reporting an incidence of between 5% and 10% of cancer deaths. Clinically significant malignant pericardial effusion is relatively rare, however. Primary malignancies with a propensity for cardiac involvement include lung cancer, breast cancer, lymphoma and leukemia, melanoma, gastrointestinal primary tumors, and sarcomas. Lung cancer is associated with the highest frequency of malignant pericardial effusion (53).

B. Clinical Manifestation

Patients with cardiac and pericardial invasion of tumor may be asymptomatic unless the pericardium accumulates more than 200 to 300 mL. Cardiac enlargement on percussion, engorgement of the cervical veins, enlargement of the liver, and increased venous pressure are common findings of pericardial effusion. Such symptoms as a precordial oppressive feeling, appetite loss, chest pain, dyspnea, nausea, easy fatigability, and epigastralgia are frequently observed in patients with pericardial effusion. The symptoms of pericardial effusion and cardiac tamponade may be similar to those of generalized carcinomatosis, and one should be cautious not to overlook them in routine follow-up after the initial treatment of malignancy. Dyspnea on exertion, edema of the lower extremities, dilatation of jugular vein, oliguria, arrhythmias, and hepatomegaly are the symptoms and signs of right-sided heart failure caused by pericardial effusion. Bilateral pleural effusion is sometimes associated with pericardial effusion as a consequence of cardiac dysfunction. Pericardial friction rub may be audible. The rapid development of a pericardial effusion can lead to cardiac tamponade. Orthopnea is frequently seen in patients with cardiac tamponade. Without emergency treatment, cardiac tamponade causes sudden death. Venous distention, distant heart sounds, paradoxical pulse, and oliguria are common findings in rapidly progressing cardiac tamponade. A paradoxical pulse is one that diminishes in amplitude during inspiration, and width of the pulse pressure is narrowed.

C. Diagnosis

1. *Electrocardiography*

About 90% of patients with symptomatic malignant pericardial effusion have abnormal electrocardiogram findings. Low voltage, sinus tachycardia, elevation of the ST segment, and T wave changes are common findings in patients with pericardial effusion. Electrical alternans with alterations in the P wave as well as the QRS-T complex is seen in pericardial effusion with a stiff pericardium.

2. *Radiography*

An enlarged cardiac silhouette (a globular or ice bag appearance) is a common finding in pericardial effusion on plain x-ray film. Serial comparison of the x-ray film with the previous film makes the diagnosis easier. In some patients, pericardial effusion may be accompanied by pleural effusion. In cardiac failure, the vascular markings of both lung fields are blurred. Using CT scan of the chest, a double contour with low attenuation around the heart is the typical finding in pericardial effusion (Fig. 5*A*). Asymptomatic pericardial effusion can be identified by thoracic CT scan.

3. *Echocardiography*

Echocardiography is a simple and sensitive method for the diagnosis of pericardial effusion with safe and noninvasive features (see Fig. 5*B*). If two distinct echoes, one from the pericardium and another from the posterior heart border, are observed, the space between these echoes indicates the presence of pericardial effusion or the pericardial thickness. Abnormal motion of the mitral leaflet may suggest the presence of cardiac tamponade. Two-dimensional echocardiography may differentiate a solid mass from pericardial effusion.

4. *Pericardiocentesis*

To clarify the cause of pericardial effusion or pericarditis in cancer patients is important because these patients may have nonmalignant effusion of various origins. The differential diagnosis between chronic radiation-induced pericarditis and progressive malignant involvement of the pericardium is difficult, especially in a patient with prior radiation therapy. Pericardiocentesis is useful for the diagnosis of malignancy. The common puncture site is the joint portion of the lowest costal cartilage and the sternum just to the left of the xyphoid process. Ultrasonography is used to find the appropriate site of puncture. All procedures should be performed under sterilized conditions. Following the insertion of the needle at the site of local anesthesia and proceeding underneath the xyphoid process, the needle should be directed toward the apex of the left shoulder. Electrocardiographic and blood pressure monitoring should be done during the pericardiocentesis. The complications of pericardiocentesis include cardiac arrythmias caused by trauma to the myocardium, hemorrhage, pneumothorax, and sudden death. Because the presence of pericardial effusion does not necessarily mean the effusion is malignant, even in patients with malignancy, it is most important to confirm the malignant origin of the pericardial effusion.

D. Treatment

Indications for initial systemic chemotherapy and radiotherapy are limited in patients with malignant pericardial effusion (Fig. 6). For chemosensitive, previously untreated tumors, such as lymphoma and breast cancer, induction chemotherapy may be effective for pericardial effusion. Radiotherapy is the only treatment choice in patients with chemorefractory and radiosensitive tumors, such as lymphoma, leukemia, testicular cancer, and small cell lung cancer. Patients at poor risk for surgery may also be candidates for radiotherapy. Such surgical approaches as the formation of a pericardial pleura window are well tolerated; however, they sometimes fail to obtain prolonged palliation. The overall survival of patients after treatment for malignant pericardial effusion is 2 to 6 months, and very limited numbers of patients have a longer life expectancy, beyond 1 year. The prognosis of patients who have malignant pericardial effusion is poor, even after the control of effusion, because there is decreased cardiac function with local and systemic disseminated tumor. It is not rare to find diffuse sclerosis of the pericardium with tumor infiltration and constrictive pericarditis in autopsy of patients who received treatment of malignant pericardial effusion.

1. Pericardiocentesis

Pericardiocentesis is performed as an emergency treatment for the palliative relief of symptoms of cardiac tamponade. If cyanosis, dyspnea, shock, or impaired consciousness develops, emergency pericardiocentesis must be performed. If definitive drainage cannot be performed immediately, isoproterenol and intravenous fluid administration are begun to improve contractility and maintain preload to

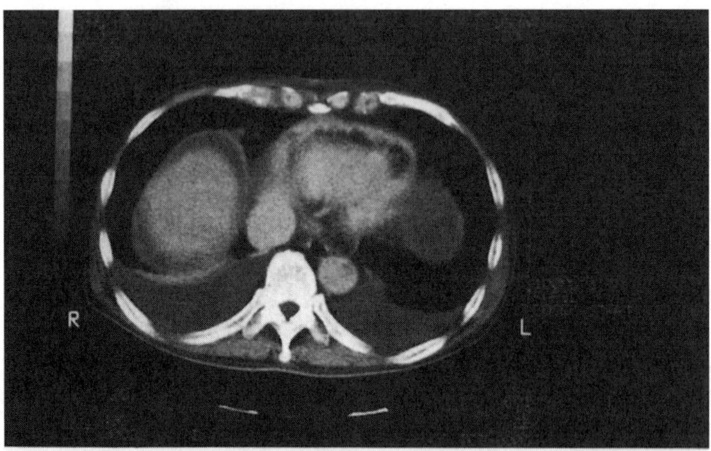

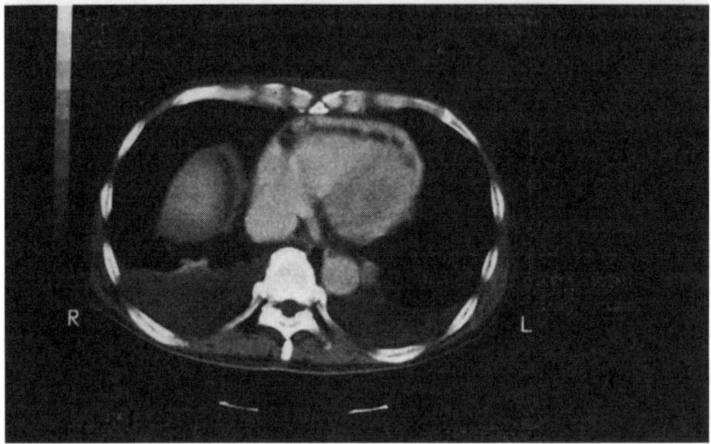

(A)

Figure 5 Diagnosis of pericardial effusion and cardiac tamponade. (A) CT findings of pericardial invasion of tumor. This patient received tube drainage through subxyphoid pericardiectomy for malignant pericardial effusion caused by advanced renal cancer. Chest CT scan reveals irregularly thickened pericardium, bilateral pleural effusion, and ascites. (B) Ultrasonographic findings of pericardial effusion: PE, pericardial effusion; LA, left atrium; LV, left ventricle, RV, right ventricle; AO, aorta.

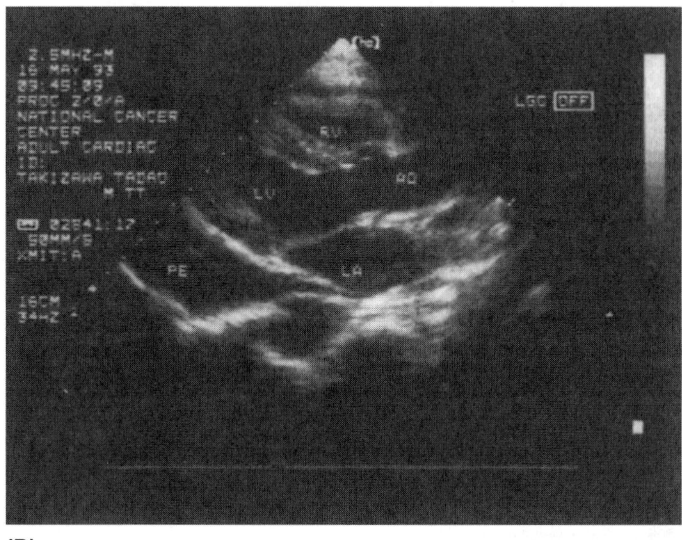

(B)

the heart. The initial removal of the effusion frequently obtains dramatic relief of circulatory symptoms, but recurrent pericardial effusion is common without additional treatment. Electrocardiographic and blood pressure monitoring are necessary during the procedure. The procedure should be performed with careful supportive treatment, such as intravenous fluid supplements and nasal oxygen, and pericardiocentesis has the risk of complications. These include cardiac arrythmias caused by trauma to the myocardium, hemorrhage, and sudden death.

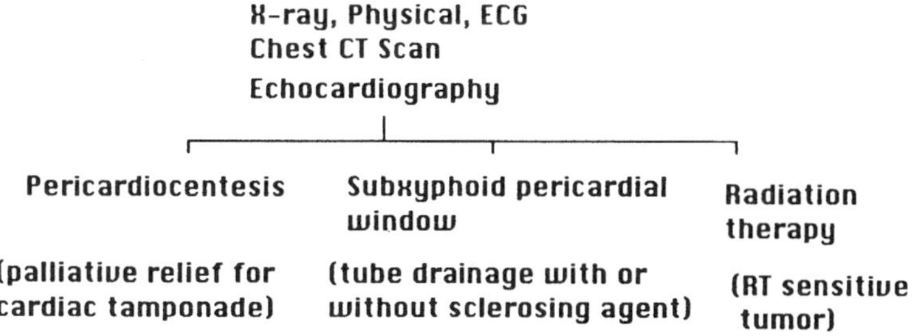

Figure 6 Diagram of the management for malignant pericardial effusion.

2. *Tube Drainage*

Tube drainage is the standard procedure for symptomatic pericardial effusion, including cardiac tamponade. Empirically, many cases of pericardial effusion can be controlled within 1 to 2 weeks using tube drainage without sclerosing agents. The recurrence rate has been reported to range from 3% to 20%. Subxyphoid pericardiectomy is a common procedure for tube drainage. The operation can be performed in 30 to 60 minutes under local anesthesia. There have been many reports of intrapericardial instillation therapy, such as with doxycycline, talc, bleomycin, and radioactive isotopes. Tetracycline hydrochloride was preferred but is no longer available. In one recent report, bleomycin and doxycycline were equally effective as sclerosing agents, but bleomycin is associated with significantly less morbidity and should be the first-line chemical sclerosing agent (54). Doxycycline, 500 to 1000 mg, or bleomycin, 10 to 20 mg, is dissolved in 10 to 20 mL normal saline and inserted through the catheter. The catheter is clamped for 1 to 2 hours and then reopened. The tube can be removed if the volume of drainage fluid decreases to less than 10 mL/day. Other agents used for sclerosing include cisplatin (55,56), vinblastine (57), and OK-432, a penicillin-treated and heat-treated lyophilized powder of the substrain of *Streptococcus pyogens* A3 (58). The disadvantages of these sclerosing and antineoplastic agents include limited efficacy despite severe local pain, fever, or myelosupression.

III. MALIGNANT ASCITES

A. Etiology

Malignant ascites occurs as a result of subdiaphragmatic lymphatic obstruction and increased production of intraperitoneal fluid. In patients with gastric, large bowel, and pancreatic cancer, a direct extension through the visceral layer of the peritoneum may occur. The affected parts of the intestine become adherent to adjacent organs. Sometimes, the affected lesion may lead to intraabdominal fistulas, volvulus formation, and complete obstruction. In patients with rapidly growing tumors, such as ovarian and gastric cancer, invasion of tumor cells tends to be transcoelomic dissemination. Small lumps of tumor cells become suspended in the ascites fluid. Increased capillary permeability caused by damaged capillary vessels, with generalized carcinomatosis and increased venous pressure from local obstruction, results in changes in the clearance of peritoneal fluid. Hypoalbuminemia associated with malignancy may also exacerbate ascites. Chylous ascites may arise as a result of disturbance of a major lymphatic drainage, such as obstruction of the thoracic duct in patients with lymphoma.

Ovarian, endometrial, breast, colonic, gastric, and pancreatic cancer are common tumors that may be associated with malignant ascites.

B. Clinical Manifestation

Ascites may result in anorexia, indigestion, heartburn, or respiratory disturbance, such as tachypnea, and orthopnea, caused by the intraperitoneal pressure and restriction of the movement of the diaphragm. The most common signs are abdominal distention, weight gain, and general discomfort. A functional or organic decrease in bowel movement may occur because of carcinomatous peritonitis, metastasis to the bowel wall, and ascites. On physical examination, a fully distended abdomen with stretched skin is common, and the shifting of fluid waves and flank dullness, depending on the position of the patient, are notable.

C. Diagnosis

Abdominal plain x-ray film reveals opacity on the outer side of the abdomen along the flank stripe and blurring of the contour of the psoas muscles and the kidneys. The gas bubbles in the bowel gather in the central portion of abdomen on the film in a supine position. Ultrasonography and abdominal CT scan are useful for discerning not only ascites but also intraabdominal and retroperitoneal tumor spread. Because the details of the ultrasonographic findings may occasionally be obscured by the gas in the intestines, an abdominal CT scan is more helpful in evaluating the extent of the disease. Because there may be a possibility of nonmalignant ascites in cancer patients, paracentesis is an important procedure to identify the origin of ascites. In malignant effusion, three-fourths of patients have ascites protein values greater than 2.5 g/mL. Tumor markers, such as CEA, are helpful in disclosing malignancy. The CEA levels greater than 12 ng/mL are suggestive of malignant ascites. Cytological examination is necessary for the definitive diagnosis of malignant effusion.

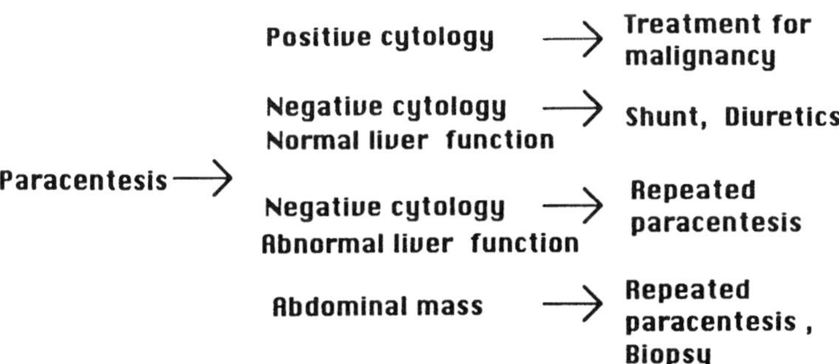

Figure 7 Management of ascites. (Modified from Ref. 66.)

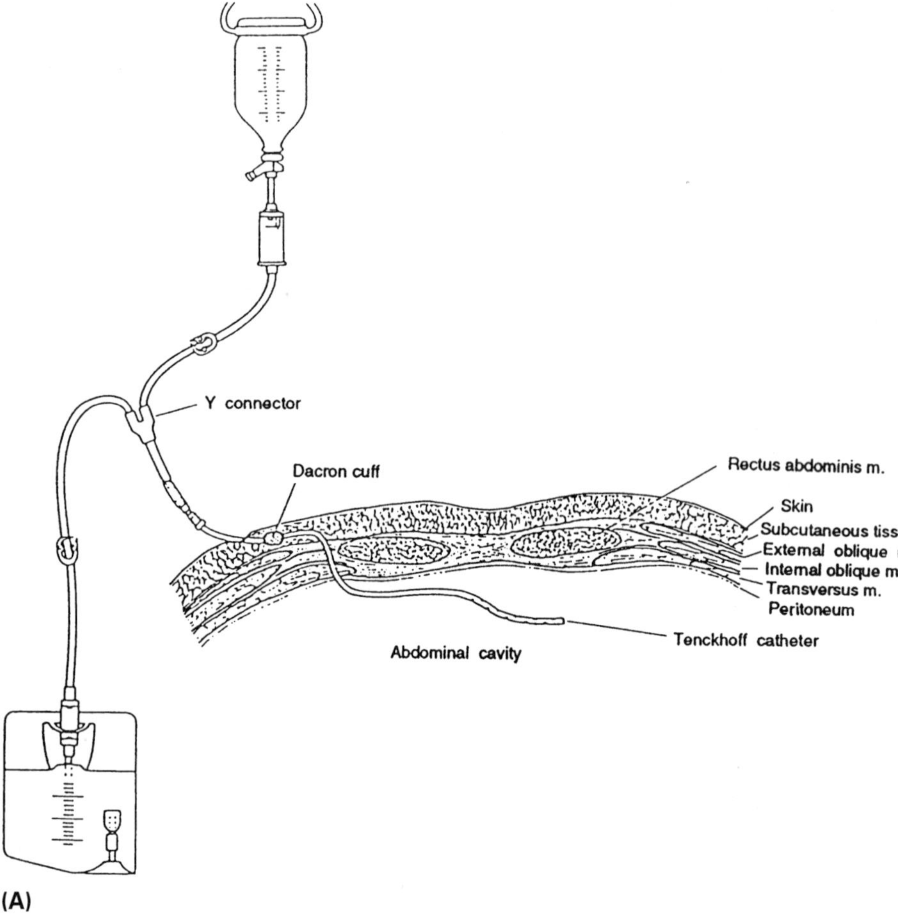

Figure 8 (A) Tenckhoff catheter and (B) Port-A-Cath. (Modified from Ref. 67.)

D. Treatment

Diuretics are ineffective for most patients with massive malignant ascites, and their use without precautions may induce water imbalance (Fig. 7). Paracentesis is also not effective in controlling ascites, and the repeated procedure causes a rapid loss of protein and progressive dehydration.

Intraperitoneal administration of radioactive isotopes, such as ^{198}Au, has been shown to be effective in controlling malignant ascites. However, these agents

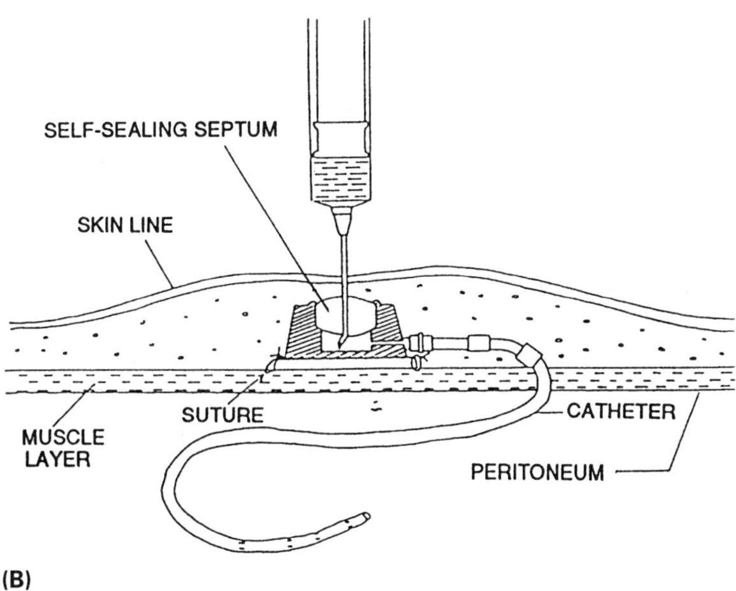

(B)

can be troublesome if leakage or spillage occurs. Intracavitary treatment with chemotherapeutic agents may be effective if the tumor is sensitive to chemotherapy, as in patients with ovarian or breast cancer. There have been trials of the intracavitary instillation of platinum-based agents. Reviewing the pathological complete remission (CR) reported in ovarian cancer patients undergoing second-line intraperitoneal therapy using various chemotherapeutic agents, about 10% of patients achieved pathological CR. The intracavitary instillation of anticancer agents, such as 5-fluorouracil, bleomycin, and thio-TEPA, resulted in about a 30% to 35% response. Mild to moderate myelosupression may occur after intracavitary treatment with anticancer agents. Devices for delivering chemotherapeutic agents have been developed, such as the Tenckhoff catheter and the Port-A-Cath (Fig. 8). The complication from implanting these devices were bowel perforation, bleeding, ileus, and leakage of fluid. The incidence was less than 10%, and even less with the Port-A-Cath. Problems with the functioning of these devices included outflow obstruction: the rate of complication was less than 30%. Intraabdominal infection was reported in 5% to 8% of the patients.

Recently, the intracavitary instillation of various immunopotentiators, including recombinant cytokines, was reported, as listed in Table 5 (59–64). Some were expected to have both a sclerosing effect for the pleura and an antitumor effect against cancer cells in the ascites through immunological reaction. How-

Table 5 New Agents for Intraperitoneal Instillation in Patients with Malignant Ascites

Number of patients	Treatment	Response (%)	Research group
14 Ovarian	rhIFN-α (5–50 × 10^6 U)	36[a]	Berek et al. 1985 (Ref. 59)
7 Ovarian	rhIL-2 (1 × 10^5 ~ 5 × 10^7 U)	None	Champman et al. 1988 (Ref. 60)
8 Gastric, uterine	OK-432 (1 × 10^6 U twice per week)	25	Kato et al. 1989 (Ref. 61)
19 Ovarian	rhIFN-α (5 ~ 15 U/m^2 twice per week)	36	Bezwoda et al. 1991 (Ref. 62)
29	rTNF-α (40–350 Âg/m^2 week)	76	Räth et al. 1991 (Ref. 63)
22	OK-432 + IL-2	81	Yamaguchi et al. 1995 (Ref. 64)

[a] Complete response.

ever, the efficacy of these agents in achieving long-term palliation have not yet been confirmed.

Portovenous shunting is a common procedure for surgical relief of malignant ascites. The LeVeen shunt drains fluid from the abdominal cavity into the superior vena cava. This kind of treatment provides long-term palliation, longer than 3 months, with minimal operative risk. The complications of the shunt are obstruction with clotting in bloody ascites and the increased risk of disseminated intravascular coagulation. The Denver shunt has a valve mechanism, and the system can be flushed and controlled by manipulation. The Denver shunt showed a lower failure rate than the LeVeen shunt; however, both were palliative treatments with the risk of fatal coagulopathy. Shunt insertion may be contraindicated in patients with malignant ascites from a gastrointestinal origin, because of the universally poor prognosis. A shunt should be used only when other treatment options have failed in a patient who is considered likely to survive for fairly long term (65).

SELECTED READING

Bartter T, Akers SM, Santarelli R, Pratter MR. The evaluation of pleural effusion. Chest 1994; 106:1209–1214.

Fentiman IS. Diagnosis and treatment of malignant pleural effusion. Cancer Treat Rev 1987; 14:107–118.

Graeber GM. Complications of therapy of malignant tumors involving the pericardium. In: Roth JA, Ruckdeschel JC, Weisenburger TH, eds. Thoracic Oncology. Philadelphia: WB Saunders, 1989:504–512.

Jones JSP. Pathology of the Mesothelium. London: Springer-Verlag, 1987.

Light RW. Pleural Diseases. Philadelphia: Lea & Febiger, 1983.

Lynch TJ. Management of malignant pleural effusions. Chest 1993; 103:385–389.

Muach P, Ultmann JE. Treatment of malignant pericardial effusion, treatment of malignant pleural effusion, treatment of malignant ascites. In: Devita VT, Hellman S, Rosenberg SA, eds. Cancer Principles and Practice of Oncology. Philadelphia: JB Lippincott, 1985:2141–2153.

Parsons SL, Watoson SA, Steele RJ. Malignant ascites. Br J Surg 1996; 83:6–14.

Press OW. Management of malignant pericardial effusion and tamponade. JAMA 1987; 257(8):1088–1092.

Reed CE. Management of the malignant pleural effusion. In: Pass HI, Mitchell JB, Johnson DH, Turrisi AT, eds. Lung Cancer: Principles and Practice. Philadelphia: Lippincott-Raven, 1996:643–654.

Richardson JD, Fenton KN, et al. Diagnosis and management of malignant pleural effusions. Am J Surg 1995; 170:69–74.

Ruckdeschel JC. Management of malignant pleural effusion; an overview. Semin Oncol 1988; 15:24–28.

Rusch VW, Harper GR. Pleural effusions in patients with malignancy. In: Roth JA, Ruckdeschel JC, Weisenburger TH, eds. Thoracic Oncology. Philadelphia: WB Saunders, 1989:594–605.

Theologides A. Neoplastic cardiac tamponade. Semin Oncol 1987; 5:181–192.

Vaitkus PT, Herrmann HC, LeWinter MM. Treatment of malignant pericardial effusion. JAMA, 1994:272:59–64.

Vladitiu AO. Pleural Effusion. Futura Pub. Co. New York 1986.

Zwischenberger JB, Bradford DW. Management of malignant pericardial effusion. In: Pass HI, Mitchell JB, Johnson DH, Turrisi AT, eds. Lung Cancer: Principles and Practice. Philadelphia: Lippincott-Raven, 1996:655–662.

REFERENCES

1. Henschke CI, Davis SD, Romano PM, Yankelevitz DF. The pathogenesis, radiologic evaluation, and therapy of pleural effusions. Radiol Clin North Am 1989; 27:1241–1255.
2. Wang N. Anatomy and physiology of the pleural space. Clin Chest Med 1985; 6: 3–16.
3. Broaddus C, Staub N. Pleural liquid and protein turnover in health and disease. Semin Respir Med 1987; 9:7–12
4. Sahn SA. The pleura. Am Rev Respir Dis 1988; 138:184–234.
5. Burgher LW, Jones FL Jr, Patterson JR, Selecky PA. Guidelines for thoracentesis and needle biopsy of the pleura. Am J Respir 1989; 140:257–258.
6. Meyer PC. Metastatic carcinoma of the pleura. Thorax 1966; 21:437–443.

7. Salyer WR, Eggleston JC, Erozan YS. Efficacy of pleural needle biopsy and pleural fluid cytopathology in the diagnosis of malignant neoplasm involving the pleura. Chest 1975; 67:536–539.
8. Winkelman M, Pfitzer P. Blind pleural biopsy in combination with cytology of pleural effusions. Acta Cytol 1981; 25:373–376.
9. Nance KV, Shermer RW, Askin FB. Diagnostic efficacy of pleural biopsy compared with that of pleural fluid examination. Mod Pathol 1991; 4:320–324.
10. Anderson C, Philpott G, Ferguson T. The treatment of malignant pleural effusions. Cancer 1974; 33:916–922.
11. Izbicki R, Weyhing BT, Baker L, Caoili EM, Vaitkevicius VK. Pleural effusion in cancer patients. A prospective randomized study of pleural drainage with the addition of radioactive phosphorus to the pleural space vs. pleural drainage alone. Cancer 1975; 36:1151–1518.
12. Mejer J, Montensen KM, Hansen HH. Mepacrine hydrochloride in the treatment of malignant pleural effusions. Scand J Respir Dis 1977; 58:319–329.
13. Bayly TC, Kisner DL, Sybert A, Macdonald JS, Tsou E, Schein PS. Tetracycline and quinacrine in the control of malignant pleural effusions: a randomized trial. Cancer 1978; 41:1188–1192.
14. Millar JW, Hunter AM, Horne NW. Intrapleural immunotherapy with *Corynebacterium purvum* in recurrent malignant pleural effusions. Thorax 1979; 35:856–858.
15. O'Neil W, Spurr C, Moss H, et al. A prospective study of chest tube drainage and tetracycline sclerosis versus chest tube drainage in the treatment of malignant pleural effusions. Proc Am Soc Clin Oncol 1980; 21:349.
16. Gupta N, Opfell RW, Padova J, et al. Intrapleural bleomycin versus tetracycline for control of malignant pleural effusion: a randomized study. Proc Am Assoc Cancer Res 1980; 21:366.
17. Zaloznik AJ, Oswald SG, Langin M. Intrapleural tetracycline in malignant pleural effusions: a randomized study. Cancer 1983; 51:752–755.
18. Fentiman IS, Rubens RD, Hayward JL. Control of pleural effusions in patients with breast cancer: a randomized trial. Cancer 1983; 52:737–739.
19. Urata A, Nishimura Y, Ohta K. Randomized controlled study of OK-432 in the treatment of cancerous pleurisy (abstr in English). Gan to Kagaku Ryohou 1983; 10:1497–1503.
20. Johonson CE, Curzon PG. Comparison of intrapleural bleomycin and tetracycline in the treatment of malignant pleural effusions. Proc Br Thoroc Soc 1984; S:6.
21. Sorenson PG, Svendson TC, Enk B. Treatment of malignant pleural with drainage with or without installation of talc. Eur J Respir Dis 1984; 65:131–135.
22. Leahy BC, Honeybourne D, Brear SG, Carroll KB, Thatcher N, Stretton TB. Treatment of malignant effusions with intrapleural *Corynebacterium parvum* or tetracycline. Eur J Respir Dis 1985; 66:50–54.
23. Kefford RF, Woods RL, Fox RM, Tatterall MH. Intracavitary adriamycin nitrogen mustard and tetracycline in the control of malignant effusions, a randomized study. Med J Aust 1986; 2:447–448.
24. Fentiman IS, Rubens RD, Hayward JL. A comparison of intracavitary talc and tetracycline for the control of pleural effusions secondary to breast cancer. Eur J Clin Oncol 1986; 22:1079–1084.

25. Kessinger A, Wigton RS. Intracavitary bleomycin and tetracycline in the management of malignant pleural effusions: a randomized study. J Surg Oncol 1987; 36:81–83.
26. Landvater L, Hix WR, Mills M, Siegel RS, Aaron BL. Malignant pleural effusion treated by tetracycline sclerotherapy: a comparison of single vs. repeated instillation. Chest 1988; 90:1196–1198.
27. Ostrowski MJ, Houston PT, Martin WNC. A randomized trial of intracavitary bleomycin and *Corynebacterium parvum* in the control of malignant pleural effusions. Radiother Oncol 1989; 14:19–26.
28. Ruckdeschel JC, Moores D, Lee JY, Einhorn LH, Mandelbaum I, Koeller J, Weiss GR, Losada M, Keller JH. Intrapleural therapy for malignant pleural effusions, a randomized comparison of bleomycin and tetracycline. Chest 1991; 100:1528–1535.
29. Hartman DL, Gaither JM, Kesler KA, Mylet DM, Brown JW, Mathur PN. Comparison of insufflated talc under thoracoscopic guidance with standard tetracycline and bleomycin pleurodesis for control of malignant pleural effusions. J Thorac Cardiovasc Surg 1993; 105:743–747.
30. Bjermer L, Gruber A, Sue-Chu M, Sandstrom T, Eksborg S, Henriksson R. Effects of intrapleural mitoxantrone and mepacrine on malignant pleural effusion: a randomized study. Eur J Cancer 1995; 31A:2203–2208.
31. Emad A, Rezaian GR. Treatment of malignant pleural effusions with a combination of bleomycin and tetracycline: a comparison of bleomycin or tetracycline alone versus a combination of bleomycin and tetracycline. Cancer 1996; 78:2498–2501.
32. Zimmer PW, Hill M, Casey K, Harvey E, Low DE. Prospective randomized trial of talc slurry vs bleomycin in pleurodesis for symptomatic malignant pleural effusions. Chest 1997; 112:430–434.
33. Frederick H, Hausheer FH, Yarbro JW. Diagnosis and treatment of malignant pleural effusion. Semin Oncol 1985; 12:54–75.
34. Lan RS, Lo SK, Chuang ML, Yang CT, Tsao TC, Lee CH. Elastance of the pleural space: a predictor for the outcome of pleurodesis in patients with malignant pleural effusion. Ann Intern Med 1997; 126:768–774.
35. Hamed H, Fentiman IS, Chaudary MA, Ruberns RD. Comparison of intracavitary bleomycin and talc for control of pleural effusions secondary to carcinoma of the breast. Br J Surg 1989; 76:1266–1267.
36. Saijo N, Eguchi K, Tominaga K, Shinkai T, Shimizu E, Shibuya M, Shimabukuro Z, Niitani H. Effect of *Nocardia rubra* cell wall skeleton against pleuritis carcinomatosa in adenocarcinoma of the lung (abstr in English). Gan to Kagaku Ryohou 1983; 10(2):290–295.
37. Yamamura Y, Sakatani M, Ogura T, Hirao H, Kishimoto S, Huruse K, Kawahara M, Hukuoka M, Takada M, Kuwabara O, Ikegami H, Nakamura S, Ogawa N. Clinical effect of *Nocardia rubra* cell wall skeleton (N-CWS) on lung cancer with malignant pleural effusion (abstr in English). Gan to Kagaku Ryohou 1983; 10:63–70.
38. Luh KT, Yang PC, Kuo SH, Chang DB, Yu CJ, Lee LN. Comparison of OK-432 and mitomycin C pleurodesis for malignant pleural effusion caused by lung cancer: a randomized trial. Cancer 1992; 69:674–679.
39. Contegiacomo A, Fiorillo L, De Placido S, Pagliarulo C, Iaffaioli RV, Genua G, Giampaglia F, Palmieri G, Bianco AR. The treatment of metastatic pleural effusion in breast cancer: report of 25 cases. Tumori 1987; 73:611–616.

40. Gravelyn TR, Michelson MK, Gross BH, Sitrin RG. Tetracycline pleurodesis for malignant pleural effusions, a 10-year retrospective study. Cancer 1987; 59:1973–1977.
41. Casali A, Gionfra T, Rinaldi M, Tonachella R, Tropea F, Venturo I. Treatment of malignant pleural effusions with intracavitary *Corynebacterium parvum*, Cancer 1988; 62:806–811.
42. Rusch VW, Figlin R, Godwin D, Piantadosi S. Intrapleural cisplatin and cytarabine in the management of malignant pleural effusions: a Lung Cancer Study Group Trial. J Clin Oncol 1991; 9:313–319.
43. Webb WR, Ozmen V, Moulder PV, Shabahang B, Breaux J. Iodized talc pleurodesis for the treatment of pleural effusion. J Thorac Cardiovasc Surg 1992; 103:881–885.
44. Rosso R, Rimoldi R, Salvati F, De Palma M, Cinquegrana A, Nicolo G, Ardizzoni A, Fusco U, Capaccio A, Centofanti R. Intrapleural natural beta interferon in the treatment of malignant pleural effusions. Oncology 1988; 45:253–256.
45. Tanaka N, Terasawa A, Matsui T, Yamada J, Hizuta A, Ichikawa J, Nakayama F, Matsuda T, Orita K. Local administration of recombinant interferon-beta to patients with cancer-associated body cavity fluids (abstr in English). Gan to Kagaku Ryohou 1988; 15(2):237–241.
46. Suzuki H. Experimental and clinical studies on intrapleural instillations interleukin-2 (IL-2) in patients with malignant pleural effusion (abstr in English). Nipping Geka Gakkaishi 1989; 90(11):1922–1931.
47. Yasumoto K, Ogura T. Intrapleural application of recombinant interleukin-2 in patients with malignant pleurisy due to lung cancer: a multi-institutional cooperative study. Biotherapy 1991; 3:345–349.
48. Tercelj-Zorman M, Mermolja M, Jereb M, Oman M, Petric-Grabnar G, Jereb B. Human leukocyte interferon alpha (HLI-a) for treatment of pleural effusion caused by non-small-cell lung cancer. Acta Oncol 1991; 30(8):963–965.
49. Astoul P, Viallat J-R, Laurent JC, Brandely M, Boutin C. Intrapleural recombinant IL-2 in passive immunotherapy for malignant pleural effusion. Chest 1993; 103: 209–213.
50. Gotoh T, Tanaka Y, Fujita Y, Hiramori N, Fujii T, Arimoto T, Iwasaki Y, Fukabori T, Nakamura T, Ono N, Nakagawa M. Intrapleural pirarubicin (4′-O-tetrahydropyranyladriamycin) for treatment of malignant pleural effusion. Jpn J Clin Oncol 1996; 26:328–334.
51. Rauthe G, Sistermanns J. Recombinant tumour necrosis factor in the local therapy of malignant pleural effusion. Eur J Cancer 1997; 33:226–231.
52. Wilkins HE, Connolly MM, Grays P, Marquez G, Nelson D. Recombinant interferon alpha-2b in the management of malignant pleural effusions. Chest 1997; 111:1597–1599.
53. Fraser RS, Viloria JB, Wang N. Cardiac tamponade as a presentation of extracardiac malignancy. Cancer 1980; 45:1697–1704.
54. Liu G, Crump M, Goss PE, Dancey J, Shephered FA. Prospective comparison of the sclerosing agents doxycycline and bleomycin for the primary management of malignant pericardial effusion and cardiac tamponade. J Clin Oncol 1996; 14:3141–3147.
55. Tomkowski W, Szturmowicz M, Fijalkowska A, Filipecki S, Figura-Chojak E. Intrapericardial cisplatin for the management of patients with large malignant pericardial effusion. J Cancer Res. Clin Oncol 120:434–436.

56. Tomkowski W, Szturmowicz M, Fijalkowska A, Burakowski J, Filipecki S. New approaches to the management and treatment of malignant pericardial effusion. Support Care Cancer 1997; 5:64–66.
57. Primrose WR, Clee MD, Johnston RN. Malignant pericardial effusion managed with vinblastine. Clin Oncol 1983; 9:67–70.
58. Imamura T, Tamura K, Takenaga M, Nagatomo Y, Ishikawa T, Nakagawa S. Intrapericardial OK-432 instillation for the managemant of malignant pericardial effusion. Cancer 1991; 68:259–263.
59. Berek JS, Hacker NF, Lichtenstein A, Jung T, Spina C, Knox RM, Brady J, Greene T, Ettinger LM, Lagasse LD. Intraperitoneal recombinant alpha-interferon for ''salvage'' immunotherapy in stage III epithelial ovarian cancer: a Gynecologic Oncology Group Study. Cancer Res 1985; 45:4447–4453.
60. Chapman PB, Kolitz JE, Hakes TB, Gabrilove JL, Welte K, Merluzzi VJ, Engert A, Bradley EC, Konrad M, Mertelsmann R. A phase I trial of intraperitoneal recombinant interleukin-2 in patients with ovarian carcinoma. Invest New Drugs 1988; 6: 179–188.
61. Kato H, Yamamura Y, Kin R, Tanigawa M, Sano H, Inoue M, Sugino S, Kondo M. Treatment of malignant ascites and pleurisy by a streptcoccal preparation OK-432 with fresh frozen plasma: a mechanism of polymorphonuclear leukocyte (PMN) accumulation. Int J Immunopharmacol 1989; 11(2):117–128.
62. Bezwoda WR, Golombick T, Dansey R, Keeping J. Treatment of malignant ascites due to recurrent/refractory ovarian cancer: the use of interferon-alpha or interferon-alpha plus chemotherapy in vivo and in vitro. Eur J Cancer 1991; 27(11):1423–1429.
63. Räth U, Kaufmann M, Schmid M, Holfmann J, Wiedenmann B, Kist A, Kempeni J, Schilick E, Bastert G, Kommerell B. Effects of intraperitoneal recombinant human tumor necrosis factor alpha on malignant ascites. Eur J Cancer 1991; 27(2):121–125.
64. Yamaguchi Y, Satoh Y, Miyahara E, Noma K, Funakoshi M, Takashima I, Sawamura A, Toge T. Locoregional immunotherapy of malignant ascites by intraperitoneal administration of OK-432 plus IL-2 in gastric cancer patients. Anticancer Res 1995; 15:2201–2206.
65. Souter RG, Tarin D, Kettlewell MG. Peritoneovenous shunts in the management of malignant ascites. Br J Surg 1983; 70:478–481.
66. Lacy JH, Shively EH. Management of malignant ascites. Surg Gynecol Obstet 1984; 159:397–412.
67. Piccart MJ, Speyer JL, Markman MM, ten Bokkel Hunink WW, Alberts D, Jenkins J, Muggia F. Intraperitoneal chemotherapy; technical experience at five institutions. Semin Oncol 1985; 12(3):58–62.

19

Neurological Complications

Jerzy G. Hildebrand
Hôpital Erasme and Université Libre de Bruxelles, Brussels, Belgium

I. INTRODUCTION

In approximately one of five patients with generalized cancer, a major neurological insult will develop and will, in many of them, shorten the patient's survival and deteriorate the patient's remaining quality of life. This chapter provides general guidelines for early diagnosis and treatment of these complications. Quite often, the outcome depends not only on what is done but also on how early a treatment is performed. This chapter also discusses paraneoplasia.

II. METASTATIC LESIONS

The main metastatic sites injuring the nervous system are brain, meninges, epidural space, and peripheral nervous system.

A. Brain Metastases

Brain metastasies (BM) occur in about 25% of cancer patients. Approximately 60% of cases originate from lung or breast. Melanoma and carcinoma of kidney or digestive tract are next common. In about 15% of patients, the primary tumor (most often a lung cancer) remains unknown. The presentation of BM is polymorphic. Symptoms and signs range from focal and sudden (seizures or strokelike events) to progressive and more diffuse (headaches, gait, and mental disorders mimicking toxic or metabolic encephalopathies). On brain computed tomography (CT) or magnetic resonance imaging (MRI), most BM present as ring-enhanced lesions surrounded by edema. This appearance, however, is not specific. In patients without known primary neoplasia and in dubious situations, such as an infectious context, a pathological confirmation is necessary.

The median survival for untreated BM is 4 to 6 weeks, and more than 50% of deaths are related to systemic lesions. Fig. 1 provides an algorithm for the treatment of BM with specific anticancer therapies. Supportive care of BM includes, in addition, the treatment of peritumoral edema and seizures, and prevention of thrombophlebitis.

1. *Brain Edema*

There are essentially three types of brain edema:

1. Vasogenic edema caused by an increased permeability of brain capillaries and thus a disturbance of the blood–brain barrier. This edema involves primarily the white matter.
2. Cytotoxic edema characterized by swelling of the cellular component and reduction in the brain extracellular space.
3. Interstitial edema, which predominates in the periventricular white matter.

Vasogenic edema is most commonly seen in neuro-oncological practice. It surrounds almost every malignant primary or metastatic brain tumor. In many cases, the symptoms and signs of the neoplasia may be hidden by the surrounding edema. As does brain tumor, brain edema may produce the following:

1. Generalized manifestations of increased intracranial pressure, such as headaches, somnolence, ataxic gait, and papilledema
2. Direct focal deficits
3. Remote focal signs resulting from displacement of intracranial structures, causing cingulate, uncal, or tonsillar herniations

Vasogenic brain edema is most effectively and most durably alleviated by glucocorticosteroids, which also reduce the water content of the compressed spinal cord. Their symptomatic effect is often dramatic and occurs within hours to a few days. The usual daily dosage is 16 mg dexamethasone in four fractions or 80 mg methylprednisolone. Higher doses are occasionally necessary, but in my experience, their benefit is often bland or transient. On the other hand, by not decreasing or discontinuing the administration of corticosteroids soon enough, one may be using unnecessarily high doses. In fact, Weissman et al. (1) showed

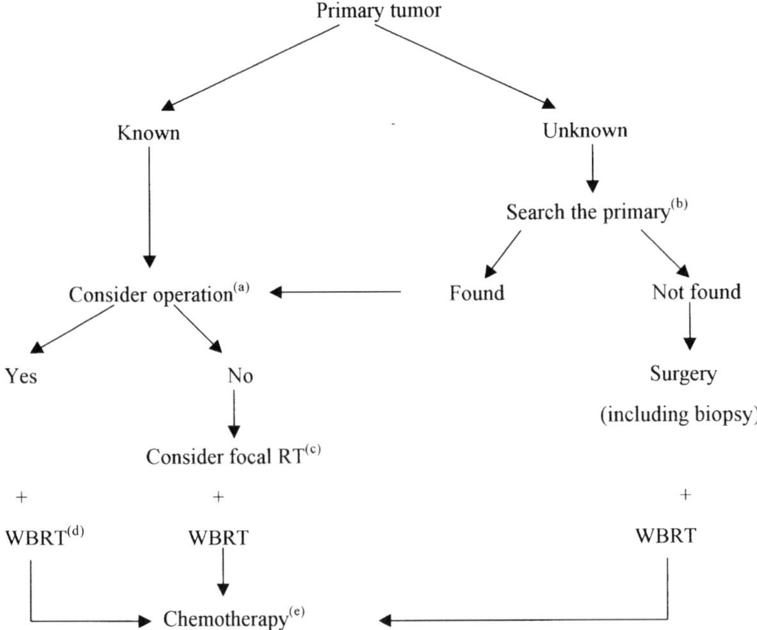

Figure 1 Algorithm for treatment of brain metastases. [a]Main operation criteria are: totally ressectable but possibly multiple lesions, minimal or controlled systemic cancer, expected survival of 6 months or more. [b]Should not delay treatment of BM. The most useful examinations are chest X-ray and chest CT. [c]Focal radiation therapy (RT) is composed of: linac, gamma knife, and possibly interstitial bradytherapy. Although neurosurgery and focal RT have their own indications, these treatment modalities are in competition. In the absence of prospective trials the choice will often be based on local expertise and available techniques. [d]Whole brain radiation therapy (WBRT) usually consists in 3000 cGy given in 10 fractions. [e]The choice of the drugs is guided by the sensitivity of the primary tumor rather that the ability of the drug to cross the blood-brain barrier.

in 20 patients with brain metastases that cerebral edema was efficiently controlled, even during radiation therapy, despite decreasing the daily dose of dexamethasone from 8 to 2 mg, and that corticosteroids could be discontinued at completion of the irradiation. Glucocorticosteroids also have salutary effects on nausea, vomiting, anorexia, and asthenia. However, the high frequency and severity of undesirable effects strongly limits their use in these circumstances.

In emergency cases, perfusions of 20% mannitol are temporarily effective in reducing brain edema. In patients who do not tolerate glucocorticosteroids, glycerol given orally at an average daily dose of 1.5 g/kg body weight in four fractions is a safe alternative.

2. Undesirable Effects of Glucocorticosteroids

Long-term administration of glucocorticosteroids is accompanied by a cohort of unwanted effects. The most important and the most common neurological manifestations are considered in this section. Except for hypoproteinemia, their occurrence is largely unpredictable. The risk factors for corticosteroid toxicity are unknown.

3. Psychiatric and Cognitic Disorders

Mental disturbances are less frequent with methylprednisolone or dexamethasone, the most communly used corticosteroids in neuro-oncology, than with natural corticosteroids or adenocorticotropic hormone (ACTH). Behavioral and personality changes, such as anxiety, nervousness, insomnia, and euphoria, are fairly common, but serious psychiatric manifestations, such as depression and acute psychotic and delirious reactions, occur in no more than 3% of cases. Depression may be seen in the early stages of corticosteroid therapy or during drug tapering. It usually vanishes after drug discontinuation. Acute psychotic and delirious reactions are characterized by paranoid behavior, often associated with visual or auditory hallucinations. In some patients, these disorders rapidly respond to drug discontinuation; in others, administration of major tranquilizers is necessary.

A decline in cognitive functions, possibly associated with cerebral atrophy, has been reported but is exceptional even in chronically treated patients.

4. Myopathy

Steroid myopathy corresponds to atrophy of type 2 muscle fibers. It is characterized by proximal wasting and weakness of the lower limbs, producing difficulties in standing up or climbing steps. In severe cases, the neck and shoulder muscles are also involved. Dropcho and Soong (2) reviewed 216 patients with primary brain tumors who received 2 weeks or more of continuous daily dexamethasone and found steroid-induced weakness in 23 (10.6%). In 15 (65%), the weakness developed between weeks 9 and 12 of treatment with a cumulative dose ranging from 580 to 1780 mg. These data suggest that treatment duration has a greater impact than the total dose of glucocorticosteroids. Furthermore, there was the protective effect of antiepileptics, especially phenytoin.

5. Lipomatosis

Long-term steroid therapy leads to the redistribution of fat tissue, including its deposition in the epidural space. Often asymptomatic, epidural lipomatosis occasionally produces spinal cord compression and paraplegia. Epidural lipomatosis also favors paraplegia in patients with vertebral collapse, which is another complication of glucocorticoid therapy. Severe cases of spinal cord compression may require surgical decompression. Lipomatosis is easily differentiated from epidural metastases by MRI because of the typical density of the fat tissue.

6. *Seizures*

The main causes of acquired seizures in cancer patients are primary or metastatic cortical tumors, metabolic encephalopathies, toxicity of chemotherapeutic agents, and central nervous system (CNS) infections.

Seizures occur in 20 to 30% of patients with metastatic or primary tumors, and may be the presenting sign leading to early diagnosis.

Seizures caused by brain tumors are essentially focal, and a careful history may help to localize both the neoplastic and the epileptogenic focus. In some cases, however, seizures generalize so quickly that their focal nature may be overlooked.

The metabolic disorders most likely to cause epilepsy are hypoglycemia, hyponatremia, hypocalcemia, hypokalemia, uremia, and hepatic failure. Their physiopathogenic mechanisms are similar to those of the metabolic encephalopathies summarized in Table 1. Seizures are a frequent complication of intracarotid chemotherapy using nitrogen mustard and, more recently, BCNU, HeCNU, and cisplatin, or etoposide (VP-16-213), and in high-dose systemic chemotherapy with methotrexate or BCNU. Besides these conditions, one must be very careful in attributing seizures to chemotherapy. In patients with generalized cancer treated by chemotherapy, brain or leptomeningeal metastases, metabolic disorders, or CNS infections are much more likely to cause epilepsy.

Determination of the cause of the disease requires a contrast-enhanced brain MRI, a search for metabolic disorders, and possibly a lumbar puncture to rule out meningeal metastases or CNS infection.

When seizures are caused by metabolic, toxic, or infectious disorders, prolonged administration of antiepileptic drugs is seldom required. On the contrary, patients with brain neoplasia suffering seizures receive anticonvulsants. I no longer use prophylaxis in patients with primary brain tumors, metastases, or even those originating from melanoma.

Carbamazepine and phenytoin appear to be the most efficient drugs to control focal seizures, including those caused by cerebral neplasia. There is a consensus to use these drugs as monotherapy at maximally tolerated doses rather than in combination. Phenytoin, which can be given intravenously (3), has the advantage that it can be used to treat status epilepticus, a severe life-threatening condition. Several factors complicate the use of antiepileptic drugs in cancer patients. First, epilepsy caused by brain tumors tends to be refractory to medical treatment. Sec-

Table 1 Acute Metabolic Encephalopathies in Cancer Patients

Metabolic disorder	Paraneoplastic production	Other causes related to cancer	Treatment
Hypercalcemia	Parathyroid hormone-related peptide, 1,25-hydroxy vitamin D	Bone metastases, multiple myeloma	Bisphosphonates, saline infusion, corticosteroids
Hypocalcemia		Malabsorption: postradiation lesions, mesenteric metastases, renal wasting of Mg and Ca caused by cisplatin	Intravenous or oral calcium
Hypophosphatemia	Deficit in 1,25-hydroxy vitamin D (?); other unknown factors	Cachexia, excessive glucose perfusion. Respiratory alkalosis	K phosphate < 60 mEq/24 h
Hypernatremia	Adeno corticotropic hormone (ACTH) (moderate)	Hemoconcentration, posterior pituitary metastases, cisplatin nephrotoxicity	Hydration, antidiuretic hormone
Hyponatremia	Inappropriate secretion of antidiuretic hormone	Vincristine, cyclophosphamide Excessive hydration + chemotherapy	NaCl, urea

Hypomagnesemia		Nephrotoxic chemotherapy (cisplatin)	
Hypoglycemia	Insulin, insulinelike products	Excessive consumption by tumor cells (?), insulinoma	Somatostatin
Hyperglycemia	ACTH	Glucocorticosteroid therapy	
Uremia		Urinary tract obstruction Nephrotoxic chemotherapy	
Anoxia, anoxemia		Severe anemia, heart failure (doxorubicin) Primary or metastatic lung tumors, lung infections or thromboemboli	
Hepatic failure		Liver primary or metastatic tumors L-Asparaginase	
Carcinoid syndrome	Serotonine ↑ in serum, ↓ in brain (?) ↑ 5 OH indol acetic acid in urine	Carcinoid tumors	Somatostatin

ond, concomitant administration of chemotherapy or glucocorticosteroids makes it difficult to maintain stable blood therapeutic drug levels. Finally, anticonvulsants are neurotoxic and may produce, especially at high levels, neurological symptoms and signs such as ataxia and nystagmus (phenytoin) or drowsiness and diplopia (carbamazepine). In addition, both drugs have been reported to increase the risk of skin reaction to brain irradiation, which can lead occasionally to a fatal Stevens-Johnson syndrome (4).

Diazepam (Valium), which is not used as chronic treatment for seizures, has two indications in neuro-oncology. Intravenous diazepam is recommended at a rate not faster than 2 mg/minute to stop seizures in status epilepticus, before starting phenytoin. Its use has also been recommended to avoid seizures in patients with brain tumors when performing contrast-enhanced CT scan, with 5 to 10 mg being given about half an hour before the procedure.

B. Leptomeningeal Metastases

Leptomeningeal metastases occur in about 5% of acute leukemias, despite prophylactic treatment. Leptomeningeal metastases also complicate lymphomas, lung and breast carcinomas, and melanomas. The clinical presentation is polymorphic, combining signs of encephalopathy, intracranial hypertension, meningeal involvement, and lesions of cranial nerves and spinal roots. The definitive diagnosis is based on the identification of neoplastic cells in the cerebrospinal fluid (CSF) found in approximately 70% of cases even after repeated lumbar punctures. The CSF is also characterized by low sugar and high protein concentration. Enhancement of meninges is seen on T_1-weighted plus gadolinium images in more than 50% of cases. Untreated leptomeningeal metastases lead to death within a few weeks. In patients with chemosensitive and radiosensitive tumors, (lymphomas, breast and small cell lung carcinomas), a median survival of 6 to 8 months may be achieved through early and aggressive therapy, combining intrathecal and systemic chemotherapy with irradiation of symptomatic areas.

C. Epidural Spinal Metastases

Epidural spinal metastases occur in 2% to 5% of cancer patients. Usually the neoplastic tissue extends from vertebral metastases originating from cancers with high ‘‘osteotropism’’: lung, prostate, breast and kidney carcinoma or lymphomas. Unlike in BM, the clinical presentation is remarkably stereotyped, differing only by the rate of progression ranging from a few days to several months. Backache and radicular pain elicited by compression, straining, or coughing is the initial and the prominent feature in at least 90% of cases. At this stage, signs of root involvement: depression of tendon reflexes, motor and sensory changes in territories of injured roots may be found. The progression to spinal cord compression may be slow (months) or rapid (few hours). Therapeutic outcome is bound to early diagnosis more than to the nature of treatment modality. The therapeutic algorithm illustrated in Fig. 2 is based on the following assumptions:

Laminectomy plus radiation therapy are not superior to radiation therapy alone, but there is no controlled trial proving this point.

The main indication for laminectomy is uncertain diagnosis.

The use of corticosteroids, which derives mainly from laboratory data, should be limited in time. They effectively relieve pain through oncolytic activity in breast carcinoma or lymphoma, and reduction of spinal cord edema in other primaries.

D. Cranial Epidural Metastases

The dominant features of cranial epidural metastases are cranial nerve palsies. Conversely, a cranial nerve lesion of unknown origin justifies a search for an underlying cancer. In relation to cancer, cranial nerve lesions may represent a potentially serious situation, justifying a careful screening for an underlying cancer schematized on Fig. 3.

Metastases involving peripheral nerves are discussed later.

III. METABOLIC AND TOXIC ENCEPHALOPATHIES

A. Physiopathogenesis and Clinical Presentation

An alteration in mental status, defined as a change in consciousness from mild confusion to coma, was, next to pain, the second most common symptom found by Clouston et al. (5) in patients referred to the Neurology Service of the Memorial Sloan-Kettering Cancer Center. Of 132 such patients, metabolic or drug-related encephalopathy was present in 80 (61%) and was the most common nonmetastatic neurological manifestation of symptomatic cancer.

Metabolic encephalopathies encountered in cancer patients are essentially of two kinds (see Table 1). The largest group is made up of metabolic encephalopathies, which are essentially due to dysfunction of vital organs, such as liver, lung, kidney or urinary tract, caused by metastatic spread or treatment toxicity. The second group represents truly paraneoplastic syndromes resulting from the production by the tumor cells, mainly small cell lung carcinoma (SCLC), of hormone or hormone-like substances.

Another cause of toxic encephalopathies in cancer patients is antineoplastic drugs, even though most of them do not readily cross the blood–brain barrier (6,7).

1. Methotrexate (MTX) produces encephalopathy after either intrathecal or

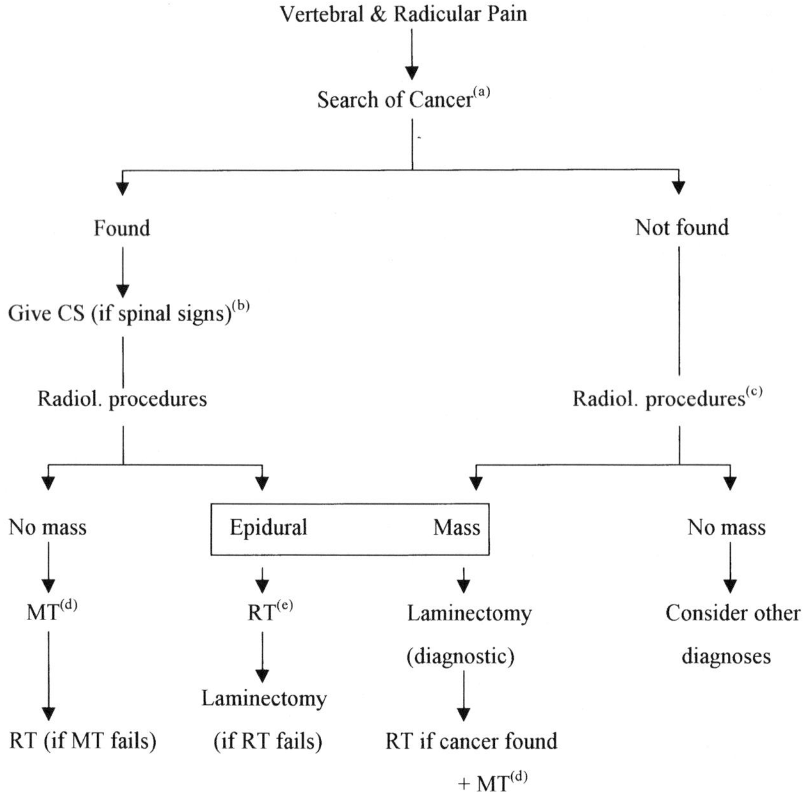

Figure 2 Algorithm for treatment for epidural metastases. [a]Even more than in brain metastases the search of the primary tumor should not delay local treatment that constitutes an emergency. [b]Doses and duration of administration of corticosteroids (CS) are not standardized. Many start with a bolus of 96 mg dexamethasone followed by 16 mg daily. [c]MRI of the entire spine is the examination of choice, showing the extension and the number of epidural metastases (multiple in about 20%), bony lesions, and neoplastic extension around the spine. [d]The choice of medical treatment (MT), including chemotherapy, hormones, and analgesics, is based on individual judgment. [e]Radiation therapy (RT) should begin as soon as possible. The usual dose is 3000 cGy in 10 fractions.

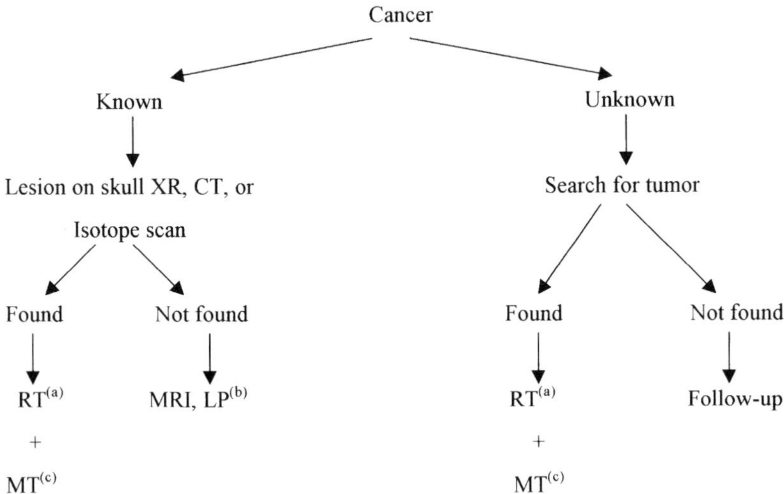

Figure 3 Diagnostic and treatment algorithm in cranial nerve lesions in relation to cancer. [a]The dose of radiation therapy (RT) and the nature of chemotherapy are related to the pathology of the primary tumor. [b]MRI and/or lumbar puncture are performed to identify leptomeningeal metastases. [c]The choice of medical treatment (MT), including chemotherapy, hormones, and analgesics, is based on individual judgment.

high-dose systemic administration. Signs of acute encephalopathy develop within hours of intrathecal administration, are often associated with a meningitic reaction, and resolve within 72 hours. Concomitant radiation therapy increases the risk of MTX encephalopathy.

2. Cortical disorders are rare after systemic therapy using cisplatin. In addition, the possible neurotoxic effect of the drug must be differentiated from the ionic disturbances induced through renal toxicity or excessive hydration combined with chemotherapy.

3. Cases of encephalopathy described in patients treated with vincristine (VCR) are rare. The physiopathogenesis of central nervous system (CNS) toxicity caused by VCR remains unclear. One mechanism is abnormal secretion of antidiuretic hormone as a result of the direct action of VCR on the hypothalamus or the peripheral volume receptors.

4. Two antipyrimidines, cytarabine and 5-fluorouracil, are primarily known to produce cerebellopathies. Occasionally, however, encephalopathy may develop.

5. Symptoms of usually mild encephalopathy, such as lassitude, sedation,

or drowsiness, may be seen when procarbazine, a monoamine oxidase inhibitor derivative, is given orally at a daily dose of 150 mg or more. The drug also has a synergistic sedation effect when combined with barbiturates or phenothiazines. Severe encephalopathy is the main limiting factor to using procarbazine intravenously.

6. The administration of L-asparaginase may produce consciousness alteration ranging from confusion to coma, caused primarily by hepatic failure or, rarely, by thrombosis of an intracranial venous sinus. The latter complication is characterized by a clinical picture consisting of headaches, papilledema, seizures, or focal signs.

7. Encephalopathy has been reported with several alkylating agents, including nitrogen mustard, chlorambucil, cyclophosphamide, and, more recently, high-dose nitrosoureas and ifosfamide.

8. Interferons, whether administered intrathecally or systemically, commonly produce signs of acute encephalopathy.

In cancer patients, the differential diagnosis of metabolic or toxic encephalopathies includes the following:

1. Multiple brain metastases, the most common CNS pathology in patients with systemic cancer. Mental changes are seen in about 30% of patients as the earliest clinical manifestation of cerebral or meningeal metastases.

2. Opportunistic CNS infections, among which *Listeria monocytogenes* and *Cryptococcus neoformans* figure prominently as causative agents, and progressive multifocal leukoencephalopathy caused by a papovavirus should be ruled out; likewise, limbic encephalitis is considered with paraneoplastic disorders.

B. Treatment

When facing recent mental disorders in a patient with generalized neoplasia, one must first rule out the possibility of multiple metastases, then meningeal seedings, CNS infections, and finally paraneoplastic disorders. This may be achieved by performing brain CT scan or preferably MRI scan with contrast enhancement of the brain and the spinal cord, and a lumbar puncture looking for evidence of leptomeningeal metastases or CNS infection. If these examinations are negative, metabolic or toxic encephalopathy becomes the most likely diagnosis.

Management of these encephalopathies combines treatment of the underlying neoplasia and a rapid symptomatic correction of the metabolic abnormality. Both the dysfunction of vital organs as a result of metastases and the paraneoplastic endocrinopathies may respond to an appropriate antineoplastic therapy. When the metabolic abnormality is attributed to chemotherapy, its administration must be discontinued. Sometimes, as in L-asparaginase–induced encephalopathy, dose reduction may suffice. Even if successful, however, these therapies do not usually produce immediate effects. Rapid symptomatic treatment is often necessary to correct the metabolic disorder.

The main treatments of metabolic encephalopathies are summarized in Table 1. Diphosphonates are the first line therapy for hypercalcemia. In addition, hypercalcemia in myeloma or lymphoma patients responds, usually after a delay of 2 to 3 days, to corticosteroids. Hyponatremia lasting for less than 48 hours may and should be corrected rapidly, but in chronic forms, the increase in serum sodium should not exceed 15 mEq/L per 24 hours to avoid brain edema and osmotic demyelinating syndrome.

In this chapter the focal cerebral toxicity count by chemotherapy administered intra-arterially is not considered because the symptoms and signs are predominantly focal and the origin is obvious.

IV. CEREBROVASCULAR DISEASE

A. Physiopathogenesis and Clinical Presentation

Graus et al. (8) published in 1985 the most comprehensive study on cerebrovascular complications in patients with cancer based on a series of 3426 complete autopsies. Cerebrovascular disease (CVD) was found in 14.5% of patients, of which half were symptomatic. The frequency of hemorrhagic and ischemic lesions was about equal. Next to heart diseases and cancer, CVD is the third cause of mortality and morbidity in the Western hemisphere and its occurrence in cancer patients, especially in the elderly, may be fortuitous. This section considers the physiopathogenesis of CVD specifically related to cancer and reviews hemorrhagic and ischemic arterial lesions, then venous occlusions. In many patients, different forms of CVD may coexist. For instance, the transformation of primary ischemic lesions into hemorrhagic lesions is common, and, in disseminated intravascular coagulation (DIC), both ischemic and hemorrhagic lesions may be found.

1. Hemorrhagic Cerebrovascular Disease

Intracerebral bleeding in cancer patients is caused primarily by coagulation abnormalities or intratumoral bleeding. The most common source of intracranial hematomas in the Graus et al. experience were abnormalities of coagulation, including hyperleukocytosis and thrombocytopenia. The underlying malignancy was acute leukemia in 69 of 88 patients; most of them had no signs of CNS leukemia. Of patients of this group, 71% were symptomatic.

Intratumoral bleeding, the second cause of massive hemorrhage, occurs in primary or metastatic brain tumors. In the series of Graus et al., in which primary CNS tumors were not included, the metastases most frequently associated with intracerebral hemorrhage originated from germ cell tumors (hemorrhagic in 59.3%) or melanomas (30.9%), whereas brain metastases of lung cancer bled rarely (5%), and those of breast carcinoma exceptionally (0.9%). In 42.6% of patients, the intracerebral bleeding caused by metastases had an acute strokelike onset.

In *subarachnoid hemorrhage*, acute nonlymphoblastic leukemia was the most common underlying neoplasia. In these patients, massive and symptomatic subarachnoid hemorrhage often leads to coma and rapid death.

Subdural hematomas were asymptomatic in three-fourths of 53 patients reported by Graus et al. Thrombocytopenia with or without DIC was present in all 25 patients with leukemia. All 27 patients with carcinoma had neoplastic infiltration of the dura. Another 10 patients had spinal subdural hematomas, all resulting from lumbar punctures; eight of them were thrombocytopenic.

2. Ischemic Cerebrovascular Disease

Nonbacterial thrombotic endocarditis (NBTE), also called *marantic endocarditis*, occurs in 0.4% to 2.4% of cancer patients, primarily lung, gastrointestinal (pancreatic), prostate, or female genital tract carcinoma. The NBTE is most likely to occur in cachetic, elderly patients with disseminated mucin-secreting cancer, but there are numerous exceptions (9). The NBTE is a major cause of cerebral embolism in patients with carcinoma. General signs of NBTE include petechiae, leukocytosis, sometimes fever mimicking infectious endocarditis, and systemic embolisms. Neurological signs are the most prominent manifestations of NBTE, not only because emboli are located in the brain more often than in many other organ but also because they are large and rarely remain asymptomatic. Neurological manifestations include focal deficits of abrupt onset and seizures, but not infrequently signs of diffuse encephalopathy are seen. Disseminated intravascular coagulation, present in about 25% of patients with NBTE, accounts for thrombocytopenia and independently produces cerebral arterial or venous occlusions and subdural and subarachnoid hemorrhages.

The etiopathogenesis of DIC may not differ fundamentally from that of NBTE, and as already mentioned, the two disorders can coexist. They differ statistically by the underlying neoplasia, however, and by the neurological presentation. Acute leukemia, lymphoma, and breast carcinoma are most commonly associated with DIC, and DIC is less often symptomatic than NBTE. Cerebral infarcts caused by DIC are multiple and small, and when symptomatic, they tend to produce a diffuse encephalopathy more often than focal deficits or seizures.

Less common causes of cerebral infarction or embolism in cancer patients include the following:

Septic infarction, which in the Graus et al. series was mainly associated with acute leukemia and was caused primarily by *Aspergillus*, *Candida*, or *Mucor* species.

Tumor emboli primarily originate from cardiac tumors, such as myxomas or sarcomas. The majority of myxomas are diagnosed in adults aged 30 to 60 years. Cerebral emboli consisting of neoplastic cells are rare.

Polycythemia, and to a *much* lesser extent *thrombocythemia* and *monoclonal gammapathies*, may lead to hyperviscosity and favor ischemic CVD.

Radiation-related lesions of large arteries may produce local thrombosis or distant emboli. These complications are seen after a delay ranging from months to more than 20 years following irradiation. Postradiation lesions of the aortic arch may account for the pathogenesis of transient ischemic attacks, such as those observed in patients with Hodgkin's disease (10).

Clinically, CVD seen in cancer patients differ from that in the general population by a much higher frequency of diffuse encephalopathy (Table 2). Thus, the differential diagnosis also includes toxic and metabolic encephalopathies and CNS infections. The differential diagnosis of CVD presenting with acute focal deficits includes brain metastases, which may mimic stroke even in the absence of intratumoral bleeding, and brain abscesses. The most helpful diagnostic procedures to be performed in different forms of CVD in cancer patients are summarized in Table 2.

3. Venous Occlusions

A hypercoagulability state is common in malignant diseases and accounts for the high rate of thrombophlebitis with or without pulmonary emboli. In turn, thrombophlebitis may produce paradoxical brain emboli, but the incidence of this complication in cancer patients is unknown. In patients with brain tumors, and possibly other cerebral lesions, paresis through immobility and blood stagnation favors the occurrence of thrombophlebitis, which develops preferentially in the limb contralateral to the brain lesion.

Thrombosis of the cerebral veins and dural sinuses is a rare event in patients with neoplasms. Symptomatic patients have signs of intracranial hypertension, headaches, seizures, and focal deficits. These complications result from metastatic infiltration or compression in most cases. The less common, nonmetastatic form may be caused by hypercoagulability or L-asparaginase treatment.

B. Treatment

The management of CVD related to cancer first requires the identification of their etiopathogenesis. Table 2 indicates that the latter is often suggested by the nature of the CNS lesion: hemorrhagic versus ischemic, the type of the underlying neo-

Table 2 Cerebrovascular Diseases in Cancer Patients

Diagnosis	Main pathogenesis	Main underlying neoplasia	Main clinical manifestation	Diagnostic procedure
Intracerebral hemorrhage	Coagulation abnormalities Hyperleukocytosis Thrombocytopenia Intratumoral bleeding Necrosis (?)	Acute leukemia (ANLL > ALL) Metastases Melanoma Germ cell tumor Lung carcinoma Glioblastoma Oligodendroglioma	Acute, strokelike in about 50%	CT, MRI Coagulation study Contrast-enhanced CT or MRI
Subdural hematoma Cerebral	Dural metastases Thrombocytopenia	Carcinoma Acute leukemia	Often asymptomatic	
Spinal	Thrombocytopenia plus LP	Acute leukemia Lymphoma	Asymptomatic or pain, paraparesis	CT, MRI
Subarachnoid hemorrhage	Meningeal, metastases Thrombocytopenia	ANLL > ALL	↓ Consciousness Headache	CT, MRI LP (angiography)
Nonbacterial thrombotic endocarditis	DIC Mucin secretion (?)	Lung carcinoma Gastrointestinal carcinoma Female genital tract and prostate carcinoma	Acute focal signs Seizures Sometimes diffuse encephalopathy	CT, MRI Cardiac echography Coagulation study

Intravascular coagulation		Acute leukemia Lymphoma Miscellaneous carcinoma	Diffuse encephalopathy Sometimes focal signs	Coagulation study
Septic emboli	*Aspergillus, Candida, Mucor*	Acute leukemia Lymphoma	Acute focal signs, diffuse encephalopathy	CT, MRI Chest, sinus x-ray study Cultures
Tumor emboli	Neoplastic emboli Sometimes DIC, thoracotomy	Cardiac myxoma, sarcoma Lung carcinoma	Acute focal signs Sometimes diffuse encephalopathy	CT, MRI Chest x-ray
Postradiation vascular lesions	Arterial occlusion Emboli	Head and neck carcinoma	Stroke Transient ischemic attacks	Angiography MRA
Hyperviscosity	Polycythemia Monogammopathy	Vaquez' disease Myeloma, Waldeström's disease	Stroke	Blood examination Protein study
Cerebral venous and sinus occlusion	Dural metastases L-Asparaginase Hypercoagulability (?)	Miscellaneous carcinoma	Subacute intracranial hypertension, focal signs, seizures	MRI MRA

Abbreviations: ANLL, acute nonlymphoblastic leukemia; ALL, acute lymphoblastic leukemia; LP, lumbar puncture; DIC, disseminated intravascular coagulation; MRA, MR angiography.

plasia (acute leukemia versus carcinoma), and the clinical presentation (focal deficits versus diffuse encephalopathy).

Evaluation of therapy of CVD in cancer patients is difficult because the outcome is related to many factors, including the spread of the underlying neoplasia, the patient's performance status, the sensitivity to antineoplastic treatment, and the severity of its toxicity, or the importance of immunodepression. In the absence of adequate prospective trials, many treatment recommendations that follow may appear controversial.

Rapid correction of coagulation disorders, thrombocytopenia, or hyperviscosity probably represents useful prophylaxis of cancer-related CVD. The prognosis of patients with massive acute cerebral hemorrhage is dismal, and neurosurgery is rarely indicated. Radiation therapy may help to stop bleeding caused by cerebral or dural metastases, especially those originating from radiosensitive neoplasia, such a germ cell tumors.

In symptomatic spinal subdural hematoma, decompressive surgery is indicated in patients with severe neurological deficit, but only after correction of the thrombocytopenia and if the general condition of the patient permits. The administration of heparin in NBTE seems useful to prevent embolic recurrence.

The occurrence of septic emboli may be prevented in leukemic patients by amphotericin B and is treated effectively by adequate antibiotics.

Postradiation vasculopathies are often segmental and amenable to surgical resection, which are recommended in symptomatic patients. Platelet antiaggregants should be used in inoperable patients. Because heparin has been shown to be effective in cranial thrombophlebitis in a general population in a prospective, randomized study (11), I also use heparin in venous and sinus occlusion, not caused by metastases, in cancer patients.

V. PERIPHERAL NEUROGENIC PAIN

The interest of early recognition and work-up of the peripheral neurogenic pain in cancer patients is of paramount importance for several reasons:

1. It may lead to discovery of a neoplastic disease.
2. It points to new neoplastic locations in patients with an already known malignancy.
3. The success of its management is related to the precocity and the accuracy of the diagnosis.

The clinical presentation of the most common and most typical peripheral neurogenic pain syndromes is summarized in Table 3. This section emphasizes the neurological presentation of these abnormalities; pain aspects and their treatment are considered in Chapter 15.

A. Pain Related to Cranial Nerve Lesions

Metastases of skull base are the main cause of pain distributed in cranial nerve territories in patients with generalized cancer. Pain location often provides useful guidance for radiological demonstration of metastatic lesions. A diagnostic and therapeutic algorithm is shown on Fig. 3.

B. Pancoast's Syndrome

The first manifestation of Pancoast's syndrome is an aching or burning pain caused by pleural involvement, reported at the anterior aspect of the chest and shoulder. Pancoast's syndrome points almost invariably to an apical pulmonary cancer. If the diagnosis is made at this early stage, an approximately 30% survival at 5 years may be expected (13). At later stages, when the eighth cervical and the first and second thoracic segments are involved, the chances for cure become dismal.

C. Plexopathies

Radicular pain is the initial manifestation of cancerous brachial or lumbosacral plexopathy in 80% to 90% of patients. Pain is rarely bilateral in early stages. The metastatic nature of plexus involvement is best confirmed by the evidence of neoplastic lesions on CT or MRI scan (14,15). These two procedures and myelography may also demonstrate epidural spread of the malignant tissue. If all these diagnostic procedures are negative and if a leptomeningeal carcinomatosis is ruled out by CSF analysis, the most likely, and the most difficult, differential diagnosis becomes postradiation plexopathy in patients previously irradiated in this area. The clinical presentation of postradiation plexopathy differs from that of neoplastic lesions in that the first symptoms are numbness, paresthesia, or weakness rather than intense radicular pain. In addition, approximately 80% of lumbosacral plexopathies caused by radiation therapy are bilateral although asymmetrical.

D. Thoracic and Lumbar Radicular Pain

Pain is the most common presentation of epidural metastases. Its characteristics and treatment algorithm have been considered earlier (see Section II C and Fig. 2).

Table 3 Main Peripheral Neurogenic Pain Syndromes Caused by Metastases

Pain location	Main associated signs	Most probable metastatic location	Structures involved
Unilateral frontal	Diplopia + exophthalmos	Orbital	Cranial nerves (12)
Unilateral frontal	Diplopia + vein turgescence	Parasellar	
Facial (pain or numbness)	Nerve V lesion	Middle fossa	
Glossopharyngeal neuralgia	Nerves IX, X, XI palsy	Jugular foramen	
Occipital	Nerve XII palsy, stiff neck	Occipital condyle	
Anterior aspect of chest and shoulder	Horner's syndrome, eighth cervical and first and second thoracic root palsy	Lung apex (Pancoast's syndrome)	Eighth cervical segment First and second thoracic segments
Upper limbs	Signs of cervicobrachial plexopathy	Epidural, cervical, axillary	Cervicobrachial plexus and/or roots
Thoracic and upper lumbar root pain	Vertebral pain Later, signs of spinal cord compression	Epidural	Thoracic roots Upper lumbar roots
Lower limbs	Signs of lumbosacral plexopathy	Epidural, pelvic	Lumbosacral plexus and/or roots

E. Peripheral Neuropathies

Three types of clinically distinct peripheral neuropathies are seen in cancer patients:

1. Sensory motor dying back polyneuropathy
2. Sensory neuropathy
3. Guillain-Barré–like polyradiculoneuritis

The two first varieties commonly manifest by burning and painful dysesthesia, whereas Guillain-Barré syndrome may be preceded by dorsal or lumbar pain. In addition to the differences in their clinical presentation, peripheral neuropathies are also diagnosed and differentiated from each other by electrophysiological features. Dying back neuropathy is characterized by a decreased amplitude of compound muscle and nerve potentials or slowing of motor and sensory nerve conduction velocities. Sensory neuronopathy is characterized by decreasing and eventually disappearance of sensory nerve potentials and Guillain-Barré syndrome by conduction blocks. The main causes of peripheral neuropathies specifically related to cancer are summarized in Table 4.

VI. FATIGUE AND WEAKNESS

According to Portenoy, quoted by Posner, fatigue is present in three fourths of cancer patients and is their most frequent complaint.

Many factors, including surgery, chemotherapy, radiation therapy, interferons, immunodepression, infections, anorexia and loss of weight, or feeling of sadness, may cause or at least aggravate the feeling of tiredness in cancer patients. Because fatigue is common in patients with generalized neoplastic diseases, several manageable conditions (Table 5) in which weakness is a prominant feature may be overlooked and their treatment unduly delayed.

These diseases include:

1. Corticosteroid myopathy, which has been considered previously.

2. Several disorders such as Lambert-Eaton syndrome, motor neuron disease, peripheral neuropathies including Guillain-Barré–like syndrome, and dermatopolymyositis, which are discussed in Section VII.

3. Hypokalemia and hypomagnesemia. In cancer patients, paraneoplastic production of ACTH, malabsorption, incoercible diarrhea and vomiting, or administration of amphotericin B (through renal tubular damage) or cisplatin (through hypomagnesemia and renal toxicity) may cause potassium depletion. Chronic corticosteroid therapy also causes hypokalemia, but corticosteroid myopathy is seldom related to ionic imbalance. Hypokalemic myopathy causes widespread weakness, which may or may not be painful, with depressed or absent tendon reflexes. Increased serum creatine kinase and myoglobinuria may be

Table 4 Cancer-Related Peripheral Neuropathies

Syndrome	Neoplastic compression or infiltration	Anticancer chemotherapy	Paraneoplasia
Dying back polyneuropathy	Very rare; seen in acute leukemias	Vinca alkaloids, procarbazine, hexamethylamine	Common form of "nontypical" neurologic paraneoplasia
Sensory neuronopathy	Posterior epidural metastases may mimic sensory neuronopathy	Cisplatin, taxol	Denny-Brown sensory neuronopathy associated with small cell lung cancer
Guillain-Barré–like syndrome	Meningeal carcinomatosis	Suramin sodium	Associated with lymphomas, mainly Hodgkin's disease

Table 5 Comparison of Selected Syndromes Causing Weakness in Cancer Patients

Syndrome	Relation to cancer	Main symptoms and signs	Main electrophysiological abnormalities	Laboratory examinations	Muscle biopsy	Treatment
Lambert-Eaton syndrome	Paraneoplastic	Proximal weakness of lower limbs, cholinergic dysfunction	Low CMAP ↑ CMAP at high-frequency stimulation	Antibodies against Ca^{2+} channel	Not contributive	Tumor reduction, immunodepression, guanidine, diaminopyridine
Hypokalemia and hypomagnesemia	Toxic, paraneoplastic	Widespread weakness	Usually not contributive	If severe, ↑ CK, myoglobinuria	Normal, vacuolar, or necrotizing myopathy	K^+ and Mg^+
Polymyositis	Paraneoplastic?	Proximal weakness dysphagia	Myopathic EMG, fibrillations	↑ Muscle enzymes, inflammatory changes	Necrotic and regenerative changes	Immunodepression
Corticoid myopathy	Prolonged treatment	Proximal lower limb weakness	Normal	Not contributive	Not contributive	Taper corticosteroids
Guillain-Barré syndrome	Paraneoplastic?	Weakness, ↓ tendon reflexes	Conduction blocks	↑ CSF protein	Not contributive	Plasmapheresis, immunoglobulins

Abbreviations: CMAP, compound muscle action potential; CK, creatinine kinase; CSF, cerebrospinal fluid.

found. Pathological studies may be either normal or show vacuolar or, in most severe cases, necrotizing myopathy. Treatment consists of restoring serum potassium and magnesium levels and correcting the abnormality that led to the ionic imbalance.

VII. PARANEOPLASIA

Paraneoplastic neurological syndromes (PNS) are neurologic disorders found in cancer patients, which are neither caused by a malignant infiltration nor by anticancer therapies, nor are due to a cause unrelated to cancer. Such an operational definition gathers under the same designation neurological insults of unidentified cause occurring in cancer patients, and disorders that are truly due to a remote effect of cancer. Paraneoplastic neurological syndromes form a group of protean diseases involving any part of the nervous system from cortex to muscle tissue; in addition, multiple lesion locations and syndromes may coexist. Paraneoplastic encephalomyelitis is the most typical example of a widespread PNS.

Not all PNS are equally suggestive of a remote effect of cancer. In his recent monography J. B. Posner rightly makes a distinction between ''classic'' PNS, which are highly evocative of an underlying cancer, and syndromes sometimes associated with cancer but more often seen in patients without malignancy (16). Most authors would regard as classic or typical PNS: Lambert-Eaton syndrome, opsoclonus occurring in children, subacute cerebellar degeneration, limbic encephalitis, sensory neuronopathy, and retinal photoreceptor degeneration. In patients with these syndromes, an extensive, even an aggressive, search for cancer is justified. Conversely, similar attitude in nontypical PNS, such as amyotrophic lateral sclerosis, sensory-motor neuropathy, or polymyositis, is often fruitless.

During the past decade, the diagnosis of PNS has been made easier by the identification, in the serum and the CSF, of specific antibodies directed toward antigens shared by the neoplasia and the nervous tissue.

The frequency of PNS is difficult to assess, but classic forms account for less than 3% of all neurological insults seen in cancer patients. For instance, in an unselected series of 1465 cancer patients, Croft and Wilkinson (17) found a high percentage of atypical PNS, whereas classic forms were very rare, with the possible exception of neuromuscular junction impairment. But even Lambert-Eaton syndrome (LES) is rare. In 150 patients with small cell lung carcinoma (SCLC) examined by Elrington et al. (18), two had LES and only one a sensory neuronopathy (95% confidence interval: 0%–4%).

The most prominent features of classic PNS are

Subacute onset progressing over weeks or few months, followed by stabilization

Severe neurological deficit, often more disabling than the malignancy itself
Inflammatory CSF changes
Neurological manifestations preceding the diagnosis of cancer in more than 50% of cases

A. Individual Syndromes

This review first describes the classic PNS with or without immunological markers, then PNS for which the relation to cancer is less certain. Not considered is myasthenia gravis, which many researchers regard as a paraneoplastic disorder because it may occur in association with thymoma and has an autoimmune marker.

1. *Classic PNS with Immunological Markers*

In general, PNS-associated antibodies are highly specific for the type of paraneoplasia and the pathology of the underlying cancer as well, but their sensitivity may be inferior to 50% (i.e., the antibodies are present in less than 50% of patients) (19). Table 6 summarizes the main clinical syndromes, the related malignancies, and their associated antibodies. These antibodies are known under different designations. The classification used herein corresponds to the initials of patients in whom they were first identified. This review is restricted to best characterized antibodies: anticalcium channels, antibodies Yo, Hu, Ri, and antiphotoreceptors. But other less well-characterized antibodies have been found in association with PNS either occasionally or in a substantial number of patients (20).

(a) Voltage-Gated Calcium Channel Antibodies

Voltage-gated calcium channel antibodies (VGCC) antibodies are found in LES, which is characterized by weakness predominating in proximal segments of the lower limbs. Typically, patients complain of difficulties in getting up or climbing stairs. On examination, strength may be increased by repetition of movements, muscle wasting is not prominent, and tendon reflexes may be depressed or absent. In severe cases, upper limbs may be involved. Respiratory distress is not rare, notably following anesthesia. Autonomic abnormalities such as dry mouth, constipation, and impotence are found in at least 50% of patients. Electromyography confirms the diagnosis. Three different patterns of repetitive nerve stimulation test have been reported. All are characterized by an initial low amplitude of compound muscle action potential (CMAP). The most typical pattern shows a striking enhancement (100%–1000%) of CMAP after high-rate stimulation and a decrease at low-rate (2–5 Hz) stimulation.

Out of 100 patients with Lambert-Eaton syndrome 60% to 70% have an underlying cancer, primarily but not exclusively, SCLC. The VGCC antibodies are

Table 6 Paraneoplastic Neurological Syndromes with Specific Antibodies

Antibody	Antigen	Clinical paraneoplastic syndrome	Associated tumor	Comments
Anti-Hu Anna-1 Type-IIa	Neuronal nuclear protein 35 to 40 kD	Limbic encephalitis, encephalomyelitis, PCD, sensory neuronopathy	SCLC Neuroblastoma (R) Non-SCLC (R) Prostate Ca (R)	Anti-Hu titers must be high
Anti-Yo PCA-1, APCA-1 Type 1	Purkinje cell cytoplasmic protein 34 kD and 62 kD	PCD	Ovarian or breast Ca Other gynecologic Ca	Antigen found in the tumors only if PNS present
Anti-Ri Anna-2 or Type IIb	Mainly nuclear neuronal protein 55 kD and 80 kD	Opsoclonus Myoclonus PCD	Breast Ca Gynecological Ca	Antigen found in the tumor only if PNS present
Voltage-gated calcium-channel antibodies	Presynaptic extracellular segment of CCA	Lambert-Eaton syndrome	SCLC	Antibodies also present in LES not associated with cancer (30%)

Abbreviations: SCLC, small cell lung carcinoma; Ca, carcinoma; PNS, paraneoplastic neurological syndrome; PCD, paraneoplastic cerebellar degeneration; (R), rare; LES, Lambert-Eaton syndrome.

found in LES associated with cancer and in patients without neoplasia as well. The VGCC determinants are expressed by SCLC cells also in patients without LES.

The VGCC antibodies are believed to cause a decrease of VGCC at nerve terminals, thus lowering presynaptic quantal release of acetylcholine (21). The LES responds to drugs that increase acetylcholine release such as guanine hydrochloride, 4-aminopyridine, which are fairly toxic, and 3,4-diaminopyridine up to 100 mg/d in three to four daily fractions, possibly combined with cholinesterase inhibitors. Occasionally, cytoreductive therapies have improved LES-symptoms. Lambert-Eaton syndrome often responds to plasmapheresis or immunodepressive drugs (22). Intravenous immunoglobulin causes a short-term improvement of strength attributed to a reduction of VGCC-antibodies (23).

(b) Anti-Yo

Anti-Yo antibodies are associated with isolated subacute paraneoplastic cerebellar degeneration (PCD). The disorder usually starts as gait ataxia, followed by limb and trunk dysmetria, dysarthria, and intentional tremor. Patients may complain of nystagmus related oscillopsia. Paraneoplastic cerebellar degeneration evolves in weeks to months and remains stable thereafter. Late CT and MRI scan may reveal cerebellar atrophy. Cerebrospinal fluid shows inflammatory changes including possible oligoclonal bands. Pathological lesions consist of diffuse and severe loss of Purkinje cells and thinning of granular and molecular layers.

Anti-Yo are directed toward cytoplasm proteins of 34 and 62 kD found only in Purkinje cells. Indirect immunostaining reveals a characteristic coarse pattern. Yo antigens are expressed in ovary and breast carcinoma only in patients with PCD (24). The main characteristics of anti-Yo are the following:

- They were found in more than 50% of PCD in women with breast or ovary carcinoma (25). Their presence in PCD associated with other cancers is exceptional.
- Anti-Yo were not found in neurologically normal individuals with cancer, in healthy controls, or in cerebellar degeneration of other causes (25).
- Anti-Yo were occasionally found in high titers in patients with ovarian carcinoma without cerebellar signs (26,27).

Paraneoplastic cerebellar degeneration does not respond to the treatment of the primary cancer and seldom to plasmapheresis or immunodepressive drugs. In most patients, however, these therapies have been given in the stable phase of the disease when the loss of Purkinje cells has already been completed. Also, intravenous immunoglobulins have been found of little value but occasional improvements have been observed in patients who received early treatment.

(c) Anti-Hu

Anti-Hu antibodies, first identified in a patient with paraneoplastic sensory neuronopathy, are in fact associated with a multifocal encephalomyelitis in which lesions can be found all the way from cortex down to sensory ganglia (28). Anti-Hu have been occasionally found in LES. The clinical presentation of the paraneoplastic encephalomyelitis (PEM) is largely determined by the most affected areas. Schematically, five clinical syndromes may be individualized; they occur either in isolation or, more commonly, in various combinations:

1. In limbic encephalitis, lesions predominate in hypothalamic and median temporal regions. Clinical presentation is characterized by mental changes (e.g., anxiety, agitation, or depression) and cognitive disorders (primarily memory disturbances). Neocortical functions are relatively preserved during the early stages of the disease. Limbic encephalitis has been reported mainly in association with SCLC but occurs occasionally in other cancers in absence of anti-Hu.
2. In patients with brain stem involvement, external ophthalmoplegia, nystagmus, and gaze paralysis are seen when the lesions predominate in the upper brain stem. Bulbar palsies are frequent when the lower brain stem is affected.
3. Clinical features of PCD may be very similar to those associated with anti-Yo when the lesions are restricted to cerebellum.
4. Spinal cord involvement that occurs as part of PEM may present with low motor neuron lesions (29) and is distinct from necrotizing myelopathy, a very rare condition described by Mancall and Rosales (30).
5. Finally, in the sensory neuronopathy first described by Denny-Brown, lesions predominate in sensory ganglia causing wallerian degeneration and demyelination of the posterior spinal columns. Patients complain of paresthesia, which may be distressing. Sensory deficits predominate in the lower limbs.

Hu antigen is a 35- to 40-kD nuclear protein expressed in all neurons of CNS and in SCLC and neuroblastoma (31).

High titers of anti-Hu are characteristic of paraneoplastic PEM and of sensory neuronopathy, but they are found in *low* titers in about 16% of patients with SCLC without paraneoplastic manifestations (32).

Treatment of PNS associated with Hu antibodies, particularly immunodepression, has been disappointing, probably for reasons previously considered for anti-Yo. Rare spontaneous improvements have been observed (33).

(d) Anti-Ri

Anti-Ri antibodies are associated with opsoclonus, myoclonus, ataxia, and occasional encephalomyelitis (34). Opsoclonus, the cardinal sign, is characterized by involuntary chaotic, multidirectional, eye saccades. Myoclonus is often evoked or enhanced by voluntary movements. Ataxia associated with anti-Ri is predominantly trancular. The onset of these signs ranges from 1 week to a few months. The most striking clinical features are fluctuations with possible recovery similar to the course of non-paraneoplastic opsoclonus-myoclonus. Favorable outcomes may be related to the paucity of pathological lesions, including in the midbrain.

Anti-Ri syndrome is associated almost exclusively with breast carcinoma.

Ri antigens are 55- and 80-kD proteins present in all neurons of CNS. Like anti-Yo, but unlike Hu or calcium channel antigens, Ri antigens were found in cancer tissue only in patients with an antibody response.

Anti-Ri antibodies have the following characteristics:

They were not found in controls nor in 87 women with breast cancer without neurological signs (35), but were found in high titers (27) in 7 of 181 women with ovarian cancer and no neurological signs of paraneoplasia.

Anti-Ri were not found in association with opsoclonus occurring in patients with SCLC or neuroblastoma.

Ri antibodies were exceptionally found in non-paraneoplastic condition.

The remitting course, spontaneous remissions, and the rarety of PNS associated with anti-Ri make it difficult to evaluate treatment.

(e) Cancer-Associated Retinopathy

Cancer-associated retinopathy (CAR) is a rare condition usually associated with SCLC. Clinically, CAR is characterized by a progressive, painless, bilateral but often asymmetrical loss of vision. The syndrome is due to loss of ganglion cells and photoreceptors. Serum antibodies react with lung cancer antigens of approximately 65 kD and with a 23-kD retinal protein (35). The antibodies were not found in sera from cancer patients without loss of vision, or from patients having retinitis pigmentosa or controls. Exposure of guinea pig optic nerve to the serum of a patient with CAR caused extensive demyelination (35).

B. Significance of Paraneoplastic Antibodies

The pathogenic role of antibodies directed against VGCC in LES is based on a body of evidence. Immunodepressive treatments (22–23) and plasmapheresis are effective. Infusion of patient's IgG reproduces experimentally the neuromuscular abnormalities. Also, the demyelination of guinea pig optic nerve after exposure to serum from a patient with CAR favors the pathogenic role of the antibodies in this syndrome (35). In most PNS, however, the significance of the antibodies found in the serum and the CSF remains uncertain.

Therapeutic trials using immunodepression are inconclusive. Negative results reported in most patients may be due to delay in treatment initiation (36). Indeed, few patients undergoing early treatment responded to immunotherapy. Additional arguments are against the hypothesis that autoantibodies cause PNS: no PNS other than LES and CAR has been consistently reproduced in experimental models through human antibodies. Classic PNS may occur in absence of specific antibodies, and high titers of autoantibodies have been observed without clinical manifestation of PNS (27).

Finally, a still unexplained and rare situation is the presence of specific antibodies in patients with a classic PNS in which no underlying cancer was found, even after a prolonged period of observation or at autopsy. Several explanations have been offered: (1) the tumor has been missed because of its small size, (2) the tumor has been rejected through the immune reaction, or (3) the antigenic stimulus is of nonneoplastic nature.

C. Paraneoplastic Neurological Syndromes Without Immunological Markers

Some disorders highly suggest the presence of a hidden neoplasia. The best example is opsoclonus-myoclonus not associated with Ri-antibody.

1. Opsoclonus-Myoclonus

Opsoclonus-myoclonus which is the cardinal feature of anti-Ri syndrome, also occurs as a paraneoplastic manifestation without marker in two main circumstances (1) in infants and children, opsoclonus is indicative of neuroblastoma in as many as 50% of cases; and (2) in adults, the likelihood of finding an underlying tumor—particularly lung cancer—is about 20%. Paraneoplastic opsoclonus, which may remit spontaneously, also responds to vitamin B_1 or clonazepam.

2. Motor Neuron Disorders

More than 95% of progressive spinal muscular atrophy (PSMA) or amyotrophic lateral sclerosis (ALS) occur in patients without cancer. These motor neuron disorders (MND) are therefore rarely paraneoplastic. However, in certain circumstances, relationship between cancer and nervous insult is highly suggestive:

1. There seems to be a disproportionate risk of MND (both PSMA and ALS) in patients with various types of lymphoproliferative disorders (37), with or without monoclonal paraproteinemia.
2. As discussed previously, in few cases MND are associated with Hu-antibodies.
3. In rare reports, signs of MND have regressed after successful treatment of the associated tumor.

3. Peripheral Neuropathies

Truly PNS are rare and peripheral neuropathies—especially of dying-back type—are common. A systematic search of an underlying malignancy when facing a peripheral neuropathy of unknown etiology is fully justified only in certain circumstances:

1. When the peripheral neuropathy presents as a sensory neuronopathy (see Section VII.A.1(c)).
2. When polyneuropathy is associated with disorders (including malignant

diseases such as multiple myeloma, lymphomas, or Waldesntröm disease [38]), producing abnormal amounts of immunoglobulins. The associated neuropathy is then often similar to the chronic inflammatory demyelinating polyneuropathy (CIDP). Whereas CIDP is in the common osteolytic form of myeloma, it is found in half of the patients with the rare osteoblastic variety where it may be part of the POEMS (polyneuropathy-organomegaly-endocrinopathy-M protein-skin changes) or CROW-FUKASE syndrome. The cause of neuropathy in myeloma remains unclear. Binding of M component to the neurological structures, particularly to myelin, has been shown only occasionally.

3. Another rare but interesting association is that of Hodgkin's disease with Guillain-Barré–like syndrome.

4. Polymyositis and Dermatomyositis

Polymyositis is a diffuse inflammatory disease of predominantly proximal skeletal muscles. The majority of cases occur in patients without malignancy, and the association between polymyositis-dermatomyositis and cancer has been questioned (39). More recently, however, this association was reasonably established in a population-based study (40), which showed that patients with polymyositis have a moderately higher risk of cancer than the general population. Thus, polymyositis may be regarded as a paraneoplastic disease, although the physiopathogenic relation to neoplasia has not been elucidated. When the characteristic skin rash is present (dermatomyositis), the diagnosis is usually made easily. In the absence of cutaneous lesions, however, the disease may be mistaken for metabolic or corticosteroid myopathy, or even LES.

REFERENCES

1. Weissman DE, Janjan NA, Erickson B, et al. Twice daily tapering dexamethazone treatment during cranial radiation for newly diagnosed brain metastases. J Neurooncol 1991; 11:235–239.
2. Dropcho EJ, Soong SJ. Steroid-induced weakness in patients with primary brain tumors. Neurology 1991; 41:1235–1239.
3. Delgado-Escueta AV, Wasterlain C, Treiman DM, Porter RJ. Management of status epilepticus. N Engl J Med 1982; 306:1337–1340.
4. Delattre JY, Safai B, Posner JB. Erythema multiforme and Stevens-Johnson syndrome in patients receiving cranial irradiation and phenytoin. Neurology 1988; 38: 194–198.
5. Clouston PD, De Angelis LM, Posner JB. The spectrum of neurological disease in patients with systemic cancer. Ann Neurol 1992; 31:268–273.
6. Posner JB. Acute encephalopathy and seizures. In: Hildebrand J, ed. Neurological Adverse Reactions to Anticancer Drugs. Berlin: Springer-Verlag, 1990:55–65.

7. Graus F. Chronic encephalopathies. In: Hildebrand J, ed. Neurological Adverse Reactions to Anticancer Drugs. Berlin: Springer-Verlag, 1990:67–73.
8. Graus F, Rogers LA, Posner JB. Cerebrovascular complications in patients with cancer. Medicine (Baltimore) 1985; 64:16–35.
9. Rosen P, Armstrong D. Non bacterial endocarditis in patients with malignant neoplastic diseases. Am J Med 1973; 54:23–29.
10. Feldman E, Posner JB. Episodic neurologic dysfunction in patients with Hodgkin's disease. Arch Neurol 1986; 43:1227–1233.
11. Einhaupl KM, Villringer A, Meister W, et al. Heparin treatment in sinus venous thrombosis. Lancet 1991; 338:597–600.
12. Greenberg HS, Deck MDF, Vikram B, Chu FCH, Posner JB. Metastasis to the base of the skull: clinical findings in 43 patients. Neurology 1981; 31:530–537.
13. Attar S, Miller JE, Satterfield J, et al. Pancoast's tumor: irradiation or surgery? Ann Thorac Surg 1979; 28:578–586.
14. Cascino TL, Kori S, Krol G, Foley KM. CT of the brachial plexus in patients with cancer. Neurology 1983; 33:1533–1557.
15. Thomas JE, Cascino TL, Earle JD. Differential diagnosis between radiation and tumor plexopathy of the pelvis. Neurology 1985; 35:1–7.
16. Neurologic complications of cancer. Posner JB, ed. Philadelphia: FA Davis, 1995: 353–385.
17. Croft PB, Wilkinson M. The incidence of carcinomatous neuropathy in patients with various types of carcinomas. Brain 1965; 88:427–434.
18. Elrington GM, Murray NMF, Spiro SG, Newsom-Davis J. Neurological paraneoplastic syndromes in patients with small cell lung cancer. A prospective survey of 150 patients. J Neurol Neurosurg Psy 1991; 54:764–767.
19. Moll JWB, Henzen-Logmans SC, Splinter TAW, van der Burg MEL, Vecht ChJ. Diagnostic value of anti-neuronal antibodies for paraneoplastic disorders of the nervous system. J Neurol Neurosurg Psychiatry 1990; 53:940–943.
20. Honnorat J, Antoine J-C, Derrington E, Aguera M, Belin M-F. Antibodies to a subpopulation of glial cells and a 66 kDa developmental protein in patients with paraneoplastic neurological syndromes. J Neurol Neurosurg Psychiatry 1996; 61:270–278.
21. Nagel A, Engel AG, Lang B, Newsom-Davis J, Fukuoka T. Lambert-Eaton myasthenic syndrome IgG depletes presynaptic membrane active zone particles by antigenic modulation. Ann Neurol 1988; 24:552–558.
22. Newsom-Davis J, Murray NMF. Plasma exchange and immunosuppressive drug treatment in the Lambert-Eaton myasthenic syndrome. Neurology 1984; 34:480–485.
23. Bain PG, Motomura M, Newsom-Davis J, Misbah SA, Chapel HM, Lee ML, Vincent A, Lang B. Effects of intravenous immunoglobulin on muscle weakness and calcium-channel autoantibodies in the Lambert-Eaton myasthenic syndrome. Neurology 1996; 47:678–683.
24. Furneaux HM, Rosenblum MK, Dalmau J, Wong E, Woodruff P, Graus F, Posner JB. Selective expression of Purkinje-cell antigens in tumor tissue from patients with paraneoplastic cerebellar degeneration. N Engl J Med 1990; 322:1844–1851.
25. Jaeckle KA, Graus F, Houghton A, Cardon-Cardo C, Nielsen SL, Posner JB. Autoimmune response of patients with paraneoplastic cerebellar degeneration to a Purkinje cell cytoplasmic protein antigen. Ann Neurol 1985; 18:592–600.

26. Brashear HR, Greenlee JE, Jaeckle KA, Rose JW. Anticerebellar antibodies in neurologically normal patients with ovarian neoplasms. Neurology 1989; 39:1605–1609.
27. Drlicek M, Bianchi G, Bogliun G, Casati B, Grisold W, Kolig C, Liszka-Setinek U, Marzorati L, Wondrusch E, Cavaletti G. Antibodies of the anti-Yo and anti-Ri type in the absence of paraneoplastic neurological syndromes: a long-term survey of ovarian cancer patients. J Neurol 1997; 244:85–89.
28. Dalmau J, Graus F, Rosenblum MK, Posner JB. Anti-Hu-associated paraneoplastic encephalomyelitis/sensory neuronopathy. A clinical study of 71 patients. Medicine (Baltimore) 1992; 71:59–72.
29. Verma A, Berger JR, Snodgrass S, Petito C. Motor neuron disease: a paraneoplastic process associated with anti-Hu antibody and small-cell lung carcinoma. Ann Neurol 1996; 40:112–116.
30. Mancall EL, Rosales RK. Necrotizing myelopathy associated with visceral carcinoma. Brain 1964; 87:639–656.
31. Tora M, Graus F, de Bolos C, Real FX. Cell surface expression of paraneoplastic encephalomyelitis/sensory neuronopathy-associated Hu antigens in small-cell lung cancers and neuroblastomas. Neurology 1997; 48:735–741.
32. Dalmau J, Furneaux HM, Gralla RJ, Kris MG, Posner JB. Detection of the anti-Hu antibody in the serum of patients with small cell lung cancer—a quantitative Western blot analysis. Ann Neurol 1990; 27:544–552.
33. Byrne T, Mason WP, Posner JB, Dalmau J. Spontaneous neurological improvement in anti-Hu associated encephalomyelitis. J Neurol Neurosurg Psychiatry 1997; 62: 276–278.
34. Luque FA, Furneaux HM, Ferziger R, Rosenblum MK, Wray SH, Schold SC Jr, Glantz MJ, Jaeckle KA, Biran H, Lesser M, Paulsen WA, River ME, Posner JB. Anti-Ri: an antibody associated with paraneoplastic opsoclonus and breast cancer. Ann Neurol 1991; 29:241–251.
35. Thirkill CE, Fitzgerald P, Sergott RC, Roth AM, Tyler NK, Keltner JL. Cancer-associated retinopathy (CAR syndrome) with antibodies reacting with retinal optic-nerve, and cancer cells. N Engl J Med 1989; 321:1589–1594.
36. Graus F, Vega F, Delattre JY, et al. Plasmapheresis and antineoplastic treatment in CNS paraneoplastic syndromes with antineuronal autoantibodies. Neurology 1992; 42:536–540.
37. Gordon PH, Rowland LP, Younger DS, Sherman WH, Hays AP, Lous ED, Lange DJ, Trojaborg W, Lovelace RE, Murphy PL, Latov N. Lymphoproliferative disorders and motor neuron disease: an update. Neurology 1997; 48:1671–1678.
38. Pollard JD, Young GAR. Neurology and the bone marrow. J Neurol Neurosurg Psychiatry 1997; 63:706–718.
39. Lakhanpal S Bunch TW, Ilstrup DM, Melton LJ. Polymyositis-dermatomyositis and malignant lesions: does an association exist? Mayo Clin Proc 1986; 61:645–653.
40. Sigurgeirsson B, Lindelof B, Edhag O, Allander E. Risk of cancer in patients with dermatomyositis or polymyositis. A population-based study. N Engl J Med 1992; 326:363–367.

20

Bone Metastases

J. J. Body
Institut Jules Bordet, Université Libre de Bruxelles, Brussels, Belgium

I. CLINICAL ASPECTS OF BONE METASTASES

According to one series, 30% to 90% of patients with advanced cancer will develop skeletal metastases. Carcinomas of the breast (47%–85%), of the prostate (33%–85%), and of the lung (32%–60%) are the tumors most commonly associated with skeletal metastases, whereas tumors of the digestive tract are only rarely (3%–13%) complicated by metastatic involvement of bone (1). The skeleton is the most common site of metastatic disease in breast cancer and the most common site of first distant relapse (2,3). These patients have a relatively long survival time after the diagnosis of bone metastases compared to patients with extraosseous metastases. Their median survival is usually beyond 20 months and about 10% of these patients are still alive 5 to 10 years after the first diagnosis of bone metastases (2). Osteolytic bone disease can thus be responsible for considerable morbidity and can markedly decrease the quality of life (Table 1) (2–5). Because of the long clinical course that breast cancer may follow, morbidity from bone metastases makes major demands on resources for health care provision. Major complications are seen in up to one-third of the patients whose first relapse is in bone (2,5).

Metastatic bone pain is traditionally attributed to various factors, notably the release of chemical mediators, increased pressure within the bone, microfractures, stretching of periosteum, reactive muscle spasm, and nerve root infiltration or

Table 1 Morbidity of Bone Metastases in Breast Cancer

Pain, functional impairment (45%–75%)
Bone fractures (10%–20% for the long bones)
Hypercalcemia (10%–15%)
Epidural compression (3%–5%)
Complications of bone marrow invasion

Source: Adapted from Refs. 2–5.

compression (6). However, as suggested by the clinical and biochemical effects of bisphosphonates, the dramatic increase in bone resorption probably plays an important contributory role as well. Pathological fractures constitute a major cause of prolonged disability in breast cancer, whereas pathological fracture is relatively unusual in prostate cancer, with its predominantly sclerotic picture. It is not rare that metastatic breast cancer remains confined to the skeleton for a long time. Sherry and collaborators studied 86 such patients in whom extraskeletal metastases developed after a mean delay of 2 years. Compared to patients who initially had metastases to other sites, these patients had a more prolonged survival (median of 48 months versus 17 months) but major complications of their skeletal disease were more often present. Thus, pathological fractures of the long bones developed in 21% and spinal cord compression in 15% (7). This relatively slow evolution of breast cancer metastasizing in bone suggests some peculiar biological properties of these tumor cells. Retrospective studies have shown that breast cancers metastasizing to the skeleton were more frequently estrogen receptor–positive and more well differentiated than the tumors metastasizing to lungs or liver (2). The presence of sclerotic lesions has been associated with a better prognosis than lytic lesions (8), but the prognostic significance of the distribution of bone metastases has been little studied. Limited data in prostate cancer suggest that the presence of bone metastases outside the pelvis and lumbar spine represents a poor prognostic factor for an equivalent tumor load and similar tumor differentiation (9).

Many authors claim that patients with metastatic bone disease have a lower response rate to antineoplastic therapy. This could reflect the slower growth rate of tumors metastasizing to bone and a lower sensitivity to cell cycle–specific tumoricidal agents, but it could also more simply reflect the relative insensitivity of current methods for evaluating the response of bone metastases to antineoplastic therapy (10). It is even more essential to obtain an early assessment of the efficacy of antineoplastic treatments that the therapy of bone metastases often relies on toxic drugs and is essentially palliative.

II. DIAGNOSIS AND MONITORING OF BONE METASTASES

The diagnosis and monitoring of bone metastases rests on clinical, scintigraphic, radiographic, biochemical, and histological techniques. The diagnosis of bone metastases is most often easy and bone biopsy is rarely necessary. However, the assessment of the response to therapy remains a continuous challenge in daily care.

A. Clinical Assessment

Pain is the most common symptom of bone metastases. A recent review indicates that pain is present at the diagnosis of neoplastic bone disease in 58% to 73% of the cases when the bone lesions are lytic or mixed but in only 42% for osteoblastic metastases (Table 2) (11).

Quantitative pain assessment is performed too rarely by the oncologists. Although none of the available pain measuring instruments has been specifically developed for bone metastases, pain intensity can be quickly assessed by visual analogue scales, verbal analogue scales, or verbal descriptor scales (list of ranked terms) (12). The most widely used pain measuring instrument is the visual analogue scale (VAS), but it reflects only the point in time when the pain assessment is performed. A combined determination of pain intensity and pain frequency appears to be more rational and has been used in recent studies on the effects of bisphosphonates on tumor bone disease (13,14). A further combination with a score for analgesic consumption and assessment of performance status deserves to be studied (11). Given the limitations and the costs of the traditional methods

Table 2 Frequency of Bone Pain at Diagnosis of Skeletal Metastases in Various Tumors

Tumor type	Number of patients with skeletal metastases	Number of patients with bone pain (%)
Myeloma	1715	1177 (69%)
Breast	364	259 (71%)
Lung	420	260 (62%)
Kidney	383	222 (58%)
Miscellaneous solid tumors[a]	226	157 (69%)
Prostate	532	224 (42%)

[a] Nasopharyngeal carcinoma, thyroid cancer, hepatoma, cervical cancer.
Source: Adapted from Ref. 11.

Table 3 Assessment of Response to Therapy of Metastatic Bone Disease

Traditional means
1. Radiographs: recalcification of lytic lesions
2. Bone scan: subjective assessment (reductions of "hot spots"); valid only after 6 months of therapy

Newer means
1. Pain relief and improved quality of life: need for reliable and simple scoring systems
2. Computed tomography and magnetic resonance imaging
3. Tumor markers
4. Biochemical markers of bone turnover: collagen cross-links, bone alkaline phosphatase, osteocalcin

for the follow-up of bone metastases, it is urgent that pain assessment and other new means for monitoring bone disease be further investigated (Table 3).

B. Bone Scintigraphy

The radionuclide bone scan remains the most widely used method for diagnosis and surveillance of bone metastatic involvement. Increased local uptake of technetium-labeled methylene diphosphonate (^{99m}Tc MDP) occurs in areas where blood flow or osteoblastic activity is increased. The bone scan is more sensitive than X-ray studies for the early detection of bone metastases. Compared to the measurement in adjacent bone, an increase in isotope uptake of 5% to 10% can be detected, whereas a loss of 30% to 50% of the bone mass is needed before being detectable by conventional X-ray techniques (15). The increased isotope uptake in pathological areas can be quantified by defining a ''region of interest,'' at which site uptake can be compared to a similar region of adjacent normal bone. This technique of ''quantitative bone scintigraphy'' could, in theory, much improve the clinical utility of the bone scan to assess the response to therapy, but several technical constraints and the poor reproducibility of the measurement account for why the method has not been widely used.

However, the relative lack of specificity of the bone scan is well known and at least one-third of solitary abnormalities detected in cancer patients are due to benign diseases (16). The appearance of one or two new abnormalities on the bone scan in cancer patients without known metastases is later confirmed to be of metastatic origin in only 11% and 24% of the cases, respectively (17). The presence of multiple focal hot spots is more specific for metastatic bone disease. Purely osteolytic lesions, as classically observed in multiple myeloma, constitute the most frequent cause of false-negative bone scans. It is rare for a bone scan to be completely normal with widespread myeloma, but radiography allows a better assessment of the extent of myeloma disease. At the other end of the spectrum, the so-called superscan can be observed in rare cases of diffuse metastatic bone disease: the increased bone to soft tissue ratio and the decreased radionuclide activity in the kidneys and the bladder avoid misclassifying such scans as normal. Whatever the sensitivity of the method used, it must be emphasized, however, that an earlier diagnosis of bone metastases by periodic bone scans, for example, will not prolong survival in patients with breast cancer, at least given the current therapeutic means (18).

Increasing scintigraphic activity does not always correspond to progressive disease. Besides the inability to quantitate these changes, which constitutes a major problem, one must be aware of the so-called flare phenomenon. This apparent worsening of the bone scan (increased scintigraphic activity in bone lesions or even the appearance of previously invisible lesions) represents the initial healing of osteolytic lesions and can thus be misinterpreted as evidence of tumor progression. A bone scan routinely performed after 3 months of therapy is frequently misleading and the appearance of new lesions is meaningful only after 6 months or more of therapy (19).

C. Radiographic Methods

Osteolytic lesions are most frequently observed, especially in cancers of the breast, the lung, the kidney, the thyroid, of the gastrointestinal tract and in melanomas. Osteoblastic lesions are typical of prostate cancer, but they can also be observed in breast cancer, in carcinoid tumors, and not rarely in lung cancers. Typically, however, most bone metastases are mixed, with an osteolytic/osteosclerotic pattern. In practice, the radionuclide bone scan may be used as a screening tool and as a guide for ordering appropriate radiographic studies.

Computed tomography (CT) is particularly useful to diagnose early metastatic involvement of bone when hot spots are detected on the radionuclide scan but corresponding radiographs are normal. This is particularly important for the spine where CT demonstrates metastatic involvement in up to 75% of cases (20). Other essential uses of CT include the diagnosis of epidural compression, the evaluation of the extent of a metastasis (e.g., in the femur), the visualization of areas difficult to image by conventional x-ray study (e.g., craniovertebral junction, sacrum, sternum), and the monitoring of a needle biopsy procedure. Magnetic resonance imaging (MRI) also appears to be able to demonstrate malignant infiltration of the thoracolumbar spine in patients who had abnormal bone scans with normal or nondiagnostic plain films (21). The MRI is more sensitive than CT for the diagnosis of bone marrow involvement and could thus be particularly useful to detect early cancellous bone lysis by tumor cells.

Bone biopsy is the theoretical "gold standard" for the diagnosis of bone metastases, but it should be reserved for difficult cases when a diagnostic doubt remains and it should be guided by CT scan. Table 3 lists the traditional and the newer methods used for the assessment of the response of skeletal metastases to therapy, which remains a daily challenge for the oncologist. According to Union Internationale Centre le Cancer (UICC) criteria, which are based on simple x-ray films, a complete response to antineoplastic therapy of a bone metastasis requires the reversal of abnormal radiographic findings, and a partial response requires some evidence of sclerosis within previously lytic lesions without any evidence of new osteolytic lesions. Response of an osteolytic lesion is seen as increasing sclerosis starting from the periphery toward the center of the lesion, whereas progression is indicated by an increase in the size of existing lesions or the appearance of new foci. However, development of new blastic lesions does not necessarily mean progression, because they can appear in previously lytic areas that were not detected on radiographs. An increase in the size of a blastic lesion can be due to the same phenomenon, signifying a favorable response to therapy, but it may also be due to tumor progression. Similarly, it is very difficult to differentiate between sclerotic metastases that progressively fade, signifying a favorable evolution, from the progressive appearance of lytic areas within the sclerotic bone, suggesting a failure of therapy. A concomitant bone scan helps in this respect, because increased isotope uptake or the appearance of new lesions usually indicates tumor progression. All the imaging techniques are actually aiming at detecting recalcification of lytic areas, which is evidently not an early phenomenon. Symptom evaluation and measurement of biochemical parameters should be more investigated for early assessment.

D. Serum Tumor Markers

The usefulness of tumor markers for diagnostic or assessment purposes is limited because of a general lack of sensitivity and specificity. Nevertheless, in prostate cancer, a serum prostate-specific antigen (PSA) concentration of $\leq$10 μg/L, in the absence of skeletal symptoms, seems to make unnecessary a staging radionuclide bone scan (22). The PSA levels also correlate with the extent of bone involvement (22).

Tumor markers are more frequently used to predict tumor recurrence before it can be detected by clinical or paraclinical means. This lead time varies between 4 and 48 months in breast cancer (23). In the series of Iwase et al., prediction of tumor recurrence, as defined by a 20% increase in tumor marker levels, was possible in 18 of 34 cases with a mean lead time of 4 months (24). In a large series of 1023 patients monitored by serial determinations of carcinoembryonic antigen (CEA), and of cancer antigen (CA) 15.3 in 533 of them, the lead time was 4 to 5 months with a sensitivity (i.e., increase in marker levels before diagnosis of recurrence) of 40%–41% (25).

More specifically for bone metastases, CA 15.3 can be assayed alongside a bone scan to confirm positive or negative results. Limited data indicate that the bone scan has more false-positive but fewer false-negative results than the CA 15.3 assay (26).

Serum tumor markers are a powerful means to obtain valuable information about the progression of malignant disease without causing any significant inconvenience to the patient and at low cost. Their main utility in metastatic disease is to distinguish between progression and nonprogression. They can thus indicate that a treatment is ineffective and should be stopped to prevent unnecessary toxicity. However, their use has been underevaluated for the assessment of bone metastases. The percentage of elevated CA 15.3 values in patients with bone metastases from breast cancer is around 69% (27). A comparison of several tumor markers in 22 patients with known bone metastases as compared to 30 patients without known metastases suggested that CA 15.3 was the most useful marker from a diagnostic point of view with an actual efficiency of 73% (28). It is difficult to conclude whether changes in CA 15.3 levels can accurately predict response of bone metastases to therapy. There are few studies but, more importantly, because changes in tumor mass are so difficult to assess in bone, it is not easy to accurately establish the predictive value of an assay for response of bone metastases. It was reported that the response to therapy is correctly indicated in approximately 70% of the patients with bone metastases and positive CA 15.3 values (29).

Tumor markers cannot distinguish between metastases to the skeleton or to other sites. Biochemical markers of bone turnover could thus complement their information.

E. Biochemical Markers of Bone Turnover

The main markers are listed in Table 4.

Total alkaline phosphatase (Alk Phos) is still the marker most often used in routine clinical practice. However, to exclude contribution from the liver and

Table 4 Biochemical Markers of Bone Turnover

Bone formation markers		Bone resorption markers
Total alkaline phosphatase	Urine:	Calcium
Bone alkaline phosphatase		Hydroxyproline
Osteocalcin (bone-GLA protein)		Collagen pyridinium cross-links (Pyr, DPyr, NTx, CTx)
Procollagen I extension peptides (PICP, PINP)	Serum:	CTx
		C telopeptide of collagen I (ICTP)

other organs, the measurement of the bone isoenzyme of Alk Phos (BAP) is required. Reproducible assays for direct BAP determination are commercially available with a cross-reactivity for liver Alk Phos between 7% and 13% (30). Osteocalcin (or bone-GLA protein; BGP) is a protein specifically made by the osteoblasts and its measurement appears to reflect more the late phases of bone formation. Assays for the peptides released during the extracellular processing of collagen, referred to as the procollagen carboxy-terminal propeptide (PICP) and the amino-terminal propeptide (PINP), might represent useful markers of bone formation because collagen is, by far, the most abundant organic component of bone matrix. However, preliminary results obtained with available assays appear to be disappointing, at least in patients with nonneoplastic diseases, and data in cancer patients are scanty.

The fasting urinary excretion of calcium and of hydroxyproline are classic markers of bone resorption. Urinary excretion of calcium is, however, not a true marker of bone resorption but rather reflects the net effects of bone formation and resorption. It lacks sensitivity and specificity. For example, in a recent series of 153 patients with bone metastases from various cancers, it has been shown that urinary calcium measurement could not differentiate patients with and without bone metastases (31). Hydroxyproline is derived from the various forms of collagen, is influenced by dietary gelatin intake, but remains a conventional and widely available parameter to assess bone resorption. When measured in fasting urinary samples, it is a reasonably valid estimate of the bone resorption rate (32).

New parameters of bone resorption have been recently introduced that will probably be more helpful because of their increased specificity for bone matrix destruction. The intermolecular cross-linking compounds of mature collagen, pyridinoline (Pyr) and deoxypyridinoline (DPyr), could be particularly well suited to monitor the breakdown of bone matrix by cancer cells, especially because they are independent from dietary intake. Their measurement requires, however, high-performance liquid chromatography (HPLC) assays and they already tend to be replaced by direct, commercially available, assays. Cross-links exist in both free (40%) and peptide-bound (60%) forms and enzyme-linked immunoassays (ELISAs) have been developed to measure the protein-bound cross-linking molecule at either the N-terminal part (NTx) or the C-terminal part (CrossLaps or CTx) and the free portions of both Pyr and DPyr. However, there are no extensive face-to-face comparisons between the classic HPLC assay and these direct telopeptide assays.

Bone markers could be useful for the diagnosis and for the monitoring of tumor bone disease.

1. *Diagnosis of Bone Metastases*

The diagnostic usefulness of biochemical markers for the diagnosis of bone metastases is limited so far. The BAP levels appear to better reflect bone metastatic involvement than total Alk Phos or BGP (33). The diagnostic sensitivity of BAP for the diagnosis of bone metastases could be superior to the one of CA 15.3, but more data are needed (34). Compared to total Alk Phos, the main advantage of measuring the bone isoenzyme appears to be a higher positive predictive value for the diagnosis of bone metastatic involvement resulting from a higher diagnostic specificity, as suggested by the study of Zaninotto et al. who found in 65 patients with metastatic prostate cancer specificities of 57% for total Alk Phos and 90% for BAP (35). Highest levels are seen in patients with multiple blastic metastases.

Limited data indicate that BAP could be superior to PSA as a marker for bone metastases and that the combination of both markers has a better diagnostic sensitivity than either marker alone (36). Compared to the upper limit of normal values, the sensitivity of BAP to detect bone metastases was 88% with a specificity of 100%. By combining BAP with PSA, the sensitivity increased to 96%.

Serum BGP levels vary widely in normocalcemic or hypercalcemic cancer patients with bone metastases. Moreover, increased BGP levels are not rarely observed in patients without bone metastases (37). In a series of 60 patients with recurring breast cancer, less than 50% of patients with bone involvement had elevated BGP levels (38). The BGP level is also less sensitive than PSA for the detection of bone metastases in prostate cancer (39).

Urinary calcium is a poor diagnostic marker for bone metastases but hydroxyproline is typically increased in patients with breast cancer metastatic to bone, although generally not at an early stage. In patients with bone metastases from breast cancer, hydroxyproline, Pyr, and DPyr are significantly increased compared to normal values but the proportion of increased values is higher for the cross-links. In a review of six studies, elevated levels of Pyr and DPyr have been found in 58%–88% and 60%–80%, respectively (40). Lipton et al. (41) have found elevated Pyr and DPyr in 66% of patients with bone metastatic involvement but also in 42% of the cancer patients without documented bone metastases. It remains unclear whether this surprisingly high percentage in patients without bone metastases reflects an excellent sensitivity or a poor specificity of these markers. Similar results have been reported by Pecherstorfer et al. (31) who found poor discrimination between patients with and without bone metastases. This could indicate subclinical involvement, or more likely a subclinical osteolysis in advanced cancer patients without overt bone metastases under the influence of parathyroid hormone-related protein (PTHrP) or other bone-mobilizing humoral tumor products. Part of the increase can also be due to artificial menopause induced by antineoplastic treatments. The diagnostic sensitivity of all markers is actually the highest for the collagen cross-links when measured by the classic HPLC method (42). Nevertheless, all available data indicate that even these markers are unsuitable for an early diagnosis of neoplastic skeletal involvement.

2. *Monitoring of Bone Metastases*

Biochemical markers of bone turnover could be useful for response assessment of bone metastases to antineoplastic therapy but also to monitor the effects of bisphosphonates. The biochemical markers of bone turnover have the potential to simplify and to improve the monitoring of metastatic bone disease, especially because it is notoriously difficult to rapidly evaluate the bone response to cancer therapy. There is, however, an urgent need for larger studies with the new markers.

Coleman et al. (43) have reported a decrease in urinary calcium 1 month after therapy in patients subsequently classified as "partial responders." In the same patients, these authors also showed a transient increase in BAP and in BGP levels (43). Limited studies indeed suggest that the BAP assay could be more useful for the follow-up of bone metastases than for an early diagnosis. Cooper et al. (44) have thus reported some patients in whom BAP levels increased before the elevation of specific tumor markers. The BAP level has been reported to correlate with the evolution of bone metastases and with bone pain (35). However, in prostate cancer, BAP and PSA changes were concordant in only 69% of 49 cases with metastatic disease (45). In short, the clinical potential of BAP for monitoring remains uncertain. The clinical interest of BGP for follow-up also remains unclear, because both decreasing and increasing serum levels are seen notably in patients with progressive multiple myeloma (46).

Limited data in breast cancer patients receiving endocrine treatment suggest that cross-links excretion increases during progressive disease but remains stable or decreases in the responders. A report of 37 well-evaluated patients suggests that NTx could be useful to reliably discriminate between patients progressing early during treatment from those with longer disease control (47). In patients with progressive disease, NTx levels steadily increased and the diagnostic efficiency of a 50% increase in NTx for identifying imminent progression was 78% (47).

In any case, even if much more work needs to be performed, biochemical markers of bone turnover appear to be better suited for the monitoring of bone metastases than for the detection of metastatic bone involvement.

Markers of bone resorption could also be especially useful to monitor the effects of bisphosphonate therapy. Markedly increased levels of Pyr and DPyr, and even more of NTx and CTx, have been found in hypercalcemic cancer patients with a reduction of 80%–90% after pamidronate therapy for NTx and CTx (32,48). In personal experience, parameters of bone matrix resorption markedly decreased after one pamidronate infusion. The decrease in CrossLaps was particularly impressive and larger than that of hydroxyproline or DPyr, indicating the potential of such new markers for delineating the optimal therapeutic schemes of bisphosphonates (Fig. 1) (42). Moreover, such markers could predict the anal-

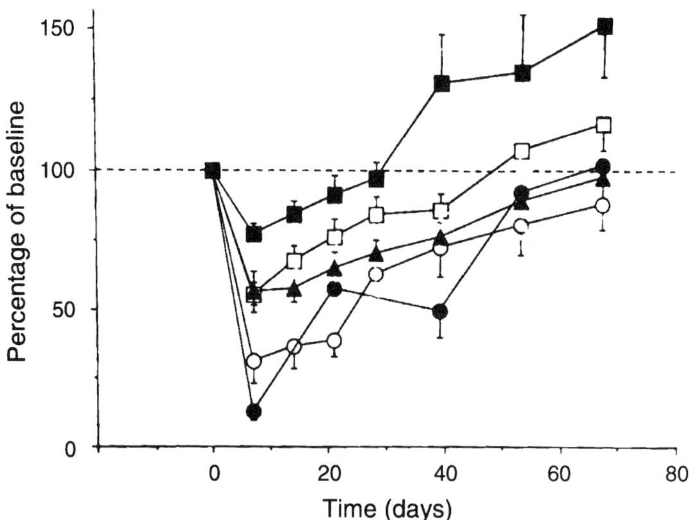

Figure 1 Relative changes in markers of bone turnover after a single pamidronate infusion. The figure indicates the changes in markers of bone resorption, either of the matrix (DPyr ▲, Pyr ■ CrossLaps ●, and hydroxyproline □) or of the mineral (uCa ○). (From Ref. 42.)

gesic response to bisphosphonate therapy. Vinholes et al. (49) showed that patients with baseline NTx levels ≥2 times the upper limit of normal responded infrequently to intravenous pamidronate (13%) compared to patients with a baseline NTx level <2 times the normal upper limit (63% response). In addition, the biochemical response was predictive of pain relief, because an analgesic response was much more frequent in the patients in whom NTx, CTx, or free DPyr remained in the normal range or returned to normal (53%–63%, dependent on the marker) than in the patients whose markers did not return to normal (0%–20% of clinical response). A high rate of bone resorption thus appears to be one of the factors underlying resistance to bisphosphonates and it is important to determine whether the frequency of skeletal events resulting from bone metastases is similarly influenced by the rate of bone resorption.

III. PATHOPHYSIOLOGY OF TUMOR-INDUCED OSTEOLYSIS

The osteotropism of breast and prostate neoplasms remains poorly understood. Preferential access of prostate cancer cells to the axial skeleton has been attributed to a passage through the vertebral venous plexus of Batson, which is a low-pressure, high-volume system of vertebral veins running adjacent to the spine. On the other hand, various properties of cancer cells, such as the production of proteolytic enzymes and the loss of specific cell adhesion molecules, can enhance their metastatic potential. More specifically, deposits into the skeleton can be due to the attraction of tumor cells by chemotactic factors released by the normal remodeling of bone matrix. These factors include fragments of type I collagen and of osteocalcin, and several growth factors (50,51).

Once breast cancer cells colonize the bone marrow, they are probably attracted to bone surfaces by the products of resorbing bone and destroy bone via osteoclast stimulation. The importance of direct osteolytic effects of metastatic cancer cells, including the effects of collagenases, is uncertain although possible in the late stages of tumor-induced osteolysis (TIO). They appear to induce osteoclast differentiation of hematopoietic stem cells or to activate mature osteoclasts already present in bone. An increased osteoclast number has been well demonstrated in the biopsies of 65 normocalcemic women with breast cancer and predominantly lytic bone metastases, whether in bone adjacent to tumor or directly in the invaded bone, indicating that increased bone resorption in metastatic breast cancer is mediated by the osteoclasts and not directly by the tumor cells themselves (52). Osteoblasts could also be important target cells for tumor secretory products. Thus, breast cancer cells have been seen to secrete factors that can inhibit the proliferation of osteoblast-like cells and of normal human osteoblasts, and to increase their second messenger response to osteolytic agents (53). Osteoblasts could thus keep the central role that they have in the regulation of osteoclast resorption activity.

The nature of the tumor-derived factors responsible for osteoclastic activation remains unknown, but recent data indicate that PTHrP could play an important role. PTHrP-like substances are expressed by about 60% of human breast cancers, and breast tumors that spread to the skeleton produce PTHrP more frequently than tumors metastasizing to non-osseous sites, but these data must be confirmed in larger series (54). PTHrP and other factors would stimulate osteoclastic bone resorption, leading to the release of bone matrix degradation products, which may be chemotactic for cancer cells. Tumor-associated factors, such as transforming growth factor (TGF)-α, could also increase the end-organ effects of PTHrP.

The following cascade of events and conditions can therefore be tentatively proposed for the genesis of TIO following invasion of bone by breast cancer. The propensity of breast cancer cells to metastasize and proliferate in bone could be explained by a ''seed and soil'' concept (50). Breast cancer cells (the ''seed'') appear to secrete factors, such as PTHrP, potentiating the development of metastases in the skeleton, which constitutes a fertile ''soil'' rich in cytokines and growth factors that stimulate breast cancer cells growth, including insulin-like growth factors (IGFs). Local production of PTHrP and of other osteolytic factors such as TGF-α by cancer cells in bone would stimulate osteoclastic bone resorption, partly through the osteoblasts, the proliferation of which may also be inhibited. Such factors probably induce osteoclast differentiation from hematopoietic stem cells and activate mature osteoclasts already present in bone. Increased osteoclast number and activity would then cause local foci of osteolysis, which could further stimulate cancer cell proliferation (50).

Prostate cancer cells stimulate osteoclast activity probably also through the osteoblasts. The precise nature of the responsible factor is unknown because various substances have been implicated, notably TGF-β, bone morphogenetic proteins, IGFs, urokinase, and PTHrP (55). Multiple myeloma is characterized by a marked increase in osteoclast activity and proliferation. This excessive resorption of bone could by itself play a contributory role to the growth of myeloma cells in bone, through the release of growth factors from resorbed bone matrix and secretion of interleukin-6 (IL-6) by the osteoclasts. Using established cell lines, it has been shown that through direct cell-to-cell contact, myeloma cells can down-regulate osteocalcin production but up-regulate IL-6 secretion, supporting the concept of the importance of the bone microenvironment in the genesis of myeloma-induced osteolysis (56).

The reasoning remains speculative, but the data summarized here indicate that bone-resorbing cells are a logical target for the treatment and perhaps the prevention of TIO.

IV. THERAPY OF BONE METASTASES

A. Traditional Therapy

An optimal use of analgesics and of physical and psychological nondrug methods constitutes an essential part of the therapeutic approach to the patient suffering from bone metastases (57). It is often claimed that nonsteroidal anti-inflammatory drugs (NSAIDs) are particularly effective for the pain of bone metastases, but a recent meta-analysis of the efficacy of NSAIDs for cancer pain could not substantiate this statement (58).

Table 5 lists the current medical therapeutic options for metastatic bone dis-

Table 5 Medical Treatment of Bone Metastases from Breast Cancer and Incidence of Bone Recalcification

Analgesics (0%)	
Antineoplastic therapy:	endocrine therapy (10%–20%)
	chemotherapy (10%–60%)
Antiosteolytic drugs:	calcitonin (unknown)
	gallium (unknown)
	bisphosphonates (up to 20%)

ease and estimations of the obtained bone recalcification rate. These figures must, however, be interpreted cautiously because the existing literature is difficult to evaluate. Many authors claim that bone metastases from breast cancer respond less well to endocrine manipulations or chemotherapy than visceral or skin metastases. As discussed previously, this could reflect biological differences but more probably reflects the relative insensitivity of current methods of assessment and patient selection. Refer to general textbooks or review articles for the hormonotherapy or chemotherapy of metastatic breast (59) or prostate cancer (60).

Even though the roles of orthopedic surgery and radiotherapy for bone metastases are not discussed in this chapter, it is important to stress that several current clinical attitudes are not based on properly conducted trials. For example, radiotherapy after orthopedic fixation of pathological fractures is generally considered to be standard therapy but the clinical benefit of this attitude has not been demonstrated. On the contrary, it seems that doses higher than 30 Gy are detrimental to bone consolidation (61). Prophylactic fixation of impending fractures is generally recommended for osteolytic lesions of at least 2.5 cm involving the femoral cortex or for any lesion having destroyed more than 50% of the cortex (61). These classic and empirical criteria have been challenged because biomechanical data indicate that they cannot accurately estimate the strength reductions or load-bearing capacity of bones such as the femur (62), but no more precise guidelines have been provided. Some authors consider that stress pain persisting despite radiotherapy is also an indication for prophylactic fixation (63). Although not evaluated prospectively, pain and performance status of these patients are often much improved after surgery and these patients are often good candidates for intensive rehabilitation programs, but maybe not if they have had a hypercalcemic episode that is actually a marker of advanced disease (64).

Concerning radiotherapy, experts state that ''the literature does not allow a definite conclusion concerning an optimal use of radiotherapy'' and that a single treatment giving doses of 5 to 8 Gy could be as effective as classic fractionated therapy in doses ranging from 25 to 40 Gy given over 2 to 4 weeks (65). Single doses or short courses over a week have similarly been advised (66). A prospective, randomized trial in 217 patients with breast cancer has convincingly shown the lack of difference for pain relief, as well as for radiological response, between a classic scheme (30 Gy in 10 fractions 5F/Wk) and a shorter, more convenient scheme (15 Gy in 3 fractions 2F/Wk) (67). In routine practice in advanced cancer patients, a single fraction of radiotherapy can be recommended for patients with localized bone pain and a limited life expectancy (68).

B. Radioisotopes

Strontium (^{89}Sr) is the bone-seeking isotope that has been most often studied. Its retention in the skeleton is a function of the degree of osteoblastic activity. In an open study including 229 men with prostate cancer treated with 40 μCi/kg, a favorable pain response was seen in approximately 80% of the patients (69). However, its efficacy has been evaluated in few prospective, randomized, double-blind trials. In 32 patients with prostate cancer metastatic to bone, there was a significant advantage for ^{89}Sr over placebo regarding pain palliation, but only a few patients had marked improvement (70). ^{89}Sr could also be useful as an adjuvant to localized external radiotherapy for bone metastases from prostate cancer. Porter et al. (71) have thus shown in a large-scale (n = 126), multicenter, randomized, placebo-controlled trial that ^{89}Sr given at the time of radiotherapy significantly reduces the appearance of new bone pain sites and the subsequent requirement for further radiotherapy. There was, however, no improvement in relief of pain at the index site or in survival, which was slightly reduced in the treated group ($p = 0.06$), perhaps because of increased hematological toxicity. On the other hand, a randomized study between ^{89}Sr and local or hemibody radiotherapy in 284 patients with metastatic prostate cancer has shown that ^{89}Sr has a comparable efficacy on the reduction of bone pain (about 30% of clear-cut improvement in all groups) and analgesic consumption, but that it is superior to conventional radiotherapy in delaying the progression of pain to new sites. Hematological toxicity is, however, more pronounced (72).

The most encouraging results have been obtained in patients with blastic bone metastases, and there is no rationale to prescribe it routinely in patients with TIO. Experts recommend to have at least two blastic metastatic deposits in bone, with pain in at least one location. A recent review of the literature indicates that as many as 80% of patients with painful osteoblastic bone metastases may experience some pain relief after ^{89}Sr and that at least 10% may become pain free. Injections can be repeated every 3 months with repeated palliative effect; repeated injections cause definite hematological toxicity but usually without serious consequences (73). However, this review also pointed to the need for larger clinical trials.

More recently, bone-seeking agents have been developed that combine radionuclides with more appropriate nuclear properties with various chelating agents to form metal complexes that localize preferentially to osteoblastic metastases after intravenous administration. Such isotopes include Samarium-153-EDTMP (=lexidronam) and rhenium-186 coupled to the bisphosphonate EHDP. A favorable pain response to Samarium-153-EDTMP has been observed in about 75% of the patients (74) and a double-blind placebo-controlled trial has been performed in 118 patients—68% had prostate cancer—comparing the doses of 0.5 or 1 mCi/kg to placebo. Patients who received 1 mCi/kg had significant reductions in pain during each of the first 4 weeks, as assessed by the patient and by the physician. There was a marked or complete relief by week 4 in 31% and two-thirds of the responders were still responding at week 16. There was also a significant reduction in opioid use, and bone marrow suppression was generally mild or moderate and reversible (75). The experience with ^{186}Re HEDP is more limited. Of all available isotopes, Sn-117m(4+) DTPA has the best combination of the percentage of bone uptake and bone-to-blood ratio (76), and human trials are underway.

C. Bisphosphonates

All bisphosphonates are characterized by a P-C-P bond in their structure, which promotes their binding to the mineralized bone matrix and their subsequent inhibitory effects on bone resorption. The rest of the bisphosphonate molecule varies according to the structural modification of the side chain, features that determine their relative potency, side effects, and probably also their precise mechanism of action. Bisphosphonates localize preferentially to sites of active bone formation and resorption. They can act directly on mature osteoclasts, decreasing their bone resorption activity, notably by lowering H^+ and Ca^{2+} extrusion and modifying the activity of various enzymes (77). Alternatively, recent findings suggest that osteoblasts, or at least those lining the bone surface, could also be essential target cells for bisphosphonates with secondary effects on the osteoclasts, probably by changing the secretion of an inhibitor of osteoclast recruitment (78). Moreover, bisphosphonates can induce osteoclast apoptosis and this effect could also be mediated through the osteoblasts. The relative importance of the osteoblast-dependent inhibitory activity of bisphosphonates compared with a direct inhibition of osteoclast activity or secretory capacity remains to be determined.

Regardless of the precise mechanisms of action, bisphosphonates have become the standard therapy for tumor-induced hypercalcemia (TIH) and a new form of medical therapy for bone metastases.

1. Tumor-Induced Hypercalcemia

Increased calcium release from bone is the main cause of hypercalcemia in cancer patients. Secretion of humoral and paracrine factors by the tumor cells stimulate osteoclast activity and proliferation. Collagen cross-links are indeed markedly increased in most patients with TIH (32). Moreover, osteoblast activity is often inhibited, leading to a characteristic uncoupling between bone resorption and bone formation. This causes a rapid increase in serum calcium, in contrast to the relatively stable levels of serum calcium seen in primary hyperparathyroidism in which bone coupling is usually maintained. Several studies have established the essential role of parathyroid hormone-related protein (PTHrP) in most types of cancer hypercalcemia (79).

Rehydration has generally mild and transient effects on calcium levels, effecting a median decrease of only 1 mg/dL (80), but it improves the clinical status and interrupts the vicious cycle of TIH by inhibiting the increased tubular reabsorption of calcium. Bisphosphonates have become the standard treatment for TIH and they have supplanted all other hypocalcemic drugs except corticosteroids for hypercalcemia of multiple myeloma. Clodronate and pamidronate are most often used.

A single-day 1500-mg infusion of clodronate is as efficient as daily 300-mg infusions for 5 days, and this therapy achieves normocalcemia in approximately 80% of cases (81). Pamidronate was first administered as daily 15-mg, 2-hour infusions that were repeated for up to 10 days. In a multicenter trial, 90% of 132 patients treated in this manner became normocalcemic after a mean interval of 3 to 4 days (82). Such a therapeutic scheme is, however, cumbersome and it was later shown that pamidronate could also be given as a single infusion over 2 to 24 hours. Large studies indicate that a dose of 90 mg achieves normocalcemia in more than 90% of patients (83). The response to lower doses of pamidronate will, however, be less in patients with humoral hypercalcemia of malignancy compared with patients with bone metastases as the importance of PTHrP becomes more evident (84).

The superiority of pamidronate over clodronate in patients with TIH has been demonstrated in a randomized trial involving 41 patients, not significantly so in terms of success rate, but quite evidently in the duration of normocalcemia. The median duration of action of clodronate was indeed 14 days compared with 28 days for pamidronate (85). Pamidronate is well tolerated, the only clinically detectable side effect being transient fever and a flu-like syndrome in about one-fourth of the cases. Oral clodronate is often prescribed after successful intravenous therapy, but the efficacy of this strategy has not been systematically examined.

Newer and more potent bisphosphonates, such as ibandronate and zoledronate, are currently being studied. A dose escalation trial with ibandronate has been conducted in 147 patients with calcium levels ≥3.0 mmol/L after rehydration, 125 of whom were evaluable for response. The success rate was 50% in the 2-mg group, which was significantly lower than the responses in the 4- and 6-mg dose groups, 76% and 77%, respectively, but the duration of response was not significantly influenced by the dose. A logistical regression analysis indicated that the response rate was also dependent on the initial calcium level and on the tumor type, because the group of patients with breast cancer or myeloma responded better than patients with other tumors. The drug was well tolerated, the only noticeable side effect being drug-induced fever in 13% of the cases (86).

2. *Metastatic Bone Pain*

External beam radiotherapy remains the treatment of choice for localized bone pain that does not respond to systemic treatment and simple analgesics. However, many patients have widespread, often previously irradiated sites of pain, and for these patients effective palliation of symptoms remains difficult. It has not been convincingly demonstrated that any of the currently available bisphosphonates administered orally can reduce metastatic bone pain. This was recently confirmed in a placebo-controlled study of oral clodronate in patients with progressing bone metastases, mainly from breast cancer (87). Compliance with the study protocol was also poor, mainly because of difficulty with swallowing the capsules.

When pooling the available data of several open phase II trials with repeated intravenous pamidronate infusions, a relief of bone pain appears to occur in one-half of the patients (51). Placebo-controlled studies have confirmed that both clodronate and pamidronate given intravenously can exert significant and rapid analgesic effects (88). The optimal dose needs to be defined, especially because it is probably a function of the disease stage. Preliminary data indicate that modern markers of bone matrix resorption, such as NTx, correlate with the analgesic effects of pamidronate and follow a similar time course (49). It remains to be seen whether higher doses of pamidronate or newer more potent compounds would then be more useful. A dose of 60 to 90 mg pamidronate every 3 to 4 weeks can, for the time being, be recommended for palliation of bone pain. Intravenous clodronate also relieves pain but its shorter duration of action would dictate a rather impractical regimen of administration, probably every 10 to 14 days.

Regular pamidronate infusions can also induce a recalcification or sclerosis of osteolytic lesions, achieving a partial objective response by conventional UICC criteria in approximately one-fifth of the patients (51). This phenomenon of recalcification appears to be similar to what can be achieved by conventional hormonotherapy or chemotherapy. Similarly, an increase in the objective bone response rate to chemotherapy has been shown in a large randomized clinical trial in which patients received chemotherapy plus pamidronate as compared to chemotherapy alone, 33% versus 18%, respectively (14).

3. Reduction of the Skeletal Morbidity Rate in Breast Cancer Metastatic to Bone

The combination of occasional poor tolerance from gastrointestinal side effects and the low absorption of oral bisphosphonates implying the need for high doses is still an obstacle to their development as oral drugs in cancer patients. However, two large-scale studies in patients with breast cancer metastatic to the skeleton, one with clodronate and one with pamidronate, indicate that the administration of oral bisphosphonates until death can nevertheless reduce the frequency of morbid skeletal events. The clodronate study was randomized, double-blind, placebo-controlled, and included 173 patients with breast cancer metastatic to bone (89). In the clodronate-treated group (1600 mg/d), there was a significant reduction in the incidence of hypercalcemic episodes, in the number of vertebral fractures, and in the rate of vertebral deformity. The combined rate of all morbid skeletal events was reduced by 28% (Fig. 2).

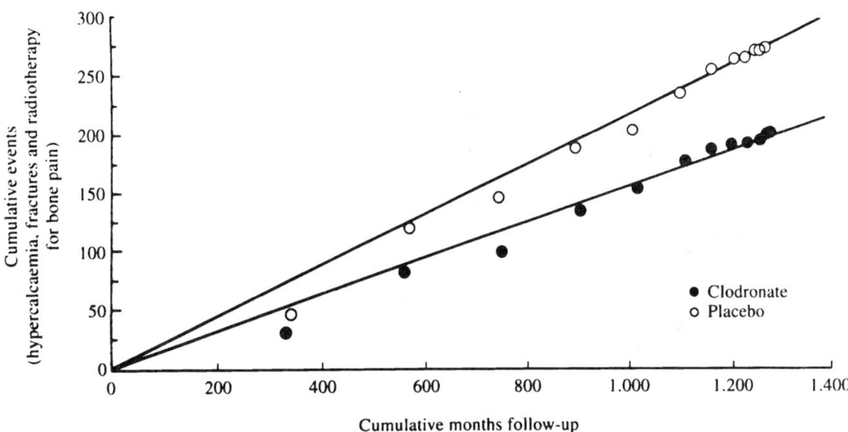

Figure 2 Cumulative skeletal events (episodes of hypercalcemia, fractures, and radiotherapy treatments for bone-related pain) in patients receiving clodronate (●) compared with placebo (○). The reduction in cumulative skeletal events for clodronate is statistically significant ($p < 0.001$). Reproduced from Ref. 89.

Three randomized studies of regular intravenous pamidronate infusions have recently been completed (90–92). There are no similar trials with clodronate, and trials with newer bisphosphonates are ongoing.

Conte and collaborators (90) randomized almost 300 patients in a multicenter open trial comparing infusions of 45 mg of pamidronate every 3 weeks plus standard first line chemotherapy or chemotherapy alone in patients with breast cancer and bone metastases. The study was stopped when the disease progressed in the skeleton. In the 224 assessable patients, there was an increase of 48% in the median time to progression in bone. Improvement in bone pain was also seen more often in the pamidronate group, but the decrease in other skeletal-related events was not significant (90). These somewhat disappointing results can be explained by the high activity of first line chemotherapy in breast cancer, by the premature cessation of bisphosphonate administration, and by the choice of too low of a dose of pamidronate. The results of double-blind, randomized, placebo-controlled trials comparing 90 mg pamidronate infusions every 4 weeks to placebo infusions for 1 or 2 years in addition to chemotherapy or hormonotherapy in large series of breast cancer patients with at least two lytic bone metastases establish that such drugs can dramatically reduce the skeletal morbidity rate. The results were particularly impressive in the chemotherapy trial that included 382 patients (14,92). Skeletal-related events were defined as pathological fractures, spinal cord compression, vertebral collapse, radiation for pain relief or for treat-

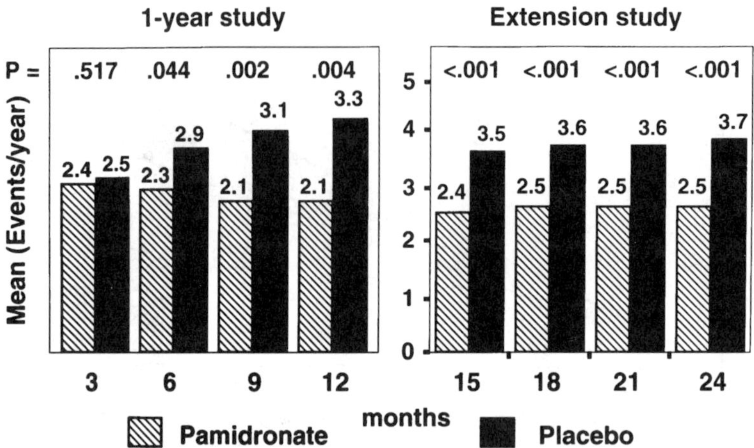

Figure 3 Skeletal morbidity rate (mean number of skeletal-related events per year) in 382 women with metastatic breast cancer and lytic bone lesions treated by chemotherapy and randomly assigned to receive either 90 mg pamidronate or placebo infusions every 3 to 4 weeks for up to 2 years in a double-blind manner. (Derived from Refs. 14 and 92.)

ment of pathological fractures or of spinal cord compression, or surgery to bone. The median time to the occurrence of the first skeletal-related event was increased by 47% in the pamidronate group (13 versus 7 months). There was a significant reduction in the proportion of patients having any skeletal-related event (43% versus 56%), in the number of nonvertebral pathological fractures (by 60%), and in the proportion of patients having radiation to bone (by 45%) or surgery on bone (by 52%) (14). The follow-up of this trial indicates that the mean skeletal morbidity rate (number of skeletal-related events per year) has been 2.1 in the pamidronate group compared to 3.3 in the placebo group for up to 2 years ($p <$ 0.005) (Fig. 3). The mean skeletal morbidity rates in the hormone therapy trial were 2.4 and 3.6 ($p < 0.01$) in the pamidronate and placebo groups, respectively (91). There were also favorable effects on the quality of life and, at the end of the evaluation, there was a significant decrease in the pain score and in the analgesic requirement in both trials.

The optimal therapeutic schedule for pamidronate is not known with certainty, but monthly infusions are clearly effective, and this schedule, although not ideal, is compatible with palliation of advanced malignancy. Criteria for when in the course of metastatic bone disease bisphosphonates should be started and stopped need to be determined. Because bisphosphonates are providing supportive care, reducing the rate of skeletal morbidity (but evidently not abolishing it), the criteria for stopping their administration have to be different from those used for classic antineoplastic drugs and they should not necessarily be stopped when metastatic bone disease is progressing. However, criteria are lacking to determine whether and how long an individual patient benefits from their administration, and the decision to continue or stop bisphosphonate therapy or increase dosage remains essentially empirical and based on personal experience. New biochemical markers of bone resorption might help identify those patients continuing to benefit from therapy.

The results obtained with the intravenous route are more impressive than the ones obtained with oral compounds. However, the choice can depend on individual circumstances. For example, the oral route is preferred for many patients on hormonal therapy, especially if the bone disease is not rapidly evolving. The cost-to-benefit ratio of such an early and prolonged intervention is unknown and will be greatly influenced by local factors. For an aggressive osteolytic disease, the choice must be the intravenous route.

The increased potency of newer agents such as ibandronate and zoledronate will allow the use of much lower doses and, of more clinical importance, their administration as rapid intravenous injections rather than slow infusions. Several studies with repeated injections or infusions of newer bisphosphonates in patients with bone metastases have just been completed. The development of oral, potent, and well-tolerated compounds should also allow more convenient therapeutic schemes. Newer bisphosphonates will perhaps also allow more efficient therapeutic schedules, in that limited data indicate that the effects of bisphosphonates on the complications of bone metastases are a function of the degree of the inhibition of bone resorption.

D. Prevention of Bone Metastases in Breast Cancer

Another potential role for bisphosphonate treatment is the prevention or at least a delay in the development of bone metastases. Trials in patients with established bone metastases suggest that long-term administration of bisphosphonates could indeed fulfill this major objective and studies in animal models of bone metastases support this exciting concept.

A secondary prevention double-blind trial continued for 3 years after extraskeletal recurrence in 133 women with breast cancer has shown a significant reduction in the number of bone metastases in the clodronate group (93). In a randomized open trial involving 302 patients with primary breast cancer and tumor cells in the bone marrow, which is an adverse risk factor for the development of metastases, it was shown that 1600 mg clodronate daily for 2 years reduced the number of bone as well as nonbone metastases by about 50% after a median follow-up of 36 months (94). Survival was also significantly prolonged. Despite the enthusiasm that these data generate, one must remain cautious and confirmation is awaited. It will be important to determine the patients at high risk of development of bone metastases before recommending a general primary preventive use of bisphosphonates. Classic prognostic factors, such as tumor size, axillary node involvement, receptor status, but also PTHrP expression by the tumor cells and selected investigational prognostic markers will probably be relevant.

Preventive therapy with bisphosphonates could also have the additional beneficial effect of preventing postmenopausal osteoporosis in a population of women for whom estrogen replacement therapy is generally avoided.

E. Multiple Myeloma

Multiple myeloma is typically characterized by a marked increase in osteoclast activity and proliferation, and an extensive osteolytic process is generally the hallmark of the disease. Moreover, this excessive resorption of bone could itself, notably through the release of interleukin-6 by the osteoclasts, play a contributory role to the growth of myeloma cells in bone. Recently performed trials support the notion that bisphosphonates are of great benefit for the treatment of multiple myeloma.

In a randomized, placebo-controlled trial in 548 patients, the efficacy of 1600 mg of clodronate given daily at the time of diagnosis was evaluated. The reduction in skeletal complication rate was not observed initially, but became apparent when the effects of chemotherapy wore off. At the time of disease progression, there were fewer patients with increased back pain or deterioration in performance status and less new vertebral fractures after the first year (95). The efficacy of regular pamidronate infusions in myeloma has also been demonstrated in a double-blind, placebo-controlled trial. The study was made up of 392 patients with at least one osteolytic lesion who received either 90 mg pamidronate or placebo infusions monthly for 9 months in addition to their antimyeloma chemotherapy regimen. The proportion of patients in whom a skeletal-related event developed was significantly smaller in the pamidronate than in the placebo group, 24% versus 41%. The mean morbidity rate was 2.1 in the placebo group versus 1.1 in the pamidronate group ($p < 0.02$). Quality of life score, performance status, pain score, incidence of pathological fractures, and the need for radiotherapy were all favorably affected by bisphosphonate therapy (13). These effects were maintained during a 1-year extension period of the trial, and follow-up data indicate a prolongation of survival in patients receiving second or subsequent lines of chemotherapy combined with pamidronate (96).

These placebo-controlled trials indicate that bisphosphonates in addition to chemotherapy are superior to chemotherapy alone for multiple myeloma. Confirmatory trials would be useful and cost-benefit analyses should be performed, but it can probably already be stated that bisphosphonate treatment should be considered for all patients with multiple myeloma and at least one osteolytic lesion. Experts state that bisphosphonates should be used early, probably in all patients, not only because of their beneficial skeletal effects but also because they may slow tumor growth (97). However, the optimal duration and doses of treatment are unknown.

F. Other Cancers

Although skeletal metastases from prostate cancer are typically osteoblastic, histomorphometric and biochemical studies have shown unequivocal evidence for an increase in bone resorption. The analgesic effect of bisphosphonates seems to parallel the inhibition of bone resorption. However, there are no large-scale, double-blind trials and there are, as yet, too few systematic data to advise the regular use of bisphosphonates in metastatic prostate cancer. There are few data on the use of bisphosphonates in patients with osteolytic bone metastases from other cancers, and no recommendations can be made at the present time.

REFERENCES

1. Galasko CSB. Skeletal metastases. Clin Orthop Rel Res 1986; 210:18–30.
2. Coleman RE, Rubens RD. The clinical course of bone metastases from breast cancer. Br J Cancer 1987; 55:61–66.
3. Kamby C, Vejborg I, Daugaard S, Guldhammer B, Dirksen H, Rossing N, Mouridsen HT. Clinical and radiologic characteristics of bone metastases in breast cancer. Cancer 1987; 60:2524–2531.
4. Bhardwaj S, Holland JF. Chemotherapy of metastatic cancer in bone. Clin Orthop Rel Res 1982; 169:28–37.
5. Elte JWF, Bijvoet OLM, Cleton FJ, van Oosterom A, Sleeboom HP. Osteolytic bone metastases in breast carcinoma: pathogenesis, morbidity and bisphosphonate treatment. Eur J Cancer Clin Oncol 1986; 22:493–500.
6. Mercadante S. Malignant bone pain: pathophysiology and treatment. Pain 1997; 69: 1–18.
7. Sherry MM, Greco FA, Johnson DH, Hainsworth JD. Metastatic breast cancer confined to the skeletal system. An indolent disease. Am J Med 1986; 81:381–386.
8. Yamashita K, Koyama H, Inaji H. Prognostic significance of bone metastasis from breast cancer. Clin Orthop Rel Res 1995; 312:89–94.
9. Yamashita K, Denno K, Ueda T, Komatsubara Y, Kotake T, Usami M, Maeda O, Nakano SI, Hasegawa Y. Prognostic significance of bone metastases in patients with metastatic prostate cancer. Cancer 1993; 71:1297–1302.
10. Body JJ. Metastatic bone disease: clinical and therapeutic aspects. Bone 1992; 13: S57–S62.
11. Pecherstorfer M, Vesely M. Diagnosis and monitoring of bone metastases. In:

Body JJ, ed. Tumor Bone Diseases and Osteoporosis in Cancer Patients. New York: Marcel Dekker. In press.
12. Grossman SA, Sheidler VR, McGuire DB, Geer C, Santor D, Piantadosi S. A comparison of the Hopkins Pain Rating Instrument with standard visual analogue and verbal descriptor scales in patients with cancer pain. J Pain Symptom Manage 1992; 7:196–203.
13. Berenson JR, Lichtenstein A, Porter L, Dimopoulos MA, Bordoni R, George S, Lipton A, Keller A, Ballester O, Kovacs MJ, Blacklock HA, Bell R, Simeone J, Reitsma DJ, Heffernan M, Seaman J, Knight RD. Efficacy of pamidronate in reducing skeletal events in patients with advanced multiple myeloma. N Engl J Med 1996; 334:488–493.
14. Hortobagyi GN, Theriault RL, Porter L, Blayney D, Lipton A, Sinoff C, Wheeler H, Simeone JF, Seaman J, Knight RD. Efficacy of pamidronate in reducing skeletal complications in patients with breast cancer and lytic bone metastases. N Engl J Med 1996; 335:1785–1791.
15. Thrall JH, Ellis BI. Skeletal metastases. Radiol Clin North Am 1987; 25:1155–1170.
16. Gold RI, Seeger LL, Bassett LW, Steckel RJ. An integrated approach to the evaluation of metastatic bone disease. Radiol Clin North Am 1990; 28:471–483.
17. Jacobson AF, Cronin EB, Stomper PC, Kaplan WD. Bone scans with one or two new abnormalities in cancer patients with no known metastases: frequency and serial scintigraphic behavior of benign and malignant lesions. Radiology 1990; 175:229–232.
18. Rosselli del Turco M, Palli D, Cariddi A, Ciatto S, Pacini P, Distante V, for the National Research Council Project on Breast Cancer Follow-up. Intensive diagnostic follow-up after treatment of primary breast cancer. JAMA 1994; 271:1593–1597.
19. Coleman RE, Mashiter G, Fogelman I, Rubens RD. Osteocalcin: a marker of metastatic bone disease. Eur J Cancer 1988; 24:1211–1217.
20. Redmond J III, Spring DB, Munderloh SH, George CB, Mansour RP, Volk SA. Spinal computed tomography scanning in the evaluation of metastatic disease. Cancer 1984; 54:253–258.
21. Jones AL, Williams MP, Powles TJ, Oliff JFC, Hardy JR, Cherryman G, Husband J. Magnetic resonance imaging in the detection of skeletal metastases in patients with breast cancer. Br J Cancer 1990; 62:296–298.
22. Haukaas S, Roervik J, Halvorsen OJ, Foelling M. When is bone scintigraphy necessary in the assessment of newly diagnosed, untreated prostate cancer? Br J Urol 1997; 79:770–776.
23. Bombardieri E, Pizzichetta M, Veronesi P, Seregni E, Bogni A, Maffioli L, Jotti GS, Bassetto MA, Zurrida S, Costa A. CA 15.3 determination in patients with breast cancer: clinical utility for the detection of distant metastases. Eur J Cancer 1992; 29:144–146.
24. Iwase H, Kobayashi S, Itoh Y, Fukuoka H, Kuzushima T, Iwata H, Yamashita T, Kaitoh A, Ithoh K, Masaoka A. Evaluation of serum tumor markers in patients with advanced or recurrent breast cancer. Br Cancer Res Treat 1994; 33:83–88.
25. Molina R, Zanon G, Filella X, Moreno F, Jo J, Daniels M, Latre ML, Gimenez N, Pahisa J, Velasco M, Ballesta AM. Use of serial carcinoembryonic antigen and CA

15.3 assays in detecting relapses in breast cancer patients. Br Cancer Res Treat 1995; 36:41–48.
26. Tomlinson IPM, Whyman A, Barrett JA, Kremer JK. Tumour marker CA 15-3: possible uses in the routine management of breast cancer. Eur J Cancer 1995; 31A: 899–902.
27. Crippa F, Bombardieri E, Seregni E, Castellani MR, Gasparini M, Maffioli L, Pizzichetta M, Buraggi GL. Single determination of CA 15.3 and bone scintigraphy in the diagnosis of skeletal metastases of breast cancer. J Nucl Biol Med 1992; 36:52–55.
28. Aydiner A, Topuz E, Disci R, Yasasever V, Dincer M, Dincol K, Bilge N. Serum tumor markers for detection of bone metastasis in breast cancer patients. Acta Oncol 1994; 33:181–186.
29. Safi F, Kohler I, Rottinger E, Beger H. The value of the tumor marker CA 15-3 in diagnosing and monitoring breast cancer. A comparative study with carcinoembryonic antigen. Cancer 1991; 68:574–582.
30. Price CP, Milligan TP, Darte C. Direct comparison of performance characteristics of two immunoassays for bone isoform of alkaline phosphatase in serum. Clin Chem 1997; 43:2052–2057.
31. Pecherstorfer M, Zimmer-Roth I, Schilling T, Woitge HW, Schmidt H, Baumgartner G, Thiebaud D, Ludwig H, Seibel MJ. The diagnostic value of urinary pyridinium cross-links of collagen, serum total alkaline phosphatase and urinary calcium excretion in neoplastic bone disease. J Clin Endocrinol Metab 1995; 80:97–103.
32. Body JJ, Delmas PD. Urinary pyridinium cross-links as markers of bone resorption in tumor-associated hypercalcemia. J Clin Endocrinol Metab 1992; 74:471–475.
33. Body JJ, Dumon JC, Blocklet D, Darte C. The bone isoenzyme of alkaline phosphatase in hypercalcaemic patients. Eur J Cancer 1997; 33:1578–1582.
34. Marchei P, Santini D, Bianco V, Chiodini S, Reale MG, Simeoni F, Marchei GG, Vecchione A. Serum ostase in the follow-up of breast cancer patients. Anticancer Res 1995; 15:2217–2222.
35. Zaninotto M, Secchiero S, Rubin D. Serum bone alkaline phosphatase in the follow-up of skeletal metastases. Anticancer Res 1995; 15:2223–2228.
36. Wolff JM, Ittel T, Boeckmann W, Reinike T, Habib FK, Jakse G. Skeletal alkaline phosphatase in the metastatic workup of patients with prostate cancer. Eur Urol 1996; 30:302–306.
37. Body JJ, Cleeren A, Pot M, Borkowski A. Serum osteocalcin (BGP) in tumor-associated hypercalcemia. J Bone Miner Res 1986; 1:523–527.
38. Kamby C, Egsmose C, Sölétormos G, Dombernowsky P. The diagnostic and prognostic value of serum bone GLA protein (osteocalcin) in patients with recurrent breast cancer. Scand J Clin Lab Invest 1993; 53:439–446.
39. Shih WJ, Wierzbinski B, Collins J, Magoun S, Chen IW, Ryo UY. Serum osteocalcin measurements in prostate carcinoma patients with skeletal deposits shown by bone scintigram: comparison with serum PSA/PAP measurements. J Nucl Med 1990; 31: 1486–1489.
40. Vinholes J, Coleman R, Eastell R. Effects of bone metastases on bone metabolism: implications for diagnosis, imaging and assessment of response to cancer treatment. Cancer Treat Rev 1996; 22:289–331.

41. Lipton A, Demers L, Daniloff Y, Curley E, Hamilton C, Harvey H, Witters L, Seaman J, Van der Giessen R, Seyedin S. Increased urinary excretion of pyridinium cross-links in cancer patients. Clin Chem 1993; 39:614–618.
42. Body JJ, Dumon JC, Gineyts E, Delmas PD. Comparative evaluation of markers of bone resorption in patients with breast cancer-induced osteolysis before and after bisphosphonate therapy. Br J Cancer 1997; 75:408–412.
43. Coleman RE, Whitaker KD, Moss DW, Mashiter G, Fogelman I, Rubens RD. Biochemical monitoring predicts response in bone to systemic treatment. Br J Cancer 1988; 58:205–210.
44. Cooper EH, Forbes MA, Hancock AK, Parker D, Laurence V. Serum bone alkaline phosphatase and CA 549 in breast cancer with bone metastases. Biomed Pharmacother 1992; 46:31–36.
45. Cooper EH, Whelan P, Purves D. Bone alkaline phosphatase and prostate-specific antigen in the monitoring of prostate cancer. Prostate 1994; 25:236–242.
46. Williams AT, Shearer MJ, Oyeyi J, Aitchison RG, Newland AC, Schey SA. Serum osteocalcin in the management of myeloma. Eur J Cancer 1992; 29A:140–142.
47. Coleman RE. Monitoring of bone metastases. Eur J Cancer 1998; 34:252–259.
48. Vinholes J, Guo CY, Purohit OP, Eastell R, Coleman R. Evaluation of new bone resorption markers in a randomized comparison of pamidronate or clodronate for hypercalcemia of malignancy. J Clin Oncol 1997; 15:131–138.
49. Vinholes JJF, Purohit OP, Abbey ME, Eastell R, Coleman RE. Relationships between biochemical and symptomatic response in a double-blind randomised trial of pamidronate for metastatic bone disease. Ann Oncol 1997; 8:1243–1250.
50. Mundy GR. Mechanisms of bone metastasis. Cancer 1997; 80:1546–1556.
51. Body JJ, Coleman RE, Piccart M. Use of bisphosphonates in cancer patients. Cancer Treat Rev 1996; 22:265–287.
52. Taube T, Elomaa I, Blomqvist C, Beneton MNC, Kanis JA. Histomorphometric evidence for osteoclast-mediated bone resorption in metastatic breast cancer. Bone 1994; 15:161–166.
53. Siwek B, Lacroix M, de Pollak C, Marie P, Body JJ. Secretory products of breast cancer cells affect human osteoblastic cells: partial characterization of active factors. J Bone Miner Res 1997; 12:552–560.
54. Vargas SJ, Gillespie MT, Powell GJ, Southby J, Danks JA, Moseley JM, Martin TJ. Localization of parathyroid hormone-related protein mRNA expression in breast cancer and metastatic lesions by in situ hybridization. J Bone Miner Res 1992; 7:971–979.
55. Goltzman D, Rabbani SA. Pathogenesis of osteoblastic metastases. In: Body JJ, ed. Tumor Bone Diseases and Osteoporosis in Cancer Patients. New York: Marcel Dekker. In press.
56. Barillé S, Collette M, Bataille R, Amiot M. Myeloma cells upregulate interleukin-6 secretion in osteoblastic cells through cell-to-cell contact but downregulate osteocalcin. Blood 1995; 86:3151–3159.
57. Twycross RG. Management of pain in skeletal metastases. Clin Orthop Rel Res 1995; 312:187–196.
58. Eisenberg E, Berkey CS, Carr DB, Mosteller F, Chalmers TC. Efficacy and safety

of nonsteroidal antiinflammatory drugs for cancer pain: a meta-analysis. J Clin Oncol 1994; 12:2756–2765.
59. Hayes DF, Henderson IC, Shapiro CL. Treatment of metastatic breast cancer: present and future prospects. Semin Oncol 1995; 22:5–19.
60. Small EJ, Vogelzang NJ. Second line hormonal therapy for advanced prostate cancer: a shifting paradigm. J Clin Oncol 1997; 15:382–388.
61. Gainor BJ, Buchert P. Fracture healing in metastatic bone disease. Clin Orthop Rel Res 1983; 178:297–302.
62. Hipp JA, Springfield DS, Hayes WC. Predicting pathologic fracture risk in the management of metastatic bone defects. Clin Orthop Rel Res 1995; 312:120–135.
63. Aaron AD. The management of cancer metastatic to bone. JAMA 1994; 272:1206–1209.
64. Bunting RW. Rehabilitation of cancer patients with skeletal metastases Clin Orthop Rel Res 1995; 312:197–200.
65. Poulsen HS, Nielsen OS, Klee M, Rørth M. Palliative irradiation of bone metastases. Cancer Treat Rev 1989; 16:41–48.
66. Hoskin PJ. Radiotherapy in the management of bone pain. Clin Orthop Rel Res 1995; 312:105–119.
67. Rasmusson B, Vejborg I, Jensen AB, Andersson M, Banning AM, Hoffmann T, Pfeiffer P, Nielsen HK, Sjøgren P. Irradiation of bone metastases in breast cancer patients: a randomized study with 1 year follow-up. Radiother Oncol 1995; 34:179–184.
68. Bates T, Yarnold JR, Blitzer P, Nelson OS, Rubin P, Maher J. Bone metastasis consensus statement. Int J Radiation Oncol Biol Phys 1992; 23:215–216.
69. Robinson RG, Preston DF, Spicer JA, Baxter KG. Radionuclide therapy of intractable bone pain: emphasis on strontium-89. Semin Nucl Med 1992; 22:28–32.
70. Lewington VJ, McEwan AJ, Ackery DM, Bayly RJ, Keeling DH, Macleod PM, Porter AT, Zivanovic MA. A prospective randomised double blind crossover study to examine the efficacy of strontium-89 in pain palliation in patients with advanced prostate cancer metastatic to bone. Eur J Cancer 1991; 27:954–958.
71. Porter AT, McEwan AJB, Powe JE, Reid R, McGowan DG, Lukka H, Sathyanarayana JR, Yakemchuk VN, Thomas GM, Erlich LE, Crook J, Gulenchyn KY, Hong KE, Wesolowski C, Yardley J. Results of a randomized phase-III trial to evaluate the efficacy of strontium-89 adjuvant to local field external beam irradiation in the management of endocrine resistant metastatic prostate cancer. Int J Radiation Oncol Biol Phys 1993; 25:805–813.
72. Quilty PM, Kirk D, Bolger JJ, Dearnaley DP, Lewington VJ, Mason MD, Reed NSE, Russell JM, Yardley J. A comparison of the palliative effects of strontium-89 and external beam radiotherapy in metastatic prostate cancer. Radiother Oncol 1994; 31:33–40.
73. Robinson RG, Preston DF, Schiefelbein M, Baxter KG. Strontium 89 therapy for the palliation of pain due to osseous metastases. JAMA 1995; 274:420–424.
74. Collins C, Eary JF, Donaldson G, Vernon C, Bush NE, Petersdorf S, Livingston RB, Gordon EE, Chapman CR, Appelbaum FR. Samarium-153-EDTMP in bone metastases of hormone refractory prostate carcinoma: a phase I/II trial. J Nucl Med 1993; 34:1839–1844.

75. Serafini AN, Houston SJ, Resche I, Quick DP, Grund FM, Ell PJ, Bertrand A, Ahmann FR, Orihuela E, Reid RH, Lerski RA, Collier DB, McKillop JH, Purnell GL, Pecking AP, Thomas FD, Harrison KA. Palliation of pain associated with metastatic bone cancer using samarium-153 lexidronam: a double-blind placebo-controlled clinical trial. J Clin Oncol 1998; 16:1547–1581.
76. Atkins HL, Mausner LF, Srivastava SC, Meinken GE, Straub RF, Cabahug CJ, Weber DA, Wong CTC, Sacker DF, Madajewicz S, Park TL, Meek AG. Biodistribution of Sn-117m(4+) DTPA for palliative therapy of painful osseous metastases. Radiology 1993; 186:279–283.
77. Zimolo Z, Wesolowski G, Rodan GA. Acid extrusion is induced by osteoclast attachment to bone. Inhibition by alendronate and calcitonin. J Clin Invest 1995; 96:2277–2283.
78. Vitté C, Fleisch H, Guenther HL. Bisphosphonates induce osteoblasts to secrete an inhibitor of osteoclast-mediated resorption. Endocrinology 1996; 137:2324–2333.
79. Grill V, Ho P, Body JJ, Johanson N, Lee SC, Kukreja SC, Moseley JM, Martin TJ. Parathyroid hormone-related protein: elevated levels in both humoral hypercalcemia of malignancy and hypercalcemia complicating metastatic breast cancer. J Clin Endocrinol Metab 1991; 73:1309–1315.
80. Singer FR, Ritch PS, Lad TE, Ringenberg QS, Schiller JH, Recker RR, Ryzen E. Treatment of hypercalcemia of malignancy with intravenous etidronate. A controlled, multicenter study. Arch Intern Med 1991; 151:471–476.
81. O'Rourke NP, McCloskey EV, Vasikaran S, Eyres K, Fern D, Kanis JA. Effective treatment of malignant hypercalcaemia with a single intravenous infusion of clodronate. Br J Cancer 1993; 67:560–563.
82. Harinck HIJ, Bijvoet OLM, Plantingh AST, Body JJ, Elte JWF, Sleeboom HP; Wildiers J, Neijt JP. Role of bone and kidney in tumor-induced hypercalcemia and its treatment with bisphosphonate and sodium chloride. Am J Med 1993; 82:1133–1142.
83. Body JJ, Dumon JC. Treatment of tumor-induced hypercalcaemia with the bisphosphonate pamidronate: dose-response relationship and influence of the tumour type. Ann Oncol 1994; 5:359–363.
84. Walls J, Ratcliffe WA, Howell A, Bundred NJ. Response to intravenous bisphosphonate therapy in hypercalcaemic patients with and without bone metastases: the role of parathyroid hormone-related protein. Br J Cancer 1994; 70:169–172.
85. Purohit OP, Radstone CR, Anthony C, Kanis JA, Coleman RE. A randomised double-blind comparison of intravenous pamidronate and clodronate in the hypercalcaemia of malignancy. Br J Cancer 1995; 72:1289–1293.
86. Ralston SH, Thiébaud D, Herrmann Z, Steinhauer EU, Thurlimann B, Walls J, Lichinitser MR, Rizzoli R, Hagberg H, Huss HJ, Tubiana-Hulin M, Body JJ. Dose-response study of ibandronate in treatment of cancer-associated hypercalcaemia. Br J Cancer 1997; 75:295–300.
87. Robertson AG, Reed NS, Ralston SH. Effect of oral clodronate on metastatic bone pain: a double-blind, placebo-controlled study. J Clin Oncol 1995; 13:2427–2430.
88. Ernst DS, Brasher P, Hagen N, Paterson AH, MacDonald RN, Bruera E. A randomized, controlled trial of intravenous clodronate in patients with metastatic bone disease and pain. J Pain Symptom Manage 1997; 13:319–326.
89. Paterson AHG, Powles TJ, Kanis JA, McCloskey E, Hanson J, Ashley S. Double-

blind controlled trial of oral clodronate in patients with bone metastases from breast cancer. J Clin Oncol 1993; 11:59–65.

90. Conte PF, Latreille J, Mauriac L, Calabresi F, Santos R, Campos D, Bonneterre J, Francini G, Ford JM. Delay in progression of bone metastases in breast cancer patients treated with intravenous pamidronate: results from a multinational randomised controlled trial. J Clin Oncol 1996; 14:2552–2559.
91. Lipton A. Bisphosphonate treatment of lytic bone metatases. ASCO Educational Book 1998:94–99.
92. Hortobagyi GN, Theriault RL, Lipton A, Porter L, Blayney D, Sinoff C, Wheeler H, Simeone JF, Seaman JJ, Knight RD, Heffernan M, Mellars K, Reitsma DJ for the Protocol 19 Aredia Breast Cancer Study Group. Long-term prevention of skeletal complications of metastatic breast cancer with pamidronate. J Clin Oncol 1998; 16: 2038–2044.
93. Kanis JA, Powles T, Paterson AHG, McCloskey EV, Ashley S. Clodronate decreases the frequency of skeletal metastases in women with breast cancer. Bone 1996; 19: 663–667.
94. Diel IJ, Solomayer EF, Costa SD, Gollan C, Goerner R, Wallwiener D, Kaufmann M, Bastert G. Reduction in new metastases in breast cancer with adjuvant clodronate treatment. N Engl J Med 1998; 339:357–363.
95. McCloskey EV, MacLennan ICM, Drayson M, Chapman C, Dunn J, Kanis JA. A randomized trial of the effect of clodronate on skeletal morbidity in multiple myeloma. Br J Hematol 1998; 100:317–325.
96. Berenson JR, Lichtenstein A, Porter L, Dimopoulous A, Bordoni R, George S, Lipton A, Keller A, Ballester O, Kovacs M, Blacklock H, Bell R, Simeone JF, Reitsma DJ, Heffernan M, Seaman J, Knight RD for the Myeloma Aredia Study Group. Long-term pamidronate treatment of advanced multiple myeloma patients reduces skeletal events. J Clin Oncol 1998; 16:593–602.
97. Bataille R. Management of myeloma with bisphosphonates. N Engl J Med 1996; 334:529–530.

21

Dermatologic Complications

Gerald P. Bodey
The University of Texas M.D. Anderson Cancer Center, Houston, Texas

I. INTRODUCTION

Patients with malignant diseases are susceptible to a variety of dermatologic complications. Antitumor agents can cause dermatologic effects either as a result of local extravasation of vesicant agents or as a result of systemic effects. Because most patients are given chemotherapy via vascular access devices, they are subject to complications such as localized infections, thrombophlebitis or, occasionally endocarditis with associated dermatologic manifestations. Skin hemorrhages develop in patients with thrombocytopenia, especially at sites of trauma. In patients with impaired host defenses, especially those with neutropenia, serious localized infections or dermatologic complications of systemic infections may develop. Primary and metastatic tumors may involve the skin. Occasionally, immunologic or allergic reactions and Sweet's syndrome develop. This discussion focuses primarily on infectious complications. The effects of local extravasation and device-related complications are discussed elsewhere in this book.

II. INFECTIONS

Most infections occur in patients with neutropenia, although a few, such as herpes zoster infection or cryptococcosis, are more common in patients with impairment

Table 1 Most Common Skin Infections in Cancer Patients

Organism	Local	Disseminated	Catheter-related
Gram-positive			
Staphylococcus aureus	x	x	x
Coagulase-negative staphylococci	x	x	x
Corynebacterium jekeium	x	x	x
Bacillus spp.	x	x	x
Clostridium spp.	x	x	
Gram-negative			
Pseudomonas aeruginosa	x	x	x
Enterobacteriaceae		x	
Aeromonas hydrophila	x	x	
Viral			
Herpes simplex	x	x	
Varicellas-zoster	x	x	
Fungal			
Candida spp.	x	x	x
Trichosporon beigelii		x	
Aspergillus spp.	x	x	x
Fusarium spp.	x	x	x
Mucorales	x	x	x

of other cellular defense mechanisms. The skin may be infected locally because of trauma or other factors, and these infections may disseminate internally in immunocompromised hosts. Tumors involving the skin, such as cutaneous lymphoma or breast cancer, may become necrotic and superinfected. Cancer patients are also subject to those skin infections prevalent in normal hosts. Table 1 lists the organisms especially likely to cause infections in cancer patients.

A. Gram-Positive Bacterial Infections

Gram-positive infections, especially those caused by *Staphylococcus aureus*, were the most common cause of infection in cancer patients before the 1960s. After the introduction of the antistaphylococcal penicillins, gram-negative bacilli emerged as the predominant pathogens, especially in neutropenic patients. During the past 15 years, gram-positive organisms have again emerged as the predominant pathogens. *Staphylococcus epidermidis* is the most prevalent pathogen, probably because of its association with vascular device infections. Other gram-positive organisms causing infections of the skin include *Clostridium* spp., *Corynebacterium jekeium* and *Bacillus* spp.

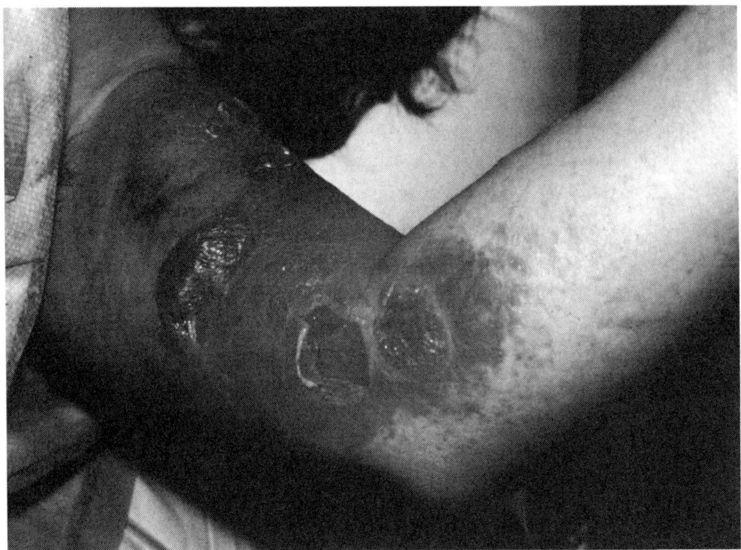

Figure 1 Scalded skin syndrome resulting from *Staphylococcus aureus* infection in a patient with acute leukemia.

1. *Staphylococcus aureus*

S. aureus causes a variety of skin infections including folliculitis, carbuncle, impetigo, hydroadenitis, cellulitis, abscess, wound infection, and scalded skin syndrome (1). It continues to be a common cause of nosocomial infections, and, consequently, is a threat to patients undergoing extensive surgery for malignant tumors. Intermittent microepidemics have occurred on some surgical services, such as head and neck services. Epidemics can be initiated by patients or hospital personnel who are nasal carriers of *S. aureus*.

In general, staphylococcal infections in cancer patients presents in a fashion similar to that in other patients and, hence, will not be discussed in detail. Staphylococcal scalded skin syndrome has occasionally occurred in cancer patients (Fig. 1). It begins with fever, skin tenderness, and a scarlatinoform rash. Large bullae appear which rupture, resulting in exfoliation with large areas of bright red skin surface. It is due to infection by a strain of *S. aureus* that produces an exfoliative exotoxin. Since a similar condition can occur due to viral infection or allergic reactions to drugs (such as fluoracil, etc.), it is important to recognize the cause expeditiously. Infection responds to penicillinase-resistant penicillins and fluid replacement.

2. *Staphylococcus epidermidis*

Several species of coagulase-negative staphylococci cause infections that are usually considered to be catheter-associated. However, some of these infections are derived from the nasopharynx, gastrointestinal tract, or other sites and at least one nosocomial epidemic on a leukemia and transplant unit has been reported (2,3).

There is nothing characteristic about *S. epidermidis* skin infections. Patients may develop cellulitis, pustular lesions, or wound infections may develop (Fig. 2). Since the organism is a common skin contaminant, it is often ignored when cultured from skin or blood specimens. This has led to failure to initiate appropriate therapy expeditiously, leading to extensive skin lesions and occasionally a fatal outcome. Many of these strains are methicillin-resistant, requiring vancomycin therapy.

3. Streptococcus *spp.*

Streptococcal toxic shock syndrome caused by *Streptococcus pyogenes* may be associated with surgical packs such as nasal packing. Progressive bacterial synergistic gangrene (Meleneys's ulcer) may develop at abdominal wound sites and, hence, can occur in patients undergoing excision of abdominal or pelvic tumors, patients with a colostomy, ileostomy, or fistulous tract (4). The infection begins as a local tender area of swelling and erythema that results in an enlarging shaggy, painful ulcer that is surrounded by gangrenous skin. The lesion is surrounded by a violaceous area with a pink border. In addition there are burrowing tracts emerging at distant sites. The infection is caused by *S. aureus* and microaerophilic or anaerobic streptococci. Gram-negative bacilli or *Entamoeba histolytica* may be involved. Therapy requires wide surgical excision of all necrotic tissue and appropriate antibiotic therapy with an antistaphylococcal penicillin plus other antibiotics. Local irrigation with bacitracin may be helpful.

Beginning in the mid-1980s, a new toxic shock–like syndrome was observed in severely neutropenic patients, caused by several species of alpha-hemolytic streptococci (5). The majority of patients in whom this syndrome has developed are bone marrow transplant recipients and children with acute leukemia, especially those with severe mucositis and those receiving antimicrobial prophylaxis and high-dose arabinosyl cytosine therapy. The syndrome may lead to the acute respiratory distress syndrome or acute renal failure. In about 60% of patients with this syndrome, flushing of the face develops and an erythematous maculopapular rash begins on the trunk and progresses to the extremities (6). Desquamation of the palms and soles occurs in 25% of these patients within 1 to 2 weeks. Vancomycin appears to be the most effective therapeutic agent because some alpha-hemolytic streptococci are tolerant or resistant to penicillin G.

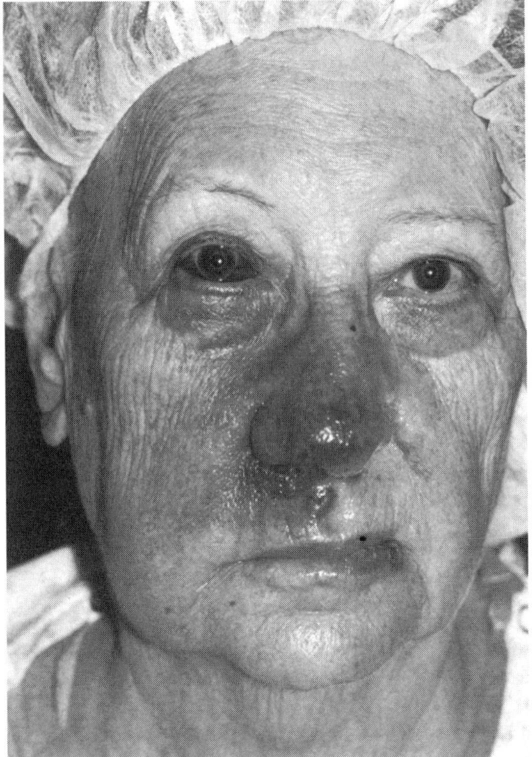

Figure 2 Cellulitis due to *Staphylococcus epidermidis* in a bone marrow transplant recipient.

4. Corynebacterium jekeium

C. jekeium is a skin organism that can cause serious infections in patients with prolonged neutropenia who have been hospitalized for a long time and have received extensive antibiotic therapy. While skin colonization by lipophilic *Corynebacterium* spp. is universal, in some series, 40% to 80% of leukemic patients are colonized by *C. jekeium* (7). *C. jekeium* skin infections include ulcers, pustules, cellulitis, and abscesses (8). Infections may arise at sites of trauma or in the groin or perianal region. Bacteremia develops in about 30% to 50% of patients with skin lesions. Some patients have multiple skin lesions, hence, skin involvement may be secondary and not always primary. If the microbiology laboratory fails to recognize the unique colonial morphology of this organism, its pathogenic potential may be overlooked. Indeed, the significance of *C. jekeium* as a cause of skin infection may only be appreciated after the organism is isolated from blood cultures. The organism is resistant to many antibiotics, including beta-lactams, but is susceptible to vancomycin. Although it does not cause fulminant infections, fatality rates of 25% have been reported in patients in whom bacteremia develops (9,10).

5. Bacillus *sp.*

Bacillus subtilis and *Bacillus cereus* have been recognized as occasional causes of skin and wound infections (11). The frequency with which these infections occur is not known but it is estimated that about half of the infections are catheter associated (12). Skin infections caused by *Bacillus* spp. include cellulitus, impetiginous lesions, ulcerations, and gas gangrene (13). All of the infections seen at the University of Texas M.D. Anderson Cancer Center have occurred in neutropenic patients (Fig. 3). It is important to identify *B. cereus* expeditiously because the organism is resistant to most beta-lactams, but is susceptible to vancomycin, imipenem, and aminoglycosides.

6. Clostridium *sp.*

Clostridial skin infections occur infrequently but they are usually fulminant and cause extensive damage. Infection may be primary or secondary to bacteremia

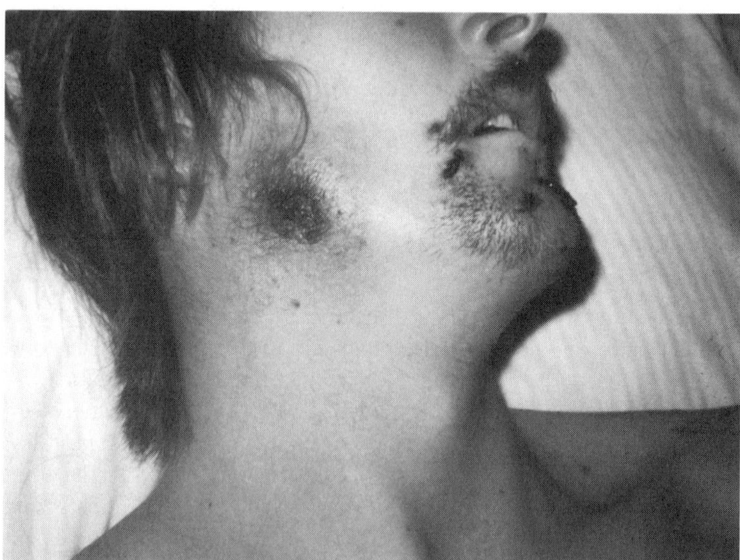

Figure 3 *Bacillus cereus* infection in a patient with acute leukemia.

(14). Most infections occur in patients with acute leukemia, other hematological malignancies, and gastrointestinal or genitourinary tumors. About 40% of infections are polymicrobial, usually associated with gram-negative bacilli, indicating a gastrointestinal source of the infection. Most infections are caused by *Clostridium perfringens* and *Clostridium septicum*, and occasionally, *Clostridium tertium* (15). Clostridial species that cause fulminant infections produce a variety of toxins that are destructive to tissues, including lecithinase, phospholipase, collagenase, protease, hyaluronidase, and desoxyribonuclease. The virulence of *C. septicum* has been attributed to its production of an alpha toxin.

The two types of skin and soft tissue infection that occur in cancer patients are gas gangrene and spreading cellulitis, both of which may occur secondary to clostridial septicemia. Currently, *C. septicum* is the most common cause of spontaneous gas gangrene (16). Gas gangrene may also occur following abdominal surgery. Gas gangrene usually presents with the sudden onset of severe pain. On initial physical examination, the site may appear normal but the disease progresses rapidly with localized tense edema, pallor, and tenderness. The skin color changes to purple or bronze with blister formation and crepitation. The organism can be detected in blister fluid with few or no leukocytes. The infection is associated with an offensive sweetish odor. Systemic symptoms include severe anxiety, dyspnea, diaphoresis, and tachycardia disproportionate to the temperature, which may be only minimally elevated. Occasionally, intravascular hemolysis, jaundice, renal failure, and metabolic acidosis develop (17).

Spreading cellulitis is a fulminant infection in neutropenic patients (Fig. 4). Typically, a small area of purplish discoloration develops on the flank or abdominal wall. The lesion rapidly enlarges over several hours associated with the appearance of new lesions. The lesions continue to enlarge and develop a brownish to blackish color with blister formation and crepitation.

Appropriate management of gas gangrene requires prompt antibiotic therapy and surgical debridement of all necrotic tissue. Hyperbaric oxygen should be used if available. The drug of choice is penicillin G, but it may be advisable to combine it with metronidazole or clindamycin because some strains have developed penicillin resistance. *C. tertium* is resistant to penicillin G but susceptible to vancomycin, ciprofloxacin, and trimethoprim-sulfamethoxazole. Spreading cellulitis in neutropenic patients has dire prognostic implications; the mortality rate is nearly 100%, regardless of therapeutic interventions.

B. Gram-Negative Bacterial Infections

Gram-negative bacteria may cause localized skin infections or metastatic skin lesions associated with bacteremia. Generally, there is nothing characteristic about these skin lesions to suggest the infecting pathogen and the diagnosis is determined from cultures of the skin lesions or blood specimens. Two gram-

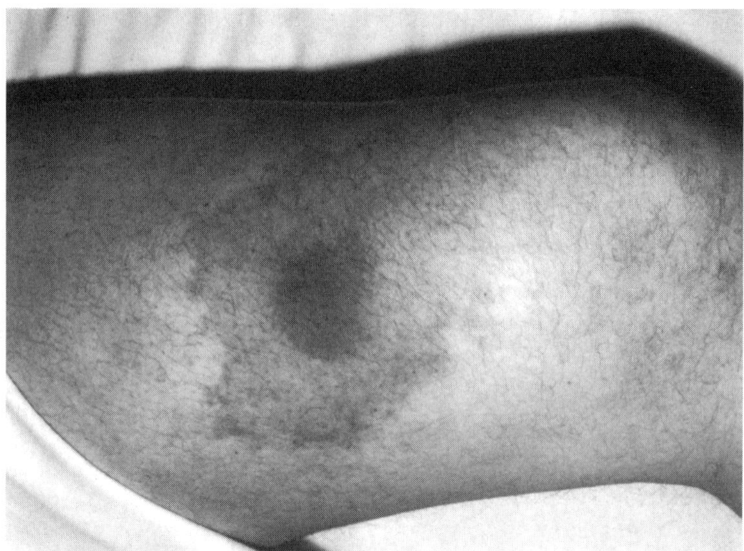

Figure 4 Spreading cellulitis on the leg in a patient with *Clostridium perfringens* septicemia.

negative bacilli that are frequently associated with skin lesions are *P. aeruginosa* and *Aeromonas hydrophila*.

1. Pseudomonas aeruginosa

Prior to the availability of effective antibiotic therapy, skin lesions occurred in about 30% of patients with *P. aeruginosa* bacteremia, but more recently skin lesions have been reported in less than 5% of patients (18,19). The most characteristic lesion in patients with *Pseudomonas* bacteremia is ecthyma gangrenosum, although this lesion may occasionally begin as a localized skin infection (Fig. 5). The vast majority of ecthymas are caused by *P. aeruginosa*, but occasionally they are due to infection by *S. aureus*, *Serratia marcescens*, *A. hydrophila*, *Aspergillus* spp., or *Mucorales*. Ecthyma gangrenosum arises most often in the groin, perianal, axillary, or inframammary area, but lesions may occur anywhere on the body, including the abdominal wall, lip, phalanx, or tongue (20). Not infrequently, lesions may arise on the eyelid and can spread to the eye, ultimately causing endophthalmitis.

Lesions begin as areas of erythema and edema that progress to a hemorrhagic bluish bulla that ruptures. Frequently, the lesions are discovered later in their evolution, at which time the typical appearance is a central bluish to blackish

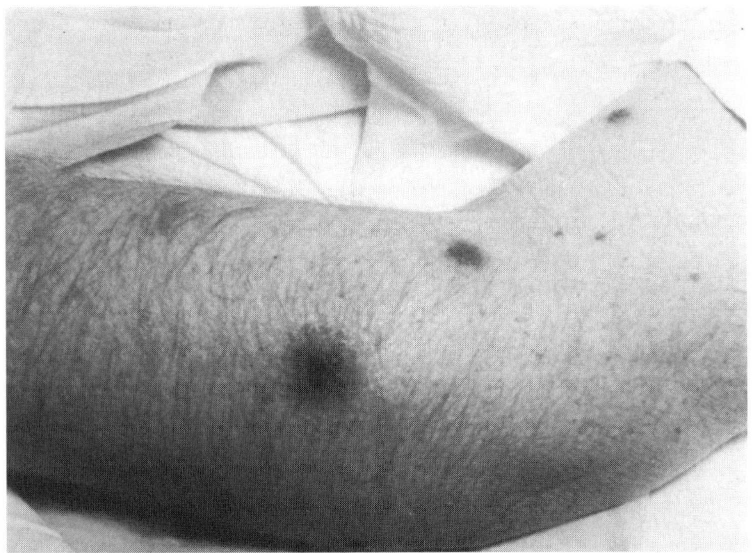

Figure 5 Multiple ecthyma gangrenosa in a patient with *Pseudomonas aeruginosa* septicema.

necrotic area surrounded by an erythematous halo. Initially, the necrotic area is not sharply defined and may enlarge rapidly over the next 12 to 24 hours. Some patients may have many small lesions throughout the body suggestive of an embolic process, whereas others may have multiple large necrotic hemorrhagic lesions. Rarely, when the infection is not treated promptly, it may progress to an extensive cellulitis and panniculitis. Once the infection is controlled, the necrotic areas become more sharply demarcated.

The pathological appearance of an ecthyma gangrenosum is characteristically prominent vasculitis, usually without thrombosis (21). With appropriate staining, numerous bacilli can be visualized in the media and adventitia, but not the intima of blood vessels. In neutropenic patients, there is a paucity of inflammatory cells in the surrounding tissues.

Several other skin lesions have been described less frequently in patients with *Pseudomonas* bacteremia. In some patients, clusters of painful vesicular lesions may develop (22). These small blebs or vesicles have an erythematous base and contain opalescent fluid from which the organism can be cultured. Occasional patients have small, pink, maculopapular plaques or nodules arising on the trunk. Painful subcutaneous nodules may occur in which the overlying skin may appear normal, erythematous, or have a bluish discoloration.

Pseudomonas infections, even in severely neutropenic patients, can usually be treated effectively with antipseudomonal beta-lactams alone or in combination with an aminoglycoside, as long as therapy is instituted promptly (19). Large ecthymas may require surgical debridement and skin grafting. Subcutaneous abscesses may be much larger than apparent on examination and require surgical drainage.

2. Aeromonas hydrophila

Most reported cases of Aeromonas bacteria have occurred in patients with acute leukemia (23). About 20% to 30% of patients with *A. hydrophila* bacteremia have skin lesions and in some cases the skin infection is the source of the bacteremia. Because the organism grows in fresh or brackish water, it may cause skin infection associated with trauma in patients swimming or fishing in contaminated waters. About 60% of infections are nosocomially acquired and the organism can contaminate solutions, sink drains, and so on (24). About one-third of skin lesions are ecthyma gangrenosa. In some patients, extensive cellulitis develops, which may become necrotic with sharply defined borders and covered by a black eschar. Other skin lesions are ill-defined, often with a purplish discoloration (Fig. 6). The organism is susceptible to extended-spectrum cephalosporins, imipenem, trimethoprim-sulfamethoxazole, and aminoglycosides but not to penicillins.

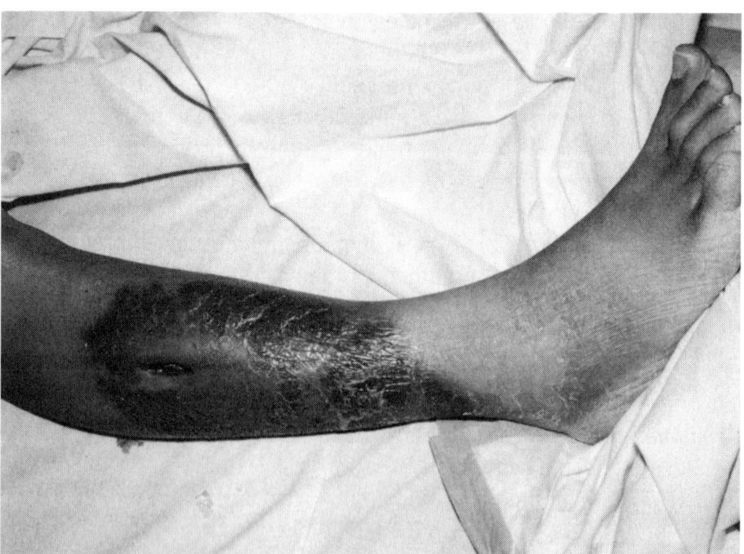

Figure 6 Nosocomially acquired cellulitis associated with *Aeromonas hydrophila* bacteremia.

C. Fungal Infection

Most fungal infections occur in neutropenic patients; however, cryptococcosis is more prevalent in patients with impaired cellular immunity, and candidiasis is an increasing cause of catheter-related infections. The most common infections in neutropenic patients are candidiasis and aspergillosis, although trichosporonosis and fusariosis are increasing in frequency. All of these infections may be associated with skin lesions.

1. *Candidiasis*

Candida spp. are capable of causing superficial nail and skin infections. Localized skin infections may be more extensive in cancer patients, but it is not clear that they are more prevalent than in the general population. However, skin lesions occur as a consequence of disseminated candidiasis, and these lesions are more prevalent in immunocompromised hosts, especially neutropenic patients. Disseminated infection caused by *C. tropicalis* seems to be most frequently associated with skin lesions; such patients may also have very painful myositis (25).

A characteristic skin lesion in disseminated candidiasis was first recognized in the early 1970s and occurs in about 5% to 10% of patients (26,27). Additionally, occasional patients may have other types of skin lesions. The characteristic skin lesions are firm nodules that may vary in size from 0.5 to 1.0 cm in diameter (Fig. 7). They are nontender, pink to red in color, and do not blanch on pressure. The lesions are discrete initially but may coalesce as the infection progresses. Most patients have widely disseminated nodules that may be confused with an allergic reaction on casual examination. Occasional patients may have only a few nodules, usually on the extremities.

Histologically, the infection is confined to the dermis with a normal overlying epidermis (27). Fibrin exudate and small hemorrhages are located in the middle and lower dermis in association with edema of blood vessel walls and surrounding perivascular tissue. Because most patients are leukopenic, there is only a minimal mononuclear inflammatory infiltrate, but with appropriate stains, the organism can be easily visualized. Unfortunately, the yeast is cultured from only 50% of skin biopsy specimens. Therapy for these patients consists of amphotericin B or fluconazole alone or in combination with flucytosine.

2. *Aspergillosis*

Aspergillosis is prevalent in patients with prolonged neutropenia or in those receiving intensive or prolonged therapy with adrenal corticosteroids (28). Skin lesions are infrequent but may occur as primary lesions or secondary to disseminated aspergillosis. Primary cutaneous infection is associated with vascular access devices and most often occurs in neutropenic patients but can occur in pa-

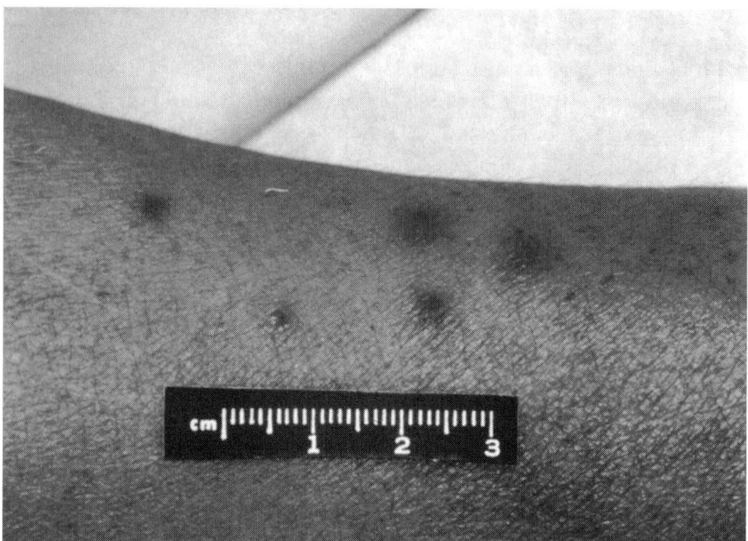

Figure 7 Skin lesions occurring in disseminated candidiasis.

tients with no discernable compromised host defenses (29). The infection may result from deposition of spores from the air during the insertion process, or the spores may be impregnated in dressing materials used to cover the insertion site. The organisms invade the skin and subcutaneous tissues, causing an erythematous to violaceous, edematous, indurated plaque that progresses to a black eschar. Lesions on an extremity may cause disseminated infection. Organisms causing lesions on the chest wall may erode into the chest and cause pulmonary infection.

Because *Aspergillus* spp. are predominantly respiratory pathogens, most infections involve the lungs or sinuses and only 30% to 40% of cases result in disseminated infection (30). Skin lesions occur in about 5% of cases of disseminated aspergillosis. The characteristic skin lesions of aspergillosis may be single or multiple and may be found anywhere on the body (31). The lesion begins as a papule that progresses to a pustule. Over several days, the lesion enlarges and develops a punched-out necrotic ulcerated center (Fig. 8). At this stage, the lesion may be confused with an ecthyma gangrenosum. Subsequently, the central ulceration becomes covered by a black eschar with sharply demarcated borders surrounded by a narrow erythematous halo. Multiple lesions in close proximity may coalesce. In patients with sino-orbital aspergillosis, similar skin lesions often develop on the bridge of the nose, anterior nares, nasal septum, or palate.

Several other uncommon types of skin lesions have been associated with disseminated aspergillosis including subcutaneous granulomas or abscesses (32).

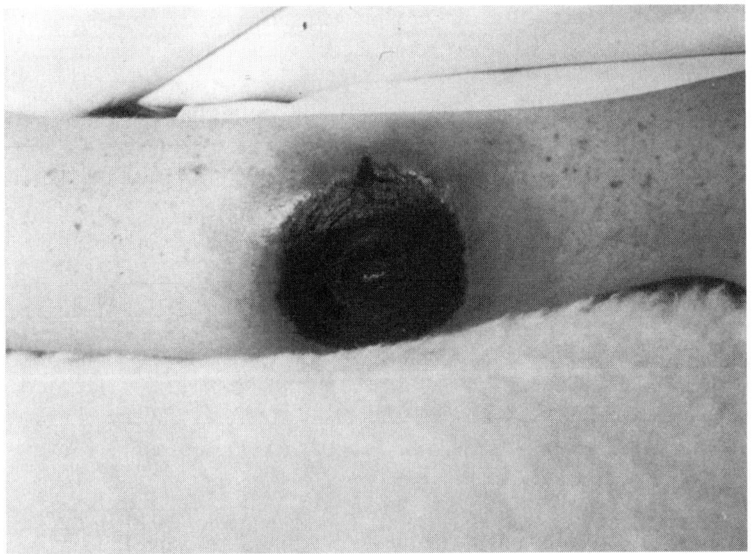

Figure 8 Black eschar on extremity of patient with disseminated aspergillosis.

Rarely, persistent, eruptive dermal macropapules with indistinct margins progress to reddish-purple granulomas. Also, confluent papules and macules with overlying scaling, crusting, or oozing of the dermis have been caused by *Aspergillus* spp.

The characteristic skin lesions are due to the propensity of *Aspergillus* spp. to invade blood vessel walls, causing thrombosis and infarction of surrounding tissues. It is usually possible to identify fungal elements in biopsy specimens of skin lesions, but it may not always be possible to identify the characteristic morphology of *Aspergillus* spp. The organism can be cultured from only about 50% of tissue specimens.

Therapy in neutropenic patients is often unsatisfactory and success is associated with neutrophil recovery (33). Therapy should be initiated with amphotericin B, but itraconazole can be substituted for long-term treatment when the patient is not neutropenic. Surgical excision of primary cutaneous lesions should not be attempted until there is evidence of response to antifungal therapy.

3. Trichosporonosis

Trichosporon beigelii, the cause of white piedra, a superficial infection of the hair shafts, can cause disseminated infection in neutropenic cancer patients (34).

Skin lesions develop in about 30% of these infected patients (35). Usually, multiple nontender erythematous nodules that are about 0.5 cm in diameter develop. These may be located anywhere on the body and may be numerous in some cases, especially on the extremities. Occasional lesions are large plaques with indistinct margins that may develop a necrotic center. Budding yeasts can be identified in skin biopsy specimens and usually can be cultured from skin specimens. In animal models, azoles are more active than amphotericin B, but response in neutropenic patients depends on recovery of the neutrophil count (36).

4. *Cryptococcosis*

Skin lesions are frequent in patients with disseminated cryptococcosis. The lesions may be nodular, pustular, vesicular, acneiform, plaquelike or ulcerated. Sometimes, areas of cellulitis or a subcutaneous abscess may develop. Lesions are most often located on the head or trunk. Biopsy of the infected area reveals aggregations of *Cryptococcus neoformans* with a minimal inflammatory response. Usually there is no difficulty in culturing the organism from skin biopsies. Amphotericin B plus flucytosine is usually used as initial therapy. Fluconazole plus flucytosine is probably as effective and less toxic.

5. *Fusariosis*

Fusarium spp. can cause superficial infections of the skin and nails. The organisms are respiratory pathogens and most infections are acquired via this route, although primary cutaneous and catheter-associated infections can occur (37). Nearly all of these infections occur in patients with acute leukemia and in bone marrow transplant recipients. About 75% of infections are disseminated and skin and soft tissue lesions are found in about 75% of these latter patients (38,39). The most characteristic lesion begins as a small rounded area of grayish discoloration about 1 cm in diameter. As the infection progresses, the central area becomes ulcerated with a sharply demarcated border, which often becomes covered by a black eschar. This lesion is surrounded by a large ill-defined area of grayish discoloration (Fig. 9). Usually, multiple lesions are present on the trunk and extremities. In some patients, extremely tender subcutaneous nodules may develop with normal appearing overlying skin. In vitro susceptibility of *Fusarium* spp. to antifungal agents is variable, but therapy is seldom effective unless the patient's bone marrow recovers.

D. Viral Infections

Cancer patients are susceptible to a variety of viral infections and these are most prevalent in patients with impaired cellular immunity such as occurs in patients with lymphoma and chronic lymphocytic leukemia and bone marrow transplant

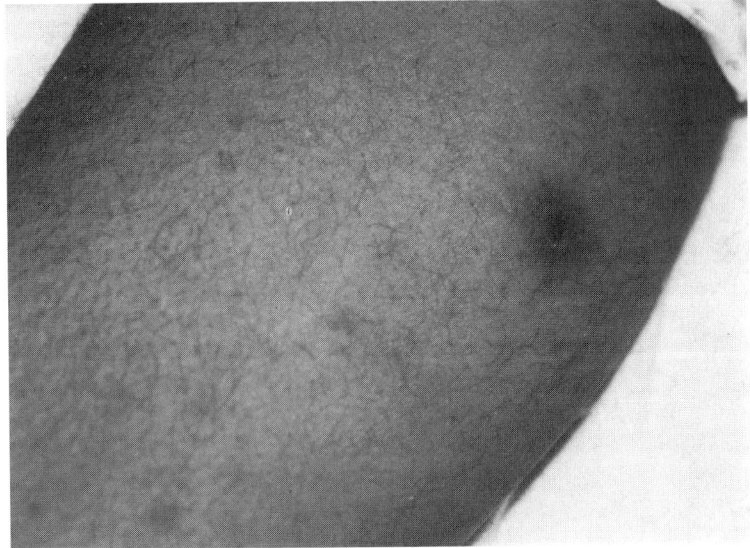

Figure 9 Skin lesion in patient with disseminated fusariosis.

recipients. The most common viral infections of the skin are herpes simplex and varicella-zoster, but cytomegalovirus, papilloma virus, and molluscum contagiosum skin lesions occur infrequently.

1. Herpes Simplex

Most herpes simplex infections represent reactivation of latent infection and are common in patients with acute leukemia and bone marrow transplant recipients (40). Most herpetic infections occur on the lips, nares, circumoral skin, and oral mucosa. Genital lesions are infrequent but may be extensive. Often, the signs of local infection are preceded by tingling, burning, or itching. Lesions begin as vesicles that rupture spontaneously, resulting in ulcerations that enlarge, coalesce, and become encrusted. Infection may pursue a chronic course with extensive necrotic lesions known as phagedena (41). Healing may require more than a month. Herpetic lesions are subject to superinfection by bacteria or fungi, and especially by *S. aureus*. Acyclovir and its congeners are effective for prophylaxis and therapy of active infections (42).

2. Varicella Zoster

Varicella is a potentially serious infection in children undergoing cancer chemotherapy, may be unduly prolonged, and has been associated with a fatality rate

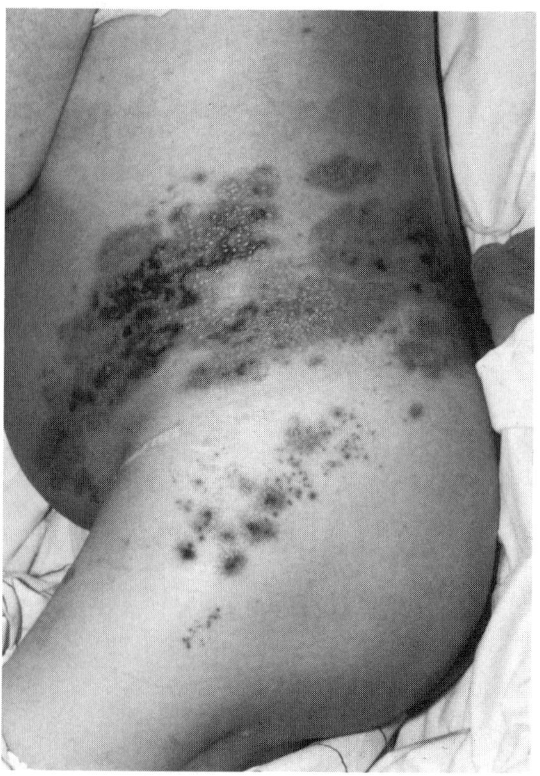

Figure 10 Patient with hemorrhagic lesions resulting from herpes zoster infection.

of about 5% (43). In patients with thrombocytopenia, the lesions may become hemorrhagic and necrotic, and bacterial superinfection may occur. Herpes zoster occurs sporadically in all cancer patients, but is more prevalent in patients with lymphoproliferative disorders (44). Lesions arise at sites where tumor is in close proximity to nerve trunks in 20% of cases and at sites of recent radiation in 20%. Infection is characterized by a painful unilateral vesicular eruption with a dermatomal distribution. In some cases, multiple dermatomes may be involved or the infection may become generalized (Fig. 10). Lesions in cancer patients may heal slowly with necrosis and scarring. Acyclovir and related antiviral agents accelerate healing of lesions. Post-herpetic pain is more common in cancer patients than in normal hosts in whom herpes zoster develops.

III. TUMORS

Primary tumors of the skin include basal cell and squamous carcinomas and malignant melanoma. Some hematological malignancies involve the skin such as cutaneous T-cell lymphoma and leukemia cutis resulting from acute leukemia. Tumors at other body sites may metastasize to the skin. These lesions may become large and necrotic and superinfected by bacteria or fungi. Often they are not amenable to surgical excision, and antimicrobial therapy is ineffective because the tumor is unresponsive to chemotherapy. Indeed, if the cancer chemotherapy causes myelosuppression, the infected skin lesion may serve as a site for hematogenous dissemination.

IV. HEMORRHAGE

Thrombocytopenia may develop in cancer patients as a consequence of their disease or its therapy. Petechiae are common in patients with prolonged thrombocytopenia, and, often, ecchmyoses develop at sites of minor trauma in these patients. Some malignancies, such as acute promyelocytic leukemia, cause disseminated intravascular coagulation that is associated with extensive cutaneous hemorrhagic lesions. This complication requires prompt therapy of the underlying disease as well as supportive therapy with heparin and transfusion of blood, frozen plasma, or cryoprecipitate and platelet concentrates.

There is a reluctance on the part of some physicians to biopsy skin lesions in patients with thrombocytopenia because of the bleeding potential. Unless patients have major hemorrhagic complications, it is unusual for skin biopsies to result in serious hemorrhage that cannot be controlled by topical measures such as ice packs, pressure dressings, topical thrombin, or epinephrine. Platelet transfusions are effective in patients failing to respond to these measures. Usually, there is greater harm to the patient from failing to identify the cause of the lesion than from the bleeding caused by a skin biopsy.

V. SIDE EFFECTS OF ANTITUMOR AGENTS

A. Alopecia

The most common dermatological side effect of antitumor agents is alopecia (45). The cells in the hair matrix proliferate more rapidly than other human cells and, hence, are more susceptible to the effects of antitumor agents. These drugs may inhibit mitosis or impair metabolic processes, causing constriction of the hair shaft, which breaks when it reaches the skin surface. Drugs most often associated with alopecia include bleomycin, alkylating agents, anthracycline antibiotics, dactinomycin, 5-fluorouracil, methotrexate, and the vinca alkaloids. Scalp tourniquets and hypothermia have led to variable success in reducing alopecia but are not recommended for patients with leukemia, lymphoma, or tumors with a high frequency of scalp metastases.

B. Nail Lesions

Chemotherapeutic agents can cause several effects on nails, including abnormal pigmentation, Muehrcke's lines and Beau's lines (45). Muehrcke's lines are hypopigmented lines across the nail that move distally with time. Beau's lines are horizontal depressions of the nail plate caused by growth arrest resulting from cessation of mitotic activity by chemotherapeutic agents.

C. Hypersensitivity and Photosensitivity Reactions

Hypersensitivity reactions resulting from antitumor agents are generally uncommon. Type I (IgE–mediated) immediate reactions, characterized by urticaria, angioedema, and anaphylaxis, are most common following L-asparaginase therapy (46). Similar reactions occur in patients receiving cisplatinol. A variety of agents are capable of causing urticaria (Table 2). Type III (immune complex–mediated) reactions characterized by urticaria, erythema multiforme, and vasculitis have been associated with hydroxyurea and mechlorethamine (45). Table 2 also lists the antitumor agents that can cause photosensitivity.

Table 2 Cutaneous Reactions to Antitumor Agents

Reaction	Antitumor agents
Photosensitivity	Mitomycin C, methotrexate, dacarbazone, 5-fluorouracil
Radiation enhancement	Methotrexate, bleomycin, anthracyclines, dactinomycin
Urticaria	Alkylating agents, platinum compounds, methotrexate, bleomycin, anthracyclines, mitomycin C, mithramycin
Hyperpigmentation	Alkylating agents, methotrexate, bleomycin, mithramycin, mitomycin C

D. Hyperpigmentation

Hyperpigmentation may be generalized or localized (Table 2). A syndrome suggestive of Addison's disease consisting of diffuse hyperpigmentation, weakness, weight loss, and diarrhea has been associated with busulfan therapy (47). Linear or flagellate streaks of hyperpigmentation have been described following bleomycin therapy (48). These lesions presumably are due to the trauma caused by scratching. Inflammation of existing actinic keratoses has followed therapy with fluorouracil, pentostatin, dactinomycin, vincristine, dacarbazine, cisplatinol, doxorubicin, and cytarabine (49). This inflammation results in pruritus and erythema.

E. Radiation and Chemotherapy Interactions

A few antitumor agents may interact synergistically with radiation to enhance the cutaneous effects of radiation therapy (45). This is due to the inhibitory effects of the antitumor agents on repair processes following radiation damage. Agents associated with this effect are listed in Table 2. Radiation recall is an inflammatory reaction following chemotherapy at sites of previous irradiation. This reaction is independent of the previous clinically apparent radiation damage and may occur years after completion of radiation therapy. It has been noted with dactinomycin and anthracycline antibiotics.

F. Miscellaneous Lesions

Neutrophilic eccrine hidradenitis is manifested by tender, erythematous macules, papules, and plaques on the trunk, neck, and extremities, which resolve over several days without specific therapy (50). Pathologically, the lesions consist of neutrophilic infiltrates around eccrine coils associated with epithelial cell necrosis and vacuolization. These lesions have most frequently been associated with cytarabine and bleomycin. Accral erythema (palmer-plantar erythrodysesthesia) begins with dysesthesias of the palms and soles, progressing over several days to pain and tenderness, especially of the distal phalanges (51). The palms and soles become swollen and erythematous progressing to bulla formation and desquamation. The condition regresses over a week after therapy is discontinued but recurs with subsequent therapy. Chemotherapeutic agents associated with this complication include cytarabine, fluorouracil, and doxorubicin.

VI. SWEET'S SYNDROME AND OTHER PARANEOPLASTIC SYNDROMES

Sweet's syndrome (acute febrile neutrophilic dermatosis) is often misdiagnosed as cellulitis, although it is not an infectious process. Even though it is associated

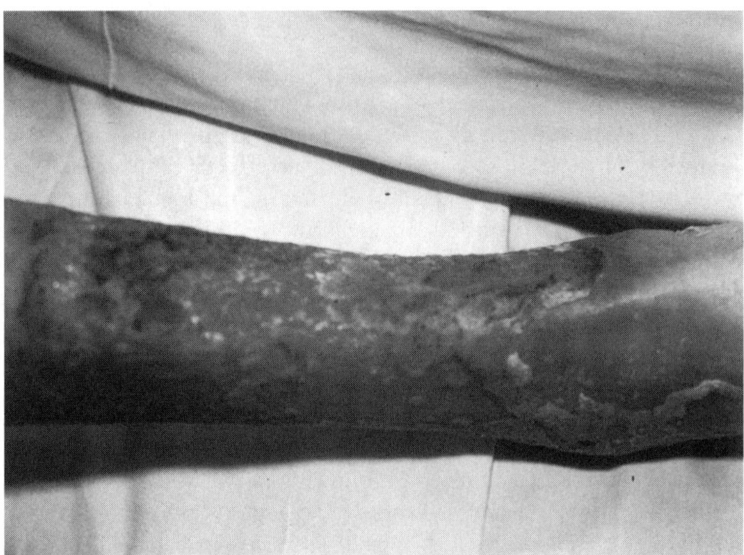

Figure 11 Patient with pre-leukemic syndrome in whom Sweet's syndrome developed.

with other underlying diseases, it often occurs in hematological malignancies (52). The predominant lesions are multiple, tender, erythematous, or violaceous plaques or nodules of acute onset. Less typical lesions include vesicles or bulla, papules, pustules, ulcers, or hemorrhagic lesions. Although lesions can occur anywhere, they most frequently involve the extremities (Fig. 11). Patients have fever and some have musculoskeletal symptoms. Histological examination of the skin reveals a dense, extensive neutrophilic infiltrate predominantly involving the mid and upper dermis. This dense neutrophilic infiltration is found even in neutropenic patients. The disease responds promptly to adrenal corticosteroid therapy and, in patients with hematological malignancies, to appropriate chemotherapy. Misdiagnosing this condition as cellulitis in neutropenic patients has led to inappropriate delays in appropriate therapy.

A variety of other skin lesions occasionally occur in patients with malignancies of internal organs (53). These include acanthosis nigricans, calcinosis cutis, dermatomyositis, tylosis, palmar erythema, and acquired ichthyosis. Because many of these lesions also occur in patients with other diseases or are familial in origin, their appearance may not indicate the presence of malignancy. If the lesions are of recent onset and there is no clinical evidence of other disease, the patient should be evaluated for the presence of cancer.

REFERENCES

1. Waldvogel FA. *Staphylococcus aureus* (including toxic shock syndrome). In: Mandell GL, Bennett JE, Dolin R, eds. Mandells, Douglas and Bennett's Principles and Practice of Infectious Diseases Vol. 2. New York: Churchill Livingstone, 1995: 1754–1777.
2. Wade JC, Schimpff SC, Newman KA, Wiernik PH. *Staphylococcus epidermidis*: an increasing cause of infection in patients with granulocytopenia. Ann Intern Med 1982; 97:503–508.
3. Oppenheim BA, Hartley JW, Lee W, Burnie JP. Outbreak of coagulase negative *staphylococcus* highly resistant to ciprofloxacin in a leukaemia unit. BMJ 1989; 299: 294–297.
4. Davson J, Jones DM, Turner L. Diagnosis of Meleney's synergistic gangrene. Br J Surg 1988; 75:267–271.
5. Ognibene FP, Martin SE, Parker MM, et al. Adult respiratory distress syndrome in patients with severe neutropenia. N Engl J Med 1986; 315:547–549.
6. Elting LS, Bodey GP, Keefe BH. Septicemia and shock syndrome due to viridans streptococci: a case-control study of predisposing factors. Clin Infect Dis 1992; 14: 1201–1207.
7. Larson EL, McGinley KJ, Leyden JJ, et al. Skin colonization with antibiotic-resistant (JK group) and antibiotic-sensitive lipophilic-diphtheroids in hospitalized and normal adults. J Infect Dis 1986; 153:701–706.
8. Dan M, Somer I, Knobel B, et al. Cutaneous manifestations of infection with *Corynebacterium* group JK. Rev Infect Dis 1988; 10:1204–1207.
9. Pearson TA, Braine HG, Rathbun HK. *Corynebacterium* sepsis in oncology patients. JAMA 1977; 238:1737–1740.
10. Stamm WE, Tompkins LS, Wagner KF, et al. Infection due to *Corynebacterium* species in marrow transplant patients. Ann Intern Med 1979; 91:167–173.
11. Pearson HE. Human infections caused by organisms of the *Bacillus* species. Am J Clin Pathol 1970; 53:506–515.
12. Banerjee C, Bustamante CI, Wharton R, et al. Bacillus infections in patients with cancer. Ann Intern Med 1988; 148:1769–1774.
13. Groschel D, Burgess MA, Bodey GP. Gas gangrene-like infection with *Bacillus cereus* in a lymphoma patient. Cancer 1976; 37:988–991.
14. Bodey GP, Rodriguez S, Fainstein V, et al. Clostridial bacteremia in cancer patients. Cancer 1991; 67:1928–1942.
15. Speirs G, Warren RE, Rampling A. *Clostridium tertium* septicemia in patients with neutropenia. J Infect Dis 1988; 158:1336–1340.
16. Stevens DL, Musher DM, Watson DA, et al. Spontaneous, nontraumatic gangrene due to *Clostridium septicum*. Rev Infect Dis 1990; 12:286–296.
17. Cabrera A, Tsukada Y, Pickren JW. Clostridial gas gangrene and septicemia in malignant disease. Cancer 1965; 18:800–806.
18. Whitecar JP Jr, Bodey GP, Luna M. *Pseudomonas* bacteremia in cancer patients. Am J Med Sci 1970; 260:216–223.

19. Bodey GP, Jadeja L, Elting L. *Pseudomonas* bacteremia: retrospective analysis of 410 episodes. Arch Intern Med 1985; 145:1621–1629.
20. Bodey GP, Bolivar R, Fainstein V, et al. Infections caused by *Pseudomonas aeruginosa*. Rev Infect Dis 1983; 5:279–313.
21. van den Brock PJ, van der Meer JWM, Kunst MW. The pathogenesis of ecthyma gangrenosum. J Infect 1979; 1:263–267.
22. Forkner CE Jr, Frei E III, Edgcomb JH, et al. *Pseudomonas* septicemia: observations on twenty-three cases. Am J Med 1958; 25:877–889.
23. Davis WA II, Kane JG, Gargusi VF. Human *Aeromonas* infections: a review of the literature and a case report of endocarditis. Medicine 1978; 57:267–277.
24. Harris RL, Fainstein V, Elting L, et al. Bacteremia caused by *Aeromonas* species in hospitalized cancer patients. Rev Infect Dis 1985; 7:314–320.
25. Jarowski CI, Fialk MA, Murray HW. Fever, rash and muscle tenderness. A distinctive clinical presentation of disseminated candidiasis. Arch Intern Med 1978; 138: 544–546.
26. Balandran L, Rothschild H, Pugh N. A cutaneous manifestation of system candidiasis. Ann Intern Med 1973; 78:400–403.
27. Bodey GP, Luna M. Skin lesions associated with disseminated candidiasis. JAMA 1974; 229:1466–1468.
28. Schaffner A, Douglas H, Braude A. Selective protection against *Conidia* by mononuclear and against *Mycelia* by polymorphonuclear phagocytes in resistance to *Aspergillus*. J Clin Invest 1982; 69:617–619.
29. Allo DM, Miller J, Townsend T, et al. Primary cutaneous aspergillosis associated with Hickman intravenous catheters. N Engl J Med 1987; 317:1105–1108.
30. Young RC, Bennett JE, Vogel CL, et al. Aspergillosis. The spectrum of the disease in 98 patients. Medicine 1970; 49:147–173.
31. Bodey GP. Dermatologic manifestations of infections in neutropenic patients. In: Pankey GA, ed. Infect Dis Clin North Am 1994; 8:655–675.
32. Findlay GH, Roux HF, Simson IW. Skin manifestations in disseminated aspergillosis. Br J Dermatol 1991; 85:94–97.
33. Bodey GP, Vartivarian S. Aspergillosis. Eur J Clin Microbiol Infect Dis 1989; 8: 413–437.
34. Anaissie EJ, Bodey GP, Rinaldi MG. Emerging fungal pathogens. Eur J Clin Microbiol Infect Dis 1989; 8:323–330.
35. Walsh TJ, Newman KR, Moodey M, et al. Trichosporonosis in patients with neoplastic disease. Medicine 1986; 65:268–279.
36. Anaissie E, Gokaslan A, Hachem R, et al. Azole therapy for trichosporonosis: clinical evaluation of eight patients, experimental therapy for murine infection, and review. Clin Infect Dis 1992; 15:781–787.
37. Bodey GP. New fungal pathogens. In: Remington J, Swartz MN, eds. Current Clinical Topics in Infectious Diseases. Malden, MA: Blackwell Science, 1997:205–235.
38. Anaissie EJ, Kantarjian H, Ro J, et al. The emerging role of *Fusarium* infection in patients with cancer. Medicine 1988; 67:77–83.
39. Rabodonirina M, Piens MA, Monier MF, et al. *Fusarium* infections in immunocom-

promised patients: case reports and literature review. Eur J Clin Microbiol Infect Dis 1994; 13:152–161.
40. Saral R, Burns WH, Laskin OL, et al. Acyclovir prophylaxis of herpes simplex virus infections. A randomized, double-blind, controlled trial in bone marrow transplant recipients. N Engl J Med 1981; 305:63–67.
41. Dreizen S, McCredie KB, Bodey GP, et al. Mucocutaneous herpetic infections during cancer chemotherapy. Postgrad Med 1988; 84:181–192.
42. Wong KK, Hirsch MS. Herpes virus infections in patients with neoplastic disease. Am J Med 1984; 76:464–478.
43. Feldman S, Hughes WT, Daniel CB. Varicella in children with cancer. Seventy-seven cases. Pediatrics 1975; 56:388–394.
44. Whitley RJ. Varicella-zoster virus infections. In: Galasso GJ, Merigan TC, Buchanan RA, eds, 2nd ed. Antiviral Agents and Viral Diseases of Man. New York: Raven Press, 1984:517–541.
45. Hood AF. Cutaneous side effects of cancer chemotherapy. Med Clin North Am 1986; 70:187–209.
46. Oettgan HF, Stephenson PA, Schwartz MK, et al. Toxicity of *E. coli*, L-asparaginase in man. Cancer 1970; 25:253–278.
47. Harrold BP. Syndrome resembling Addison's disease following prolonged treatment with busulfan. BMJ 1966; 1:463–464.
48. Guillet G, Suillet M-H, de Meaux H, et al. Cutaneous pigmented stripes and bleomycin treatment. Arch Dermatol 1986; 122:381–382.
49. Kerker BJ, Hood AF. Chemotherapy-induced cutaneous reactions. Semin Dermatol 1989; 8:173–181.
50. Scallan PJ, Kettler AH, Levy ML, Tschen JA. Neutrophilic eccrine hidradenitis: evidence implicating bleomycin as a causative agent. Cancer 1988; 62:2532–2536.
51. Lokich JJ, Moore C. Chemotherapy-associated palmar-plantar erythrodysesthesia syndrome. Ann Intern Med 1984; 101:798–800.
52. Cohen PR, Talpaz M, Kurzrock R: Malignancy-associated Sweet's syndrome: review of the world literature. J Clin Oncol 1988; 6:1887–1897.
53. Dreizen S, McCredie KB, Bodey GP, Keating MJ. External expressions of internal malignancy. Postgrad Med 1987; 82:91–98.

22

Intensive Care and Oncological Emergencies

Jean-Paul Sculier
Institut Jules Bordet, Université Libre de Bruxelles, Brussels, Belgium

I. INTRODUCTION

Intensive care is becoming more and more important in the management of cancer patients and major cancer hospitals have developed intensive therapy units not only for surgical patients but also for medical patients. There is, however, limited information in the medical literature about intensive care in oncology, especially concerning description (1–3) of the types of patients admitted in such units. A recent international inquiry performed in anticancer centers (4) showed that 70% of the cancer hospitals have at least one intensive care unit (ICU) that is specially devoted to patients with neoplastic diseases. Whether general, surgical, or medical, such units do not depart from the recommended guidelines for intensive care, as far as the number of beds, the nursing staff, and the main critical care techniques performed are concerned.

II. MAIN INDICATIONS FOR INTENSIVE CARE IN ONCOLOGY

Admission of patients in an ICU is usually based on the following three principles (5). First, the patients have to be "salvageable." That is, patients whose chances of being cured or having their disease put into remission are minimal should not be admitted or should not stay in an ICU. Second, the patient's "autonomy" must be respected. That is, a patient who refuses intensive supportive therapy because he or she understands the potential poor prognosis of the underlying neoplastic disease should not be admitted in the ICU. Third, because medical resources are limited, even in highly developed countries, ''distributive justice'' should be taken into account. That is, patients with the best chances of benefiting from intensive therapy should be admitted in priority.

The assumption that patients with active malignant disease should not be admitted to an ICU often predominates in general hospitals, making it difficult for oncologists to collaborate with intensivists for the management of the critically ill cancer patients. This negative opinion is not supported by scientific data; rather, it results from a bias of many physicians who refuse critical care to cancer patients even though they are willing to provide such care to patients with serious nonneoplastic diseases, such as advanced heart failure or liver cirrhosis, and who do not have a better short- or long-term prognosis (6).

There are four main reasons to admit a cancer patient to the intensive care unit:

1. Postoperative recovery (7,8) just as for any high-risk postoperative patient (availability of continuous hemodynamic monitoring, early identification of cardiovascular and respiratory disturbances, facilities for respiratory support, and constant skilled nursing care)
2. Critical complications of the cancer disease and its treatment. These are various and can be specific for oncology. Their management must take into consideration the presence of a severe chronic underlying disease.
3. Intensive anticancer treatment administration and monitoring, which is useful in various situations such as increased risk for treatment administration related to the patient's condition, administration of intensive chemotherapy requiring patient monitoring, treatment of unknown toxicity in phase I trial requiring optimal safety conditions of surveillance, and administration of treatment that frequently results in acute severe toxicity.
4. Acute disease (such as myocardial infarction or asthmatic crisis), possibly unrelated to the neoplastic disease or its treatment.

This chapter focuses on the problems that are specific to oncological critical care and reviews recent literature on the topic, giving practical guidelines based mainly on personal experience.

III. PROGNOSIS AND MORTALITY RATE OF THE CANCER PATIENT IN INTENSIVE CARE

Cancer patients who are admitted in an ICU have a higher mortality rate than those with other diseases: 55% (22 of 40) versus 17% (118 of 864) in the experience of a medical critical care unit (9) and 91% (20 of 22) versus 64% (37 of 58) in a series of patients with acute respiratory failure (10). These data must be considered cautiously, however, because of the small number of cancer patients in the series and because of the potential biases in referral of cancer patients to the ICU, making it possible that cancer patients in the ICU are at a more severe stage of the complication than noncancer patients. Moreover, in cancer centers, the ICU mortality rate is usually similar to that reported in general ICUs: 22% in a medical surgical unit (1), 23% and 22% in two consecutive series of a medical critical care unit (2,3), 3% in a surgical ICU where the patients were principally admitted for short postoperative care (11), and 50% of the patients with hematological malignancies and 41% of those with solid tumors admitted for nonoperative intensive care in a general ICU (12).

The combined impact of age and type of malignancy on ICU use and outcome has been retrospectively studied at the Memorial Sloan-Kettering Cancer Center (13). The care provided to all 1,212 patients admitted over a 2-year period was reviewed with respect to use of total parenteral nutrition, mechanical ventilation, pulmonary artery catheterization, dialysis, and blood product transfusion. Also reviewed were mean length of stay in the ICU, primary diagnosis, outcome and average daily severity of illness scores. Older patients (75 years and older) represented 14% of all intensive care unit patients and younger (between 65 and 74 years) represented 28%. The ICU mortality rate of those two groups was significantly lower than that of the youngest (younger than 65 years) patients (17%, 27%, and 30%, respectively). The use of nutritional support, pulmonary artery catheters, and dialysis was similar for all three groups but older patients used less mechanical ventilation and needed fewer blood transfusions. The two older groups had more solid tumors, similar mean length of stay in the ICU, and lower average daily therapeutic intervention scoring system (TISS) scores compared with the younger cohort. Mortality rate was not significantly different between the three groups. This study suggests that age should not be considered a determining factor in the allocation of ICU beds to patients with malignancies, similar to a report on patients undergoing craniotomy for neoplastic disease in which age was not found discriminant for ICU stay length, final outcome, or costs (14).

Scoring systems have been proposed to determine the prognosis in critically ill patients, such as APACHE II (acute physiologic and chronic health evaluation), which consists of acute physiological measures, patient's age, and chronic health status. A retrospective analysis of 451 ICU oncology admissions in a community hospital (15) has been performed to determine the role of APACHE II as a predictor of outcome in critically ill cancer patients. A direct relationship between severity of physiological derangement and the risk of death was demonstrated. Patients with scores of 30 or greater had hospital mortality rates of 100% for postoperative and 92.6% for nonoperative conditions. In a small retrospective study performed in 52 patients with breast cancer at the M.D. Anderson Cancer Center (16), a higher APACHE II score was also found significantly associated with higher mortality rate. Other factors associated with a poorer outcome were the number of metastatic sites and the presence of respiratory failure. APACHE II has also been shown to be a successful prognostic score in granulocytopenic patients with hematological malignancies (17) in both ward and ICU settings. Of the 26 ICU patients, six survived with a mean APACHE II of 18 and 20 died with a mean score of 27.5. All 14 patients with APACHE II scores exceeding 27 on the day of maximal illness died. In a retrospective study of 107 consecutive neutropenic cancer patients admitted to the ICU of a cancer hospital (18) with a multivariate analysis on prognostic factors including SAPS II (simplified acute physiological score) and number of organ system failures (OSFs), only the number of OSFs and respiratory failure were found to be independent predictors of mortality.

More data are available for patients with hematological malignancies (19–25). In-ICU mortality rate ranged between 43% and 76%; 12% to 43% of the patients could be discharged alive from the hospital. Table 1 summarizes the underlying disease, the types of organ failure, the frequency of mechanical ventilation support, and the results. Some of the reported series contain a few patients with aplastic anemia. The physiological score of the APACHE system was found to be a significant predictor for short-term outcome (20,23,25). Brunet et al. (23) reported that survivors had a SAPS (simplified acute physiologic score) calculated at admission of 11.2 ± 4.7 whereas nonsurvivors had a SAPS of 16.1 ± 6.3. The number of organ failures was also found to be a significant predictor (20,22) for in-ICU mortality. However, there seems to be no relationship between the severity of the acute illness phase as assessed by the APACHE II and the duration of long-term survival after hospital discharge (24). The number of failed organs appears also to be not a good predictor of long-term prognosis (24).

Oncology pediatric patients admitted to an ICU have been evaluated for outcome (26,27). Severity of illness measured by the physiological stability index and quantity of care measured by the TISS were both predictors of in-ICU mortality (26), but the authors emphasized that these methods are not sufficient to decide withdrawal of support in individual cases. This point is also true for all the studies discussed herein. The pediatric risk score for mortality (PRISM) was also found to be predictive of survival but with the same limitations (27).

Causes of death were analyzed in a medical oncology ICU (28). Among 330 admissions, 55% were for a medical complication and 47 patients (28%) died in the ICU. Only one death was reported among the 150 patients admitted for monitoring during administration for an intensive or potentially toxic treatment. Autopsy was performed in 34 cases. The clinical diagnosis of the immediate cause of death was correct in only 41% of the cases, probably because uncomfortable investigations were often not performed when the survival estimation became

Table 1 Prognosis of Patients with Hematologic Malignancies in Intensive Care

Reference	Schuster 1983 (19)	Lloyd-Thomas 1986 (20)	Butt 1988 (21)	Torrecilla 1988 (22)	Brunet 1990 (23)	Yau 1991 (24)	Paz 1997 (25)
Number of patients	77	22	133 (children)	25	260	92	36
Underlying disease							
Lymphoma	26	7	21	2	54	28	10
Leukemia	48	15	75	23	144	61	24
Bone marrow transplant	—	—	—	25	?	—	all
Organ failure							
Respiratory	41	20	41	18	175	?	25
Renal	?	?	?	?	49		?
Cardiac-circulatory	15	?	36	12	106		5
Bone marrow	?	15	?	8	123		?
Cerebral	7	?	29	2	51		1
Hepatic	?	?	?	2	?		?
Septic shock/sepsis	14	?	28	12	235	?	10
Mechanical ventilation	52	17	67	16	111	?	28
Postoperative care	—	—	27	—	—	?	—
In intensive care unit mortality rate	59%	55%	48%	76%	43%	65%	67%
In hospital mortality rate	80%	82%	?	88%	57%	77%	?
Survival rate	20%	18%	?	12%	43%	23%	?

poor. Authors found an unexpected high frequency of pathological evidence of pulmonary edema (68% of the cases in which autopsies were done). No predictive factor for this phenomenon could be determined, but a tentative explanation was the existence of an enhanced immune response working on pulmonary capillaries sensitized by the metastatic process, making cancer patients more "fragile."

IV. CARDIOPULMONARY RESUSCITATION

Cardiopulmonary resuscitation (CPR) of the cancer patient is a controversial procedure, particularly if metastases are present. A review (29) of all the studies published from 1980 to 1989 dealing with survival after CPR showed that far fewer patients with cancer survived to discharge compared with patients with other diagnoses. Of nine studies of outcome after CPR, only two found patients with cancer who survived and were discharged (total of seven patients of 243 resuscitated), and all these patients had localized disease; there were no survivors among patients with metastatic disease. These data, from which it could be recommended not to resuscitate metastatic cancer patients, are not supported by other experiences, reported by intensivists from cancer centers.

The effectiveness of cardiopulmonary resuscitation in medical and surgical cancer patients was evaluated at Memorial Sloan-Kettering Cancer Center in New York (30). During a 3-year period, 750 patients suffered from cardiopulmonary arrest (1.53% of all admissions) and 114 underwent resuscitative procedures because of their good general conditions and the absence of a no-code status (not-for-resuscitation) order. Seventy-five patients (66%) were successfully resuscitated but only 12 of these (16%), including patients with metastatic disease, survived long enough to be discharged from the hospital, after an average stay of 11.3 days in the ICU and with an overall mean survival after discharge of 223 days (median: 150 days; range: 3 to 350 days). A statistical analysis showed that performance status on admission was the single significant and independent factor that predicted the likelihood of being discharged alive before cardiopulmonary arrest and after successful CPR. Age, interval from diagnosis of cancer to the arrest, sex, underlying malignancy, and cause of arrest were not significant prognostic factors in the study.

A retrospective analysis of the patients admitted to a medical ICU was conducted at the Jules Bordet Institute in Brussels (31) to determine the effectiveness and potential indications of CPR. During a 6-year period, cardiac arrest occurred in 49 nonsurgical cancer patients (Table 2). Cardiopulmonary resuscitation was successful in 19 (39%) but only five (10%) were discharged alive from the hospital. Cardiopulmonary resuscitation was successful in all eight patients in whom cardiac arrest was the consequence of an acute cardiovascular drug toxicity, even

Table 2 Results of Cardiopulmonary Resuscitation According to Patient's Clinical Characteristics in a Medical Oncology Intensive Care Unit

	Category			
	A	*B*	*C*	*D*
n	30	12	2	5
Mean age (years)	50	56	57	52
Range	20–77	26–77	54–60	42–63
Type of tumor				
Solid	13	7	2	5
Locoregional	3	2	—	1
Metastatic	10	5	2	4
Hematological	17	5	—	—
Functional stage				
Diagnosis	2	—	—	—
Treatment for cure	14	4	—	—
Treatment for control	11	5	1	5
Candidate for palliative care	3	3	1	—
Cause of admission to ICU				
Cardiac arrest	5	5	2	2
Anticancer treatment	—	—	—	3
Medical complications	25	7	—	—
Cause of cardiac arrest				
Drug cardiovascular toxicity	—	2	1	5
Other causes	30	10	1	0

Abbreviations: Category A, patients who failed to respond to cardiopulmonary resuscitation (CPR); category B, patients who had a successful CPR but died later in the ICU; category C, patients who had a successful CPR but died in the hospital after discharge from the ICU; category D, patients who had a successful CPR and were discharged from the hospital; ICU, intensive care unit.
Source: Ref. 31.

if the cancer was metastatic and the purpose of the treatment not curative. Five of these patients could be discharged alive from the hospital. Cardiopulmonary resuscitation was only effective in 25% of the patients in whom cardiac arrest was an ultimate complication of various problems such as septic shock or respiratory failure complicating a neoplastic disease; none of these patients could be discharged alive from the hospital. The results of this study suggest that, in cancer, like in other types of disease, CPR is mainly indicated when cardiac arrest is the consequence of an acute insult, as stated in the initial report in 1960 by Kouwenhoven et al. on closed-chest massage that was used with a high success rate to resuscitate victims of insults such as drowning, electrical shock, drug overdose, anesthetic accident, heart block, acute myocardial infarction, or surgery.

V. CRITICAL CARE OF PATIENTS WITH COMPLICATIONS OF CANCER OR ITS TREATMENT

Complications of cancer or its treatment are multiple, as illustrated in Table 3 by data obtained during a 28-month period in the medical ICU at Jules Bordet Institute in Brussels. These complications have specific characteristics related to their particular frequency (e.g., coronary acute events are rare but hypercalcemia is frequent), to the occurrence of complications only seen in oncological patients (e.g., acute tumoral lysis or leukostasis), and to the presence of a severe underlying disease (i.e., cancer). Management of the patient must take into account the underlying neoplastic disease making the patient more fragile because of the presence of immunosuppression, neutropenia, hemostatic disorders, metastatic process, or paraneoplastic syndromes. Treatment must integrate critical care support, anticancer therapy, and preventive or supportive care of related toxic effects. The toxicity of neoplastic drugs often is increased in critically ill cancer patients because of their poor general condition, with a low performance status making them ineligible for regular cancer treatment protocols. In this section, the focus is on points specific to intensive care; other complications are discussed in more detail in other chapters of this book and in other books (32,33).

A. Respiratory Problems

Among all the potential complications of cancer or its treatment, respiratory problems are the only ones for which relatively consistent data are available from the point of view of critical care medicine, particularly concerning adult respiratory distress syndrome (ARDS), outcome of respiratory failure, and results of mechanical ventilation.

In addition to the usual causes (e.g., infections), ARDS can rarely be due to specific complications of cancer. As the result of a direct neoplastic infiltration of the lungs (34–36), initial presentation of cancer can be ARDS in solid tumors and lymphomas as well as in leukemia. This picture may be indistinguishable from ARDS from other causes. Anticancer treatment can also cause ARDS by various mechanisms; it can induce lung damage by tissue factors released from necrotic leukemic cells following chemotherapy (37). In the ''retinoic acid syndrome,'' all-trans retinoic acid induces a capillary leak syndrome with fever, weight gain, and episodic hypotension as well as a respiratory failure syndrome resulting from lung interstitial infiltration with maturing myeloid cells (38). Cyto-

Table 3 Types of Medical Complications Requiring Admission in a Medical Intensive Care Unit[a]

I. Respiratory problems *(58)*	
Upper respiratory failure	3
Pleural effusion	10
Pneumothorax	5
Pneumonia	14
Diffuse pneumonitis	8
ARDS	4
Various	14
II. Cardiovascular problems *(82)*	
Syncope	4
Cardiac arrest	7
Thromboembolic disease	15
Arrhythmias	26
Cardiac failure	8
Myocardial infarction	7
Thoracic pain	4
Pericardial disease	8
Superior vena cava obstruction	3
III. Renal and metabolic problems *(58)*	
Acute renal failure	9
Schwarz-Bartter syndrome	6
Hypercalcemia	33
Diabetes mellitus	2
Tumoral lysis and/or leukostasis	8
IV. Neurological problems *(28)*	
Encephalopathies	5
Infectious meningitis	1
Neoplastic meningitis	1
Intracranial hypertension	3
Convulsions	8
Paralysis and stroke	6
Drug intoxication	4
V. Digestive problems *(13)*	
Acute abdomen	5
Ascitis	2
Liver failure	3
Digestive bleeding	3
VI. Infections hematological and shock problems *(63)*	
Fungal infections	2
Bacteremia	3
Febrile neutropenia	5
Septic shock	31
Hypovolemic shock	5
Other types of shock	2
Allergic reactions	2
Various types of bleeding	8
Coagulopathies	2
Severe anemia	3

[a] Experience obtained at the Jules Bordet Institute between October 1989 and January 1992.

static drugs, cytokines (e.g., interleukin-2), and chest irradiation may also have a direct toxic effect on the lungs leading to an increased alveolar capillary permeability and noncardiogenic pulmonary edema (39–41). Some of the new drugs recently introduced for treatment of common solid tumors have been the object of pulmonary toxicity with fatal pulmonary edema in the case of gemcitabine, with a clinical picture similar to that reported with Ara C (42), or with severe interstitial pneumonia associated with lymphocytopenia when paclitaxel and radiotherapy are used (43).

Neutropenia induced by chemotherapy does not protect the patient against ARDS (44). The frequency of neutropenia in bacteremic patients who had ARDS was compared with that in a control group who had bacteremia alone (45); 3 of 18 patients in the ARDS group were neutropenic as opposed to 1 of 18 in the control group. Histological examination of the lungs from two of these patients with ARDS and neutropenia demonstrated the absence of neutrophils. A frequent cause of ARDS in febrile neutropenic patients given appropriate standard empirical antibiotherapy is septicemia caused by streptococcal species such as *Streptococcus mitis* (46).

Patients with severe thrombopenia and hematological malignancies, particularly in case of bone marrow transplantation, may have diffuse alveolar hemorrhage and major respiratory distress (47). This complication usually requires intubation and artificial ventilation; the prognosis is significantly improved if high-dose corticosteroids are administered.

Consider the following etiologies and specific treatment:

1. Pneumocystis carinii: high-dose cotrimoxazole
2. Cytomegalovirus: ganciclovir plus immunoglobulins
3. Aspergillosis: amphotericin B
4. Carcinomatous lymphangitis: chemotherapy, steroids
5. Leucostasis: chemotherapy, leukapheresis
6. Diffuse alveolar hemorrhage: high-dose corticosteroids
7. Leucoagglutinines (transfusions): corticosteroids
8. Capillary leak syndrome resulting from interleukin 2: stop IL-2 therapy and consider corticotherapy

The following practical recommendations can be given for the management of ARDS in the cancer patient:

1. Perform, if indicated, sputum culture, bronchoalveolar lavage, transbronchial biopsy.
2. Control thrombopenia, particularly in case of bleeding.
3. Try, if possible, continuous positive airway pressure (CPAP) with a facial mask before intubation.

4. Prefer oral over nasal tracheal intubation and consider early tracheotomy.
5. Choose artificial ventilation continuous positive pressure ventilation (CPPV) with a positive end-expiratory pressure or permissive hypercapnia.
6. Maintain an adequate circulation status with fluids and vasopressors but avoid fluid overload facilitated by the frequent presence of a capillary leak syndrome.
7. Provide adequate sedation and analgesia to the patient.
8. Consider corticotherapy if no improvement is observed after a few days to prevent lung fibrosis.

Respiratory distress can also be due to obstruction of the major airways by tumors involving the tracheobronchial tree. Because conventional treatment such as radiation therapy or chemotherapy is often too slow to reopen the airway, endoscopic Nd:YAG laser therapy should be used without delay and may allow rapid relief of dyspnea (48). Another life-threatening emergency is massive hemoptysis for which the cause must be rapidly identified to provide appropriate treatment such as surgery, endobronchial laser therapy, bronchial artery embolization (49), or corticotherapy in cases of diffuse alveolar damage (47).

Pleural effusion is a common complication of lung cancer and metastatic malignancies (50). It can be life-threatening and was significantly present in about half of the patients with solid tumors managed by artificial ventilation in the series reported by Snow et al. (51). A pleural effusion in a cancer patient is not always malignant but can result from therapy (irradiation or chemotherapy), lymphatic obstruction, superior vena cava syndrome, bronchial obstruction with pneumonia or atelectasis, pulmonary embolism, or hypoproteinemia. In the case of malignant effusion, long-term control often requires pleurodesis with a sclerosing agent such as bleomycin or iodized talc. Talc is probably the most effective agent in this indication and can be instillated during thoracoscopy or through a tube thoracostomy (52).

Table 4 summarizes the data available about the outcome of cancer patients with respiratory failure (19,20,22,23,51,53–57). All the studies except that by Snow et al. (51) have been performed in patients with hematological malignancies or bone marrow transplantation. Most of the patients (85% to 100%) have received mechanical ventilation. The causes of respiratory failure are often not explained and the classifications used are heterogeneous, preventing the reader from getting a good knowledge of the frequencies of the various complications requiring ventilation support. In-ICU mortality rates range between 60% and 82%, with a rate of discharge from the hospital between 4% and 20%. The only study including patients with solid tumors (51) has shown that patients with breast cancer who received mechanical ventilation have a better survival outlook than

Table 4 Outcome of Cancer Patients with Respiratory Failure

Reference	Snow (51)	Schuster (19)	Estopa (53)	Lloyd-Thomas (20)	Torrecilla (22)	Peters (54)	Denardo (55)	Brunet (23)	Crawford (56)	Todd (57)
Number of patients	180	52	30	20	18	116	50	111	348	54
Patient selection	no	Hematological	Hematological	Hematological	BMT	Hematological	BMT	Hematological	BMT	BMT in children
Percent with mechanical ventilation	100%	100%	87%	87%	89%	100%	88%	100%	100%	100%
In ICU mortality rate	74%	77%	80%	60%	83%		82%	85%	79%	
Hospital discharged		8%	7%	20%		18%	18%	13%	4%	11%
6-Month survival	7%		7%					79%	66%	
Median survival time						12 months	124 days			

Abbreviations: BMT, bone marrow transplantation.

those with hematological or other solid malignancies. However, no multivariate analysis has been done to confirm this observation. In the study performed in Seattle on 348 patients with respiratory failure complicating bone marrow transplantation and requiring artificial ventilation (56), 72 (21%) were extubated and 15 (4%) were discharged from the hospital with 10 (3%) surviving 6 months after transplantation. All the survivors were physically functional. Older age, active malignancy at the time of transplantation, and donor-recipient marrow HLA-nonidentity were found to be risk factors for subsequent respiratory failure in this population of 1482 patients, of whom 23% required mechanical ventilation.

B. Cardiovascular Problems

As shown in Table 3, the main cardiovascular problems requiring intensive care in cancer patients are arrhythmias and thromboembolic complications. For other problems such as myocardial infarction or cardiac failure, the treatment is basically the same as in nonneoplastic diseases. There are no studies supporting a more specific approach for cancer patients.

Intensivists should be aware of the potential cardiotoxicity of a series of anticancer drugs such as anthracyclines, high-dose cyclophosphamide, amsacrine, 5-fluorouracil, taxol, and interleukin-2 (58). Anthracyclines—doxorubicin and epirubicin—can rarely cause acute and subacute cardiac toxicity, consisting of arrhythmias, acute failure of the left ventricle, and pericarditis or a fatal pericarditis-myocarditis syndrome. The cardiotoxicity of anthracyclines is mainly chronic, related to the cumulative dose received and resulting in cardiac failure (59). High doses of cyclophosphamide, usually in the context of bone marrow transplantation, can induce particularly severe cardiac toxicity: myocardial necrosis with fatal failure, pericardial effusions with or without tamponade, life-threatening arrythmias, or conduction blocks. Total doses of more than 200 mg/kg should not be administered (60). This toxicity appears to be directly related to the dose expressed by body square meter (61) and to the drug pharmacokinetics (62). Another commonly used cytostatic agent, 5-fluorouracil, can cause various and frequent cardiac side effects: angina, supraventricular or ventricular tachycardia, congestive heart failure, reversible cardiomyopathy, myocardial infarction, and sudden death (63). The toxicity results probably from a direct toxic effect of the drug on the myocardial cell (64). Besides the hemodynamic consequences of the capillary leak syndrome, interleukin-2 can induce fatal noninfectious myocarditis or acute myocardial infarction (65).

Cardiac tamponade is a common cause of shock in cancer patients. Diagnosis of pericardial effusion is performed by echography. Treatment requires drainage (66); systemic anticancer therapy is effective in controlling the malignant effusion in cases of tumors that are very sensitive to chemotherapy, and local intrapericardial sclerosis with tetracycline or bleomycin can avoid effusion relapses (67).

Surgery with creation of a pleuropericardial or pleuroperitoneal window is highly effective in preventing fluid reaccumulation and has little morbidity (68).

The superior vena cava obstruction syndrome, although spectacular in some cases, should not be considered as an emergency for radiotherapy. With careful surveillance and work-up a pathological diagnosis can be obtained (69).

Pulmonary embolism is a common complication in the oncological patient. It is usually caused by a thrombus formation in a peripheral vein, giving the classic clinical picture of thromboembolic disease and which must be treated with the same approach as in the noncancer patient. However, the differential diagnosis should be performed with pulmonary tumor embolism (70), in which neoplastic cells cause a direct obstruction of the pulmonary capillaries, giving a picture of respiratory distress. When analyzing the cytology of blood aspirated from a wedged pulmonary catheter, neoplastic cells must be differentiated from megacaryocytes by an experienced pathologist. Treatment of pulmonary tumor embolism consists mainly of anticancer chemotherapy. When occurring at a slow rate, this complication leads to the picture of carcinomatous lymphangitis.

Nonbacterial thrombotic endocarditis is another typical complication of cancer. It is the source of systemic embolism and is associated with disseminated intravascular coagulation with increased levels of circulating D-dimers. Diagnosis is suggested by a clinical picture of repeated systemic embolisms and can be demonstrated by echocardiography showing valvular vegetations. This problem is not rare, as suggested by a study performed in 200 nonselected ambulatory patients with a solid tumor, in which the presence of cardiac valvular vegetations was found in 19% of the patients by the routine performance of echocardiography (71). Thromboembolism was significantly more frequent in those patients in comparison to those with a normal test. Treatment is based on the specific control of the neoplastic disease.

C. Renal and Metabolic Problems

Hypercalcemia, in our experience, is the most frequent metabolic complication related to cancer (see Table 3). Management has changed in the past decade because there has been progress made in therapy; rehydration and biphosphonates are the standard treatment (72). Pamidronate (APD) has been shown by randomized trials to be more effective than another biphosphonate—etidronate (73)—and more effective than plicamycin, priorly called mithramycin (74). Extensive research has been performed to develop more potent biphosphonates such as ibandronate (75). It is unclear, however, whether hypercalcemia is a direct cause of death in cancer patients or simply a marker of advanced disease. A retrospective study (76) of 126 consecutively studied patients with cancer-associated hypercalcemia attempted to answer that question. Despite effective antihypercalcemia treatment (mainly biphosphonates), which resulted in a significant decrease in serum calcium levels and in an improvement of all symptoms (including renal and central nervous system manifestations) except pain, the overall median survival was poor (30 days). Follow-up measurement of serum calcium was done in 40 patients until death; recurrent or persistent hypercalcemia was present in 11 and contributed to death in 7. Those data suggest that hypercalcemia is a marker of advanced cancer rather than the actual cause of death in many cases. Moreover, the availability of specific anticancer treatment was an important prognostic indicator for survival. The median survival was 135 days for the 26 patients who underwent such treatment, compared with 30 days in the remainder. From the critical care point of view, patients with severe hypercalcemia should probably not be admitted to an ICU if specific cancer therapy is not available. Practically, treatment consists of rehydration by 3 to 4 liters per day with normal saline for 24 to 48 hours followed by a 4-hour pamidronate (1 mg/kg or 60 mg) infusion. A randomized trial has recently established that a 4-hour infusion duration is as effective as a 24-hour duration (77). In cases of severe and symptomatic hypercalcemia with neurological or cardiovascular symptoms, calcitonin or calcium-free hemodialysis (78) can be proposed to obtain a more rapid control of the calcemia.

Other metabolic emergencies include hyponatremia (often in the context of inappropriate secretion of antidiuretic hormone), ectopic adrenocorticotropic syndrome, adrenal failure, hypoglycemia, lactic acidosis, and tumoral lysis syndrome (79,80). Lactic acidosis may be a rare complication of extensive cancer, particularly in cases of metastatic hepatic lesions. Chemotherapy against the neoplastic disease is the only effective treatment of this type of lactic acidosis (81). Tumor lysis syndrome is rarely spontaneous, but it is often induced by chemotherapy. This clinical picture is made of various metabolic derangements: hyperkalemia, hyperuricemia, and hyperphosphatemia resulting from massive cell lysis and being a potential cause of severe renal failure. The release of several active enzymes by the lysed cells can induce lung damage and ARDS (82). One practical approach to this syndrome is as follows:

1. Initial phase (before anticancer treatment administration). Take measures against hyperuricemia:
   Hyperdiuresis with saline and bicarbonate: maintain a diuresis of >2.5 L/m^2/24 h with a urinary pH of 7.5.
   Urate-oxydase: 1000 U IV q6–8h (Uricozyme).
2. Cytotoxic therapy. Initiate as soon as hyperuricemia is controlled and a correct diuresis is obtained.
3. Postanticancer therapy phase:
   Stop urine alkalinization as soon as hyperuricemia is controlled.
   Maintain saline hyperdiuresis, eventually with the help of furosemide or dopamine at low dosage.
   Control hyperkalemia with oral exchange resins.

4. Extrarenal epuration. Perform early in cases of massive fluid retention, systemic acidosis, uncontrolled hyperkalemia, acute renal failure, or symptomatic hypocalcemia.

Hyponatremia is another frequent metabolic complication that can be related to cancer (83) or its treatment (84). The syndrome of inappropriate secretion of antidiuretic hormone (SIADH), also called Schwarz-Bartter syndrome, is a classic clinical presentation for small cell lung cancer. In a context of asthenia, nausea, anorexia, headaches, confusion, somnolence, convulsions, or coma, diagnosis is performed by the following clinical and biological signs: hyponatremia, maintained natriuresis, no evidence of fluid depletion, plasmatic hypo-osmolality, relatively increased urinary osmolality, and normal renal, adrenal, and thyroid functions. Treatment consists of fluid restriction or administration of urea (30–40 g/d without fluid restriction).

Renal failure has various causes in cancer patients (e.g., tumor invasion of the kidney or of the urinary tract [ureteral obstruction]; acute tumor lysis syndrome; nephrotoxic drugs including high-dose methotrexate, cisplatin, and mitomycin; hypercalcemia; multiple myeloma; infections; renal hypoperfusion). When a cancer patient is admitted to the ICU with renal failure, the first step is to exclude by an echographic examination a postrenal cause. If bladder retention or ureteral obstruction is diagnosed, an adequate catheterization must be performed. In some patients, the procedure is followed by an osmotic hyperdiuresis resulting from renal recovery, which can lead to severe metabolic disorders if not appropriately managed. In other patients, differential diagnosis should be performed by biological tests between functional and organic renal failure. Management is similar to that of noncancer patients.

D. Neurological Problems

Neurological complications are a less frequent source of admission of cancer patients to the ICU. This does not mean that neurological emergencies are rare, but they are usually not life-threatening. For example, epidural carcinomatosis (85) complicates about 1% of the cancers and can benefit from early corticotherapy (86). Encephalopathies, convulsions, and some paralytic presentations are the principal types of problems that are referred, in my experience, to intensive care. These problems may be due to direct neoplastic involvement such as meningeal carcinomatosis (87); antineoplastic drug toxicity (88) (e.g., ifosfamide is responsible for frequent encephalopathies [89] that are potentially reversible by methylene-blue [90], or high-dose cytosine arabinoside is responsible for acute polyneuropathies with quadriparesis and need for ventilation support [91]), paraneoplastic syndromes such as myasthenic crisis associated with thymoma (92);

or severe central nervous system infections (93). Drug intoxication occurs rarely in the cancer patient population of a cancer hospital and is usually iatrogenic.

E. Digestive Problems

Digestive complications of the cancer patients are not frequent in a medical ICU because many of them are treated in surgical ICUs. Acute abdomen, particularly in neutropenic patients, is a difficult problem. A retrospective analysis of 50 neutropenic patients (mainly with hematological malignancies) with abdominal pain (94) revealed that abdominal distention was the only sign associated with mortality. The study failed to find pivotal signs or symptoms for the decision for or against surgical intervention. Overall, 60% of the patients in this series died, confirming the results of prior reports. Care of patients with neutropenic enterocolitis (also called typhlitis) should be individualized (95,96): nonsurgical management with bowel rest, decompression, nutritional support, and broad-spectrum antibiotics is recommended initially. Surgery is indicated for those with perforation or those whose condition deteriorated clinically during close, frequent observation.

Hepatic veno-occlusive disease (VOD) is a major complication of intensive therapy associated with bone marrow transplantation, with a potential high risk of death by liver insufficiency (97). It is frequently associated with a multiorgan failure with renal and cardiopulmonary insufficiencies (98). It can be reversed by rt-PA (99,100) with a major risk of fatal hemorrhage. Otherwise, management of established VOD is essentially symptomatic, including careful monitoring of electrolyte balance.

F. Infectious, Hematological, and Shock Problems

Because of the effects of the neoplastic disease and its treatment, coagulation disorders, neutropenia, and immunosuppression are often present in the same patient, predisposing him or her to development of infections (101) and septic or hypovolemic (by bleeding) shocks. As shown in Table 3 (and as expected), septic shock is a main cause of admission for cancer patients in the ICU. A retrospective analysis of causes of death in febrile granulocytopenic cancer patients receiving empirical antibiotic therapy (102) has shown that infection was the main cause of death with two-thirds of the cases presenting with septic shock, followed by bleeding complications (diffuse or cerebromeningeal hemorrhage). The management of the cancer patients with septic shock and other types of shock is mainly standard without major critical care specific measures. (Antibiotics are discussed elsewhere in this book.) A practical approach for the management of the patient with septic shock is the following:

1. Anti-infectious treatment:
   - Perform blood culture and search for a source: Lung? Urine? Skin? Neuromeningeal? Abdominal? Endocarditis?
   - Start, as soon as possible, antibiotics on an empirical basis: combination of a β-lactamine and an aminoside, with a glycopeptide when staphylococcal infection is suspected.
2. Anti-shock therapy. In addition to oxygenotherapy and ventilation support:
   - 1st phase: fluid resuscitation with colloid or starch, and CVP monitoring.
   - 2nd phase (in case of nonadequate response): vasopressor, i.e. dopamine (5 to 20 γ/kg/min).
   - 3rd phase (in case of presisting shock): perform echocardiography or right cardiac catheterization:
   - If hyperdynamic syndrome persists: infusion of norepinephrine.
   - In hypovolemia: further fluid resuscitation and exclude a specific cause (e.g., ex. bleeding).
   - In left ventricular dyfunction: add to dopamine the inotrope dobutamine.

Allergic reactions to cytotoxic drugs are multiple and can be seen with many agents (102,103). Type I hypersensitivity reactions predominate. The drugs with the highest risks of such complications are L-asparaginase and taxans, followed by teniposide and etoposide, cisplatin and its analogues, and cytarabine. The exact mechanism by which a cytostatic drug induces an allergic reaction has rarely been investigated and it is probable that ancillary drugs and excipients sometimes play an important role. In cases in which anaphylactic reactions are frequent, a prophylaxis by antihistamines and corticoids may be administered and patients monitored in ICU. In any case, the drug should not be given in the absence of a physician.

Severe, potentially lethal bleeding is another frequent problem in oncology, especially in patients with leukemia or undergoing chemotherapy. In a retrospective analysis of 438 patients with acute leukemia (104), there was bleeding on admission in 38% of the patients and during the first month in 11%. Twenty-six fatal bleedings were documented, mainly at the intracranial level followed by the gastrointestinal tract.

VI. INTENSIVE CARE FOR ANTICANCER TREATMENT ADMINISTRATION AND SURVEILLANCE

Anticancer treatment administration and surveillance is a new activity for intensive care medicine resulting from the progress made in medical oncology requiring sophisticated support for some types of new therapies (4). Data about these indications are still limited.

A. Risk for Treatment Administration Related to the Patient's Condition

Anticancer treatment administration can be at special risk in some patients because of their own health condition or of the clinical situation. The problems to be managed are multiple and, when suspected, patients can be admitted in the ICU for the treatment surveillance. A severe risk of acute toxicity can be expected from drug interactions and from interactions between the patient and the treatment because of the patient's poor general condition or to more specific problems such as comorbidity or prior reactions to therapy. An anticancer treatment should be administered in such a patient only if the potential benefit for the patient is high and if the patient has provided appropriate informed consent.

B. Administration of Intensive Chemotherapy Requiring Patient Monitoring

Intensive or high-dose chemotherapy, often performed in the context of bone marrow transplantation, can induce various severe nonhematological toxicities (105). Whereas with standard-dose chemotherapy, limiting toxicity is usually hematological (leukopenia or thrombopenia), in high-dose chemotherapy, limiting toxicity can be multiple according to the drugs used: gastrointestinal (mucositis, diarrhea), cardiac (arythmias, necrosis, tamponade), pulmonary (fibrosis), neurological (encephalopathy, coma, brain necrosis), renal (renal failure), urothelial (hemorrhagic cystitis), or hepatic (acute hepatitis, fibrosis).

The rigorous schedules for administering chemotherapy, infusion of large volumes of fluid and management of the side effects, may require close monitoring of the patient as optimally provided in an ICU. Two drugs can be particularly dangerous when given at high doses without appropriate expertise: methotrexate (106) and cyclophosphamide (60). Methotrexate can induce particularly severe renal failure and cyclophosphamide can induce cardiac necrosis and arrythmias.

C. Treatment of Unknown Toxicity in Phase I Trial Requiring Optimal Safety Conditions of Surveillance

New phase I trials of anticancer drugs have to be performed directly in patients with cancer, because of their important carcinogenic properties. These drugs are usually given in patients who have good performance status and no major other disease, but for which cancer cannot be treated with effective curative or palliative antineoplastic treatment. If a severe toxic effect occurs, patients have to be treated by adequate supportive care, including critical care techniques such as resuscitation. It is thus recommended to administer these new drugs in optimal safety conditions such as those present in ICUs. One example of the life-threatening complications that might occur during phase I trials is the potentiation of chemotherapy by drugs inhibiting the multiple drug resistance expression in cancer cells, for example, high-dose verapamil, which has induced acute cardiac side effects (e.g., heart blocks) that have been appropriately managed by the ICU team (107).

D. Administration of Treatment Frequently Resulting in Acute Severe Toxicity

Administration of some anticancer treatments is regularly associated with a high risk of acute complications, because of the immediate toxicity of the drug or with the complexity of the care to be provided. Thus, it should preferably be managed in an ICU. Recent developments in medical oncology have produced an application for this indication: adoptive immunotherapy with interleukin-2 (IL-2).

Interleukin-2 is the cytokine that has allowed a renewal of immunotherapy and has become part of the standard management of renal carcinoma. However, IL-2 is associated with complex and potentially severe toxicity, particularly when given at high dose (108). These side effects are mainly related to the occurrence of a capillary leak syndrome with a hemodynamic pattern similar to that of septic shock (109), which can evolve to a multiple organ failure syndrome (40). Patients given high-dose IL-2 require appropriate cardiac rate and rhythm, blood pressure, urinary output, body weight, respiratory rate, temperature, and consciousness and mental status surveillance. Treatment of complications may require critical care techniques including vasopressor agents and mechanical ventilation.

VII. CRITICAL CARE TECHNIQUES IN CANCER PATIENTS

Critical care techniques performed in cancer patients are basically the same as in noncancer patients. This section reviews specific data and considerations that can be useful in the management of critically ill oncological patients.

A. Central Venous Catheters

Cancer patients, mainly those undergoing chemotherapy, often have permanent central venous catheters. Totally implantable injection ports (110) are increasingly being used, and they appear to be safer than classic external indwelling catheters (111). Those catheters cannot be used for correctly measuring central venous pressure, and, in the case of infection, the policy is to provide treatment to the patient with the catheter to save it (in that situation, antibiotics should be administered through the suspected lumen). If the catheter is obstructed by a thrombus, low-dose urokinase can be used to restore its function (112). Streptokinase should not be used repetitively to avoid potential allergic reactions. Furthermore, the prolonged presence of a central venous catheter predisposes to the development of superior vena cava syndrome, a new iatrogenic entity (113).

Interleukin-2 induces defects in neutrophil chemotaxis, facilitating the occurrence of staphylococcal infections, with catheters being a common source. A randomized trial performed in 92 patients has shown a significant reduction in triple-lumen catheter-related sepsis when prohylactic antibiotics were administered (114).

The profoundly thrombocytopenic patient is particularly exposed to hemorrhagic complications resulting from central line placement. With appropriate precautions, including using platelet transfusions and experienced personnel, the bleeding risk is minimal (115).

B. Invasive Monitoring and Right Cardiac Catheterization

The risks of invasive procedures are likely to be high in cancer patients, particularly when they have neutropenia or thrombopenia. With appropriate management, including administration of platelets and fresh frozen plasma, these techniques can, however, be performed without major complications (20,115) and can be helpful. In a series (23) of 54 patients with septic shock requiring a right heart catheterization to adjust a treatment combining inotropic or vasoactive agents and volume expansion, 15 were discharged from the ICU (mortality rate, 73%) and four were still alive 1 year later.

A pulmonary artery catheter can be useful to obtain blood to perform pulmonary microvascular cytology and to contribute to the diagnosis of neoplastic pulmonary embolism lymphangitic carcinomatosis (116).

C. Renal Replacement Therapy

Renal replacement therapy includes peritoneal dialysis, hemodialysis, and hemofiltration. In a series of 31 patients with hematological malignancy and acute renal failure (117), a combination of hemofiltration and hemodialysis was applied to 22 patients and recovery of renal function occurred in six. In another study (23), hemodialysis was performed in 34 patients, also with hematological malignancies, for sepsis-related anuria (22 cases) or acute hydroelectrolytic disease (12 cases). Eleven of these patients were discharged from the ICU (mortality rate, 67%) and five were still alive 1 year later. In a series (118) of 30 pediatric patients requiring dialysis early after bone marrow transplantation, seven recovered a normal renal function and all long-term survivors were among them. These results show that renal replacement therapy can be effective in critically ill cancer patients.

For the cancer-associated hemolytic-uremic syndrome, immunoperfusion over staphylococcal patients A column appears to be the most successful treatment (119).

D. Respiratory Assistance and Mechanical Ventilation

In patients requiring respiratory assistance and in sufficiently compliant patients, continuous positive airway pressure (CPAP) by face mask can be a good means to avoid endotracheal intubation, particularly when respiratory failure is due to diffuse pulmonary infiltrates such as *Pneumocystis carinii* pneumonia (120,121). If tracheal intubation is necessary, the oral route is more advisable than the nasal one, in order to prevent infection of nasal sinuses.

If thrombocytopenia is associated with neutropenia, some authors recommend early tracheostomy to reduce the risk of occurrence of bleeding gums, nasal bleeding, and fungal infections of the oropharynx (122). Tracheostomy using electrocautery and careful technique can be performed without major complications in those patients (123). Furthermore, it allows easier tracheal aspirations, better oropharyngeal care, and more facile weaning (124) and can be performed early, without increased mortality rate (125).

Leukopenic patients with severe respiratory failure are usually ventilated by volume-controlled procedures. A recent comparative study (126) has established that they can perfectly tolerate biphasic positive airway pressure ventilation, allowing the application, for example, of permissive hypercapnia in ARDS cases.

Results of treatment of respiratory failure by mechanical failure have been reported in adult patients with solid tumors (51,126a) and with hematological malignancies (19,20,22,23,53–56), and in children (21,26,57,127). They are summarized in Table 5: survival rates (with extubation and ICU discharge) range between 0% and 35%. Some authors have reported that mechanical ventilation for more than 5 to 7 days was associated with uniformly fatal prognosis (19,20,22), but this statement is not supported by the results of larger series (23,54) showing that long-term survival can be obtained after prolonged survival.

E. Multiple Life Support Techniques

The need for multiple life support techniques is associated with poor prognosis as described by Brunet et al. (23). In their study, 62 patients had multiple life support techniques performed. Few of those patients were discharged from the ICU: four of 31 required both mechanical ventilation and hemodynamic monitoring of shock, one of eight required both ventilation and hemodialysis, and one of 12 required all three techniques.

Table 5 Results Obtained in Cancer Patients with Respiratory Failure Treated by Mechanical Ventilation

Reference	Type of cancer	Number of patients	Survivors
Snow (51)	Any type	180	26%
Ewer (126)	Lung cancer	46	15%
Schuster (19)	Hematological malignancy	52	23%
Estopa (53)	Hematological malignancy	26	7%
Lloyd-Thomas (20)	Hematological malignancy	17	35%
Torrecilla (22)	Hematological malignancy	16	6%
Peters (54)	Hematological malignancy	116	18%
Denardo (55)	Bone marrow transplant (BMT)	40	2.5%
Brunet (23)	Hematological malignancy	111	15%
Crawford (56)	BMT	348	21%
Butt (21)	Children	15	0%
Sivan (26)	Children	27	26%
Todd (57)	BMT children	54	11%
Bojko (127)	BMT children	43	12%

VIII. ETHICAL CONSIDERATIONS

The decision for admission of a cancer patient into an ICU depends not only on the prognosis of the complication requiring intensive care support but also and mainly on the prognosis of the neoplastic underlying disease that is a function of the effective therapeutic possibilities and on the role of an experimental therapy in the life-threatening complication requiring critical care. In the latter situation, the critical care oncologist is confronted with a difficult problem: to provide intensive care to a patient with an initial good health status but with an incurable cancer and who has received an investigational therapy resulting in a severe complication (5). This patient should receive appropriate treatment to avoid iatrogenic consequences, including toxic death, but the patient's autonomy must be respected, and the patient's agreement is necessary for performing critical care techniques.

To avoid unnecessary invasive resuscitation procedures, Australian authors (128) have proposed a staging system of the neoplastic disease to determine when resuscitation is appropriate in a given case:

1. Stage 1, or diagnosis, when the patient's disease is assessed and appropriate treatment goal and treatment are negotiated
2. Stage 2, or potential cure, when the goal of treatment is cure with the risks of associated morbidity

3. Stage 3, when disease in controllable but not curable, when a temporary remission that will significantly prolong life may be achievable
4. Stage 4, when specific treatment aimed at cure or control has failed (this is the most critical point in the disease for many cancer patients)
5. Stage 5, or palliative management

In the two latter stages, a not-for-resuscitation order should be given because the chances that a patient will benefit from cardiopulmonary resuscitation are minimal in such very rarely reversible situations, regardless of the acute precipitating event, and cardiac arrest is usually the end result of generalized multisystem failure. For the same reasons, invasive life support methods such as mechanical ventilation or hemodialysis should not be performed, except in case of experimental therapy, as already discussed.

In addition to the patient's salvageability and autonomy, distributive justice has also to be considered because resources are limited in terms of ICU space availability. A difficult task for many physicians with these patients is to be free from prejudices. In a survey of physicians of different subspecialities with carefully designed clinical vignettes of patients with different chronic medical illnesses (129), decisions for resuscitation were less frequent for cancer vignettes than for vignettes of other chronic medical illnesses before and after mortality information was given. However, when looking to attitudes according to medical subspecialties, this difference was present in cardiologists, pulmonologists, and neurologists but not in hematologists and oncologists. Another study (6) performed in a general hospital showed that 47% of lung cancer patients had ''do not resuscitate'' orders, 16% of those with cirrhosis had such orders, and 4% of those with heart failure had them. In-hospital mortality rate was, respectively, 14%, 18%, and 3%; 6 months' survival estimate was 54%, 64%, and 47%; and 5-year survival estimate was 6.6%, 21.9%, and 11.1%. None of these differences were statistically significant. Physicians' judgment should be based on more scientific data, allowing appropriate decisions in a precise context.

IX. PERSPECTIVES

Critical care medicine and oncology are at the beginning of a collaboration that should become more and more important. Providers of critical care medicine will be required to administer anticancer treatment and to support the complications of treatment. Like in infectious diseases, therapy against cancer has, as its objective, the destruction of the pathological process with the intention to cure, even if it is not currently the case for every patient. Treatment goals are thus not palliative as it is in the case of many degenerative diseases such as cardiovascular disease or chronic obstructive pulmonary disease, in which the restoration of a normal healthy situation is practically impossible. With the development of new therapies, more cancer patients will have the opportunity to receive curative treatment, a major reason to be actively managed in case of life-threatening situations. Distributive justice will require that these patients be admitted to the ICU with a higher priority than those with incurable chronic degenerative diseases.

There is another reason for which both critical care and oncological disciplines should work together. In invasive cancer as in multiple organ system failure (MOSF), a cascade of immune cells and cytokines is activated (in a more chronic way in cancer). During its development, cancer induces a kind of chronic MOSF syndrome. In both critical care medicine and oncology, a lot of research is performed to understand this immune cascade and to find tools to control its consequences. A better collaboration between researchers of both fields at the clinical as well at the laboratory levels is needed.

SELECTED READINGS

Chevrolet JCl, Jolliet Ph: An ethical look at intensive care for patients with malignancies. Eur J Cancer 1991; 27:210–212. Reflection on the intersections between oncology and intensive care. The first part is a review of the basic principles of patient admission to the intensive care unit: salvageability, respect of patient autonomy, and distributive justice. In the second part, the authors plead that a cancer patient be considered like any other patient, because major progress has been made in both supportive and clinical cancer treatment.

Brunet F, Lanore JJ, Dhainaut JF, Dreyfus F, Vaxelaire JF, Nouira S, Giraud T, Armaganidis A, Monsallier JF. Is intensive care justified for patients with haematological malignancies? Intensive Care Med 1990; 16:291–297. The authors reviewed their 4-year experience in the intensive care unit management of hematological malignancies. Among adults admitted, the overall mortality rates in the intensive care unit and in the hospital were 43% and 57%, respectively. Among survivors, 44% (35 patients) were still alive 1 year after admission. The impact of the life support techniques such as hemodialysis or mechanical ventilation was studied and the authors conclude that such supportive therapies should be initiated for this type of patient.

Sculier JP, Markiewicz E. Cardiopulmonary resuscitation in medical cancer patients: the experience of a medical intensive care unit of a cancer centre. Support Care Cancer 1993; 1:135–138. This retrospective study aimed to determine the effectiveness and potential indications of cardiopulmonary resuscitation (CPR) in medical cancer patients. During a 6-year period, cardiac arrest occurred in 49 cancer patients. Cardiopulmonary resuscitation was successful in 19 (39%), but only five (10%) were discharged alive from the hospital. Cardiopulmonary resuscitation was successful in all eight patients in which cardiac arrest was the consequence of an acute cardiovascular drug toxicity, even if the cancer was metastatic and the purpose of treatment not curative. It was only effective in 25% of those in whom cardiac arrest was an ultimate complication of various problems such as septic shock or respiratory failure complicating the neoplastic disease. The results suggest that, in cancer as in other types of disease, CPR is mainly indicated when cardiac arrest is the consequence of an acute insult.

Groeger JS. Critical care of the cancer patient. 2d ed. St. Louis: Mosby–Year Book, 1991. The only textbook in English on critical care of cancer patient available in 1998. It reflects the practice at the Memorial Sloan-Kettering Cancer Center in New York. Chapters are mainly devoted to oncological emergencies. Some invasive procedures are discussed in the context of a neoplastic disease, as well as perioperative care, pain control, and sedation.

Crawford SW, Petersen FB. Long-term survival from respiratory failure after marrow transplantation for malignancy. Am Rev Respir Dis 1992; 145:510–514. This study, performed at the Fred Hutchinson Cancer Research Center in Seattle, aimed to determine the effectiveness of assisted mechanical ventilation in patients with respiratory failure after marrow transplantation. Of 348 patients (23%) who required mechanical ventilation, 72 (21%) were extubated and 15 (4%) were discharged from the hospital, with 10 (3%) surviving 6 months after transplantation. All of these survivors are physically functional. Older age, active malignancy at time of transplantation, and donor-recipient marrow HLA-non-identity were risk factors for subsequent respiratory failure.

REFERENCES

1. Turnbell A, Goldiner P, Silverman D, Howland W. The role of an intensive care unit in a cancer center. Cancer 1976; 37:82–84.
2. Sculier JP, Ries F, Verboven N, Coune A, Klastersky J. Role of intensive care unit in a medical oncology department. Eur J Cancer Clin Oncol 1988; 24:513–517.
3. Sculier JP, Markiewicz E. Medical cancer patients and intensive care. Anticancer Res 1991; 11:2171–2174.
4. Sculier JP, Markiewicz E. Intensive care in anticancer centers: an international inquiry. Support Care Cancer 1995; 3:130–134.
5. Chevrolet JCl, Jolliet Ph. An ethical look at intensive care for patients with malignancies. Eur J Cancer 1991; 27:210–212.
6. Wachter RM, Luce JM, Hearst N, Lo B. Decisions about resuscitation: inequities among patients with different diseases but similar prognoses. Ann Intern Med 1989; 111:525–532.
7. Filshie J, Robbie DS. Anaesthesia and malignant disease. London: Edward Arnold, 1989.
8. Howland WS, Rooney SM, Goldiner PL. Manual of anesthesia in cancer patients. New York: Churchill Livingstone, 1986.
9. Hauser M, Tabak J, Baier H. Survival of patients with cancer in a medical critical care unit. Arch Intern Med 1982; 142:527–529.
10. Cox SC, Norwood SH, Duncan CA. Acute respiratory failure: mortality associated with underlying disease. Crit Care Med 1985; 13:1005–1008.
11. Polansky M, Fromm RE Jr, Keenan CH, Varon J. Outcome of cancer patients in a surgical intensive care unit. Intensive Care World 1996; 13:146–149.
12. Schapira DV, Studnicki J, Bradham DD, Wolff P, Jarrett A. Intensive care, survi-

val, and expense of treating critically ill cancer patients. JAMA 1993; 269:783–786.
13. Chalfin DB, Carlon GC. Age and utilization of intensive care unit resources of critically ill cancer patients. Crit Care Med 1990; 18:694–698.
14. Layon AJ, George BE, Hamby B, Gallagher TJ. Do elderly patients overutilize healthcare resources and benefit less from them than younger patients? A study of patients who underwent craniotomy for treatment of neoplasm. Crit Care Med 1995; 23:829–834.
15. Abbott RR, Setter M, Chan S, Choi K. APACHE II: prediction of outcome of 451 ICU oncology admissions in a community hospital. Ann Oncol 1991; 2:571–574.
16. Headley J, Theriault R, Smith TL. Independent validation of APACHE II severity of illness score for predicting mortality in patients with breast cancer admitted to the intensive care unit. Cancer 1992; 70:497–503.
17. Johnson MH, Gordon PW, Fitzgerald FT. Stratification of prognosis in granulocytopenic patients with hematologic malignancies using the APACHE-II severity of illness score. Crit Care Med 1986; 14:693–697.
18. Blot F, Guiguet M, Nitenberg G, Leclercq B, Gachot B, Escudier B. Prognostic factors for neutropenic patients in an intensive care unit: respective roles of underlying malignancies and acute organ failures. Eur J Cancer 1997; 33:1031–1037.
19. Schuster DP, Marion JM. Precedents for meaningful recovery during treatment in a medical intensive care unit. Outcome in patients with hematologic malignancy. Am J Med 1983; 75:402–408.
20. Lloyd-Thomas AR, Dhaliwal HS, Lister TA, Hinds CJ. Intensive therapy for life-threatening medical complications of haematological malignancy. Intensive Care Med 1986; 12:317–324.
21. Butt W, Barker G, Walker C, Gillis J, Kilham H, Stevens M. Outcome of children with hematologic malignancy who are admitted to an intensive care unit. Critical Care Med 1988; 16:761–764.
22. Torrecilla C, Cortès JL, Chamorro C, Rubio JJ, Galdos P, Dominguez De Villota E. Prognostic assessment of the acute complications of bone marrow transplantation requiring intensive therapy. Intensive Care Med 1988; 14:393–398.
23. Brunet E, Lanore JJ, Dhainaut JF, Dreyfus F, Vaxelaire JF, Nouira S, Giraud T, Armaganidis A, Monsallier JF. Is intensive care justified for patients with haematological malignancies? Intensive Care Med 1990; 16:291–297.
24. Yau E, Rohatiner AZS, Lister TA, Hinds CJ. Long term prognosis and quality of life following intensive care for life-threatening complications of haematological malignancy. Br J Cancer 1991; 64:938–942.
25. Paz HL, Crilley P, Weinar M, Brodsky I. Outcome of patients requiring medical ICU admission following bone marrow transplantation. Chest 1993; 104:527–531.
26. Sivan Y, Schwartz PH, Schonfeld T, Cohen IJ, Newth CJL. Outcome of oncology patients in the pediatric intensive care unit. Intensive Care Med 1991; 17:11–15.
27. Van Veen A, Karstens A, van der Hoek ACJ, Tibboel D, Hählen K, van der Voort E. The prognosis of oncologic patients in the pediatric intensive care unit. Intensive Care Med 1996; 22:237–241.
28. Gerain J, Sculier JP, Malengreaux A, Rykaert C, Thémelin L. Causes of deaths in

an oncologic intensive care unit: a clinical and pathological study of 34 patients. Eur J Cancer 1990; 26:377–381.
29. Faber-Langendoen K. Resuscitation of patients with metastatic cancer. Is transient benefit still futile? Arch Intern Med 1991; 151:235–239.
30. Vitelli CE, Cooper K, Rogatko A, Brennan MF. Cardiopulmonary resuscitation and the patient with cancer. J Clin Oncol 1991; 9:111–115.
31. Sculier JP, Markiewicz E. Cardiopulmonary resuscitation in medical cancer patients: the experience of a medical intensive care unit of a cancer centre. Support Care Cancer 1993.
32. Dutcher JP, Wiernik PH. Handbook of hematologic and oncologic emergencies. New York: Plenum, 1987.
33. Groeger JS. Critical care of the cancer patient. 2d ed. St. Louis: Mosby–Year Book, 1991.
34. McGowan MP, Pratter MR, Nash G. Primary testicular choriocarcinoma with pulmonary metastases presenting as ARDS. Chest 1990; 97:1258–1259.
35. Ravid M, Shapira J, Lang R, David R. Acute respiratory distress syndrome: a presenting syndrome of malignant lymphoma. JAMA 1979; 241:2191–2192.
36. Vernant JP, Brun B, Mannoni P, Dreyfus B. Respiratory distress of hyperleukocytic granulocytic leukemias. Cancer 1979; 44:264–268.
37. Hewlett RI, Wilson AF. Adult respiratory distress syndrome (ARDS) following aggressive management of extensive acute lymphoblastic leukemia. Cancer 1977; 39:2422–2425.
38. Frankel SR, Eardley A, Lauwers G, Weiss M, Warrell RP Jr. The ''retinoic acid syndrome'' in acute promyelocytic leukemia. Ann Intern Med 1992; 117:292–296.
39. Haupt HM, Hutchins GM, Moore GW. Ara-C lung: noncardiogenic pulmonary edema complicating cytosine arabinoside therapy of leukemia. Am J Med 1981; 70:256–261.
40. Sculier JP, Bron D, Verboven N, Klastersky J. Multiple organ failure during interleukin-2 administration and LAK cells infusion. Intensive Care Med 1988; 14: 666–667.
41. Fulkerson WJ, McLendon RE, Prosnitz LR. Adult respiratory distress syndrome after limited thoracic radiotherapy. Cancer 1986; 57:1941–1946.
42. Pavlakis N, Bell DR, Millward MJ, Levi JA. Fatal pulmonary toxicity resulting from treatment with gemcitabine. Cancer 1997; 80:286–291.
43. Reckzeh B, Merte H, Pflüger KH, Pfab R, Wolf M, Havemann K. Severe lymphocytopenia and interstitial pneumonia in patients treated with paclitaxel and simultaneous radiotherapy for non-small-cell-lung cancer. J Clin Oncol 1997; 14:1071–1076.
44. Ognibene FP, Martin SE, Parker MM, Schlesinger T, Roach P, Burch C, Shelhamer JH, Parrillo JE. Adult respiratory distress syndrome in patients with severe neutropenia. N Engl J Med 1986; 315:547–551.
45. Laufe MD, Simon RH, Flint A, Keller JB. Adult respiratory distress syndrome in neutropenic patients. Am J Med 1986; 80:1022–1026.
46. Arning M, Gehrt A, Aul C, Runde V, Hadding U, Schneider W. Septicemia due to *Streptococcus mitis* in neutropenic patients with acute leukemia. Blut 1990; 61: 364–368.
47. Metcalf JP, Rennard SI, Reed EC, Haire WD, Sisson JH, Walter D, Robbins RA,

the University of Nebraska Medical Center Bone Marrow Transplant Group. Corticosteroids as adjunctive therapy for diffuse alveolar hemorrhage associated with bone marrow transplantation. Am J Med 1994; 96:327–334.

48. Dedhia HV, Le Roy N, Jain PR, Thompson AB, Withers A. Endoscopic laser therapy for respiratory distress due to obstructive airway tumors. Crit Care Med 1985; 13:464–467.
49. Spain RC, Whittlesey D. Respiratory emergencies in patients with cancer. Semin Oncol 1989; 16:471–489.
50. Sahn SA. Pleural diseases related to metastatic malignancies. Eur Respir J 1997; 10:1907–1913.
51. Snow RM, Miller WC, Rice DL, Ali MK. Respiratory failure in cancer patients. JAMA 1979; 241:2039–2042.
52. Webb WR, Ozmen V, Moulder PV, Shabahang B, Breaux J. Iodized talc pleurodesis for the treatment of pleural effusions. J Thorac Cardiovasc Surg 1992; 103: 881–886.
53. Estopa R, Marti AT, Kastanos N, Rives A, Agusti-Vidal A, Rozman C. Acute respiratory failure in severe hematologic disorders. Crit Care Med 1984; 12:26–28.
54. Peters SG, Meadows JA III, Graley DR. Outcome of respiratory failure in hematologic malignancy. Chest 1988; 94:99–102.
55. Denardo SJ, Oye RK, Bellamy PE. Efficacy of intensive care for bone marrow transplant patients with respiratory failure. Crit Care Med 1989; 17:4–6.
56. Crawford SW, Petersen FB. Long-term survival from respiratory failure after marrow transplantation for malignancy. Am Rev Respir Dis 1992; 145:510–514.
57. Todd K, Wiley F, Landow E, Gajewski J, Bellamy PE, Harrisson RE, Brill JE, Feig SA. Survival outcome among 54 intubated pediatric bone marrow transplant patients. Crit Care Med 1994; 22:171–176.
58. Allen A. The cardiotoxicity of chemotherapeutic drugs. Semin Oncol 1992; 19: 529–542.
59. Shan K, Lincoff AM, Young JB. Anthracycline-induced cardiotoxicity. Ann Intern Med 1996; 125:47–58.
60. Buckner CD, Rudolph RH, Fefer A, Clift RA, Epstein RB, Funk DD, Neiman PE, Slichter SJ, Storb R, Thomas ED. High-dose cyclophosphamide therapy for malignant disease. Toxicity, tumor response, and the effects of stored autologous marrow. Cancer 1972; 29:357–365.
61. Goldberg MA, Antin JH, Guinan EC, Rappeport JM. Cyclophosphamide cardiotoxicity: an analysis of dosing as a risk factor. Blood 1986; 68:1114–1118.
62. Ayash LJ, Wright JE, Tretyakou O, Gonin R, Elias A, Wheeler C, Eder JP, Rosowsky A, Antman K, Frei E III. Cyclophosphamide pharmacokinetics: correlation with cardiac toxicity and tumor response. J Clin Oncol 1992; 10:995–1000.
63. Gradishar WJ, Vokes EE. 5-fluorouracil cardiotoxicity: a critical review. Ann Oncol 1990; 1:409–414.
64. de Forni M, Malet-Martino MC, Jaillais P, Shubinski RE, Bachaud JM, Lemaire L, Canal P, Chevreau C, Carrié D, Soulié P, Roché H, Boudjema B, Mihura J, Martino R, Bernadet P, Bugat R. Cardiotoxicity of high-dose continuous fluorouracil: a prospective clinical study. J Clin Oncol 1992; 10:1795–1801.

65. Kragel AH, Travis WD, Steis RG, Rosenberg SA, Roberts WC. Myocarditis or acute myocardial infarction associated with interleukin-2 therapy for cancer. Cancer 1990; 66:1513–1516.
66. Vaitkus PT, Herrmann HC, LeWinter MM. Treatment of malignant pericardial effusion. JAMA 1994; 272:59–64.
67. Liu G, Crump M, Goss PE, Dancey J, Shepherd FA. Prospective comparison of the sclerosing agents doxycycline and bleomycin for the primary management of malignant pericardial effusion and cardiac tamponade. J Clin Oncol 1996; 14:3141–3147.
68. Wilkes JD, Fidias P, Vaickus L, Perez RP. Malignancy-related pericardial effusion. Cancer 1995; 76:1377–1387.
69. Sculier JP, Feld R. Superior vena cava obstruction syndrome: recommendations for management. Cancer Treat Rev 1985; 12:209–218.
70. Bassiri AG, Haghighi, Doyle RL, Berry GJ, Rizk NW. Pulmonary tumor embolism. Am J Respir Crit Care Med 1997; 155:2089–2095.
71. Edoute Y, Haim N, Rinkevich D, Brenner B, Reisner SA. Cardiac valvular vegetations in cancer patients: a prospective echocardiographic study of 200 patients. Am J Med 1997; 102:252–258.
72. Mundy JR, Guise TA. Hypercalcemia of malignancy. Am J Med 1997; 103:134–145.
73. Gucalp R, Ritch P, Wiernik PH, Sarma PR, Keller A, Richman SP, Tauer K, Neidhart J, Mallette LE, Siegel R, VandePol CJ. Comparative study of pamidronate disodium and etidronate disodium in the treatment of cancer-related hypercalcemia. J Clin Oncol 1992; 10:134–142.
74. Thürlimann B, Waldburger R, Senn HJ, Thiébaud D. Plicamycin and pamidronate in symptomatic tumor-related hypercalcemia: a prospective randomized crossover trial. Ann Oncol 1992; 3:619–623.
75. Pecherstorfer M, Herrmann Z, Body JJ, Manegold C, Degardin M, Clemens MR, Thürlimann B, Tubiana-Hulin M, Steinhauer EU, van Eijkeren M, Huss HJ, Thiébaud D: Randomized phase II trial comparing different doses of the biphosphonate ibandronate in the treatment of hypercalcemia of malignancy. J Clin Oncol 1996; 14:268–276.
76. Ralston SH, Gallacher SJ, Patel V, Campbell J, Boyle IT. Cancer-associated hypercalcemia: morbidity and mortality. Ann Intern Med 1990; 112:499–504.
77. Gucalp R, Theriault R, Gill I, Madajewicz S, Chapman R, Navari R, Ahmann F, Zelenakas K, Heffernan M, Knight RD. Treatment of cancer-associated hypercalcemia. Double-blind comparison of rapid and slow intravenous infusion regimens of pamidronate disodium and saline alone. Arch Intern Med 1994; 154:1935–1944.
78. Camus C, Charasse C, Jouannic-Montier I, Seguin P, Tulzo YL, Bouget J, Thomas R. Calcium free hemodialysis: experience in the treatment of 33 patients with severe hypercalcemia. Intensive Care Med 1996; 22:116–121.
79. Ebie N, Ryan W, Harris J. Metabolic emergencies in cancer medicine. Med Clin North Am 1986; 70:1151–1166.
80. Odell WD. Endocrine/metabolic syndromes of cancer. Semin Oncol 1997; 24:299–317.
81. Sculier JP, Nicaise C, Klastersky J. Lactic acidosis: a metabolic complication of extensive metastatic cancer. Eur J Cancer Clin Oncol 1983; 19:597–601.

82. Tobias JD. Tumour lysis pneumopathy. Clin Intensive Care 1991; 2:305–308.
83. Sorensen JB, Andersen MK, Hansen HH. Syndrome of inappropriate secretion of antidiuretic hormone (SIADH) in malignant disease. J Intern Med 1995; 238:97–110.
84. Berghmans T. Hyponatremia related to medical anticancer treatment. Support Care Cancer 1996; 4:341–350.
85. Boogerd W, van der Sande JJ. Diagnosis and treatment of spinal cord compression in malignant disease. Cancer Treat Rev 1993; 19:129–150.
86. Sorensen PS, Helweg-Larsen S, Mouridsen H, Hansen HH. Effect of high-dose dexamethasone in carcinomatous metastatic spinal cord compression treated with radiotherapy: a randomised trial. Eur J Cancer 1994; 30A:22–27.
87. Jayson GC, Howell A. Carcinomatous meningitis in solid tumours. Ann Oncol 1996; 7:773–786.
88. Tuxen MK, Hansen SW. Neurotoxicity secondary to antineoplastic drugs. Cancer Treat Rev 1994; 20:191–214.
89. Cerny T, Küpfer A. The enigma of ifosfamide encephalopathy. Ann Oncol 1992; 3:679–681.
90. Küpfer A, Aeschlimann C, Wermuth B, Cerny T. Prophylaxis and reversal of ifosfamide encephalopathy with methylene-blue. Lancet 1994; 343:763–764.
91. Openshaw H, Slatkin NE, Stein AS, Hinton DR, Forman SJ. Acute polyneuropathy after high dose cytosine arabinoside in patients with leukemia. Cancer 1996; 78: 1899–1905.
92. Berrouschot J, Baumann I, Kalischewski P, Sterker M, Schneider D. Therapy of myasthenic crisis. Crit Care Med 1997; 25:1228–1235.
93. Carpentier AF, Bernard L, Poisson M, Delattre JY. Infections du système nerveux central chez les patients atteints d'une pathologie maligne. Rev Neurol (Paris) 1996; 152:587–601.
94. Wade DS, Douglass H Jr, Nava HR, Piedmonte M. Abdominal pain in neutropenic patients. Arch Surg 1990; 125:1119–1127.
95. Wade DS, Nava HR, Douglass HO Jr. Neutropenic enterocolitis. Clinical diagnosis and management. Cancer 1992; 69:17–23.
96. Williams N, Scott ADN. Neutropenic colitis: a continuing surgical challenge. Br J Surg 1997; 84:1200–1205.
97. Bearman SI. The syndrome of hepatic veno-occlusive disease after marrow transplantation. Blood 1995; 85:3005–3020.
98. McDonald GB, Hinds MS, Fisher LD, Schoch HG, Wolford JL, Banaji M, Hardin BJ, Shulman HM, Clift RA. Veno-occlusive disease of the liver and multiorgan failure after bone marrow transplantation: a cohort study of 355 patients. Ann Intern Med 1993; 118:255–267.
99. Yu LC, Malkani I, Regueira O, Ode DL, Warrier RP. Recombinant tissue plasminogen activator (rt-PA) for veno-occlusive liver disease in pediatric autologous bone marrow transplant patients. Am J Hematol 1994; 46:194–198.
100. Espigado I, Rodriguez JM, Parody R, Carmona M, Digon J, Olloqui E. Reversal of severe hepatic veno-occlusive disease by combined plasma exchange and rt-PA treatment. Bone Marrow Transplantation 1995; 16:313–316.
100a. Sculier JP. Indications for intensive care in the management of infections in cancer

patients. In: Klastersky J, ed. Infectious complications of cancer. Dordrecht: Kluwer, 1995:233–244.
101. Sculier JP, Weerts D, Klastersky J. Cause of death in febrile granulocytopenic cancer patients receiving empiric antibiotic therapy. Eur J Cancer Clin Oncol 1984; 20:55–60.
102. O'Brien MER, Souberbielle BE. Allergic reactions to cytotoxic drugs—an update. Ann Oncol 1992; 3:605–610.
103. Weiss RB. Hypersensitivity reactions. Semin Oncol 1992; 19:458–477.
104. Törnebohm E, Lockner D, Paul C. A retrospective analysis of bleeding complications in 438 patients with acute leukaemia during the years 1972–1991. Eur J Haematol 1993; 50:160–167.
105. Armitage JO, Antman KH. High-dose cancer therapy. Pharmacology, hematopoietins, stem cells. Baltimore: Williams & Wilkins, 1992.
106. Ackland SP, Schilsky RL. High-dose methotrexate: a critical reappraisal. J Clin Oncol 1987; 5:2017–2031.
107. Pennock GD, Dalton WS, Roeske WR, Appelton CP, Mosley K, Plezia P, Miller JP, Salmon SE. Systemic toxic effects associated with high-dose verapamil infusion and chemotherapy administration. J Natl Cancer Inst 1991; 83:105–110.
108. Siegel JP, Puri RK. Interleukin-2 toxicity. J Clin Oncol 1991; 9:694–704.
109. Diana D, Sculier JP. Haemodynamic effects induced by intravenous administration of high doses of R-Met Hu IL-2 [ala-125] in patients with advanced cancer. Intensive Care Med 1990; 16:167–170.
110. Gyves JW, Ensminger WD, Niederhuber JE, Dent T, Walker S, Gilbertson S, Cozzi E, Saran P. A totally implanted injection port system for blood sampling and chemotherapy administration. JAMA 1989; 251:2538–2541.
111. Carde P, Cosset-Delaigne MF, Laplanche A, Chareau I. Classical external indwelling central venous catheter versus totally implanted venous access systems for chemotherapy administration: a randomized trial in 100 patients with solid tumors. Eur J Cancer Clin Oncol 1989; 25:939–944.
112. Horne McDK III, Mayo DJ. Low-dose urokinase infusions to treat fibrinous obstruction of venous access devices in cancer patients. J Clin Oncol 1997; 15:2709–2714.
113. Bertand M, Presant CA, Klein L, Scott E. Iatrogenic superior vena cava syndrome. A new entity. Cancer 1984; 54:376–378.
114. Bock SN, Lee RE, Fisher B, Rubin JT, Schwartzentruber DJ, Wei JP, Callender DPE, Yang JC, Lotze MT, Pizzo PA, Rosenberg SA. A prospective randomized trial evaluating prophylactic antibiotics to prevent triple-lumen catheter-related sepsis in patients treated with immunotherapy. J Clin Oncol 1990; 8:161–169.
115. Barrera R, Mina B, Huang Y, Groeger JS. Acute complications of central line placement in profoundly thrombocytopenic cancer patients. Cancer 1996; 78:2025–2030.
116. Masson BG, Krikorian J, Luki P, Evans GL, McGrath J. Pulmonary microvascular cytology in the diagnosis of lymphangitic carcinomatosis. N Engl J Med 1989; 321: 71–76.
117. Harris KPG, Hattersley JM, Feehally J, Walls J. Acute renal failure associated with

haematological malignancies: a review of 10 years experience. Eur J Haematol. 1991; 47:119–122.

118. Lane PH, Mauer SM, Blazar BR, Ramsay NKC, Kashtan CE. Outcome of dialysis for acute renal failure in pediatric bone marrow transplant patients. Bone Marrow Transplant 1994; 13:613–617.
119. Lesesne JB, Rothschild N, Erickson B, Korec S, Sisk R, Keller J, Arbus M, Wooley PV, Chiazze L, Schein PS, Neefe JR. Cancer-associated hemolytic-uremic syndrome: analysis of 85 cases from a national registry. J Clin Oncol 1989; 7:781–789.
120. Schlemmer R, Dhainaut JF, Bons J, Mathiot C, Varet B, Sylvestre R, Monsallier JF. Pneumopathies aiguës au cours des hémopathies malignes en aplasie: nouvelle approche nosologique et thérapeutique. Ann Méd Interne 1982; 133:174–177.
121. Gregg RW, Friedman BC, Williams JF, McGrath BJ, Zimmerman JE. Continuous positive airway pressure by face mask in *Pneumocystis carinii* pneumonia. Crit Care Med 1990; 18:21–24.
122. Turnbull AD, Carlon G. Airway management in the thrombocytopenic cancer patient with acute respiratory failure. Crit Care Med 1979; 7:76–77.
123. Blot F, Nitenberg G, Guiguet M, Casetta M, Antoun S, Pico JL, Leclercq B, Escudier B. Safety of tracheotomy in neutropenic patients: a retrospective study of 26 consecutive cases. Intensive Care Med 1995; 21:687–690.
124. Schlemmer B. Aplasie médullaire et ventilation artificielle. Revue de Praticien 1990; 23:2152–2153.
125. Blot F, Guiget M, Antoun S, Leclercq B, Nitenberg G, Escudier B. Early tracheotomy in neutropenic, mechanically ventilated patients: rationale and results of a pilot study. Support Care Cancer 1995; 3:291–296.
126. Kiehl M, Schiele C, Stenzinger W, Kienast J. Volume-controlled versus biphasic positive airway pressure ventilation in leukopenic patients with severe respiratory failure. Crit Care Med 1996; 24:780–784.
126a. Ewer MS, Ali MK, Atta MS, Morice RC, Balakrishnan PV. Outcome of lung cancer patients requiring mechanical ventilation for pulmonary failure. JAMA 1986; 256: 3364–3366.
127. Bojko T, Notterman DA, Greenwald BM, De Bruin WJ, Magid MS, Godwin T. Acute hypoxemic respiratory failure in children following bone marrow transplantation: an outcome and pathologic study. Crit Care Med 1995; 23:755–759.
128. Haines IE, Zalcberg J, Buchanan JD. Not for resuscitation orders in cancer patients—principles of decision-making. Med J Austr 1990; 153:225–229.
129. Lawrence VA, Clark GM. Cancer and resuscitation. Does the diagnosis affect the decision? Arch Intern Med 1987; 147:1637–1640.

23

Outpatient Management of Chemotherapy Treated Patients

Edward B. Rubenstein and Charlotte C. Sun
The University of Texas M.D. Anderson Cancer Center, Houston, Texas

I. INTRODUCTION

Originally, the underlying premise of modern oncology emphasized interdisciplinary care; cancer patients benefited from the progressive management of surgeons, medical oncologists, radiation oncologists, and oncology nurses in the form of coordinated cancer therapy. Recently, the American Society of Clinical Oncology (ASCO) recommended that subspecialty medical training include an emphasis on patient management in the outpatient setting. Specifically, ASCO urged that trainees learn to manage patients in a longitudinal fashion and be able to participate in multidisciplinary ambulatory cancer care (1). Similarly, nurses in oncology outpatient settings encounter many challenges, including high volumes of patient business fluctuating census, increasingly complex chemotherapy regimens, higher patient acuity, and a diversified case mix of patients (2). Recognizing that the role of ambulatory care in oncology is increasing in importance, the International Union Against Cancer (UICC) recommended that comprehensive cancer centers carefully examine resources allocated to ambulatory care (3). This chapter explores some of the factors influencing the development of outpatient cancer care and provides a theoretical and practical framework for selecting appropriate patients for outpatient care. Applications of these selection criteria and benefits of outpatient care are outlined.

II. FACTORS INFLUENCING OUTPATIENT CARE

A. Technology

During the past 30 years, several remarkable transformations have occurred in medicine, which have greatly altered both the standard and delivery of cancer care. These transformations include the development of newer medical technologies based on advances in basic science at the molecular and genetic level. An explosion in drug development has led to major advances in chemotherapy and its supportive care byproducts. These include newer antineoplastic agents, biologic response modifiers, growth factors, potent broad-spectrum antibiotics (including oral agents), widespread use of more effective antiemetics, and availability of effective narcotic analgesics (4–10). Medical devices such as the endoscope with its laser technology along with advances in infusion technology allow physicians to screen, diagnose, and treat cancer in patients as outpatients in ways never imagined just 2 decades ago (11–13). Anesthetic and surgical techniques allow for more rapid recovery of patients and an ability to treat shift operative and postoperative care more quickly to the outpatient setting (14).

B. Economics

Economic changes in health care have greatly influenced the general shift from inpatient to outpatient cancer care. The National Cancer Institute estimates the overall annual costs for cancer to be $107 billion, with $37 billion for direct medical costs (15). Although cancer involves a complex array of clinical diagnoses and subspecialty care with its treatment and supportive care resources, reimbursement policies in oncology often drive resource utilization patterns. Since the introduction of prospective payment mechanisms, providers have attempted to deliver care in the outpatient setting, because inpatient care is more resource intensive than outpatient care, particularly in terms of more hotel, medical, and clinical resource use (16).

C. Policy

Along with advances in medical technologies, changes in reimbursement policies can be traced as the other major impetus for the increase in outpatient cancer visits. Fig. 1 illustrates the various factors that have contributed to increases in outpatient delivery of cancer care. The Omnibus Reconciliation Act of 1980 eliminated the requirement that patients spend 3 days as inpatients to qualify for outpatient care services reimbursable by Medicare. The act also discontinued the cap on reimbursed home nursing visits at 100 visits per year. The Social Security Act of 1983 effectively ended retrospective cost reimbursement by Medicare and introduced the diagnosis-related groups (DRGs) (17). Hospitals responded by

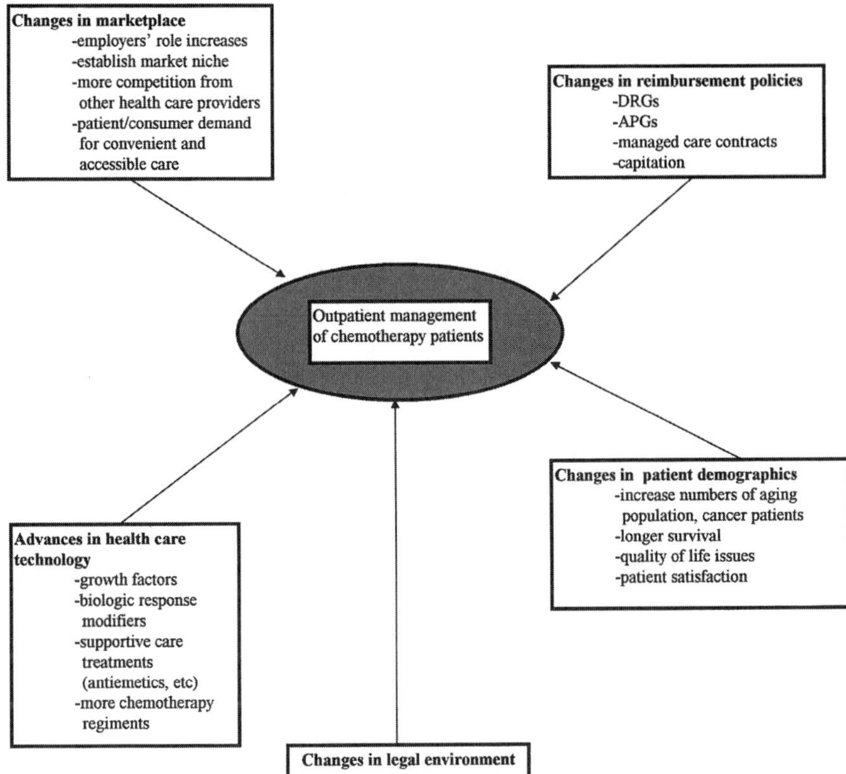

Figure 1 Factors influencing the trend in outpatient treatment of cancer patients.

shifting much of their inpatient care delivery to outpatient settings. Fig. 2 demonstrates the changing patterns in health care delivery for the United States (18). Fig. 3 illustrates how these trends also exist in a comprehensive cancer center.

The DRGs use a fixed payment structure, wherein core diagnosis groups receive standardized reimbursement for a specific coded diagnosis or procedure. Currently, the ambulatory patient groups (APGs) are the parallel reimbursement mechanism to the inpatient DRGs. Like DRGs, APGs consist of a fixed payment for a core procedure, in addition for any associated laboratory and minor radiological services, drugs, and supplies (19). Viewed another way, fixed payments essentially cost-shift the risk to the providers of care. Cost-shifting also occurs in capitated reimbursement systems; physicians must decide how many dollars to allocate to their covered populations. Reimbursements for inpatient visits are

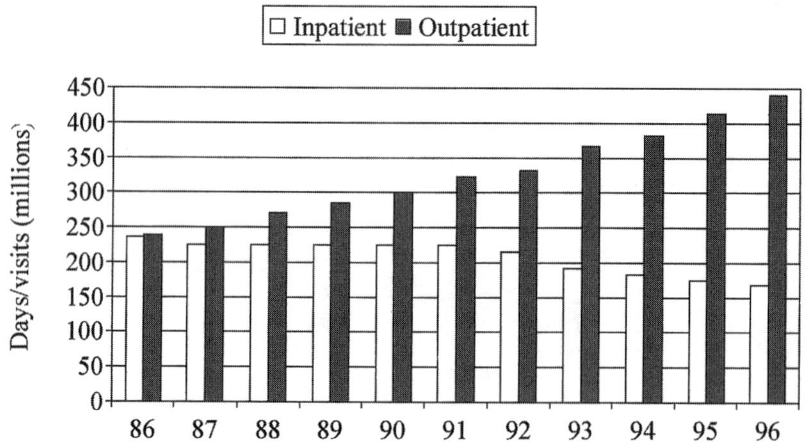

Figure 2 Community hospital inpatient days compared to outpatient visits during 1986–1996.

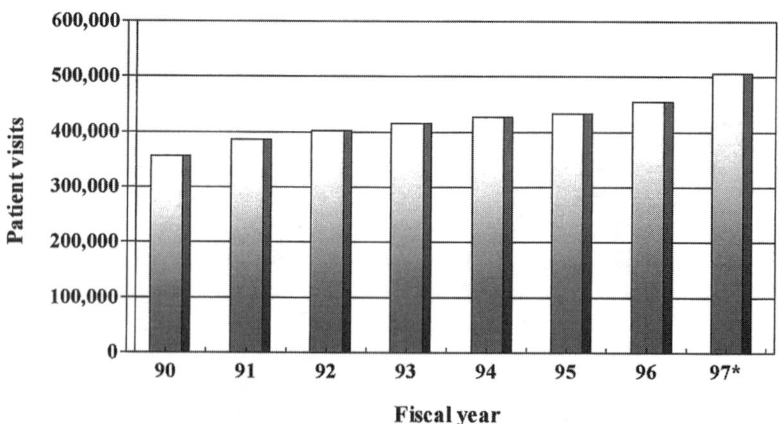

Figure 3 Outpatient visits, M.D. Anderson Cancer Center.

steadily decreasing, whereas outpatient visits are viewed as the more cost-effective way of delivering cancer care. The challenge for both hospitals and clinicians will be in deciding how to incorporate the use of new medical technologies and cancer treatments in APGs. As health care costs continue to increase and reimbursement dollars continue to decrease, hospitals and physicians face intensified competition for limited resources (20).

D. Societal Demographics

Increasing numbers of outpatient visits are also a response to consumer/patient demand for convenient and accessible cancer care (21). As the United States population ages, oncologists can expect a substantial increase in the number of cancer patients. Consequently organization and prospective planning will be required to effectively meet the growing demand for cancer care. Cancer care and supportive care should be viewed as a continuous spectrum of care, encompassing everything from cancer prevention to aggressive supportive care for patients undergoing intent-to-cure surgical therapy as well as chemotherapy and includes palliative and terminal care for patients with advanced disease (22). Managing patients across this continuum requires an understanding of the various factors that are integral to successful outpatient supportive care.

III. IDENTIFYING PATIENTS SUITABLE FOR OUTPATIENT CARE

A. Risk Assessment and Outcomes

To deliver the most effective and efficient care to cancer patients in ambulatory care settings, it is particularly important to be able to determine which patients are most appropriate for outpatient treatment. Ideally, outpatients would have the ability to travel back and forth to the clinic without limitations, never miss appointments, always respond to treatment, never develop complications of therapy, and never require hospitalization. Unfortunately, this ''ideal subject'' does not exist. Therefore, clinicians must rely on a strategy for identifying patients who are close to this ideal. This process can be simple and experiential or more quantitative and complex.

The concept of risk assessment has been used in oncology care to assist in identifying subgroups of patients who may have different outcomes of experiences when treated in similar fashions. It is important to recognize that risk implies ''risk of what?'' (23). The outcome associated with risk must be explicitly defined. In terms of outpatient treatment of chemotherapy-treated patients, it is meant to be risk of experiencing major medical complications in the outpatient setting rather than risk of not responding to chemotherapy. Risk for outcomes (both good and bad) is often a function of patient factors (such as age and performance status), disease factors (limited versus extensive malignancy), comorbid conditions (diabetes mellitus or congestive heart failure), and treatment factors (intensity of chemotherapy, surgery, or radiotherapy). How these variables interact to influence patient outcomes is an important area of research and not easily apparent enough to apply at the patient's bedside. As a consequence, a variety of patient classification strategies is often used to help distinguish between subgroups of patients.

B. Patient Classification Systems

1. Performance Status

Many methods are used to distinguish which individuals should be treated as inpatients as opposed to outpatients. For many years, the physician's judgment was the sole criterion used to determine site of care; the physician's judgment was rarely, if ever, documented or questioned. Oncology, like many areas of medicine, is moving away from an experiential approach to care and shifting toward an evidence-based or explicit way of making many decisions, both for individual patients and for setting health care policy.

As investigators in oncology began to explore factors predictive of survival, ambulatory status and performance status emerged as routinely reproducible predictors of better outcomes compared to patients with poorer performance status and those who were already hospitalized.

Developed in 1948, the Karnofsky Performance Status Scale (KPS) was one of the first numerical attempts to measure patients' level of activity and medical care requirements (Table 1) (24). The KPS has been used as an indicator of patients' functional status and as a marker of their ability to tolerate antineoplastic therapies. Although widely used, there are little data exploring its prospective validity using other measures as a control.

In one of the few studies conducted that formally evaluated the reliability and validity of this indicator of patient's functional status, the KPS was compared to other measures as part of the National Hospice Study (NHS). The NHS was a nationwide evaluation of the impact of hospice care on the quality of life and cost of caring for terminally ill cancer patients. Interviewers underwent extensive orientation and training before conducting initial interviews with patients and their families. Three to 10 days after admission to the NHS, information was gathered on patients' pain, symptoms, satisfaction with care, satisfaction with life, and services being used. The KPS was recorded during the initial interview and during regularly scheduled visits until the patient's death. The KPS scores in the clinic as assessed by nurses and physicians were compared to KPS scores of the same patients as assessed in their homes by social workers (25). Overall, the correlation coefficients were high with a tendency for patients to be rated 5

Table 1 Karnofsky Performance Status Index

General category	Index	Specific criteria
Able to carry on normal activity; no special care needed.	100	Normal, no complaints; no evidence of disease.
	90	Able to carry on normal activity; minor signs or symptoms of disease.
	80	Normal activity with effort; some signs or symptoms of disease.
Unable to work; able to live at home and care for most personal needs; varying amount of assistance needed.	70	Cares for self; unable to carry on normal activity or to do work.
	60	Requires occasional assistance from others but able to care for most needs.
	50	Requires considerable assistance from others and frequent medical care.
Unable to care for self; requires institutional or hospital care or equivalent; disease may be rapidly progressing.	40	Disabled; requires special care and assistance.
	30	Severely disabled; hospitalization indicated; death not imminent.
	20	Very sick; hospitalization necessary; active supportive treatment necessary.
	10	Moribund.
	0	Dead.

points higher by clinic staff than by social workers. This suggests that patient setting may influence KPS. As a predictor of survival, low KPS was strongly associated with death; only 1 of 104 patients with an initial KPS less than 50 lived longer than 6 months. The converse was not true because many of the patients with high initial KPS scores died quickly. Using KPS as a single measure may not adequately describe patients well enough to separate those who can safely receive care in the outpatient setting from those who require hospital-based care for management of acute medical illnesses.

The construct validity of the KPS was evaluated by comparing it with two other observations made regarding the patients' ability to perform other activities of daily living Table 2 shows data from the NHS concerning performance level of activities of daily living (ADL) by KPS. The differences in performance level for each KPS score are significant. The proportion of patients able to function independently across a variety of indicators of functionality increases as the patients' KPS scores increase.

Using the functional variables from Table 2, Mor et al. (26) developed a

Table 2 Performance Level of Activities of Daily Living by Karnofsky Status

	Karnofsky performance status (%)					
Functional variables[a]	10	20	30	40	50	Total
Continence						
Unable	28.6	28.3	15.3	7.1	.9	12.0
With help	50.0	55.4	59.4	50.6	27.0	50.6
Independent	21.4	16.3	25.3	42.3	72.2	37.4
Transferring in/out of bed/chair						
Unable	42.9	45.7	20.3	7.1	0.0	16.0
With help	57.1	44.6	60.2	58.4	27.0	52.5
Independent	0.0	9.8	19.5	34.5	73.0	31.5
Walking						
Unable	50.0	57.6	36.4	18.4	.9	27.4
With help	50.0	33.7	48.3	49.8	32.2	44.6
Independent	0.0	8.7	15.3	31.8	67.0	28.0
Dressing						
Unable	71.4	64.1	52.9	21.0	1.7	35.4
With help	28.6	31.5	40.2	60.7	49.6	47.7
Independent	0.0	4.3	6.9	18.4	48.7	17.0
Bathing						
Unable	57.1	60.9	52.5	24.0	4.3	36.0
With help	42.9	35.9	41.0	59.6	56.6	49.4
Independent	0.0	3.3	6.5	16.5	39.1	14.6
Climbing stairs						
Unable	78.6	87.0	71.3	51.7	10.4	57.0
With help	21.4	10.9	24.1	40.8	61.7	34.2
Independent	0.0	2.2	4.6	7.5	27.8	8.8
Mobility outside home						
Unable	78.6	83.7	63.6	43.1	16.5	51.8
With help	21.4	15.2	34.5	52.4	66.1	43.1
Independent	0.0	1.1	1.9	4.5	17.4	5.1
Overall	1.9	12.3	34.8	35.6	15.4	100.0

[a] No. = 685.

Table 3 Severity Index by Karnofsky Performance Status[a]

	Severity index	Karnofsky performance status (%) 10	20	30	40	50	Total
Most functional	0–2	0.0	2.2	5.7	11.6	40.0	12.5
	3–5	0.0	5.4	9.6	18.7	30.4	15.4
	6–8	28.6	8.7	21.4	31.5	22.6	23.7
Least functional	9–11	21.4	31.5	31.4	26.2	6.9	25.5
	12–14	50.0	52.2	31.9	12.0	0.0	22.9
Total		1.9	12.3	34.8	35.6	15.4	100.0

[a] No. = 685.

severity index, which is shown in Table 3. A score of 0 was assigned if the patient could perform the activity independently; a score of 1 was assigned to the patient if he or she required assistance; a score of 2 indicated that the patient was unable to perform the activity. There is a very strong relationship between increasing KPS scores and higher functional status. The majority of patients with low KPS scores are in the least functional severity grouping.

Although patients may not be able to function independently without assistance, there is little evidence that hospitalization is of benefit. Patients with advanced disease who are less functional and in a terminal phase of their illness may actually derive more quality of life benefit by being at home with family where their emotional and spiritual needs can be met rather than in the sterile environment of the inpatient cancer ward. Similarly, patients with acute limitations of their functional status who are recovering from surgery may actually benefit more from outpatient rehabilitation programs than from prolonged hospitalizations. The KPS is not adequate as a single measure to discriminate between those patients who need and will benefit from hospitalization and those who can best be treated in the outpatient setting.

As an overall predictor of survival, however, KPS has been found to be an extremely important factor and in some studies has been more important than number of metastatic sites. In a study that examined the relationship between dose intensity and outcome in patients receiving CMF chemotherapy for treatment of breast cancer, Brufman and Biran (27) stratified their analysis by performance status using the KPS. Fig. 4 demonstrates 3-year survival rate according to performance status and shows that, for patients with a KPS >80%, more than half the patients are alive at 3 years compared to a 14% survival rate for patients with poor performance status ($p < .0001$).

The Zubrod score was developed in 1960 and is similar to the KPS (28). Zubrod, as part of a system to track data for clinical trials, developed a 5-point

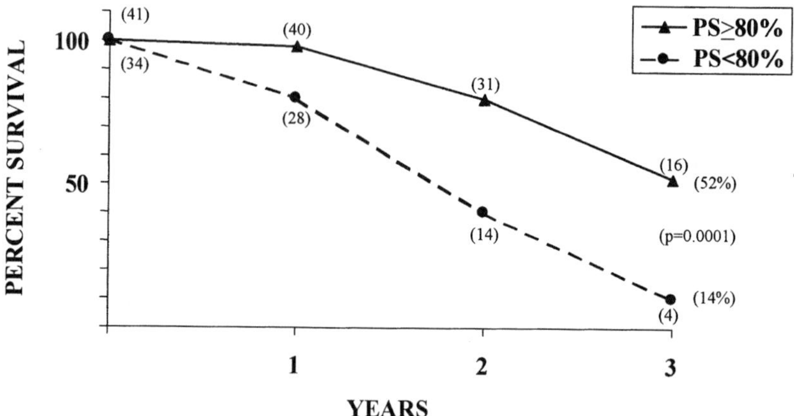

Figure 4 Actuarial 3-year survival rate according to performance status.

scale that focused only on patient's functional status. Table 4 demonstrates the original Zubrod scoring system and illustrates how other symptoms such as pain, nutrition, and nausea should be measured as part of the global assessment of patients' performance. Both the KPS and Zubrod scores have been used as proxy measures for rating quality of life. Because they only assess one dimension of the many constructs in quality of life, they should no longer be considered adequate as quality of life scores.

Performance status remains one of the most powerful predictive tools for selecting patients who are likely to benefit from chemotherapy. Performance status can also be used as a predictor of complications of febrile neutropenia and other common symptoms in outpatients receiving chemotherapy.

2. Severity of Illness

Another strategy for selecting patients who are suitable for outpatient treatment is to examine their severity of illness and choose patients according to a preset threshold value. In general, severity of the illness scoring systems have been used outside the field of oncology and are helpful in predicting short-term morbidity and mortality. One of the best known severity of illness systems is known as APACHE. The Acute Physiology and Chronic Health Evaluation (APACHE) scoring system was developed as a mechanism to correlate the risk of hospital death with intensive care unit (ICU) status (29). The APACHE II uses a point score based on initial values of 12 routine physiological measurements, previous health status, and age to provide a general measure of severity of disease (30). The APACHE II scores can range from 0 to 71 with a higher number indicating

Table 4 Original Zubrod Scoring System

Performance—Record in this section the performance that the patient is capable of. For example, a patient in the hospital for metabolic studies may be fully capable of normal activities, but will remain in bed through his own choice. Such a patient should be coded 0, "normal."
- 0 Normal activity
- 1 Symptoms, but nearly fully ambulatory
- 2 Some bed time, but needs to be in bed less than 50% of normal daytime
- 3 Needs to be in bed greater than 50% of normal daytime
- 4 Unable to get out of bed

Pain
- 0 None
- 1 Mild
- 2 Moderate
- 3 Severe

Food intake—Give calories of food intake if available, otherwise list patient's appetite as
- 3 Poor
- 2 Fair
- 1 Good

Nausea
- 0 None
- 1 Some
- 2 Marked

more severe illness. A variety of studies have been conducted using the scoring system to compare outcomes in the intensive care unit (31–33). The relationship between APACHE II score and hospital mortality is shown in Fig. 5. Although this system was developed in the general medical population, it can be used to discriminate between patients who have a high risk of dying in-hospital and those who are at very low risk of death. This scoring system can be used in oncology patients to select a low-risk population who might be suitable for an outpatient approach to therapy. Because this system was developed for use in the intensive care unit, it must be considered a research technique and undergo appropriate study and validation before it is routinely used outside the ICU in the oncology setting.

Another scoring system, which has been developed for case-mix adjustment, is known as MedisGroups (Medical Illness Severity Grouping System) (34). This proprietary system can be used upon admission to classify patients into one of five severity groupings. It uses key clinical information to help predict which patients will respond to therapy and those who will deteriorate and die in-hospital.

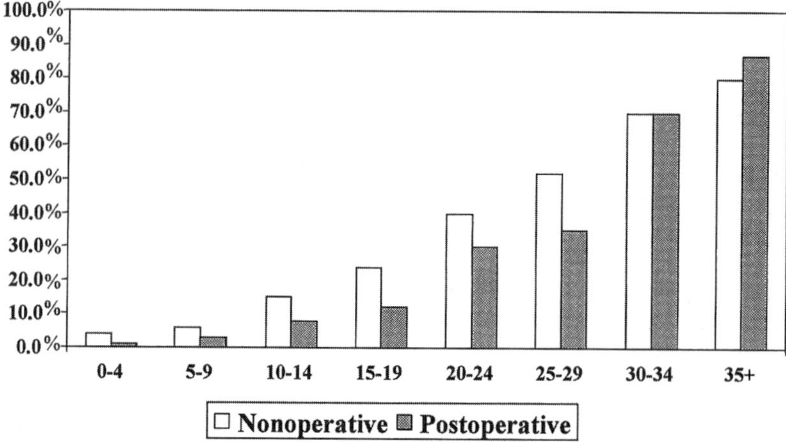

Figure 5 The relationship between APACHE II scores and hospital mortality among 5815 intensive care unit admissions.

Because it has not been used exclusively in patients with cancer, its generalizability to the oncology setting is unclear. Nevertheless, it provides a mechanism by which to identify patients at a high risk of death who are not suitable for outpatient treatment strategies.

Severity of illness systems are attractive to use because they provide the clinician with an objective measure that can be correlated with prospectively defined outcomes. As opposed to clinical judgment, which varies from practitioner to practitioner and is hard to define, severity of illness scores indicate that the higher the severity, as measured by the scoring system, the greater the patients' risk of experiencing major complications or death during their episodes of care. Most systems have been developed in the general medical population and have focused on complications of inpatient care. An objective system totally developed and validated in an oncology population would be of great value because it would enhance clinicians' ability to focus outpatient resources on the appropriate ambulatory population.

3. *Stability*

When choosing patients for outpatient care, it would be useful if clinicians could identify patients who were clinically stable and unlikely to undergo development of major medical complications or to die imminently. Acute clinical stability is a dimension of the patient's clinical status, which reflects his or her ability to handle physiological stress. The more stable a patient, the less likely it is that he or she will experience a major complication, such as shock or respiratory distress when faced with a new or added insult. The variables that make up stability are generally indicators of the patient's underlying organ function and metabolic status (23). These include the patient's vital signs (pulse, respiratory rate, blood pressure, temperature), serum electrolytes, renal function, liver function, arterial pH and level of oxygenation, hemoglobin, white blood cell count, level of consciousness, and nutritional status.

Generally, these variables are routinely measured in patients both in the hospital and the clinic setting. It is intuitive to clinicians that major derangements in these physiological parameters are predictive of bad outcomes in patients. It is easy to understand that a patient with a hemoglobin of 5.0 gs/dL and a serum creatinine of 13 mg/dL is likely to experience a short-term major medical complication or die unless there's an effective intervention. A complex scale or multiple variable model is not needed to help the clinician understand the importance of severe anemia and renal insufficiency as important indicators of stability. What is needed, however, is an understanding of the influence of some of these parameters on the patient's underlying condition to choose which patients can be safely treated outside the hospital setting. For example, a 33-year-old patient with carcinoma of the breast who has a new painful bone metastasis and who has a heart rate of 120 beats per minute may well be clinically stable and effectively treated as an outpatient with narcotic analgesics. The very same patient 1 month later who has an emergency department visit with fever and a pulse of 120 beats per minute may or may not be stable, depending on other parameters such as absolute neutrophil count or the presence or absence of hypotension. The ability to distinguish with certainty which patient is acceptable to treat as an outpatient depends on many factors and to a certain extent on interactions between factors. In the cases under discussion, other conditions might influence the physician's decision to admit these patients to the hospital for care, for example, another illness besides cancer.

4. Comorbidity

Patients with cancer often have other diseases besides their malignancies. These comorbid conditions often influence treatment decisions for the patients as well as their doctors. A patient with chronic obstructive lung disease who has active wheezing may be selected for inpatient chemotherapy treatment, whereas another patient with small cell carcinoma of the lung and of similar age and stability but without active bronchospasm may receive chemotherapy in the clinic. In addition to recognizing that comorbid conditions exist, it is also important to comprehend the extent of these conditions. Patients with chronic comorbidities, some of which are poorly controlled, may have much higher complication rates and lower response rates to treatment with higher mortality rates than similar patients without comorbid conditions. Many times, these comorbid conditions influence the types of chemotherapy that the patient receives or increases the patient's risk of having complications from chemotherapy. Common chemotherapeutic regimen, such as CHOP and ASHAP for lymphoma, may cause diabetics to decompensate because of the effects of steroids on glucose control. It is not unusual for patients with type II diabetes mellitus whose conditions are well controlled on oral hypoglycemic agents to temporarily require insulin during chemotherapy that contains high-dose steroids. Starting patients on insulin may be the reason for hospitalization in some settings, whereas, in others that have an infrastructure in place to handle diabetic education, the same situation can be handled in the outpatient environment.

Comorbidity scores have also been developed that examine the influence of multiple common chronic conditions on outcomes. Charlson et al. (35), in a population of 604 general medical patients admitted to the hospital in 1984, developed a weighted comorbidity index that takes into account both the number and seriousness of comorbid diseases in order to predict 1-year mortality rate.

Using this index, which is shown in Table 5, they demonstrated an increase

Table 5 Weighted Index of Comorbidity

Assigned weights for diseases	Conditions
1	Myocardial infarct
	Congestive heart failure
	Peripheral vascular disease
	Cerebrovascular disease
	Dementia
	Chronic pulmonary disease
	Connective tissue disease
	Ulcer disease
	Mild liver disease
	Diabetes
2	Hemiplegia
	Moderate or severe renal disease
	Diabetes with end organ damage
	Any tumor
	Leukemia
	Lymphoma
3	Moderate or severe liver disease
6	Metastatic solid tumor
	Acquired immunodeficiency disease

Table 6 Percentage 1-Year Mortality Rate According to Severity, Reason, and Scores from the Weighted Index of Comorbidity

Severity and reason for admission	Weighted index of comorbidity[a]			
	0	1–2	3–4	>5
Not ill to mildly ill				
Low risk	7 (82)	14 (68)	29 (14)	60 (20)
High risk	5 (18)	21 (19)	100 (3)	100 (5)
Moderately ill				
Low risk	7 (30)	19 (44)	38 (13)	91 (11)
High risk	16 (19)	28 (22)	50 (14)	73 (11)
Severely ill				
Low risk	26 (19)	33 (39)	36 (11)	100 (14)
High risk	38 (13)	58 (33)	94 (16)	100 (21)
Total	12 (181)	26 (125)	52 (71)	85 (82)

[a] The number in each cell represents the % dead followed in parentheses by the sample size.

in 1-year mortality rate as severity and comorbidity scores increased (Table 6). Charlson et al. then validated the comorbidity index in a cohort of 588 breast cancer patients who had a lower prevalence of comorbid disease than that of the derivation group. One-year survival rates were higher in the breast cancer cohort than in the general medical population, which demonstrates the difficulty in developing predictive classification systems in dissimilar populations. Nevertheless, the risk of death increased in stepwise fashion as the weighted index increased in both the general medical and breast cancer groups. Other systems currently in use are designed to evaluate short-term outcomes such as probability of 30-day mortality and risk of rehospitalization.

Our research program has explored, using performance status, severity of illness and stability scores to predict emergency center length of stay and disposition from the emergency center (admit versus discharge). In a study of 136 consecutive patients who presented to our emergency center with a variety of symptoms, including fever, pain, and dyspnea, those who were admitted to the hospital tended to have worse sickness scores than those patients sent home (36). Patients with pain who were admitted to the hospital tended to have worse severity of illness scores than those who could be managed without hospitalization. Performance status scores were less predictive of disposition from the emergency center, suggesting that patient severity of illness or stability may be a more important determinant that correlates with the clinical judgment to admit patients to the hospital. The use of these measures is displayed in Fig. 6 and demonstrates how

VISUAL ANALOG SCALE

How sick is the patient at presentation?
(Estimate the burden of illness considering all comorbid conditions. Make a vertical mark through the line corresponding to the assessment).

No signs or symptoms	Mild signs or symptoms	Moderate signs or symptoms	Severe signs or symptoms	Moribund

How stable is the patient at presentation?
(Estimate the patient's physiological reserve and his/her ability to compensate for the stress of an acute illness, invasive testing or rigorous treatment regimens. Make a vertical mark across the line corresponding to the assessment).

Can tolerate extreme stress	Can tolerate most stress	May have trouble with moderate stress	Trouble with mild stress	Trouble without stress

ZUBROD SCALE

Circle the appropriate score:

0	Fully active, able to carry out all pre-disease activities without restrictions (Karnofsky 90-100)	**3**	Capable of only limited self-care, confined to bed or chair 50% or more of waking hours. (Karnofsky 30-40)
1	Restricted in physically strenuous activity but ambulatory and able to carry out work of a light or sedentary nature, for example, light housework or office work. (Karnofsky 70-80)	**4**	Completely disabled, cannot carry on any self-care, totally confined to bed or chair. (Karnofsky 10-20)
2	Ambulatory and capable of all self-care but unable to carry out work activities. Up and about more than 50% of waking hours. (Karnofsky 50-60)		

Figure 6 Physician's record.

incorporating these instruments into routine practice may facilitate analysis of population-based data for improvement of clinical and administrative processes. Future studies are needed to assess how these measurements can be used to rapidly assess which patients require hospitalization, how these measurements correlate with short-term outcomes (e.g., hospital length of stay and inpatient complication rates), and whether they correlate with readmission rates when assessed before hospital discharge.

C. Risk Assessment Prediction Models and Receiver Operating Characteristic Curves

As previously discussed, a variety of methods exist to identify specific subsets of patients. However, single measures such as performance status, severity of illness, stability, or comorbidity are often inadequate in helping clinicians and policy makers decide which patients can be safely and effectively treated with outpatient strategies.

More complex methods using formal statistical modeling techniques may be used. These methods evaluate and weight various patient, disease, and treatment factors to discriminate between low and non-low risk patients. The process of statistical modeling usually involves selecting the population of interest and determining which outcomes of interest the investigator is trying to predict. To identify patients appropriate for outpatient care, we would like to predict those patients who are able to complete their therapy in the outpatient setting with a low rate of complications (defined in advance of the study) and a low incidence of hospitalization (or rehospitalization if early discharge is being considered). These patients are defined as low-risk cancer patients. A preliminary prediction model or derivation model can be developed using multivariate statistical techniques with either a retrospective data set or a prospective observational group. The resulting model is then validated using a separate prospective data set. Once derived and validated, the characteristics of the model can be evaluated using strategies that have evolved from the development of diagnostic tests. The model is then used to predict or prospectively distinguish low-risk cancer patients from all other cancer patients (defined here as non-low risk cancer patients).

In health promotion and disease prevention, clinicians use a variety of screening tests. The validity of a screening test is gauged by its performance, that is, to correctly identify individuals who have the disease or condition in question as ''test positive'' and to classify those without the disease or condition of interest as ''test negative'' (37). The sensitivity of a test, also known as the true positive, describes the probability of a ''test positive'' individual given that he or she truly has the disease. The false positive is simply 1-sensitivity, or the probability of a test being positive given that the individual truly does not have disease. Similarly, the specificity of a test, also known as the true negative, describes the probability of a ''test negative'' individual given that he or she truly does not have the condition of interest. Finally, false negative refers to 1-specificity, or the probability of a test being negative given that the person truly does have the condition of interest.

Using the principles of screening test validity, this same framework can be

Table 7 Screening Test Results Applied to a Prediction Model that Identifies Low-Risk Cancer Patients Who Can Be Appropriately Treated as Outpatients

	True underlying risk status		
Prediction model results	Truly low risk	Truly non–low risk	Total
Low-risk cancer patients	a	b	a + b
Non–low-risk cancer patients	c	d	c + d
Total	a + c	b + d	a + b + c + d

1. Sensitivity of clinical prediction model (defined as the probability or proportion of cancer patients correctly identified by prediction model as low risk) = true positive rate = a/(a + c).
2. Specificity of clinical prediction model (defined as the probability or proportion of cancer patients correctly identified by model as non–low risk) = true negative rate = d/(b + d).

applied to the identification of low-risk cancer patients who may be appropriately treated as outpatients. Table 7 shows a modification of the traditional 2 × 2 screening test table to reflect the operating characteristics of a clinical prediction model. If the clinical prediction model can be constructed such that low-risk patients can be prospectively identified, then resources can be efficiently used by assigning these patients to ambulatory treatment strategies. Likewise, those patients who have more likelihood of developing clinical morbidity can be treated in the inpatient setting where early intervention can be implemented once complications develop, and overall morbidity and mortality of treatment (with hopefully a lower cost of treatment) can be minimized. Viewed another way, prospective identification of patients with higher acuity and higher risk of complications who then are initially treated as inpatients minimizes the number of individuals who would be inappropriately undertreated with initial therapy in the outpatient setting. The number of individuals who would be overtreated (e.g., patients who should be outpatients but instead are kept in the inpatient setting) would also be minimized.

The receiver operating characteristic curve (ROC) can also be used to represent the results of a screening or diagnostic test or clinical prediction model. The ROC is constructed by graphing the sensitivity and 1-specificity for all possible cutoff values of a diagnostic test. One advantage of this technique is that ROC graphs provide a visual comparison of the tradeoffs between the true-positive rate (or sensitivity) and the false-positive rate (1-specificity) of a test. The ROC curves are most often used for three purposes: 1) to determine the discriminative ability of a diagnostic test, 2) to compare several diagnostic tests to each other, and 3) to determine the optimal cut-off point of a diagnostic test. In medicine, clinical judgment involves the synthesis of subjective data such as symptoms, objective signs, laboratory values, and diagnostic tests, all of which are amassed into specific diagnoses.

An ROC is a useful graphical technique, because it allows clinicians to measure the performance of a screening or diagnostic test to discriminate between diseased and nondiseased individuals within a given population (38). Among the many applications in oncology, ROC analysis has been used in evaluating the diagnostic performance in breast cancer, prostate cancer detection, and radiotherapy for cancer (38–43).

Fig. 7 shows a hypothetical ROC graph for the clinical prediction model. Following the framework introduced in Table 7, the sensitivity (or the proportion of true positives) of the model is measured along the ordinate; this is the proportion of cancer patients correctly identified by the model as being low risk. Similarly, the proportion of patients incorrectly identified by the prediction model as

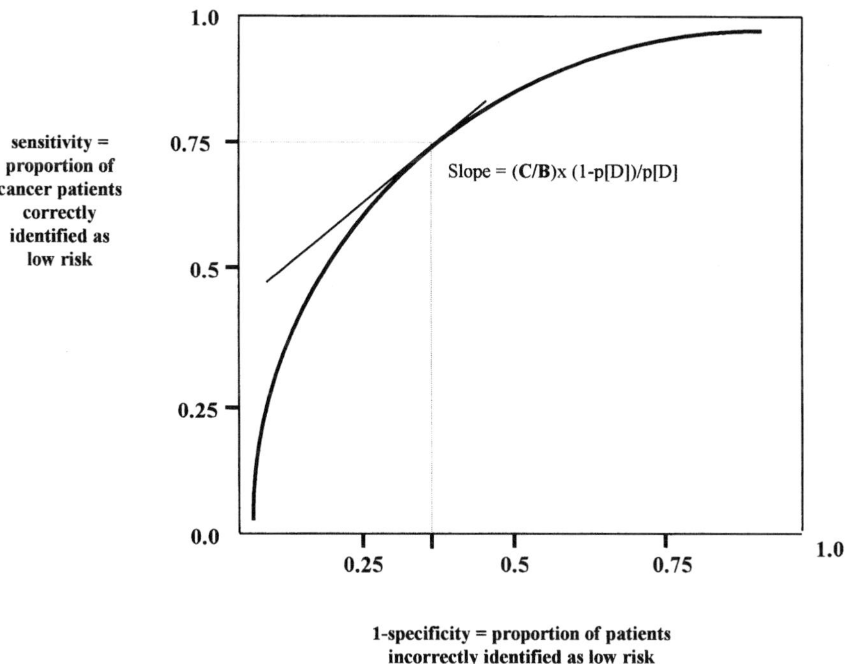

Figure 7 An example of a receiver operating curve for a prediction model that identifies low-risk cancer patients who can be appropriately treated as outpatients.

low risk (proportion of false positives) is plotted along the abscissa. The greater the area under the receiver operating curve, the better the discriminative ability of the test. This is easily visualized, because (although technically impossible) the ideal test would have both 100% sensitivity and 100% specificity. In other words, clinicians generally prefer those tests that have the greatest area under the curve. In real life, however, sensitivity is usually maximized by a trade-off for lower specificity.

The selection of an appropriate cut-off point to distinguish positive tests from negative tests may also be chosen from the ROC graph. Typically, when test results are expressed as continuous variables, clinicians can select which results will be deemed ''abnormal'' (this is usually the ''upper limit of normal''). The ROC provides a different strategy for the selection of a cut-off point. This technique incorporates two characteristics of the patient: the pretest probability of testing positive (or the likelihood that the patient is a low-risk cancer patient) and the importance to the patient (or clinician) of avoiding false-positive and false-negative results; that is, minimizing overtreatment and undertreatment. The appropriate cut-off point is the point at which the slope of the ROC curve equals the following: $(C/B) \times (1\text{-}p[D])/p[D]$, where C is costs or burden of overtreating; B is benefits of appropriate treatment; and p[D] is the prevalence of the condition of interest. Thus, selecting the cut-off point for a test using the ROC method allows for the explicit incorporation of tradeoffs between overtreatment and undertreatment.

The threshold or cut-off point that separates cancer patients who are likely to be low risk from those patients who are likely to be high risk relies on the ratio between the net ''costs'' of treating individuals who are truly low risk on an inpatient basis (rather than the more appropriate outpatient setting) and the net ''benefits'' of treating cancer patients who are truly high risk on an inpatient basis. In other words, the threshold point encompasses the relative costs or burdens of overtreatment to the net benefits or gains of appropriate treatment. Costs and benefits can be measured in dollars or in a metric that incorporates the quality of life or patient preferences.

As a result, the challenge for clinicians is to identify the point on the ROC curve where the relative sensitivity (or true-positive rate) and specificity (or true-negative rate) are acceptable in the clinical setting. Put another way, clinicians (and patients) must decide what costs or burdens of overtreatment they are willing to accept for a given level of benefit of appropriate treatment. If the condition of interest is a matter of life and death and has a reasonably high probability of occurring (and hospitalization with early intervention and treatment is effective), then clinicians would be most likely to accept a higher rate of overhospitalization rather than undertreating high-risk patients as outpatients; that is, it is better to hospitalize a few extra low-risk patients who do not need hospitalization rather than let high-risk patients be treated initially in the outpatient setting.

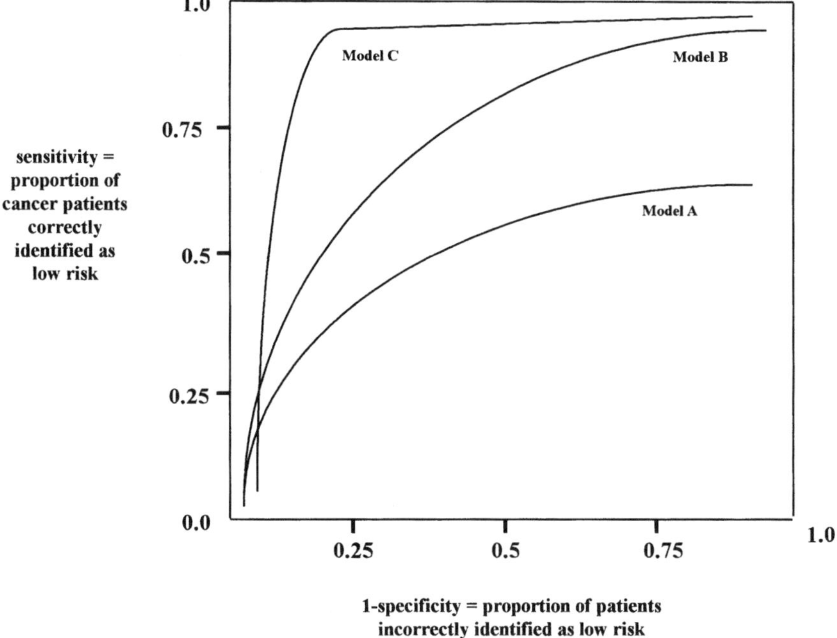

Figure 8 An example of receiver operating curves to compare several clinical presentation models.

Finally, if several diagnostic tests exist to test for the same clinical condition, ROC analysis allows clinicians to visually compare the operating characteristics of each test. For example, suppose three different clinical prediction models exist. The superior prediction model is the one that encompasses the greatest area under the curve (AUC). Fig. 8 illustrates this example. The ROC of prediction model C clearly encompasses the greatest AUC; therefore, prediction model C demonstrates the greatest level of sensitivity and specificity and is the superior model.

This approach using formal statistical methods is being used by the Multinational Association for Supportive Care in Cancer Study Section for Infectious Disease to develop a model to predict outcomes in patients with febrile neutropenic episodes. Preliminary data suggest that important factors that predict a low risk of developing complications during a febrile neutropenic episode include outpatient status at the onset of fever, $p < .001$, absence of dehydration, $p < .0001$, normal renal function, $p < .02$, solid tumor or lymphoma, $p < .01$, age younger than 60 years, $p < .003$, normal respiratory rate at presentation with fever, $p < .03$, and clinical stability at presentation, $p < .001$ (44).

D. Nonmedical Criteria

Patients may be clinically eligible for outpatient chemotherapy or other treatment for complications of chemotherapy yet still not be able to be effectively managed outside the hospital setting. Local institutional practices may be insufficient to support technically feasible therapeutic approaches. Outpatient services may not be available 24 hours a day; these services are essential for programs such as outpatient treatment of febrile neutropenia.

1. *Psychosocial Factors*

Family or caregiver support systems are often necessary to implement effective outpatient treatment programs. Patients often require assistance with transportation back and forth to the clinic. Some treatment regimens are associated with sedating side effects or other symptoms such as nausea and vomiting, which may make it unsafe for the patient to drive himself or herself to appointments.

Patient compliance is another factor that influences the decision to admit a patient to the hospital for treatment or to try outpatient therapy. Patients who have a history of being noncompliant with their appointments for tests or follow-up visits are considered to be unreliable subjects for complex outpatient treatment strategies. In some situations, patients who have difficulty taking their medications as prescribed are hospitalized so that medicines that are ''time-dependent'' (e.g., leucovorin) can be given with certainty.

Patients who have some degree of functional disability may need caregiver support to handle complex outpatient treatment protocols, which are common in comprehensive cancer centers. Programmable outpatient infusion devices, often used for chemotherapy, hydration, antibiotics, and pain control, can be difficult for some patients to manage by themselves. Family and caregiver burden associated with these needs may place additional stress on a social network that already may be struggling to deal with the psychological effects of having a patient with a potentially catastrophic illness.

Little is known about the role functioning effects of being an outpatient undergoing cancer chemotherapy (45). Is the patient expected to fulfill the usual family role of spouse, parent/provider and maintain the vigor needed to battle illness? Many patients experience depression, anger, grief, and social isolation as part of their illness. The ability to handle the psychological effects of the cancer experience in many ways is influenced by patients' premorbid state of mental health and that of their family. At times, patients and their families need some respite to handle the stress of outpatient cancer care (45).

Some patients prefer being hospitalized for their care, and in certain situations, these preferences are the sole reason for hospitalization. As decisions to hospitalize patients are subject to greater scrutiny and case management, these nonmedical criteria for admission are likely to be underreported and justified using different, ''more medically appropriate'' reasons.

2. Socioeconomic Factors

Reimbursement factors are some of the most common nonmedical reasons to admit patients to the hospital for treatment. In the United States, some insurance plans do not pay for outpatient care, whereas they do pay for the same treatment if administered inside the hospital. Many years ago, the Health Care Financing Administration (HCFA) changed its policies for reimbursement for outpatient intravenous antibiotic therapy, allowing for some diagnoses to be treated in the outpatient setting under the Medicare program. Patients with endocarditis and osteomyelitis can be treated with outpatient intravenous antibiotics and providers can receive reimbursement for these services. Common treatments for cancer patients, such as intravenous antibiotic therapy for febrile neutropenic episodes, are not reimbursable under federally sponsored Medicare and Medicaid programs. This leads to routine hospitalization when other ambulatory approaches have been demonstrated to be safe and effective (46,47). The costs of certain drugs such as colony-stimulating factors are reimbursed when administered in doctors' offices or hospital-based outpatient treatment infusion centers but not when dispensed directly to the patient, thereby imposing extra transportation burdens for patients and their families.

In addition to the transportation burdens, there may be increased motel and hotel costs of visits when the cancer center is located far from home. As a result, outpatient chemotherapy or treatment for complications become difficult for patients and their caregivers. In these situations, patients are frequently hospitalized for care when, from a medical and technical standpoint, they theoretically could receive their treatment on an outpatient basis. Some outpatient treatment programs are technically feasible and patients are medically suitable, but the therapies are complex, requiring extensive patient education and surveillance. In these situations, telephone follow-up is frequently useful so that patients can call clinic personnel for advice. Outpatient research protocols are facilitated when research nurses can call the patient at home to collect symptom response data and assess compliance with therapy. Unfortunately, some patients may not have access to a telephone at their residence, raising concerns about the appropriateness of ambulatory care in these situations.

IV. BENEFITS OF OUTPATIENT CARE

Cancer care should be viewed as a continuum that intersperses episodic events with cycles of treatment. From the onset of symptoms that prompt the diagnostic evaluation to the initiation of therapy, 85% to 90% of all cancer care occurs on an outpatient basis. It has been estimated that, on average, all cancer patients will undergo one surgical procedure, two cycles of chemotherapy, and 0.6 courses of radiation therapy in their lifetime.

The influence of outpatient cancer care on outcomes such as quality of life, cost of care, productivity, and other benefits are poorly documented. Because most of these benefits are intuitive, they are not empirically studied and are therefore open to question. Our own research has suggested that it is possible to shift traditionally inpatient-based care, such as the treatment of febrile neutropenia, to the outpatient setting. We have documented the cost-effectiveness of outpatient management of febrile neutropenia compared to the traditional approach of inpatient intravenous antibiotic therapy (48). We have preliminary data suggesting that quality of life in patients with febrile episodes can be measured and that quality of life improves as the fever decreases in response to antibiotic therapy (49). Assuming that this treatment occurs in the outpatient setting, one can conclude that outpatient treatment of febrile episodes in neutropenic cancer patients is associated with an improvement in quality of life. We do not know whether outpatient cancer care lowers colonization rates with resistant microbial flora, but this is theoretically possible.

Using the techniques of risk assessment, it is possible to identify other populations of low-risk patients who are commonly admitted to the hospital for complications of chemotherapy or other problems associated with their malignancy. Treatment strategies for these low-risk patients can be designed and tested. If proven to be safe and effective, these strategies can be implemented while improvements in outcomes are evaluated. Other areas where research seeking to identify particular subgroups of patients for various treatment strategies have been conducted. These include high-dose chemotherapy and peripheral blood stem cell infusion in patients with non-Hodgkin's lymphoma, management of febrile neutropenic pediatric cancer patients at low risk of bacteremia, development and validation of prediction rules for bacteremia in patients with sepsis syndrome, outpatient treatment of patients with community-acquired pneumonia, inpatient treatment of patients with community-acquired pneumonia, and prevention of deep vein thrombosis in high-risk patients (50–57).

The psychological benefits to patients and their families of outpatient cancer care should not be underestimated. Many patients view cancer therapy as a life-changing event that calls into question their spiritual beliefs and challenges them to reassess what they value. Outpatient cancer care may give patients faced with catastrophic ailments such as cancer an opportunity to maintain some control over what they believe is a situation in which their bodies are out of control. Patients often view hospitalization as an indication that the severity of the cancer is worsening. Outpatient care maximizes the amount of time patients can spend with their family and loved ones, particularly for patients who have progressive disease with little hope for cure. It is not known how patients value outpatient cancer care as compared to inpatient therapy. Incorporating patient preferences into medical decision making is an important area of future research.

The issue of how outpatient cancer care influences overall cost of care is a complex economic question. Many economists view outpatient therapy as simply cost shifting with the hotel costs and other caregiver costs transferred to the patients or their families.

V. CONCLUSIONS AND FUTURE RESEARCH

The practice of medicine is shifting from an age of empiricism to an era of evidence-based process/outcomes driven care. How we use population-derived data to make individual patient decisions will be important. Clinical judgment is still very important and caring for patients should be driven by what is best for them rather than what is permissible. Outpatient cancer care, whether it is chemotherapy, biological/molecular medicine, surgery or radiation therapy, is highly complex, inherently multidisciplinary, and costly. We should focus our research efforts in many areas as part of the ''quest for the cure.'' Efficient use of limited health care resources benefits the practice of medicine and outcomes research as it relates to outpatient cancer care and should assist in helping to define ''the right procedure, in the right setting, at the right time.''

REFERENCES

1. American Society of Clinical Oncology. Training resource document for curriculum development in medical oncology. J Clin Oncol 1998; 16(1):372–379.
2. Hotchkiss SM. Nurses must provide effective teaching and support in oncology outpatient settings. Oncol Nursing Forum 1997; 24(8):1330–1331
3. International Union Against Cancer. Guidelines for Developing a Comprehensive Cancer Center and Other Clinical Cancer Facilities. 3rd ed. Geneva, Switzerland: UICC, 1990.
4. Einzig AI, Wiernik PH, Sasloff J, et al. Phase II study and long-term follow up of patients treated with Taxol for advanced ovarian adenocarcinoma. J Clin Oncol 1992; 10:1748–1753.
5. The Italian Cooperative Study Group on Myeloid Leukemia. Interferon alfa-2a as compared with conventional chemotherapy for the treatment of chronic myeloid leukemia. N Engl J Med 1994; 330:820–825.
6. Crawford J, Ozer H, Stoller R, et al. Reduction by granulocyte colony-stimulating factor of fever and neutropenia induced by chemotherapy in patients with small-cell lung cancer. N Engl J Med 1991; 325:164–170.
7. Rolston K, Berkey P, Bodey G, et al. A comparison of imipenem to ceftazidime with or without amikacin as empiric therapy in febrile neutropenic patients. Arch Intern Med 1992; 152:283–291.

8. Haron E, Rolston KVI, Cunningham C, Holmes F, Umsawasdi T, Bodey GP. Oral ciprofloxacin therapy for infections in cancer patients. J Antimicrob Chemother 1989; 24:955–962.
9. De Mulder PHM, Seynaeve C, Vermorker JB, et al. Ondansteron compared with high dose metoclopramide in prophylaxis of acute and delayed cisplatin-induced nausea and vomiting: a multicenter, randomized, double-blind, crossover study. Ann Intern Med 1990; 113:834–840.
10. Foley KM, Inturrisi CE. Analgesic drug therapy in cancer pain: principles and practice. Med Clin North Am 1987; 71:207–231.
11. Garnick MB. Prostate cancer: screening, diagnosis, and management. Ann Intern Med 1993; 118:804–818.
12. Davidsohn I. Early immunologic diagnosis and prognosis of carcinoma. Am J Clin Pathol 1972; 57:715–730.
13. Peters W, Ross M, Vredenburgh J, et al. The use of intensive clinic support to permit outpatient autologous bone marrow transplantation for breast cancer. Semin Oncol 1994; 21(suppl):25–31.
14. Hunt KK, Feig BW, Ames FC. Ambulatory surgery for breast cancer. The Cancer Bulletin 1995; 47(4):292–297.
15. American Cancer Society. Cancer Facts and Figures—1998. New York: American Cancer Society, 1998.
16. Inglehart J. Early experience with prospective payment of hospitals. N Engl J Med 1986; 22:1460–1464.
17. Rubenstein EB. Costs and benefits of outpatient therapy. Supportive Care Cancer 1994; 2:307–311.
18. American Hospital Association. Hospital trends, U.S. community hospitals. Chicago: AHA Hospital Statistics, 1998:9.
19. Bailes JS. Current issues in oncology reimbursement. Oncology 1995; 9(11 suppl): 185–189.
20. Stoline A, Weiner J. The new medical marketplace. Baltimore: The Johns Hopkins University Press, 1993:5–116.
21. Thomas S, Glynne-Jones R, Chait I. Is it worth the wait? A survey of patients' satisfaction with an oncology outpatient clinic. Eur J Cancer Care (English Language Edition) 1997; 6(1):50–58.
22. Klastersky J, Razavi D. Supportive care: editorial review. Curr Opin Oncol 1994; 6:333–334.
23. Iezzoni LI. Dimensions of risk. In: Risk Adjustment for Measuring Health Care Outcomes. Health Administration Press, Ann Arbor, Michigan 1994:29–118.
24. Karnofsky DA, Burchenal JH. The clinical evaluation of chemotherapeutic agents in cancer. In: Macleod CM, ed. Evaluation of Chemotherapeutic Agents. New York: Columbia University Press, 1948:191–205.
25. Yates JW, Chalmer B, McKegney FP. Evaluation of patients with advanced cancer using the Karnofsky Performance Status. Cancer 1980; 45:2220–2224.
26. Mor V, Laliberte L, Morris JN, Wiemann M. The Karnofsky Performance Status Scale: an examination of its reliability and validity in a research setting. Cancer 1984; 53:2002–2007.
27. Brufman G, Biran S. Prognostic factors affecting treatment results with combina-

tion chemotherapy in metastatic breast cancer. Anticancer Research 1986; 6:733–736.

28. Zubrod C, Schneiderman M, Frei E, Brindley C, Gold GL, Shnider B, et al. Appraisal of methods for the study of chemotherapy of cancer in man: comparative therapeutic trial of nitrogen mustard and triethylene thiophosphoramide. J Chron Dis 1960; 11(1):7–33.
29. Knaus WA, Zimmerman JE, Wagner DP, et al. APACHE—acute physiology and chronic health evaluation: a physiologically based classification system. Crit Care Med 1981; 9:591.
30. Knaus WA, Draper EA, Wagner DP, Zimmerman JE. Apache II: a severity of disease classification system. Crit Care Med 1985; 13(10):818–829.
31. Knaus WA, Draper EA, Wagner DP, Zimmerman JE. An evaluation of outcome from intensive care in major medical centers. Ann Intern Med 1986; 104:410–418.
32. Brannen AL, Godfrey LJ, Goetter WE. Prediction of outcome from critical illness: A comparison of clinical judgment with a prediction rule. Arch Intern Med 1989; 149:1083–1086.
33. Dragsted L, Jorgensen J, Jensen N, Bonsing E, Jacobsen E, Knaus WA, et al. Interhospital comparisons of patient outcome from intensive care: Importance of lead-time bias. Crit Care Med 1989; 17:418.
34. Brewster AC, Karlin BG, Hyde LA, Jacobs CM, Bradbury RC, Chae YM. MEDISGRPS: a clinically based approach to classifying hospital patients at admissions. Inquiry 1985; 22(4):377–387.
35. Charlson ME, Pompei P, Ales KL, MacKenzie CR. A new method of classifying prognostic comorbidity in longitudinal studies: development and validation. J Chronic Dis 1987; 40(5):373–383.
36. Bratka C, Elting L, Martin C, Chau Q, Rubenstein EB. Patients' ratings of illness and stability: correlation with clinicians' ratings and emergency center outcomes (abstract 71). Supportive Care Cancer 1997; 5(2):173
37. Hennekens CH, Buring JE. Epidemiology in medicine. Mayrent SL, ed. Boston: Little, Brown, 1987.
38. Rombach JJ, Collette BJA, de Waard CF, Slotboom BJ. Analysis of the diagnostic performance in breast cancer screening by relative operating characteristics. Cancer 1986; 58:169–177.
39. Dominguez-Gadea L, Martin-Curto LM, Crespo A, Avila C. MCA serum determination in breast carcinoma patients for the diagnosis of bone metastases. Int J Biol Markers 1993; 8:203–207.
40. Littrup PJ, Kane RA, Mettlin CJ, Murphy GP, Lee F, Toi A, Badalament R, Babaian R. Cost-effective prostate cancer detection: reduction of low-yield biopsies. Cancer 1994; 74:3146–3158.
41. Catalona WJ, Hudson MA, Scardino PT, Richie JP, Ahmann FR, Flanigan RC, deKernion JB, Ratliff TL, Kavoussi LR, Dalkin BL, Waters WB, MacFarlane MT, Southwick PC. Selection of optimal prostate specific antigen cutoffs for early detection of prostate cancer: receiver operating characteristic curves. J Urol 1994; 152: 2037–2042.
42. Maciejewski B, Zajusz A, Rota L. ROC analysis of benefit and limitation in radiotherapy for cancer of the oral cavity. Neoplasma 1993; 40:181–184.

43. Andrews JR. Benefit, risk, and optimization by ROC analysis in cancer radiotherapy. Int J Radiation Oncol Biol Phys 1985; 11: 1557–1562.
44. Klastersky J. Prognostic factors for outcome in cancer patients with febrile neutropenia: a multinational survey from the Infection Committee of the Multinational Association for Supportive Care in Cancer (17:419A, abstract 1617). In: Program Proceedings of the American Society of Clinical Oncology, Los Angeles, CA, May 16–19, 1998.
45. Frisbee-Hume S. Ambulatory treatment of oncology patients: impact on caregivers. The Cancer Bulletin 1995; 47(4):330–334.
46. Rubenstein EB, Rolston K, Benjamin RS, Loewy J, Escalante C, Manzullo E, et al. Outpatient treatment of febrile episodes in low-risk neutropenic patients with cancer. Cancer 1993; 71(11):3640–3646.
47. Rubenstein EB, Rolston K. Outpatient management of febrile episodes in neutropenic cancer patients. Supportive Care Cancer 1994; 2:369–373
48. Cantor SB, Rubenstein EB, Elting LS, Frisbee-Hume S, Bratka CS, Stedman D, et al. Economic evaluation of management strategies for low risk febrile neutropenic cancer patients (16:419a, abstract 1498). In: Program/Proceedings of the American Society for Clinical Oncology, Denver, CO, May 17–20, 1997.
49. Elting LS, Rubenstein EB, Frisbee-Hume S, Kurtin D, Deng Y. Quality of life assessment in cancer patients receiving supportive care (abstract P-44). In: Proceedings of the 6th International Symposium Supportive Care in Cancer. New Orleans, LA, March 2–5, 1994.
50. Weaver Ch, Schwartzberg L, Zhen B, Mangum M, Leff R, Tauer K, Rosenberg A, Pendergrass K, Kaywin P, Hainsworth J, Greco FA, West WH, Buckner CD. High dose chemotherapy and peripheral blood stem cell infusion in patients with non-Hodgkin's lymphoma: results of outpatient treatment in community cancer centers. Bone Marrow Transplantation 1997; 20(9):753–760.
51. Mustafa MM, Aquino VM, Pappo A, Tkaczewski I, Buchanan GR. A pilot study of outpatient management of febrile neutropenic children with cancer at low risk of bacteremia. J Pediatr 1996; 128(6):847–849.
52. Rackoff WR, Gonin R, Robinson C, Kreissman SG, Breitfeld PB. Predicting the risk of bacteremia in children with fever and neutropenia. J Clin Oncol 1996; 14(3):919–924.
53. Bates DW, Sands K, Miller E, Lanken PN, Hibberd PL, Graman PS, Schwartz JS, Kahn K, Snydman DR, Parsonnet J, Moore R, Black E, Johnson BL, Jha A, Platt R. Predicting bacteremia in patients with sepsis syndrome. Academic Medical Center Consortium Sepsis Project Working Group. J Infect Dis 1997; 176(6):1538–1551.
54. Minogue MF, Coley CM, Fine MJ, Marrie TJ, Kapoor WN, Singer DE. Patients hospitalized after initial outpatient treatment for community-acquired pneumonia. Ann Emerg Med 1998; 31(3):376–380.
55. Fine MJ, Hough LJ, Medsger AR, Li YH, Ricci EM, Singer DE, Marrie TJ, Coley CM, Walsh MB, Karpf M, Lahive KC, Kapoor WN. The hospital admission decision for patients with community-acquired pneumonia: results from the pneumonia Patient Outcomes Research Team cohort study. Arch Intern Med 1997; 157(1):36–44.
56. Agnelli G, Sonaglia F. Prevention of venous thromboembolism in high-risk patients. Haematologica 1997; 82(4):496–502.
57. Anand SS, Wells PS, Hunt D, Brill-Edwards P, Cook D, Ginsberg JS. Does this patient have deep vein thrombosis? JAMA 1998; 279(14):1094–1099.

24

Infusion, Access Devices, and Complications of Extravasation

J. C. Pector

Institut Jules Bordet, Université Libre de Bruxelles, Brussels, Belgium

I. INTRODUCTION

Vascular access is one of the most commonly used techniques in the care of the patient with cancer. Long-term management of cancer requires reliable vascular access for delivery of cytotoxic drugs, analgesics, antiemetics, antibiotics, fluids, blood products and nutritional support. Moreover, frequent blood sampling is needed for monitoring of the effects of treatment upon cell counts and serum chemistries. Often treated as a routine matter, venous access can have serious consequences and therefore must be taken seriously by physician and patient.

Formerly, cytotoxic drugs were delivered intravenously through peripheral cannulas placed in veins of the hand or forearm or through temporary central lines inserted in the brachial or subclavian vein. Serious problems were associated with these methods, including drug extravasation into soft tissue, phlebitis, vein exhaustion, pneumothorax, hemothorax, and significant patient discomfort.

New techniques and catheters for venous access in cancer patients have been devised, resulting in greater comfort and improved quality of life during therapy. The indwelling venous access devices provide safe and comfortable delivery of cytotoxic drugs in patients who previously had to endure multiple painful attempts at peripheral and central venous cannulation. However, the insertion of vascular access devices is technically demanding and should not be underestimated as "minor surgery." An indwelling venous access device is not without potential for morbidity and even mortality. As such, the benefit of placing such a device needs to be carefully measured against the potential risks associated with it. Factors contributing to this decision include access availability, type and length of therapy, and patient compliance.

II. VASCULAR ACCESS DEVICES

Several systems are devised for obtaining chronic central venous access in the cancer patient. Each of these systems has its own relative indication as well as advantages and disadvantages in regard to placement, care, and management of potential complications.

A. Percutaneous, Short-Term Central Venous Catheters

Placement of a stiff plastic central venous catheter provides a more secure route of access than a peripheral cannula and avoids extravasation. It is a temporary method only, however, and suitable for use in an acute inpatient setting over 2 to 3 weeks at most. A triple-lumen catheter is available when multiple drugs are to be administered simultaneously.

A theoretical advantage of this kind of catheter is that it can be replaced at the bedside over a guide wire. Although routine changing of these catheters is often practiced, studies have failed to demonstrate the effectiveness of this to prevent infection, and exchanging catheters using a guide wire actually increases the risk of development of bacteremia (1).

B. Long-Term, Silastic, Tunneled Right Atrial Catheters

Initially implemented by Broviac (2) in 1973 and subsequently modified by Hickman (3) in 1979, long-term indwelling Silastic venous access devices have numerous advantages over short-term peripheral or central venous catheters: they eliminate discomfort and anxiety from multiple venipunctures and their larger lumen permits more rapid infusion. The Silastic material is associated with a low rate of vein thrombosis and a low rate of catheter obstruction, compared to devices made from other materials or with smaller internal diameters.

To reduce the risk of infection, the catheter is brought out to the skin via a subcutaneous tunnel at least 10 cm from the site of venous implantation. Burying the catheter in a subcutaneous tunnel reduces pathogen transfer by increasing the distance between the skin/catheter junction and vein. A Dacron cuff is added to the midportion of the catheter; this cuff produces a fibrotic reaction with the subcutaneous tissues forming a barrier to the upward migration of bacteria along the route of the catheter.

Because some length of the catheter protrudes from the skin, it is susceptible to damage and dislodgement. Both the catheter and the site must routinely be maintained to decrease the risk of infection. Not to be underestimated are the alterations in self-image and the limitations in activities of daily living and lifestyle imposed by this type of device.

C. Long-Term, Double-Lumen, Silastic Right Atrial Catheters

Patients who are receiving multiple-agent chemotherapy or bone marrow transplantation may require intensive intravenous (IV) support through more than one route of venous access. This need can be met by a double-lumen, Silastic right atrial catheter, which allows simultaneous infusion of several, possibly incompatible agents. The double-lumen catheter is also useful for patients during the perioperative period, allowing both intensive IV support and total parenteral nutrition. Each lumen of the Quinton double-lumen catheter has a D-shaped configuration but the outer catheter contour is round, allowing an easy percutaneous placement through a peel-away introducer.

D. Subcutaneous, Totally Implanted Venous Access Ports

The totally implanted venous access port consists of a plastic, stainless steel, or titanium chamber connected to a standard silicone right atrial catheter. The port is implanted subcutaneously against the chest wall just superficial to the pectoralis major muscle, in an infraclavicular position. The Silastic septum of the port is designed for penetration by a needle that is introduced through the skin, through the septum, and into the port chamber. The ''Huber'' needle used to access ports has a side hole designed to minimize coring of the Silastic septum.

More than 25 companies manufacture totally venous access ports, which have gained increasing popularity.

Drugs may be infused or blood samples withdrawn through the access port. It has a cosmetic advantage over percutaneous catheters in that it does not compromise the patient's normal physical appearance and does not interfere with daily activities when the catheter is not in use.

E. P.A.S. Port

The P.A.S. Port (Pharmacia-Deltec, St. Paul, MN) is subcutaneously inserted peripherally in the arm. The catheter is introduced via a vein in the antecubital region and then advanced to its central venous location. Because it is peripherally placed, operative complications such as pneumothorax and hemothorax are avoided. However, many patients may not have adequate antecubital venous access as a result of, for example, previous chemotherapy or obesity.

F. Infusion Pumps

Many types of pumps have been devised to deliver chemotherapy and other drugs intra-arterially or intravenously. For example, to deliver floxuridine to a tumor in the liver by hepatic artery infusion, a catheter is inserted surgically in the gastroduodenal artery and connected to a subcutaneously implanted device such as the Infusaid Pump (Infusaid Corp., Norwood, MA), which contains a two-phase charging fluid that compresses a collapsible bellows reservoir when heated to body temperature.

Some chemotherapy is delivered by continuous infusion rather than by bolus IV injection. A variety of portable pumps that can be connected easily to the venous access system have been developed, providing greater simplicity, miniaturization, or sophistication of delivery. The simplest ''pumps''—such as the Travenol Infusor (Travenol Laboratories, Deerfield, IL)—consist of a balloon reservoir (in a plastic case) that contracts at a relatively constant rate of 2 mL/h.

The CADD-plus (Pharmacia Deltec, St. Paul, MN) is a battery-driven, portable external pump, which may be used to deliver a 100-mL infusion over 1 to 4 days. Electronically controlled pumps offer the possibility of patient-activated bolus doses of pain medication, simply by pressing a button. A PCA (patient-controlled analgesia) pump delivers a preprogrammed amount of analgesic intravenously into the epidural space or subcutaneously. A programmed lock-out time prevents overdosage. Continuous infusion of the pain medication may be used in addition to bolus self-injection.

III. OPERATIVE TECHNIQUES

Most of the devices can be placed with local anesthesia. General anesthesia is rarely needed. Central venous access is usually obtained by accessing the superior vena cava via the internal or external jugular, subclavian, or cephalic veins. Because the upper central circulation may be obliterated as a result of thrombus or contraindicated by tumor impingement or by future surgery or radiotherapy, the inferior vena cava may be accessed through the saphenous or femoral veins when needed (4).

Percutaneous placement is simple and rapid, made possible by the development of the peel-away introducer. Although venous cutdown is usually somewhat more time-consuming, it is advocated by some authors (5,6) as the procedure of choice, on the basis of certainty of placement and a very low risk of pneumothorax. However, most studies suggest that the insertion technique requiring minimal dissection is more beneficial in terms of excessive bleeding, hematoma formation, and subsequent infection (7,8).

Often treated as a routine matter, the procedure requires that the operating surgeon must be well versed in vascular anatomy, the more experienced operators having the lower complications rate (9).

IV. MANAGEMENT OF VASCULAR ACCESS COMPLICATIONS

A. Intraoperative Morbidity and Complications

The potential intraoperative complications include bleeding, brachial plexus injury, cardiac arrhythmia, cardiac tamponade, hematoma, hemothorax, hydrothorax, vessel laceration or perforation, pneumothorax, and thoracic duct injury. The most common complications include hemorrhage, pneumothorax, and an inability to gain central venous access.

1. Hemorrhage

Inadvertent puncture of the carotid artery may cause a hematoma. Should artery entry occur, the needle is immediately withdrawn and compression applied.

In many cancer patients, intraoperative or postoperative bleeding is exacerbated by preexisting hematological defects, mainly thrombocytopenia. Preoperative platelet transfusion is recommended for patients with absolute platelet counts of less than 40,000/mm^3 to minimize the risk of significant intraoperative hemorrhage (10,11). Persistent bleeding from the subcutaneous tunnel or pocket can often be controlled with direct pressure.

2. Pneumothorax

Puncture of the pleura is likely to lead to pneumothorax. This complication results mainly from percutaneous placement of a central venous access device via the subclavian approach and less frequently via the internal jugular approach. At our institution, the incidence of pneumothorax is about 2%.

In many instances, a small pneumothorax requires no definite treatment and spontaneously resorbs; a larger or symptomatic pneumothorax requires the placement of a closed tube thoracostomy.

B. Postoperative Complications

1. Infection

Although reduced by rigorous aseptic nursing care, infection remains the most frequent complication of chronic venous access (12–14). Infection or suspicion of catheter-related infection is the cause of 75% of early removal of the devices at our institution. Infectious complications can be categorized as port pocket infections or catheter-associated bacteremias. They are especially important because many cancer patients are spontaneously or therapeutically immunosuppressed. To determine whether bacteremia is related to an ''infected'' catheter, quantitative bacterial blood cultures can be drawn through the catheter and from a peripheral vein. A high bacterial count in blood drawn through the catheter compared with the peripheral count is convincing evidence that the catheter is contaminated. Infection is cleared in most patients with bacteremia after infusion of systemic antibiotics directly into the catheter. Although it was suggested that the addition of urokinase as a thrombolytic agent to lyse any accumulated thrombus or fibrin would increase the successful catheter clearance by antibiotics, this was not confirmed by a recent randomized study (15). Failed antimicrobial therapy imposes the catheter replacement. The use of a new site can lead to central venous stenosis and compromise future long-term upper extremity access. In selected patients, when the tunnel tract is clinically not infected, the replacement of the catheter through preexisting subcutaneous tunnel with guide wire exchange provides a save option for prolonging tunneled catheter access sites (16,17).

Skin erosion and ulceration over the port is usually associated with either toxic drug extravasation resulting from needle dislodgement or port pocket infection.

2. *Withdrawal Occlusion*

The implantable venous access devices are designed for both the administration of therapeutic agents and the withdrawal of blood. However, it is sometimes impossible to withdraw blood, although infusion continues without difficulty. Such a catheter usually is ''one way,'' because of malposition of its tip against the wall of the vena cava or right atrium. In other cases, this situation may be the consequence of a flap-valve or sheath of fibrin at the catheter tip, preventing withdrawal of blood but allowing infusion. The use of the Groshong catheter designed to prevent the reflux of blood into the catheter does not seem to significantly reduce the incidence of this complication (18,19). Instillation of urokinase or streptokinase can restore a normal patency. Withdrawal occlusion is not necessarily an indication for device removal although it has been suggested that this complication was associated with a higher risk of subsequent development of port-related venous thrombosis (20).

3. *Venous Thrombosis*

Any factor of Virchow's triad—hypercoagulability, stasis, and endothelium injury—may be present alone or in combination in a cancer patient with a central venous access. Many thromboses associated with central venous access devices are asymptomatic. When symptomatic, the clinical presentation is either catheter malfunction or pain and swelling associated with the affected venous system. The incidence of pulmonary embolism is very low.

When venous thrombosis is suspected, venography is performed to evaluate the extent of the thrombus and the degree of venous collateralization. Intravenous heparin is used to prevent propagation of the thrombus. The venous access device can often be left in place. However, in case of persistent symptoms or notable propagation of the clot despite anticoagulation, the device must be explanted.

4. *Catheter-Related Complications*

Catheter-related complications include malposition of the tip, dislocation, embolization, rupture, and compression of the catheter.

Rupture of the catheter and subsequent extravasation may be the consequence of an excessive pressure in an attempt to restore the patency of an occluded system. In other cases, the catheter may be injured by friction on bony structures such as the clavicle or the first rib. Embolization requires extraction of the catheter fragment via invasive radiological techniques.

V. EXTRAVASATION

Extravasation of vesicant agents may cause significant morbidity and force major delays in subsequent chemotherapy treatments. Infiltration injuries generally occur in subcutaneous sites related to percutaneously placed intravenous needles or catheters. The most common sites are the dorsum of the hand, the wrist, and the forearm, which, when considered together, account for approximately 90% of extravasation injuries (21).

The use of permanent central venous access catheters and ports has probably decreased the incidence of drug extravasations, which can occur as a consequence of specific mechanisms. They include displacement of the Huber needle from the silicon septum of subcutaneous ports, lacerations or tears in the Silastic catheter in the subcutaneous tunnel, retrograde tracking of the vesicant along the catheter outside of the vein as a result of thrombosis, and separation of the port from the catheter with infusion into the subcutaneous pocket (22).

If extravasation of a cytotoxic drug (e.g., anthracyclines or mitomycin C) is suspected, the infusion should be discontinued immediately and the cannula removed. Usually, the amount of extravasated agent is small, resulting in no reaction except erythema. An ice compress may be applied to the site and the extremity elevated. Extravasation of larger amounts of drug may lead to necrosis, which becomes evident with demarcation of a necrotic area of skin, persistent pain, and eventually tissue slough. Prompt surgical excision of the area with debridement and placement of a meshed skin graft is usually recommended (23). However, a more conservative management was recently proposed (24), consisting of early liposuction and saline flushout to remove extravasated material while conserving the overlying skin. A majority of patients treated with this procedure healed without any soft tissue loss.

REFERENCES

1. Cobb DK, High KP, Sawyer RG, Sable CA, Adams RB, Lindley DA, Pruett TL, Schwenzer KJ, Farr BM. A controlled trial of scheduled replacement of central venous and pulmonary-artery catheters. N Engl J Med 1992; 327:1062–1068.
2. Broviac JW, Schribner BH. Prolonged parenteral nutrition in the home. Surg Gynecol Obstet 1974; 139:24–28.
3. Hickman RO, Buckner CD, Clift RA, Sanders JE, Stewart P, Thomas ED. A modified right atrial catheter for access to the venous system in marrow transplant recipients. Surg Gynecol Obstet 1979; 148:871–875.
4. Curtas S, Bonaventura M, Meguid MM. Cannulation of the inferior vena cava for long-term central venous access. Surg Gynecol Obstet 1989; 168:121–124.
5. Hoch JR. Management of the complications of long-term venous access. Semin Vasc Surg 1997; 10:135–143.
6. Raaf JH, Heil D. Open insertion of right atrial catheters through the jugular veins. Surg Gynecol Obstet 1993; 177:295–298.
7. Ahmed Z, Mohyuddin Z. Complications associated with different insertion techniques for Hickman catheters. Postgrad Med J 1998; 74:104–107.
8. Sabel MS, Smith JL. Principles of chronic venous access: recommendations based on the Roswell Park experience. Surg Oncol 1998; 6:171–177.
9. Nightingale CE, Norman A, Cunningham D, Young J, Webb A, Filshie J. A prospective analysis of 949 long-term central venous access catheters for ambulatory chemotherapy in patients with gastrointestinal malignancy. Eur J Cancer 1997; 33:398–403.
10. Eastridge BJ, Lefor AT. Complications of indwelling venous access devices in cancer patients. J Clin Oncol 1995; 13:233–238.
11. Stellato T, Gauderer W, Lazarus H, Herrzig R. Percutaneous Silastic catheter insertion in patients with thrombocytopenia. Cancer 1985; 56:2691–2693.
12. Kock HJ, Pietsch M, Krause U, Wilke H, Eigler FW. Implantable vascular access systems: experience in 1500 patients with totally implanted central venous port systems. World J Surg 1998; 22:12–16.
13. Ray S, Stacey R, Imrie M, Filshie J. A review of 560 Hickman catheter insertions. Anaesthesia 1996; 51:981–985.
14. Schwarz RE, Groeger JS, Coit DG. Subcutaneously implanted central venous access devices in cancer patients: a prospective analysis. Cancer 1997; 79:1635–1640.
15. Atkinson JB, Chamberlin K, Boody BA. A prospective randomized trial of urokinase as an adjuvant in the treatment of proven Hickman catheter sepsis. J Pediatr Surg 1998; 33:714–716.
16. Duszac R Jr, Haskal ZJ, Thomas-Hawkins C, Soulen MC, Baum RA, Shlansky-Goldberg RD, Cope C. Replacement of failing tunneled hemodialysis catheters through pre-existing subcutaneous tunnels: a comparison of catheter function and

infection rates for de novo placements and over-the-wire exchanges. J Vasc Interv Radiol 1998; 9:321–327.

17. Robinson D, Suhocki P, Schwab SJ. Treatment of infected tunneled venous access hemodialysis catheters with guidewire exchange. Kidney Int 1998; 53:1792–1794.
18. Biffi R, Corrado F, de Braud F, de Lucia F, Scarpa D, Testori A, Orsi F, Bellomi M, Mauri S, Aapro M, Andreoni B. Long-term, totally implantable central venous access ports connected to a Groshong catheter for chemotherapy of solid tumours: experience from 178 cases using a single type of device. Eur J Cancer 1997; 33: 1190–1194.
19. Tolar B, Gould JR. The timing and sequence of multiple device-related complications in patients with long-term indwelling Groshong catheters. Cancer 1996; 78: 1308–1313.
20. Young C, Gould JR. The timing and sequence of multiple device-related complications in patients with indwelling subcutaneous ports. Am J Surg 1997; 174:417–421.
21. Rudolph R, Larson DL. Etiology and treatment of chemotherapeutic agent extravasation injuries. A review. J Clin Oncol 1987; 5:1116–1126.
22. Ettinghausen SE. Management of chemotherapy extravasation. In: Lefor AT, ed. Surgical Problems Affecting the Patient with Cancer. Interdisciplinary Management. Philadelphia: JB Lippincott, 1996:211–222.
23. Raaf JH, Heil D, Rollins DL. Vascular access, pumps, and infusion. In: McKenna RJ, Murphy GP, eds. Cancer Surgery. Philadelphia: JB Lippincott, 1994:47–62.
24. Gault DT. Extravasation injuries. Br J Plast Surg 1993;46:91–96.

25

Practical Guide to Chemotherapy and Hormonal Therapy Administration for Physicians and Nurses

Nathalie Cornez, Ahmad Awada, and Martine J. Piccart
Institut Jules Bordet, Université Libre de Bruxelles, Brussels, Belgium

I. INTRODUCTION

Chemotherapy and endocrine therapy have been the milestones of cancer treatment for the past 3 decades.

Various combinations are used, and ways of administering the drugs and the number of potentially active new drugs are continually increasing, adding to the complexity of the treatments.

This chapter provides a practical and easy way to use chemotherapeutic and hormonal agents: they are presented by families, which include, in tables, their major indications, useful pharmacokinetic data for clinical practice, details about their ways of administration, and selected important information. Only the "standard drugs" and the drugs in "late phase of development" are reviewed.

Some doses and schedules of drugs are in constant evolution; therefore, we strongly advise the reader to check the notice included in the package of each drug. Recommended reading is indicated at the end of this chapter as references.

II. CHEMOTHERAPEUTIC AGENTS (see Tables 1–7)

III. CHEMOPROTECTORS (see Table 8)

IV. HORMONAL AGENTS (see Tables 9–13).

Table 1 Antimicrotubule Agents

Agents	Registered and useful indications	Pharmacokinetics and drug interactions	Drug administration (doses in mg/m²)	Comments
Paclitaxel (P)	Ovarian, breast cancers (advanced disease)	CDDP → P : elimination of P reduced by one-third → severe neutropenia. P → doxo: more mucositis than the reverse sequence.	*Single agent* 135 (24 h)–175 (3 h) q 3 wk Minimally pretreated breast cancer patients: 200 (3 h) *Combinations*[(1)] P (135, 24 h) → CDDP (75)[(2)] (ovarian cancer) P (175, 3 h) → CDDP (75)[(3)] (ovarian cancer) Doxo (50) → P (150, 24 h) + G-CSF (breast cancer) 0.3 to 1.2 mg/mL solution in 5% dextrose or normal saline. PVC materials should be avoided. *Premedication:* DXM 20 mg orally 6 and 12 h before P Diphenhydramine 50 mg IM and ranitidine 50 mg (or cimetidine 300 mg) *IV* 30 to 60 min before P	[(1)] Toxicities are sequence-dependent. [(2)] Severe neurotoxicity: 4% of patients [(3)] Severe neurotoxicity: 24% of patients Premedication used to reduce the incidence and severity of hypersensitivity reactions

Docetaxel (D)	Breast cancer (Anthracycline-failures) Lung cancer (2nd line)	Metabolized in the liver. Patients with elevated liver function tests (LFTs) tend to eliminate the drug slower than patients with normal LFTs. Ketoconazole and erythromycin may interact with D.	*Single agent* 100[4] (1 h), q 3 wk *Combinations* Doxo (50), D (75) or doxo (60), D (60) (breast cancer) Diluted in 250 mL 5% dextrose or normal saline *Premedication*[5]: several schemes are in use, such as methylprednisolone 32 mg at 12, 3, and 1 h before (D) and 12, 24, and 36 h following (D).	[4] 75 should be used in case of elevated LFTs or if 100 induces febrile neutropenia [5] Intended to reduce and to delay fluid retention problems
Vinorelbine (NVB)	Non-small cell lung cancer; advanced breast cancer	Metabolized in the liver. Bioavailability of oral form is about 20%.	*Single agent* 30/wk *Combinations* NVB has been combined with different drugs using multiple doses and schedules (most frequent: d1 + 8 or d1 + 5) in several tumor types. Diluted in 50 to 150 mL normal saline or 5% dextrose. Infusion in 5 to 10 min. Flushing the vein with 150 mL normal saline or 5% dextrose after NVB decreases the risk of phlebitis.	NVB is vesicant. Oral capsules are investigational.

Table 1 Antimicrotubule Agents (Continued)

Agents	Registered and useful indications	Pharmacokinetics and drug interactions	Drug administration (doses in mg/m^2)	Comments
Vincristine (VCR)	Leukemia, lymphoma, rhabdomyosarcoma, neuroblastoma, Wilms' tumor, Ewing's sarcoma. Useful in the treatment of other tumors.	Metabolized in the liver. Elimination half-life ~85 h. Incompatibilities: furosemide, idarubicin.	0.5 to 1.4 q 1 to 4 weeks (total individual dose: 2 mg) IV bolus (in 5% dextrose or normal saline) Continuous infusion regimens have also been used.	VCR is vesicant.
Vinblastine (VLB)	Lymphoma, testis, Kaposi's sarcoma, histiocytosis X, choriocarcinoma, breast cancer. Useful in the treatment of other tumors.	Metabolized in the liver. Elimination half-life ~20 h. Incompatibilities: heparin, furosemide.	6 to 10 q 2 to 4 wk IV bolus (1 mg/mL solution in 5% dextrose or normal saline) Continuous infusion regimens have also been used.	VLB is vesicant.
Vindesine (VDS)	Lymphoma, non-small cell lung cancer, leukemia, breast cancer	Metabolized in the liver	2 to 4 q 1 to 3 wk IV bolus (1 mg/mL solution in 5% dextrose or normal saline)	VDS is vesicant.

Abbreviations: CDDP, cisplatin; doxo, doxorubicin; DXM, dexamethasone; IV, intravenous; IM, intramuscular; G-CSF, granulocyte colony-stimulating factor.

Table 2 Antitumor Antibiotics

Agents	Registered and useful indications	Pharmacokinetics and drug interactions	Drug administration (doses in mg/m^2)	Comments
		1. Anthracyclines		
Doxorubicin (A)	Leukemia; Wilms' tumor; neuroblastoma; soft tissue and bone sarcomas; breast, ovarian, bladder, thyroid, stomach, small cell lung cancers; lymphoma. Useful in the treatment of other tumors.	Metabolized in the liver Elimination half-life ~18 to 30 h. A does not penetrate into the cerebrospinal fluid. Incompatibilities: heparin, fluorouracil, aminophylline, methotrexate, dexamethasone, furosemide.	*Single agent* 60 to 75 q 3 to 4 wk or 20 weekly IV bolus (2 mg/mL solution in normal saline or sterile water) Continuous infusion regimens have also been used. Total cumulative dose should not exceed 500 to 550 to avoid cardiomyopathy. *Combinations* 40 to 60 q 3 to 4 wk (± G-CSF)	Monitoring of LVEF is recommended during treatment. Cardiac risk is reduced with weekly schedule or continuous infusion and when used with dexrazoxane. Cardiac risk is increased in case of mediastinal irradiation, preexisting cardiac disease (e.g., hypertension), old age, and concomitant administration with paclitaxel (3-h infusion) and herceptin. A is vesicant. Bilirubin 1.2 to 3 mg/dL: reduce dose by 50%. Bilirubin >3 mg/dL: reduce dose by 75% or omit.

Table 2 Antitumor Antibiotics (continued)

Agents	Registered and useful indications	Pharmacokinetics and drug interactions	Drug administration (doses in mg/m^2)	Comments
Caelyx (C) (doxorubicin hydrochloride liposomal injection)	AIDS-related Kaposi's sarcoma. Ongoing studies in breast and ovarian cancers.	Elimination half-life ~50 h.	20 q 3 wk (Kaposi's sarcoma) 40 to 50 q 4 wk (breast and ovarian cancer) Diluted in 250 mL of 5% dextrose, in 30 min	C is not vesicant. In comparison with doxorubicin: Reduced risk of cardiomyopathy (<1%), gastrointestinal, hematological, and alopecia with Caelyx Increased risk of mucositis and skin toxicity especially if patients receive high doses at short intervals (e.g., ≥40 mg/m^2 q 3 wk)

Epirubicin (E)	Leukemia, soft tissue sarcomas, breast, ovarian, small cell lung cancers, lymphoma. Not registered in the United States.	Metabolized in the liver. Elimination half-life ~30 to 40 h.	60 to 120 q 3 wk IV bolus (2 mg/mL solution in normal saline or sterile water)	Cardiomyopathy is related to total cumulative dose (that should not exceed 800 to 1000 mg/m^2). E is vesicant. E 90 mg/m^2 produces an equivalent degree of myelosuppression as doxorubicin, 60 mg/m^2.
Daunorubicin (DNR)	Leukemia. Useful in the treatment of other tumors. Daunoxome (liposomal formulation) is approved for HIV-associated Kaposi's sarcoma.	Metabolized in the liver. Elimination half-life ~18 to 20 h. Incompatibilities: heparin, 5-fluorouracil and dexamethasone.	45 to 60, per day, for 3 d IV bolus (5 mg/mL solution in sterile water) Liposomal DNR: 40 mg/m^2 q 2 wk (over 60 min)	Cumulative cardiotoxicity (mainly after a total dose of 500 mg/m^2). LVEF monitoring is recommended. Liposomal DNR is less cardiotoxic. DNR is vesicant.

Table 2 Antitumor Antibiotics (continued)

1. Anthracyclines				
Agents	Registered and useful indications	Pharmacokinetics and drug interactions	Drug administration (doses in mg/m^2)	Comments
Idarubicin (I)	Acute non lymphocytic leukemia. Oral form of I: breast cancer.	Metabolized in the liver. 20% of I penetrates into the cerebrospinal fluid. Elimination half-life of I ~13 to 26 h. Elimination half-life of idarubicinol (active metabolite) ~38 to 63 h. Bioavailability of oral form is about 20% to 30%. Incompatibilities: etoposide, dexamethasone, heparin, methotrexate, and vincristine.	12, per day, for 3 d IV bolus (1 mg/mL solution in normal saline or sterile water) Oral form of I: 45 daily × 3 days q 4 wk (breast) Oral form of I in combination with oral CPM: I (35 d1) + CPM (200 d3–6) q 4 wk (elderly breast cancer patients)	Cumulative cardiotoxicity At cumulative doses of 150 to 290 mg/m^2, cardiomyopathy occurs in 5% of the patients. I is vesicant.

Mitoxantrone (M)	Acute nonlymphocytic leukemia. Useful in the treatment of non-Hodgkin's lymphoma, breast, prostate, and hepatocellular tumors.	Metabolized in the liver. Elimination half-life of 2.3 to 13 days. Elimination of M in patients with serum bilirubin concentrations of 1.3 to 3.4 mg/dL is similar to that observed in patients with normal bilirubin levels. Incompatibilities: heparin (immediate precipitation)	10 to 12 q 3 wks (solid tumors) 10 to 12 per day, for 2 to 5 days (hematological tumors) IV bolus or slow IV infusion (diluted in 50 mL 5% dextrose or normal saline, in 15 to 30 min) Continuous IV regimens have also been used.	Cumulative cardiomyopathy but less than doxorubicin and daunorubicin. Monitoring of LVEF is recommended. Total cumulative dose = 140 mg/m^2 in patients without any risk factors for development of cardiomyopathy. M is vesicant.

Table 2 Antitumor Antibiotics (continued)

Agents	Registered and useful indications	Pharmacokinetics and drug interactions	Drug administration (doses in mg/m^2)	Comments
2. Other Drugs				
Bleomycin (B)	Squamous cell carcinoma (head and neck, skin, penis, cervix, vulva), lymphoma, sarcoma. Germ cell tumors	Mainly excreted by the kidney as nonmetabolized drug (50% to 70%). Elimination half-life of 2 to 5 h (normal renal function) and up to 30 h (renal failure). Approximately 45% of B is observed into the systemic circulation after intracavitary administration. B is inactivated by methotrexate, mitomycin, and ascorbic acid.	10 to 20 IU/m^2 weekly or twice weekly IM, subcutaneously, slow IV infusion, or IV infusion over a period of 3 to 7 d (5 IU/mL solution in 5% dextrose or normal saline is suggested) *Test dose* (risk of anaphylactic reactions: 1% to 8% incidence in lymphoma) 2 IU, IV (in 50 mL 5% dextrose or normal saline over 15 min) before the first treatment followed by an observation period of 1 to 2 h.	Total cumulative dose = 300 IU (risk of pulmonary fibrosis). The dose should be reduced in patients with reduced creatinine clearance (CrCl) (e.g., a 25% reduction for a CrCl of 10 to 50 mL/min). Fever with or without chills is common (25%). Bleomycin must be used with caution in patients receiving hyperbaric oxygen as from anesthesic gas delivery.

Mitomycin (MMC)	Stomach, pancreatic cancers (in combination with other drugs). Useful in the treatment of breast, cervix, and lung tumors.	Inactivated by microsomal enzymes in the liver and metabolized in the kidneys. Elimination half-life of 0.5 to 1 h.	10 to 20, q 6 to 8 wk 6 q 3 wk (in combination) IV bolus (0.5 mg/mL solution in sterile water) Instillation into the bladder, 20 to 40 mg MMC (mixed with 20 to 40 mL of water or saline) is given weekly for 8 wk	Total cumulative dose = 50 mg/m^2 (risk of HUS increases beyond this level). Interstitial pneumonitis is rare but can be severe.
Dactinomycin (ACTD)	Wilms' tumor, sarcomas, testicular and uterine cancers.	Metabolized in the liver. Elimination half-life of 30 to 40 h.	1 to 2, q 3 wk or 0,25 to 0,6/d, for 5 d q 3 to 4 wk IV bolus or IV infusion (in 50 mL 5% dextrose or normal saline, in 20 to 30 min). Final concentration is 0.5 mg/mL. The drug has been administered by isolated perfusion (extremities).	ACTD is vesicant.

Abbreviations: C, cyclophosphamide; CDDP, cisplatin; LVEF, left ventricular ejection fraction; AIDS, acquired immunodeficiency syndrome; IV, intravenous; G-CSF, granulocyte colony-stimulating factor; HIV, human immunodeficiency virus; IU, units; HUS, hemolytic uremic syndrome; IM, intramuscularly; IV, intravenously.

Table 3 Platinum Compounds

Agents	Registered and useful indications	Pharmacokinetics and drug interactions	Drug administration (doses in mg/m²)	Comments
Cisplatin (CDDP)	Testicular, ovarian, bladder cancers. CDDP may be a useful treatment for cancers of the uterus, head and neck, esophagus, lung, bone, and non-Hodgkin's lymphoma.	20% to 45% of CDDP is eliminated unchanged via the kidneys. Elimination half-life of 60 to 90 h. Approximately 50% to 100% of cisplatin is absorbed into the systemic circulation after intraperitoneal administration.	INTRAVENOUS *Single agent* 50 to 100, as a single dose, or divided in 3 or 5 d, q 3 to 4 wk IV infusion, in 250 mL of normal or hypertonic (3%) saline, in 30 min (5% dextrose to be avoided) *Hydratation* If doses ≥ 40, as a short infusion *Prehydratation:* – 1 to 2 L of normal saline (+ 20 mEq KCl + 8 mEq MgSO4 per L) In general, hydration should be adequate to maintain a urine output of 100 to 150 mL/h before administration of CDDP. *Posthydratation:* same as prehydration. Furosemide may be added to increase diuresis and to prevent fluid overload. *Combinations* 50 to 75 q 3 wk (e.g., with doxorubicin or paclitaxel) INTRAPERITONEAL (ovarian cancer) CDDP (100) q 3 wk (in combination with cyclophosphamide [600, IV] if first line therapy for optimally debulked ovarian cancer)	CDDP is vesicant (if ≥ 0.75 mg/mL solution) Nephrotoxicity (hypomagnesemia, decrease in CrCl), peripheral sensory neuropathy and ototoxicity are frequent when the cumulative CDDP dose exceeds 400 mg/m². These toxicities may be reduced by amifostine. Aggressive antiemetic regimen (e.g., anti 5H3 + dexamethasone) is necessary during CDDP treatment. Monitoring of creatinine clearance and magnesemia and neurological examination are essential during CDDP treatment.

Carboplatin (CBDCA)	Ovarian cancer. Useful in the treatment of neuroblastoma, refractory leukemia, bladder, head and neck, and lung cancers.	60% to 70% of the drug is eliminated unchanged in the urine. Elimination half-life of ~2.5 to 6 h.	360 to 400 q 3 to 4 wk Other CBDCA dosing calculations: AUC method: total dose (mg) = target AUC × (CrCl + 25) Platelet nadir adjustment method dose (mg/m²) = 0.091 × (CrCl/BSA) × (Pre PC − desired nadir PC/Pre PC × 100)[a] + 86 Chatelut formula: total dose (mg) = CrCl × target AUC [CrCl = [0.134 × weight] + [218 × weight × (1 − 0.00457 × age) × (1 − 0.314 × sex)]/Cr IV infusion, in 250 mL 5% dextrose or normal saline, in 30 min Higher doses have been used with hematopoietic support	CBDCA is vesicant. Target AUC as monotherapy = 4 to 6 in previously treated patients; = 6 to 8 in previously untreated patients. [a] − 17 in previously treated patients. Target AUC in combination = 4 to 5 in previously untreated patients.
Oxaliplatin (OXA)	Useful in the treatment of colon and ovarian cancers.	In vitro synergism with fluorouracil has been observed in preclinical studies.	*Single agent:* 130 q 3 wk (ovary) In combination with 5-fluorouracil (5-FU): OXA (130) + 5FU (2600) + folinic acid (500) (colon cancer) IV infusion, in 250 mL 5% dextrose in 2 hr Other schedules of both oxaliplatin and 5-FU are equally active	Less gastrointestinal toxicity than cisplatin. No nephrotoxicity. Minimal hematological toxicity. Peripheral neuropathy and (sometimes) pharyngolaryngeal dysesthesia triggered and enhanced by cold.

Cr = creatinine (micromolar concentration); weight in kg; age in year; sex: 0 if male and 1 if female.
Abbreviations: BSA, body surface area; AUC, area under the curve (= 4 to 8 mg/mL/min); PC, platelet count; CPM, cyclophosphamide; Pre PC, pretreatment platelet count; CrCl, creatinine clearance (in ml/min); IV, intravenous.

Table 4 Topoisomerase I Inhibitors

Agents	Registered and useful indications	Pharmacokinetics and drug interactions	Drug administration (doses in mg/m^2)	Comments
Irinotecan (CPT-11)	Metastatic colorectal carcinoma following fluorouracil exposure. Useful in carcinoma of the lung and cervix.	Metabolized to SN-38, which is 40 to 200 times more potent than CPT-11. Elimination half-life of SN-38 ~7 to 14 h.	*Single agent* Several regimens have been evaluated, e.g., 100 to 125/wk × 3 wk q 4 wk or 350 q 3 wk *Combination* CDDP (80 q 4 wk) + CPT-11 (60-wk × 3 wk q 4 wk) IV infusion in 500 mL of 5% dextrose or normal saline over a period of 60 to 90 min.	Neutropenia and delayed diarrhea are dose-limiting. At the first sign of diarrhea: loperamide 4 mg followed by 2 mg every 2 h (4 mg every 4 h during the night) until there are no signs of diarrhea for a period of at least 12 h (maximum 48 h).
Topotecan	Advanced ovarian cancer after failure of first or second line chemotherapy. Useful in the treatment of small cell lung cancer.	22% to 48% of topotecan is eliminated unchanged in the urine. Elimination is delayed in patients with compromised renal function. Elimination half-life of 2 to 3 h.	1.25 to 1.5 daily × 5 days q 3 wk 0.75 daily × 5 days (if CrCl 20–40 mL/min) IV infusion, in 250 mL normal saline or 5% dextrose, in 30 min. Continuous infusion regimens have also been used. An oral form is being developed.	Neutropenia is dose-limiting.

Abbreviations: IV, intravenous; CDDP, cisplatin; CrCl, creatinine clearance.

Table 5 Antimetabolites

Agents	Registered and useful indications	Pharmacokinetics and drug interactions	Drug administration (doses in mg/m^2)	Comments
1. Pyrimidine Antimetabolites				
Fluorouracil (5-FU)	Stomach, colon, rectal, breast, and pancreatic cancers. Useful for the treatment of cancers of the esophagus and head and neck.	22% to 45% of 5-FU is metabolized by the liver. Elimination half-life of 10 to 20 min. New oral forms combined with compounds inhibiting 5-FU degradation are under investigation. Incompatibilities: doxorubicin, daunorubicin, idarubicin, cytarabine, and diazepam.	*Most frequently used regimens* 400 to 600, day 1 and day 8 q 4 wk, IV bolus (breast cancers, in combination with other drugs) 750 to 1000, day 1 to day 3, day 4 or day 5, continuous IV infusion (in combination with CDDP) 200 to 300, per day, indefinitely, continuous IV infusion (breast and colorectal cancers) *Regimens used in colorectal cancer* • de Gramont FA (200, IV in 2 h) → 5-FU (400, IV bolus) → 5-FU (600, IV infusion in 22 h), day 1 and day 2, q2 wk • Mayo FA (20, IV) → 5-FU (425, IV bolus), day 1 to day 5 q 4 wk • Machover FA (500, IV in 2 h) → 5-FU (2600, IV infusion in 24 h), weekly × 6 q 8 wk • NSABP FA (500, IV in 2 h) → 5-FU (500, IV bolus), weekly × 6 q 8 wk Diluted in 5% dextrose or normal saline	Toxicities of 5-FU are more severe in patients with dihydropyrimidine dehydrogenase deficiency

Table 5 Antimetabolites (continued)

1. Pyrimidine Antimetabolites

Agents	Registered and useful indications	Pharmacokinetics and drug interactions	Drug administration (doses in mg/m^2)	Comments
Floxuridine (FUDR)	Gastrointestinal adenocarcinoma metastatic to the liver	Metabolized in the liver to the active metabolite FUDR-MP. FUDR is preferred over 5-FU for intrahepatic therapy. Elimination half-life of 0.3 to 6 h. Combined with uracil.	0,1 to 0,6 mg/kg/d intrahepatic infusion, usually over a period of 7 to 14 d 60 mg/kg/wk, IV infusion in 5% dextrose or normal saline over 15 min	Severe diarrhea = 26% of patients (continuous infusion). Biliary toxicity (may be reduced by dexamethasone).
Tegafur (UFT)	Colorectal (investigational)	Metabolized to 5-FU after oral administration. Peak serum levels of 5-FU occur ~1 h after oral administration of UFT.	300 daily × 28 q 5 wk Orally, given in 3 divided doses	Oral FA is often used (15 to 150 mg/d, in 3 doses).

2. *Thymidylate Synthase Inhibitor*

Agents	Registered and useful indications	Pharmacokinetics and drug interactions	Drug administration (doses in mg/m^2)	Comments
Tomudex (ZD)	Advanced colorectal cancer.	Elimination half-life varies widely from 8 to 105 h.	3 q 3 wk IV infusion (diluted in 50 to 250 mL 5% dextrose or normal saline, in 15 min)	Neutropenia is dose-limiting.

3. *Ribonucleotide Reductase Inhibitors*

Agents	Registered and useful indications	Pharmacokinetics and drug interactions	Drug administration (doses in mg/m^2)	Comments
Gemcitabine (G)	Pancreatic cancer. Useful in the treatment of ovarian, breast, and lung cancers.	The pharmacokinetics of G are influenced by age, gender (younger patients and men tend to eliminate the drug more rapidly) and the length of the IV infusion. Eliminated almost entirely in the urine.	1000 weekly × 3 weeks q 4 weeks (a) 1000 weekly × 7 weeks q 8 weeks and then as (a) IV infusion (40 mg/mL solution normal saline), in 30 min	Doses should be reduced in older patients, heavily pretreated patients, and patients with renal function impairment (e.g., 800 mg/m^2).

Table 5 Antimetabolites (continued)

3. Ribonucleotide Reductase Inhibitors

Agents	Registered and useful indications	Pharmacokinetics and drug interactions	Drug administration (doses in mg/m^2)	Comments
Hydroxyurea (H)	Chronic myelogenous leukemia. Useful for the treatment of polycythemia vera. Previously used in combination with radiation in head and neck cancer.	Oral absorption >80%. 50% metabolized in the liver; 50% eliminated unchanged in the urine.	Orally, 60 to 80 mg/kg as a single dose every third day in combination with radiation in head and neck cancer patients (investigational) Orally, 20 to 30 mg/kg daily (hematological tumors)	Doses should be reduced in patients with renal function impairment (i.e., 50% reduction for a CrCl of 10 to 50 mL/min).

4. Purine Analogues

Agents	Registered and useful indications	Pharmacokinetics and drug interactions	Drug administration (doses in mg/m^2)	Comments
Fludarabine (FAMP)	B-cell chronic lymphocytic leukemia. Useful in the treatment of low-grade non-Hodgkin's lymphoma and hairy cell leukemia.	Active metabolite (2-FLAA), eliminated primarily by the kidneys (elimination half-life of 9 to 10 h).	25 daily × 5 days q 4 weeks IV infusion in 50 to 100 mL 5% dextrose or normal saline, in 15 to 30 min.	A 30% decrease in dose is suggested for patients with renal impairment. Severe cellular immunosuppression.

Cladribine (2-CdA)	Hairy cell leukemia. Useful for treatment of chronic lymphocytic leukemia, low-grade non-Hodgkin's lymphoma.	Phosphorylated metabolites of 2-CdA accumulate in cells with high deoxycytidine kinase activity such as lymphocytes. 37% to 55% of 2-CdA oral form is absorbed. Eliminated half-life of 5 to 7 h. Incompatibilities: 5% dextrose (increases 2-CdA degradation).	0.12 mg/kg daily × 5 d (maximum 2 cycles if no response) Continuous 24-h infusion, in 500 to 1000 mL normal saline (in 2 h in 100 mL if outpatient)	Lymphopenia is observed in 100% of patients. 2-CdA has been detected in significant concentrations in the cerebrospinal fluid after doses of 0.15 mg/kg/d.

5. *Cytidine Analogue*

Agents	Registered and useful indications	Pharmacokinetics and drug interactions	Drug administration (doses in mg/m^2)	Comments
Cytarabine (Ara-C)	Leukemia. May be useful in treatment of lymphoma.	High concentration of ara-CTP may be reached in case of renal insufficiency, resulting in CNS toxicities. Elimination half-life of 1 to 3 h.	*Common doses* 60 to 200 daily × 5 or 10 d, continuous IV infusion 100 IV twice a day × 5 days q 4 wk 10 to 30 intrathecally up to 3 times per week 1000 to 3000 IV (1 to 3 h) q 12 h for 3 to 6 d 10 SC q 12 h for 15 to 21 d Dissolution in 5% dextrose or normal saline	"Ara-C syndrome" can be controlled by corticosteroids. Neurological (usually cerebellar) toxicity is dose-dependent. Keratitis is frequent with >3 $g/m^2/d$.

Table 5 Antimetabolites (continued)

Agents	Registered and useful indications	Pharmacokinetics and drug interactions	Drug administration (doses in mg/m^2)	Comments
		6. Antifolates		
Methotrexate (MTX)	Choriocarcinoma, hydatidiform mole, leukemia, breast, head and neck, lung cancers, lymphoma, osteosarcoma. Useful in treatment of bladder cancer.	90% of unchanged MTX is eliminated via the kidneys. Elimination half-life of 3 h. Incompatibilities: bleomycin, doxorubicin, idarubicin, droperidol, metoclopramide, and ranitidine.	*Intravenous* 20 to 40, q 1 to 2 wk (solid tumors) 12,000 to 15,000 + folinic acid rescue (sarcomas) 200 to 500, q 2 to 4 wk (hematological tumors) IV bolus if doses ≤100 mg IV infusion if doses >100 mg (in 50 mL or more 5% dextrose or normal saline over 30-min period or longer) *Intrathecal* 10 to 15 mg (2.5 mg/mL solution in *preservative-free saline*)	Folinic acid rescue if doses >80 mg/wk or following intrathecal administration (see Folinic Acid). Patients with renal impairment should receive an attenuated dose of MTX with folinic acid rescue. Aspirin and nonsteroidal anti-inflammatory drugs may prolong MTX clearance and increase toxicity.

Abbreviations: Ara-CPT, cytosine arabinoside triphosphate; CNS, central nervous system; IV, intravenous; SC, subcutaneous; CrCl, creatinine clearance (in ml/min); FA, folinic acid; IV, intravenous.

Table 6 Alkylating Agents

Agents	Registered and useful indications	Pharmacokinetics and drug interactions	Drug administration (doses in mg/m^2)	Comments
Cyclophosphamide (CPM)	Lymphoma, myeloma, neuroblastoma, ovarian, breast cancers. Useful in the treatment of Ewing's sarcoma, lung (SCLL), and endometrial cancers.	Oral absorption ~75% CPM is activated by hepatic microsomal enzymes. Elimination half-life of 3 to 10 h.	500 to 1500, q 3 wk, IV (bolus or infusion in 100 mL, of 5% dextrose or normal saline in 15 min) 50 to 200 daily × 15 d q 4 wk, orally 60 mg/kg, D1 and D2, IV (with hematological support) *Hydratation* 500 to 1000 mL of normal saline if doses CPM > 1000 mg	Avoid late administration in view of the increased risk of bladder toxicity (stagnation of metabolites overnight). Hydration and treatment with mesna if high doses of CPM (i.e., 50 to 60 mg/kg) to avoid hemorrhagic cystitis.
Ifosfamide (IFO)	Testicular cancer. Useful in the treatment of lymphoma, Ewing's sarcoma, osteosarcoma, lung cancer.	Must be activated by hepatic microsomal enzymes. Metabolized by the liver to inactive metabolites. 15% to 56% of IFO is excreted unchanged in the urine.	1000 to 1200 daily × 5 d q 3 to 4 wk or 2500 to 4000 daily × 2 or 3 d q 3 to 4 wk IV infusion, in 500 mL 5% dextrose or normal saline, in 3 h (30 min to 24 h) *Concomitant hydration* is recommended (at least 2 to 3 L/d) *Uroprotective* therapy with mesna must be used (see Chemoprotectors)	Chloroacetaldehyde metabolite is responsible for neurotoxicity (risk increases with renal dysfunction). Hydration and mesna are used to avoid hemorrhagic cystitis.

Table 6 Alkylating Agents (continued)

Agents	Registered and useful indications	Pharmacokinetics and drug interactions	Drug administration (doses in mg/m^2)	Comments
		Pharmacokinetics differ if IFO is given as a single dose or divided in 5 days. Single dose of drug "activates" microsomal enzymes to activate subsequent doses.		
Busulfan (BSF)	Chronic myelogenous leukemia.	Good oral absorption. Metabolites excreted into the urine. Elimination half-life of ~2.5 h.	4 to 8 mg/d (induction) 1 to 2 mg/d (2 mg/wk to 4 mg/d) (maintenance) Has been used as a part of high-dose therapy with hematological support (4 mg/kg/d × 4 days)	Interstitial pulmonary fibrosis is a complication of BSF. Neurological (CNS) toxicity is associated with high-dose therapy (for this reason, prophylactic antiepileptic therapy is recommended).

Chlorambucil (CHL)	Chronic lymphocytic leukemia, lymphoma.	Good oral absorption (85% to 90%). Almost entirely metabolized by the liver to some active metabolites. Elimination half-life of 1 to 2 h.	0.1 to 0.2 mg/kg/d PO for 3 to 6 wk (leukemia induction) 0.4 mg/kg, q 2 to 4 wk PO 16 daily × 5 days q 4 wk (lymphoma) PO	Neurological (seizures) toxicity has been observed in patients with impaired renal function.
Melphalan (L-PAM)	Myeloma, ovarian cancer. Has been used in isolated limb perfusion (for melanoma) and as a part of high-dose therapy.	Variable oral absorption (25% to 90%). L-PAM undergoes hydrolysis in the bloodstream. 10% to 15% of L-PAM is eliminated in the urine. Elimination half-life of 15 min.	*Oral form of L-PAM* 0.25 mg/kg/d, in combination with prednisone 2 mg/kg/d × 4 days q 6 wk (in myeloma) 0.2 mg/kg daily × 5 days q 4 wk (in ovarian carcinoma) *IV administration* 100 to 200 in single dose or divided among 3 d (high-dose therapy) *Limb perfusion* 10 mg/L of limb volume or 0.45 mg/kg (upper extremity) and 0.9 mg/kg (lower extremity) have been given. Solution of no greater than 0.45 mg/mL in normal saline, over 15 to 30 min	Infusion durations longer than 60 minutes are not recommended because of drug instability. A 50% dose reduction of IV L-PAM has been advocated for patients with a serum BUN of 30 mg/dL or higher.
Dacarbazine (DTIC)	Melanoma, Hodgkin's disease. Useful treatment for sarcomas.	DTIC is activated by microsomal hepatic enzymes. 30% to 50% of the active metabolite is excreted unchanged in the urine. Elimination half-life of 3 to 5 h.	150 to 250 daily × 5 days q 3 to 4 wk 650 to 1450 q 3 to 4 weeks 375, D1 and D15 (ABVD regimen for Hodgkin's disease) IV infusion, in 100 mL normal saline or 5% dextrose, in 30 min Continuous infusion regimens have also been used. Solution should be protected from light.	Pain along injection site if DTIC is perfused quickly. A change in the color of the solution from pale yellow to pink is indicative of decomposition of the drug.

Table 6 Alkylating Agents (continued)

Agents	Registered and useful indications	Pharmacokinetics and drug interactions	Drug administration (doses in mg/m²)	Comments
Temozolomide (T)	Brain tumors, melanoma (investigational).	Prodrug. Active metabolite (monomethyl triazenoimidazole carboxamide) is formed by chemical degradation at physiological pH.	150 to 200 daily × 5 d q 4 wk Oral (empty stomach; entire capsule)	Hematological toxicity usually occurs 2 to 8 wk after the start of treatment.
		NITROSOUREA		
Carmustine (BCNU)	Brain tumors, myeloma, lymphoma. Useful in treatment of melanoma.	Penetration in cerebrospinal fluid (up to 70% of plasma concentrations). Metabolized in the liver. 80% of BCNU and its metabolites are eliminated via the kidneys. Incompatibilities: polyvinyl chloride infusion bags and sodium bicarbonate.	150 to 200 as a single dose, or divided in 2 d, q 6 wk 300 to 600 (high-dose therapy with hematological support) IV infusion, in 100 to 250 mL 5% dextrose or normal saline, in 30 to 120 min (not longer than 120 min because of incompatibility with the IV tubing)	Total cumulative dose ≤1400 mg/m² (risk of pulmonary fibrosis).

		Cimetidine may slow the metabolism of BCNU and result in enhanced myelosuppression.		
Lomustine (CCNU)	Brain tumors, Hodgkin's disease. Useful in treatment of melanoma.	Good oral absorption. Penetration in cerebrospinal fluid. Metabolized by the liver to active metabolites that are eliminated by the kidneys. Elimination half-life ~72 h.	100 to 130, q 6 wk, orally	Total cumulative dose ≤1100 to 1400 mg/m^2 (risk of pulmonary toxicity). Dose reductions are recommended if renal function is impaired.
Fotemustine	Melanoma	Penetration in cerebrospinal fluid. Metabolized in the liver. Eliminated via the kidneys.	100 q 1 wk IV infusion, in 250 mL 5% dextrose, in 1 h IA, in 4 h	Normal saline should be avoided (instability).

Abbreviations: IV, intravenous; CNS, central nervous system; PO, by mouth; BUN, blood urea nitrogen; SCLC, small cell lung cancer; IA, intraarterial; ABVD, doxorubicin, bleomycin, vinblastin, dacarbazine.

Table 7 Miscellaneous

Agents	Registered and useful indications	Pharmacokinetics and drug interactions	Drug administration (doses in mg/m^2)	Comments
Etoposide (VP-16)	Testicular, small cell lung cancers. Useful treatment for leukemias, lymphoma, sarcomas, non-small cell lung cancer.	Topoisomerase II inhibitor. Variable oral absorption (25% to 75%). Metabolized in the liver. Eliminated in the bile (10% to 15%) and urine (30% to 40%) as unchanged drug. Etoposide phosphate is rapidly converted to etoposide in plasma after IV administration. Incompatibilities: idarubicin.	50 to 120 daily × 3 or 5 d q 3 wk 400 d × 3 (high-dose therapy with hematological support) *IV infusion:* 0.2 to 0.4 mg/mL solution 5% dextrose or normal saline, over *at least* 30 min (risk of hypotension) *Oral form:* 50 to 100 daily × 21 days.	VP-16 doses should be reduced if renal function is impaired. It has been recommended that doses of VP-16 be reduced by 33% if serum albumin <3.5 g/dL. In high-dose therapy, the use of etoposide phosphate may shorten the time necessary to administer the drug and reduce the necessary volume of fluid.

Amsacrine (AMSA)	Acute leukemia.	Intercalating agent and topoisomerase II inhibitor. Metabolized in the liver and excreted in the bile (50% of unchanged drug and metabolite) and urine (22% to 42% are unchanged drug). Elimination half-life of 6 to 7 h.	90 to 150 daily × 5 days Slow IV infusion, in 500 mL 5% dextrose, in 1 or more hours Chloride-containing solutions should be avoided (risk of precipitation). Plastic syringes or bottle should not be used.	Potassium level should be normal before AMSA infusion (cardiac arrest risk). AMSA is vesicant.
Asparaginase (ASP)	Acute lymphocytic leukemia	*Escherichia coli* (or PEG-modified *E. coli*) or *Erwinia carotovara*-derived enzyme. Hydrolyzes the amino acid asparagine (protein synthesis inhibitor).	*Dose test* (risk of hypersensitivity reactions): 2 IU of *E. coli*-derived ASP intradermal, 1 h before the therapeutic dose (must be repeated if more than 1 week separates successive doses) 200 IU/kg daily × 28 d, IV infusion (in 100 mL 5% dextrose or normal saline, in 30 min) 6000 to 10,000 UI/m^2, IM injection, for 9 injections, q 3 d (after cytotoxic therapy)	Toxicities: prolonged thrombin, prothrombin times. Decrease of fibrinogen and depression of clotting factors (antithrombin III), resulting in thrombosis and/or pulmonary embolism.

Abbreviations: IV, intravenous; IM, intramuscular.

Table 8 Chemoprotectors

Agents	Registered and useful indications	Pharmacokinetics and drug interactions	Drug administration (doses in mg/m^2)	Comments
Amifostine (AMI)	Reduces the nephrotoxicity and neurotoxicity of cisplatin given to patients with ovarian and non-small cell lung carcinomas. May also reduce the toxicity of CPM and radiation.	Organic sulfhydril compound. Prodrug. Cytoprotection against chemotherapeutic agents related to the differential distribution in normal and malignant tissues. Rapidly metabolized.	910, IV infusion in 15 min, in 50 mL normal saline (or 5% dextrose) (for cisplatin doses $\geq$100 mg/m^2) 740 (for cisplatin doses $<$100 mg/m^2) 340 daily $\times$ 5 d (for cisplatin doses of 20 mg/m^2 daily $\times$ 5 d) 340 daily in combination with radiotherapy (radioprotective effect) Starting 30 min before chemotherapy *Antiemetics* Dexamethasone 20 mg, IV 5 HT3 receptor antagonist before AMI	Close monitoring of blood pressure is required (T_0, T_{+5}, T_{+10}, T_{+15}, $T_{+20\ min}$): The infusion of AMI should be interrupted and a hydration with normal saline should be initiated in case of important hypotension during AMI infusion.
Dexrazoxane (DEX)	Protective agent for doxorubicin-induced cardiotoxicity (metastatic breast cancer).	Intracellular chelating agent that prevents iron from combining with doxorubicin to form free oxygen radicals. Metabolized by the liver. 35% to 50% is eliminated unchanged in the urine. Elimination half-life of 2 to 4 h.	500 of DEX by 50 of doxorubicin, IV infusion in 100 mL 5% dextrose or normal saline, in 15 to 30 min, 30 min before doxorubicin	DEX enhances leukopenia slightly when administered with doxorubicin.

Folinic acid (FA)	Rescue agent after high-dose methotrexate (MTX) therapy (osteosarcoma). Also used following intrathecal MTX.	Tetrahydrofolic acid derivative Good oral absorption (~75% to 97%) Two forms of folinic acid: 1 mg Elvorine = 2 mg Ledervorin.	10 to 25, orally or IV, q 6 h (for 6 to 8 doses), starting 6 to 24 h after MTX	Dose adjustments are made based on MTX serum levels and serum creatinine levels (high-dose MTX therapy). Also used to potentiate the effects of fluorinated pyrimidine (doses ranging from 20 to 500 mg/m^2).
Mesna	Prevention of ifosfamide-induced hemorrhagic cystitis. Protection seen also with high-dose cyclophosphamide.	Mesna binds with acrolein (urotoxic metabolite). Incompatibilities: cisplatin.	20% of the ifosfamide dose, just before and then t_{+4} and t_{+8h} (total mesna dose is 60% of the ifosfamide dose) IV infusion, in 50 mL 5% dextrose or normal saline, in 5 min Continuous infusion mesna has been used concurrently with ifosfamide (a total dose of mesna equal to the total dose of ifosfamide is given, proceded by a loading dose of 6% to 10% of the total ifosfamide dose).	

Abbreviations: CPM, cyclophosphamide.

Table 9 Antiestrogens

Agents	Registered and useful indications	Pharmacokinetics and drug interactions	Drug administration (doses in mg/m^2)	Comments
Tamoxifen (TAM)	Breast cancer (adjuvant and metastatic). Also prescribed for endometrial cancer, malignant melanoma, and hepatocarcinoma.	Good oral absorption. Metabolized by the liver. Elimination half-life = 7 d (TAM) and 14 d (major metabolite). Potentiate the anticoagulant effect of warfarin.	Oral 20 mg/day	Well tolerated. Risk of endometrial cancer with prolonged therapy.
Toremifen	Metastatic breast cancer.	High affinity for estrogen receptor. Good oral absorption. Metabolized by the liver to 2 active metabolites. Nonsteroidal antiestrogen.	Oral 60 to 200 mg/day	
Faslodex	Metastatic breast cancer.	Pure antiestrogen, high affinity for estrogen receptor. No agonist effect.	125 to 250 mg (optimal dose under investigation) IM, slowly (at least 2 min) 1 ×/month	Local discomfort following injection.

Abbreviations: IM, intramuscular.

Table 10 Aromatase Inhibitors

Agents	Registered and useful indications	Pharmacokinetics and drug interactions	Drug administration (doses in mg/m^2)	Comments
1. Nonsteroidal Aromatase Inhibitors				
Aminoglutethimide	Metastatic breast cancer.	Good oral absorption. Metabolized by the liver to several metabolites. Elimination half-life ~7 to 9 h. Induces metabolism of warfarin, theophylline, digoxin. Blocks adrenal steroid biosynthesis.	Oral 250 mg × 2/day Hydrocortisone 2 × 20 mg/d should be added if doses >500 mg/d	Transient cutaneous rash, reversible. Somnolence. FT4 and TSH should be monitored regularly (risk of hypothyroidism).
Anastrozole	Metastatic breast cancer.	Good oral absorption. Metabolized by the liver (inactive metabolite). Elimination half-life ~50 h.	Oral 1 mg/day	
Letrozole	Metastatic breast cancer.		Oral 2.5 mg/day	

Table 10 Aromatase Inhibitors (continued)

2. Steroidal Aromatase Inhibitors				
Agents	Registered and useful indications	Pharmacokinetics and drug interactions	Drug administration (doses in mg/m^2)	Comments
Exemestane	Metastatic breast cancer.		Oral 25 mg/d	

Abbreviations: TSH, thyroid-stimulating hormone; FT4, free T_4.

Table 11 Progestational Agents

Agents	Registered and useful indications	Pharmacokinetics and drug interactions	Drug administration (doses in mg/m^2)	Comments
Medroxyprogesterone acetate	Breast, endometrial, renal, and prostate cancers (palliative therapy).	Oral bioavailability ~10%. Elimination half-life ~14 to 60 h. Metabolized by the liver.	Oral; 2 × 250 mg/d IM; 400 to 1000 mg/wk (induction), 400 mg/mo (maintenance)	Risk of thromboembolism
Megestrol acetate	Breast, endometrial cancers. Anorexia associated with cancer or HIV infection.	Well absorbed. Metabolized by the liver. Elimination half-life ~15 to 20 h.	80 mg b.i.d. or 160 mg/d Anorexia: 320 mg/d	Risk of thromboembolism

Abbreviations: IM, intramuscular; LH, luteinizing hormone; HIV, human immunodeficiency virus.

Table 12 LH and RH Analogues

Agents	Registered and useful indications	Pharmacokinetics and drug interactions	Drug administration (doses in mg/m^2)	Comments
Goserelin	Advanced prostatic or breast cancer (often associated with antiestrogen or antiandrogen).	Eliminated unchanged in the urine. Released over 28-day period from the implant.	SC; once every 28 d (into abdominal fat)	Hot flushes.
Buserelin	Advanced prostatic cancer.		SC; 500 μg × 3/d (for the first week); 200 μg/d (for the next weeks) IN, alternatively; 800 μg × 3/day followed by 400 μg × 3/day	Hot flushes.
Eriptorelin	Advanced prostatic cancer.		SC; 3.75 mg once every 28 d (into abdominal fat)	Hot flushes.
Leuprorelin acetate	Advanced prostatic cancer.		SC; 3.75 mg once every 28 d (into intra-abdominal fat)	Hot flushes.

Abbreviations: IN, intranasal inhalation; SC, subcutaneous.

Table 13 Antiandrogens

Agents	Registered and useful indications	Pharmacokinetics and drug interactions	Drug administration (doses in mg/m^2)	Comments
Flutamide	Prostate cancer (in combination with LH-RH agonist)	Nonsteroidal antiandrogen. Good oral absorption. Metabolized by the liver. Elimination half-life ~8 to 10 h.	Oral 250 mg × 3/day Can be mixed in soft food	Toxicities: gastrointestinal disturbances, loss of libido.
Bicalutamide	Prostate cancer (in combination with LH-RH agonist)	Nonsteroidal antiandrogen. Slow oral absorption (not affected by food). Metabolized by the liver to inactive metabolites. Elimination half-life ~6 d. Increase prothrombin time when warfarin is given.	Oral 50 mg/day	Toxicities: gastrointestinal disturbances, loss of libido.
Cyproteron acetate	Prostate cancer (in combination with LH-RH agonist)	Steroidal antiandrogen. Elimination half-life ~40 h.	Oral 100 to 300 mg/d (100 mg per dose)	Toxicities: gastrointestinal disturbances, loss of libido.

SUGGESTED READING

1. Fisher DS, Knobf MT, Durivage HJ. The Cancer Chemotherapy Handbook. 4th Edition, Mosby, 1993.
2. Fisher DS, Knobf MT, Durivage HJ. The Cancer Chemotherapy Handbook. 5th Edition, Mosby, 1997.
3. Awada A, Piccart M. New agents in development for cancer therapy. An ongoing challenge to improve patient care. In Consultant Series No. 18, 1997.
4. De Vita VT, Hellman S, Rosenberg SA. Cancer: Principles and Practice of Oncology, 5th ed. L.B. Lippincott Company, 1997.
5. de Valeriola D, Awada A, Roy J-A, Di Leo A, Biganzoli L, Piccart M. Breast cancer therapies in development. A review of their pharmacology and clinical potential. Drugs 1997; 54(3):385–413.
6. Dorr RT, Van Hoff DD. Cancer Chemotherapy Handbook, 2d ed. 1994.

26

Ostomy Care

Debra Broadwell Jackson
Clemson University, Clemson, South Carolina

I. INTRODUCTION

The major advances in cancer detection and treatment and the identification through genetic research of people at risk for cancer have changed many aspects of cancer care. As the success rate of earlier diagnosis and more effective cancer therapy increases, more individuals are finding that they are living with a cancer diagnosis. These same advances mean that fewer and fewer individuals will require an ostomy as part of their overall cancer management plan. For the individual who must have an ostomy, it becomes critical that the skills and techniques developed over the past decades continue to progress. The expertise of doctors in creating good stomas in ideal locations, the expertise of nurses in teaching patients and families fundamental care, the availability of support and self-help groups, and the development of state-of-the-art pouching systems are essential components to continued, improved quality care.

Cancer, as a chronic illness, requires that health care professionals view the patient from a perspective of a person with functional abilities rather than as a person with a disease process. Patients and families may not realize that the impact of cancer will require coping with change over an extended period of time and that cure may be possible for some types of cancer.

An ostomy is a surgical procedure that may be indicated when a person has colon or bladder or gynecological cancer that cannot be managed by less body-altering surgeries. It is this feeling of ''last resort'' that most greatly affects the person's rehabilitation and ability to live with an ostomy. The surgery results in the creation of a stoma and is performed for curative reasons, although occasionally a stoma is done for palliative treatment. Adjuvant therapy may precede or follow surgery.

A common public myth is that cancer of the colon or bladder automatically results in an ostomy. The fear of ostomy often delays diagnosis or treatment for people who fear having diversional procedures. Whereas the number of ostomies that are performed each year have decreased as new, sphincter-sparing procedures are developed, each person undergoing ostomy surgery deserves a comprehensive and caring approach to learning self-care. This chapter focuses on the care of patients who have had cancer of the bowel, bladder, or gynecological systems that necessitate the surgical creation of a permanent stoma or ostomy. While recognizing that stomas for feeding, esophagostomy, and drainage gastrostomy are used for supportive care, this chapter deals with the care of the person with a colostomy, ileostomy, or ileal conduit (urinary diversion, urostomy). However, the pouching and skin care techniques discussed may be applied to all stomas.

II. SIGNIFICANCE OF THE PROBLEM

Cancer is second to heart disease as the leading cause of death in the United States. The number of new cases of cancer involving the colon and rectum, urinary bladder, and female genital organs has shown signs of decreasing. The American Cancer Society estimates 131,200 new cases per year of colon and rectal cancer (1). The incidence of colorectal cancers has declined in recent years from a high of 53 per 100,000 cases in 1985 to 45 per 100,000 in 1993. The public is becoming more aware of signs and symptoms of cancer and carcinogens associated with the development of certain cancers, and health screenings are widely publicized to encourage early diagnosis. Research has suggested that the recent decline may have been due to increased sigmoidoscopic screening and polyp removal, preventing progression of polyp to invasive cancers (1).

The 1997 World Health Report reports that the number of cancer cases is expected to at least double in most countries over the next 25 years. At present, cancer in all forms is responsible for 6.3 million deaths a year. Fifty percent of all cancer deaths are from lung, stomach, colorectal, liver, and breast cancers. Colorectal cancer was associated with 495,000 people in 1996 (2).

A major concern for health professionals is the delay between recognizing symptoms and diagnosis. Hurney and Holland reported that early symptoms of bladder and colon cancers may be present for months before a person seeks medical help (3,4). The vague signs and symptoms often associated with cancer may delay the diagnosis even more. An average lag time from recognizing symptoms to diagnosis of colorectal cancer was 8.25 months in a study of 200 patients conducted in England (5). Ignorance, denial, fear of mutilation, and excessive modesty were associated with delays in seeking diagnosis. Holland reports that fear of having an ostomy may also cause a delay in diagnosis (6).

A. Colon and Rectal Cancer

Several strategies identified for the management of colon cancer include identification of carcinogens and protection of the bowel from these substances, screening of the general population older than 50 years of age, follow-up of high-risk individuals, adequate primary surgical management in conjunction with adjuvant therapy, and aggressive therapy for localized recurrence (7). The risk factors for colorectal cancer are listed in Table 1. A personal or family history of colorectal cancer or polyps, as well as a history of inflammatory bowel disease, indicates a need for regular screening protocols by family physicians (1,4). Colon cancer has received increased publicity recently as new research has indicated a DNA defect associated with familial cancer of the colon (8). More importantly, recent studies indicate that stool for occult blood may be an important screening tool despite the number of false-positive results. Other risk factors associated with colorectal cancer are physical inactivity, high-fat, and diets low in fruits and vegetables. Estrogen replacement therapy and nonsteroidal anti-inflammatory drugs are being considered for reduction of colorectal cancers.

The World Health Organization reports that, although colorectal cancers are more common in richer countries, the incidence is increasing in some developing countries (2). The incidence increases rapidly in first generation migrants moving from a country of low risk to a country of high risk. The shift in diet from high to low contents of vegetables, legumes, and whole grains at the same time the diet of red meats increases has been associated with increased risk (2).

The American Cancer Society and the National Cancer Institute recommend

Table 1 Colorectal Cancer Risk Factors

- Older than 40 years of age
- Low-fiber and high-fat diets
- Family history of colon cancer
- History of colon cancer
- Adenomatous polyps
- Family history of familial polyposis coli
- Ulcerative colitis
- Crohn's disease
- Previous pelvic radiation

that men and women older than age 50 years be screened with fecal occult blood tests to detect early colorectal cancers (1,9). Digital rectal examination, fecal occult blood tests, and sigmoidoscopy can be used to detect asymptomatic patients. Positive screening results indicate the need for a complete diagnostic evaluation including colonoscopy or barium enema x-ray study, plus flexible sigmoidoscopy.

Community-based patients may not receive a complete evaluation of abnormal test results (9–11). The low rate of complete evaluations following screenings reduces the potential benefits of performing community screening programs. Morbidity and mortality rates are not reduced through early identification of colorectal lesions if follow-ups are inadequate or absent (9). The American Cancer Society reports 1-year survival rates of 82% and a 5-year survival rate of 61% (1). When the cancer is detected early and it is localized, the 5-year survival rate increases to 91%. Most colorectal cancers are not found in early stages, however.

Colon and rectal cancers are categorized as primary if they develop from the bowel, and metastatic when the cancer spreads from adjacent or distant sites. Metastatic colorectal cancers can develop from lymphoma, leiomyosarcoma, malignant melanoma, and cancer of the breast, ovary, prostate, and lung (12). Once the cancer has spread to adjacent organs and lymph nodes, the survival rates decrease to 63% at 5 years (1).

The primary treatment for adenocarcinoma of the colon and rectum is surgical resection with the approach determined by the site of the lesion and the presence of adjacent organ involvement. Permanent colostomy is seldom recommended for colon cancer and is infrequently required for rectal cancers.

B. Bladder Cancers

Bladder cancers are more common in men than women, and even though bladder cancers may occur at any time, the tumors are more common after 60 years of age. The incidence of bladder cancer is lower than colorectal cancer, with approximately 57,000 new cases occurring in the United States each year (1). The cause of bladder cancers remains unknown, even though several environmental agents have been implicated (Table 2). Repeated exposure to risk factors increases the incidence of bladder cancer. Whereas occupational exposure often leads to bladder cancer 40 to 50 years after exposure to chemicals and aniline dyes, toxins from cigarette smoking may be a greater risk. Smokers experience twice the risk of bladder cancer than nonsmokers. Approximately half of bladder cancers are in smokers (13). Smoking has been associated with 47% of bladder cancer deaths in men and 37% of women (1). The more a person smokes increases the risk significantly.

Transitional cell carcinomas account for 95% of all bladder cancers, followed by squamous cell (3%), and adenocarcinoma (2%) (14). Most bladder tumors

Table 2 Risk Factors for Bladder Cancer

Category	Specific agent
Occupational toxins	
Aromatic amines	Dyes, leather tanning
Organic chemicals	
Cigarette smoking	2-naphthylamine and nitrosamine
Artificial sweeteners	Cyclamates
Foods	Coffee
Infectious agents	Schistosomiasis
Drugs	Phenacetin, cyclophosphamide

originate from epithelial cells. The exposures to toxic substances over time are associated with these lesions. Chronic irritation of the bladder seems to be associated with squamous cell cancers of the bladder. In Egypt, approximately 70% of bladder cancers are squamous cell carcinomas and are secondary to schistosomiasis infections. The organisms may be found in contaminated water. When a person becomes infected, the eggs are laid in the muscle wall of the bladder and intestine. The irritation of the ova in the bladder wall progresses to squamous cell carcinoma (13).

Bladder tumors recur more frequently when they invade the layers of the bladder wall. This predictable pattern influences the treatment programs provided to patients. The tumors recur in the same stage and grade as the original tumor (13). Solid tumors are more likely to invade the muscle wall of the bladder and to metastasize early.

The key to diagnosis is painless hematuria: gross or microscopic. The first symptom may be an increase in frequency of urination. Patients may complain of altered patterns of elimination with urinary frequency and flank pain associated with ureteral obstruction or metastasis.

Noninvasive bladder tumors are treated with transurethral resections, laser fulguration, and intravesical chemotherapy. Surgery is limited to invasive tumors and may include partial or radical cystectomy or cystoprostatectomy, urinary diversion, adjunct chemotherapy, and adjunct radiation therapy (14). The urinary diversion may be incontinent or the continent diversion (Kock pouch, Indiana pouch, Mainz pouch, UCLA pouch).

C. Pelvic Malignancy

Pelvic exenteration surgery is performed in both sexes for a variety of pelvic malignancies, including colorectal carcinoma and occasionally for radiation necrosis. The most frequent indication for this procedure is radioresistant, recurrent, or advanced cervical cancer. Anterior pelvic exenteration involves the removal of the urinary bladder and the distal segments of the ureters with a resultant urinary diversion. In women, the female reproductive organs are removed, including all or part of the anterior vagina. Posterior pelvic exenteration includes the removal of the colon, rectum, uterus, vagina, and adnexa. A colostomy is required, but the bladder is intact. A total pelvic exenteration includes the removal of all reproductive organs, bladder, colon, and rectum with resultant colostomy and urinary diversion (15). The physician and family must carefully weigh the indications for this high-risk surgery.

III. SURGICAL PROCEDURES

A. Colostomy

Colostomy means an opening into the colon and can be surgically created anywhere along the length of the large intestine. (Ileostomy refers to small intestinal ileum.) Three types of primary colostomies are end, loop, or double-barrel and refer to overall surgery required (Figs. 1 and 2).

An end colostomy is the most common procedure for colorectal cancer involving the low rectum and anus. The surgeon brings the bowel through a small opening in the abdominal wall and cuffs the lumen back upon itself, suturing the skin at the base to create the stoma, the externalized bowel that remains (16). The innermost mucosal layer of the bowel wall is exposed when the stoma is created. The distal diseased colon, rectum, and anus are removed in a procedure called abdominoperineal resection, or Miles resection. The abdominoperineal resection involves an abdominal incision, used to free up part of the bowel and create the stoma, and a perineal incision, through which the distal portion, rectum, and anus are removed. A large defect is left during the surgery. Three types of closures may be used for the perineal area: primary closure, partial closure, or open and packed. A primary closure, which heals much faster, is indicated if there is adequate hemostasis, no infection, and no fecal contamination. A partially closed wound includes the use of a Penrose drain in the midline perineal incision to facilitate drainage. The open and packed management is used when necessary to control bleeding (17).

When the distal colon or rectum is not removed, two procedures may be selected. The rectal stump is oversewn and left in situ, called a Hartmann's pouch. The patient has an end colostomy and the rectum and anus are intact. Mucus drainage from the rectum is expected. A Hartmann's pouch is indicated when the surgeon does not want to do an anastomosis and the patient is unable to tolerate the larger, more traumatic perineal resection (16).

The distal bowel may be brought through the abdominal wall and a second stoma created. This procedure is called a ‘‘double-barrel’’ stoma. The stoma

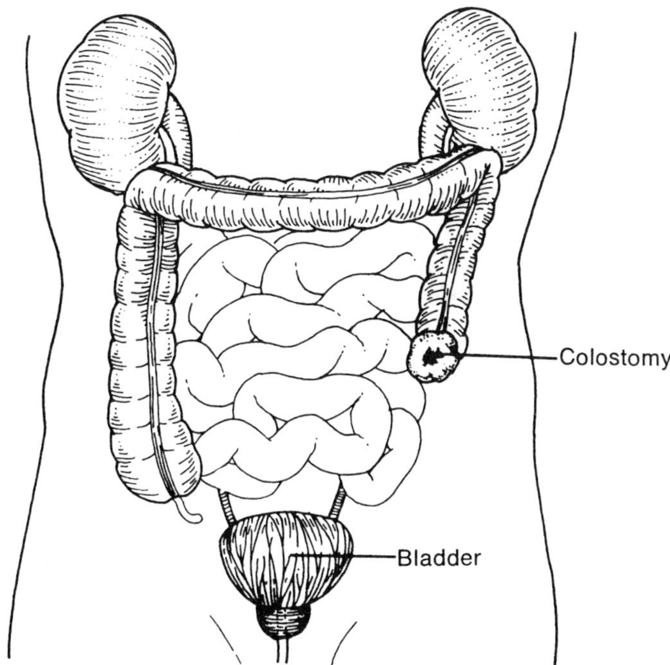

Figure 1 Resection of the rectosigmoid colon with construction of a sigmoid colostomy. (From Ref. 19.)

leading to the functional bowel is the functioning colostomy stoma. The stoma leading to the distal bowel is nonfunctioning, except to drain mucus. Mucus may drain from the rectum as well. This surgery is most effective from the patient's point of view when enough distance separates the stomas on the abdomen that the functioning stoma can be pouch, and the nonfunctioning stoma is covered with a nonsterile dressing or pad (18).

Bringing a loop of bowel through an abdominal incision forms a loop stoma. The posterior wall of the bowel is supported for 5 to 7 days by a rod or bridge. The anterior wall of the loop is opened transversely and forms one stoma with two distinct openings. The surgery results in a larger, oval-shaped stoma. The loop stoma is indicated in the case of emergency surgery or palliative surgery. Most loop colostomies are performed for blunt trauma and perforating injuries rather than for cancer (16).

Many surgeons have developed techniques to be used to save the sphincter mechanism and normal bowel elimination whenever possible. Colon resections are much more common than colostomies, particularly permanent colostomies

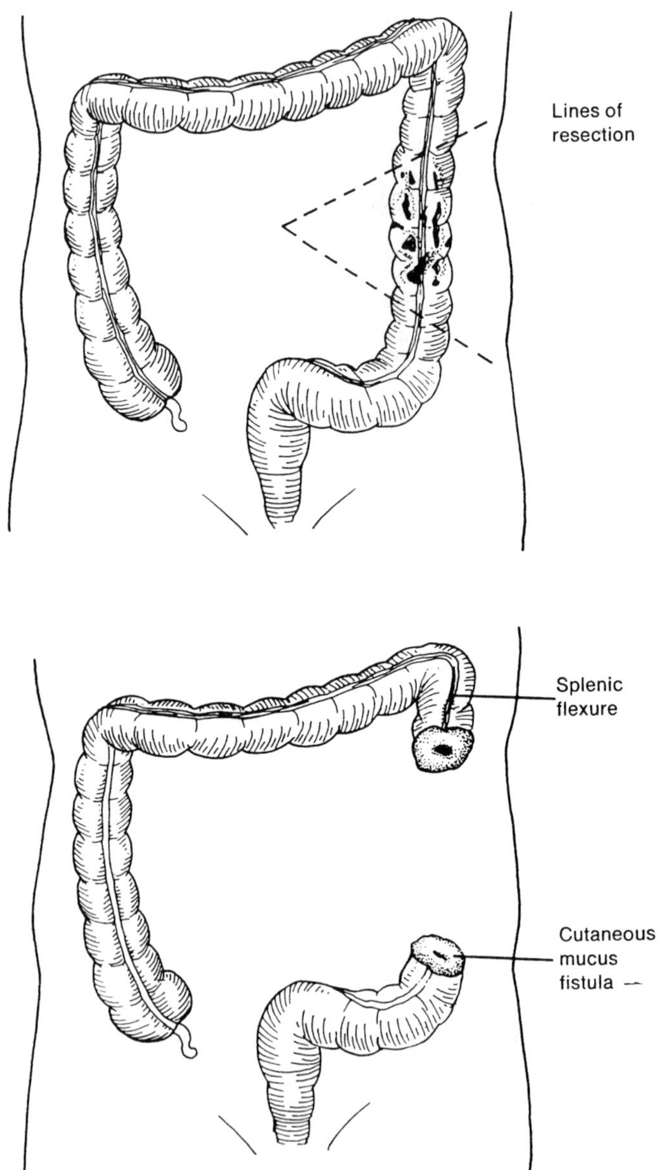

Figure 2 Disease or injury to a colon segment requires resection of the segment and may result in a double-barrel colostomy. (From Ref. 19.)

with abdominoperineal resections. Continent procedures for persons requiring total colectomy, decreasing the number of permanent ileostomies, are available including the Kock pouch and ileoanal reservoirs that preserve the anal sphincters.

B. Urinary Diversion

A urinary diversion is a general term that refers to the diversion of the urine away from the urethra or bladder. A urinary diversion may be necessary for a number of clinical reasons. When the bladder is removed for cancer, the most common type of diversion is the ileal conduit (Figs. 3 and 4). A ureterostomy can be performed, but is not as common. Bricker first described the ileal conduit in the early 1950s (19). Until the refinement of the continent urinary diversion in the late 1980s, the Bricker procedure was the standard diversion for bladder cancer that did not respond to other nonsurgical methods of treatment. A 6-inch segment of ileum is removed from the small intestine with its mesentery intact. The intestinal tract is reanastomosed. One end of the segment is closed, and the other end is brought through the abdominal wall to form the stoma. The ureters are implanted into the ileal segment, which becomes a conduit for the passage of urine. The conduit should empty freely and easily without residual urine remaining in the segment. An excessively long conduit may result in urinary stasis, which is associated with increased urinary tract infections and electrolyte imbalance caused by urine reabsorption by the ileum.

Continent urinary diversions are gaining favor in many major medical centers over the traditional ileal conduit. The continent procedures lower the long-term negative consequences associated with ileal conduits. As survival rates increase, Pernet and Jonas (20) report a high rate of renal deterioration following ileal conduit. In addition, continent procedures eliminate the need for an external collecting device or pouch that may leak unexpectedly and require regular maintenance and care. The major reason that continent procedures are done more often is that clean intermittent catheterization can be done, which allows a clean procedure to be used for emptying the internal reservoir rather than a sterile procedure (21).

Two types of urinary continent procedures are discussed in this chapter: Kock pouch and Indiana pouch. The Kock urinary reservoir is a variation of the Kock continent ileostomy. Approximately 60 to 80 cm of ileum are used to create an internal pouch with two intussuscepted nipple valves. The afferent limb prevents reflux of urine from the internal pouch back toward the ureters that are anastomosed to the distal portion of the limb. The efferent limb is brought out through the abdominal wall to form a stoma; the nipple valve prevents leakage from the Kock pouch. The time of surgery is lengthened for the patient by one to two hours. The most serious complication of this surgery is the loss of continence.

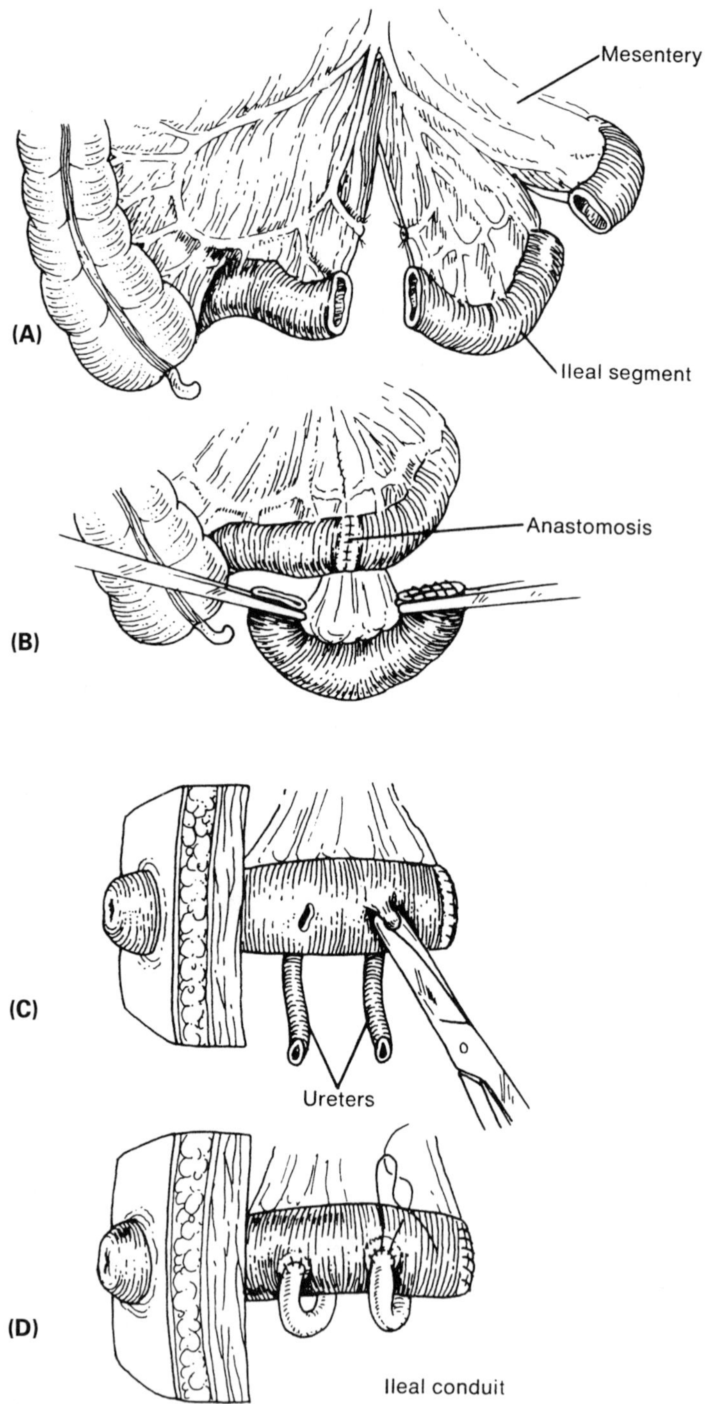
Mesentery
(A)
Ileal segment
Anastomosis
(B)
(C)
Ureters
(D)
Ileal conduit

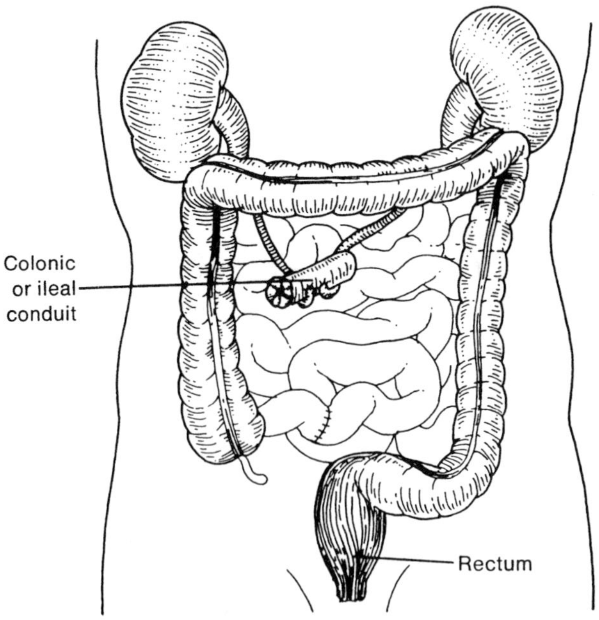

Figure 4 Completed ileal conduit. Note reanastomosed ileum. (From Ref. 19.)

The Indiana, or ileocecal, pouch uses 20 cm of cecum and 15 cm of terminal ileum, plus an additional segment of ileum or colon is used as a patch to complete the pouch construction. The distal portion of the ileum is anastomosed to the colon to reestablish bowel continuity. The cecum and the patch segment are opened and connected to form a pouch. The ureters are tunneled into the taeniae of the colonic segment, creating an antireflux mechanism. The ileal segment is brought through the abdominal wall to form a stoma. Continence is achieved by the ileocecal valve and the plication of the ileum to form a long outflow tract (21). Several surgical variations have been reported and address different methods for

---

Figure 3 Construction of ileal conduit. (A) Segment of ileum is isolated from the gastrointestinal (GI) tract with its mesenteric blood flow. (B) GI tract is reanastomosed. (C) Ureters, which are located retroperitoneally, are brought into the abdominal cavity. Incisions are made in the conduit for ureteral implantation. (D) Abdominal stoma is mature, and the ureters are anastomosed to the ileum segment in an end-to-side fashion. (From Ref. 19.)

providing continence. The care and management of the continent urinary diversions are similar.

IV. PATIENT OUTCOMES

Rehabilitation is a dynamic, goal-directed process designed to help individuals function at their maximal level within the limitations and constraints of the disease and treatment protocols (22). The physical, mental, emotional, social, sexual, and economic potential of the individual is used to design a comprehensive rehabilitation program. The first phase of rehabilitation begins at the time of diagnosis and is enhanced by a comprehensive team approach to cancer therapy.

The success of the rehabilitation following ostomy procedures depends on five major factors:

1. The surgical construction of the stoma and the location of the stoma on the abdomen;
2. The identification of a planned rehabilitation program, which has a key individual to coordinate the activities within and among team members;
3. The commitment of the health care team to provide ongoing evaluation and planning for changes as the person lives with cancer and a stoma;
4. The involvement of patient and family in the process from the initial screening; and
5. The effectiveness of communications between team members that will directly impact the success of the rehabilitation program in general and for the individual patient.

Throughout the phases of the disease—treatment, remission, cure, or palliative care and death—cancer rehabilitation must be individualized. Whereas certain responses and coping behaviors are seen in persons faced with life-threatening illness, each individual has unique responses and personal interpretations of the meaning of illness and its treatment (19). Patient and family education is essential. The patient and family need to have an understanding of the trajectory of the disease, treatment, and outcome. The doctor and nurse have many opportunities to explain to the patient and family what will happen. Health care professionals, who have worked with numerous people undergoing diversions for cancer, have knowledge of the stages families can expect. The experience can be made easier if a person understands what he or she can expect to have happen or what others have experienced. For example, if patients have a nasogastric tube inserted, the caregiver should explain how it feels, what the tube is for, and when it will be removed.

A person with an ostomy experiences many changes in functional ability.

Teaching the patient and family about the disease, the treatment and side effects, and the procedures to improve, maintain, or support changes in functions is integral to successful rehabilitation (23). The International Ostomy Association (IOA) approved a charter of rights for a person undergoing ostomy surgery and includes preoperative counseling, well-constructed stoma, full and impartial information, and availability of resources (Table 3).

Nurses use clinical pathways or care maps as management tools to organize, sequence, and time interventions to provide quality care based on standards of practice across the continuum of care settings (24). A person with an ostomy has different needs from preoperative to postoperative to home care. Goals vary for each setting. Patient education is highly individualized. Adults learn best when they are respected, when the information is useful to them, and learning is related to life experiences (25). The educational plans for teaching people about ostomy management should incorporate the knowledge and skills for caring for the ostomy and the support necessary for adjustment.

Table 3 International Ostomy Association Charter of Ostomates' Rights

It is the declared objective of the International Ostomy Association that all ostomates shall have the right to a satisfactory quality of life after their surgery and that this charter shall be realized in all countries of the world.
Receive preoperative counseling to ensure that they are fully aware of the benefits of the operation and the essential facts about living with a stoma.
Receive experienced and professional medical support and stoma nursing care in the preoperative and postoperative period both in the hospital and in their community.
Receive full and impartial information about all relevant supplies and products available in their country.
Have the opportunity to choose from the available variety of ostomy management products without prejudice or constraint.
Be given information about their National Ostomy Association and the services and support which can be provided.
Receive support and information for the benefit of the family, personal carers, and friends to increase their understanding of the conditions and adjustments which are necessary for achieving a satisfactory standard of life with a stoma.
Receive assurance that personal information regarding ostomy surgery will be treated with discretion and confidentiality to maintain privacy.

From the International Ostomy Association (IOA) Coordination Committee, June 1993, revised June 1997, and made available on the IOA web site.

A. Ostomy Adjustment

Making the adjustment to ostomy surgery requires time: time to grieve for the loss and changes resulting from surgery, time to adapt to a new method of elimination, time to learn that others are accepting of you, the individual, and time to have new experiences and successes. Patients often discuss retirement at the time of their diagnosis. The health care team can assist people in waiting to make major life decisions until the treatment is completed. Ambulatory patients diagnosed and undergoing treatment for cancer identified three physical parameters that changed during the course of the treatment: level of physical activity, sleeping habits, and weight. Body image, a psychosocial dimension, and economic status also changed over time (26). The research by Frank-Stromborg and Wright (26) did not support the assumption that a diagnosis of cancer produces a marked change in lifestyle. In a study of 289 individuals with colostomies, ileostomies, and urinary diversions, 75% of colostomy subjects and 80% of urinary diversion subjects were not employed or were retired, as compared to 50% of ileostomy subjects. The average age of both the colostomy and urinary diversion samples was 17 years older than the ileostomy sample, which probably accounted for the difference in employment (27).

B. Diagnosis and Decision for Surgery

Cancer of the colon and rectum has often been referred to as the ''cancer no one talks about'' (18). Societal impressions related to living with a colostomy or a urinary diversion are a major consideration in educating the public, and they play an important role in the preoperative education of persons with bladder or rectal cancer. An ostomy creates a physical change in the body, alters normal elimination patterns, and impacts sexual functioning. The quality of life is of considerable importance. However, quality of life is a daily question for a person with an abdominal stoma who is confronted with bowel and bladder function daily (28). To a considerable extent, the quality of life following ostomy surgery is dependent upon the surgeon to create a stoma that is well placed, of proper length, and pouchable. Druckerman (29) reviewed six key areas in the management of permanent colostomies: diet, medication, irrigation and training, use of appliances and dressings, care of the skin, and general measures. This classic study conducted in 1938 is still relevant. Current research (27) suggests that these areas continue to be of importance and general measures have been refined to include sexual functioning, emotional adaptation and adjustment, management of complications, and living with an ostomy issue.

C. Preoperative Teaching

People who need to have ostomy surgery benefit from an enterostomal therapy (ET) nurse, ostomy nurse, or oncology nursing specialist visit as soon as the decision is reached that an ostomy is necessary. The nurse is able to augment what the physician has explained. Some patients and families are in shock and hear little if anything the physician has said. Patients and families need to know that their feelings and reactions are normal and expected (18).

The patient wants to know everything and nothing. For the most part, the patient's questions can guide the discussion and the depth of the answers provided. A quiet, unhurried environment is necessary, and the language should be down-to-earth lay language. Handouts and patient materials are helpful, but only if the material is related to the patient and the institution. Written material does not substitute for the nurse's time in answering questions and concerns. Topics that should be included in the preoperative discussions are listed in Table 4.

Questions can be managed in general rather than specific terms. A person may want to know how he or she will go to the bathroom, but the answer does not have to include every step in the process of emptying a pouch. The answer may simply be ''While sitting on the toilet, you can open the bottom of the pouch and empty the stool/urine into the toilet.''

Patients are interested in the sensations that they can expect before, during, and after surgery: what will happen when. How will this influence me? Will it hurt and for how long? When will I go home? Following colostomy surgery, a person can expect to have a nasogastric tube until bowel sounds return and will be on intravenous fluids until tolerating food.

The preoperative teaching session is the time to define terms for use, for example, stool and feces. *Bowel movements* is a term for discussing colostomy output. Colostomy output and urinary output may be appropriate terms for nurses or doctors, but patients need more comfortable, familiar terms. The health care provider can help by providing patients with acceptable words.

The preoperative visit provides an opportunity for patient and family assessments that can guide the health team in planning a comprehensive teaching and rehabilitation program. For example, what is the patient's and family's level of understanding concerning the disease and treatment protocol? Any preconceived ideas or misunderstandings can be clarified immediately. Does the patient know that he or she has cancer? Sometimes, the physician uses the word cancer, tumor, or growth. The patient does not hear cancer and the patient decides that the ''tumor'' is not cancer, not realizing that the terms are being used interchangeably. It is always helpful to ask if the patient and family know anyone with an ostomy and determine whether the experience was positive or negative. Physical limitations that may interfere with a person's ability to manage the ostomy may be identified and methods for adaptation can be initiated. Social and family networks are essential to successful rehabilitation and assessments of support groups should be included. Personal concerns include sexual functioning, and these should be addressed openly and honestly. The nurse needs to know what the physician has

Table 4 Preoperative Teaching Guidelines

Common patient questions	Suggested response
What is an ostomy?	Define in lay terms what type of surgery is planned and the reason for the surgery. Drawings are helpful for explaining the anatomy and the surgical alterations planned.
What will a stoma look like?	Describe the normal red color of the intestinal stoma, the peristaltic movement that can be seen, and the lack of sensory nerve endings.
Will the ostomy be hard to take care of?	Discuss in general terms the management based on the type of ostomy planned. If possible, link the discussion to the patient's ability to do and to learn new activities.
What does a pouch or bag look like?	Show a pouch that is likely to be used at discharge as well as a pouch applied at the time of surgery if they differ. Discuss selection of a pouching system that is not visible under clothing and that fits the person's body.
Will my diet have to change?	Discuss the return to a normal diet.
Will I be able to manage at work? At play?	Identify with the patient his or her current employment activities, hobbies, and other activities enjoyed and explore with the patient any anticipated management issues and how the concerns can be handled successfully.
Can I bathe or shower?	Discuss general activities of daily living and how having an ostomy does not necessarily lead to any changes.
Will I be sick or disabled?	Explore the patient's fears and concerns about the outcome of surgery and the cancer diagnosis and treatment plan. Be as supportive and encouraging as possible.
What else should I know?	Some patients are hesitant to ask relationship and sexual questions. Initiate the discussion with the patients.
Should I keep the ostomy a secret?	Help the patient explore his or her concerns about others knowing about the ostomy and then assure him or her that no one will know unless the patient decides to provide the information.
Will I smell?	Describe the types of pouching systems available that help to prevent odors. Odor-proof pouching systems are very effective.

said regarding potential nerve damage and to build on this information as she or he discusses alternatives.

In summary, people with ostomies eat normal diets, wear the clothes they wish to wear, and resume all the presurgical activities they enjoyed. Unless they tell others that they have had surgery, no one can know by just looking at them. Many patients and family ask whether they should tell others. An ostomy should not be a secret that a person keeps from everyone, and an ostomy is not something to be ashamed of, but the patient should decide who he or she informs and make those decisions based on relationships and comfort level.

D. Stomal Construction and Placement

The most important predictor of successful rehabilitation is a well-constructed stoma that is properly located on the abdomen (30). The quality of life following ostomy surgery is linked directly with the person's ability to maintain a pouch seal, avoiding unplanned leakage of stool or urine and odors, regardless of his or her physical activities. A study evaluating the impact of stoma site marking and preoperative education on the outcomes of ostomy surgery compared early and late complications of ostomy surgery (31). The authors found that between 1978 and 1996, 292 of 593 patients received stoma site markings by ET (enterostomal therapy) nurses. Early complications were defined as occurring within 30 days of surgery, and late complications developed after the first 30 days. The researchers concluded that patients who received stoma site markings and preoperative teaching by ET nurses experienced fewer ostomy-related complications. The results should have been expected based on anecdotal data by surgeons, ET nurses, and patients. The stoma construction and its site on the abdomen are essential to successful rehabilitation (Figs. 5 and 6). A stoma that is retracted below the skin level or at the skin level is difficult to pouch; leakage of stool or urine and skin irritation is common. Stomas located in folds or dimples, near scars or bony prominences, or too low for the patient to see create difficult pouching situations.

The doctor or ET nurse trained in stoma marking should select, before surgery, the appropriate placement or site for the stoma (Table 5). Stoma marking is not difficult in ambulatory adults of normal weight and good abdominal musculature. The patient is observed in standing, sitting, and bending positions as well as supine. Bending at the waist and hips shifts the abdomen and should be observed carefully. Flexing the legs at the hips while standing also is observed. The patient should sit in a chair and slowly bend forward as if to touch the floor. Careful observation of the abdomen during this step of stoma marking detects troublesome folds or creases. Running a finger along a fold may lengthen the crease and bring attention to a potentially difficult area.

The method for marking the stoma varies. The use of methylene blue injec-

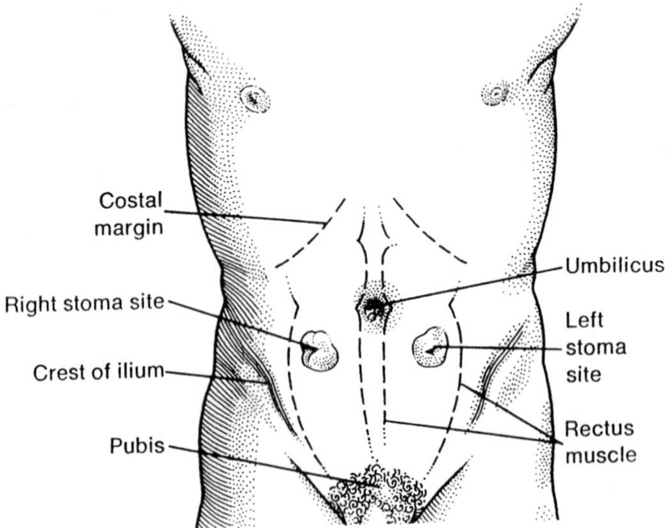

Figure 5 Right and left lower quadrant abdominal stoma sites for an ambulatory adult of normal weight. (From Ref. 19.)

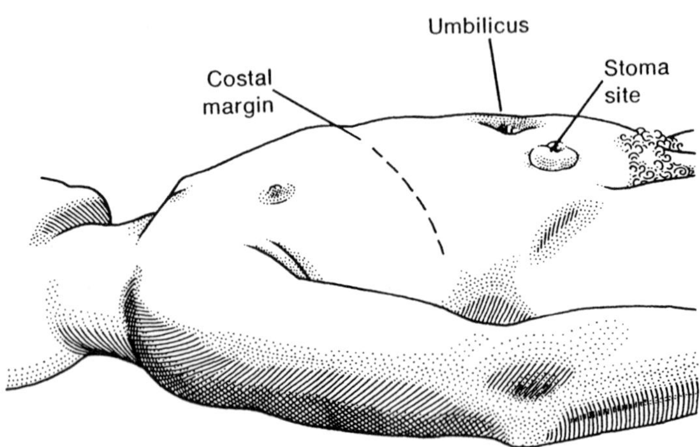

Figure 6 Lower quadrant stoma sites for a supine adult of normal weight. (From Ref. 19.)

Table 5 Criteria for Stoma Site Selection

- The patient is able to see the stoma when sitting or standing.
- The stoma avoids abdominal scars, folds, and creases when the patient is sitting, standing, and supine.
- The site allows for a 2-inch diameter of smooth skin surrounding the stoma.
- The stoma site avoids costal margins, superior iliac crest, and symphysis pubis.
- The stoma is located over the rectus abdominis.

tions (0.01 mL) forms a permanent tattoo; if for some reason the marked stoma site is not used during surgery, the patient retains the tattoo (30). The scratching of the skin with a sterile needle to mark the location is uncomfortable for the patient and could lead to a localized infection. A black waterproof felt marker is neither permanent nor painful, but may fade during the surgical preparation. A compromise used by many physicians and ET nurses is to mark the site preoperatively with a waterproof marker. The patient can darken the spot before and after presurgical scrubs or showers the night before surgery. Once the patient is in the operative suite, and asleep, the doctor scratches the marked skin with a needle.

E. Special Considerations to Stoma Marking

1. *Obesity*

If the patient is obese, the stoma may be sited in the upper quadrant or level with the umbilicus to allow for adequate visualization after surgery. Otherwise, the patient has great difficulty in changing the pouch without assistance. The location of the inferior costal margin and the iliac crest are carefully noted while the person is sitting. The stoma site should be at least 2 inches below the inferior costal margin, above and lateral to the umbilicus (Figs. 7 and 8).

2. *Two Stomas*

When a patient requires two stomas, such as a double-barrel colostomy, the functioning stoma is positioned for effective pouching and should be in an ideal abdominal location. Even when the surgery is considered temporary, the placement of the functioning stoma is a critical decision and affects skin care and leakage of stool and odor. The nonfunctioning mucus fistula is placed approximately 3 inches away from the functioning stoma to prevent interference with the pouch (Fig. 9).

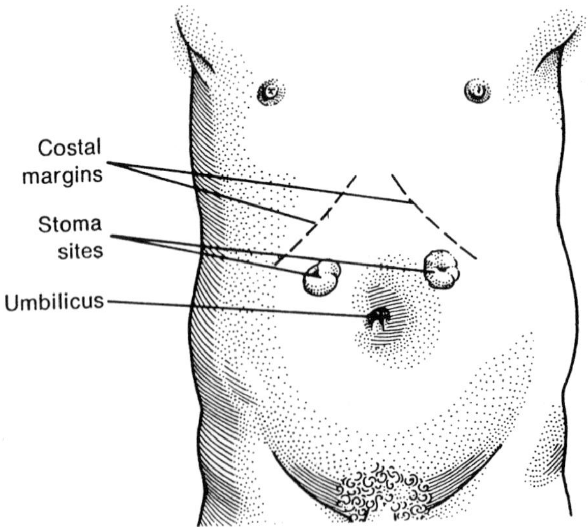

Figure 7 Right and left upper quadrant abdominal stoma sites for an ambulatory adult with an obese or enlarged abdomen. (From Ref. 19.)

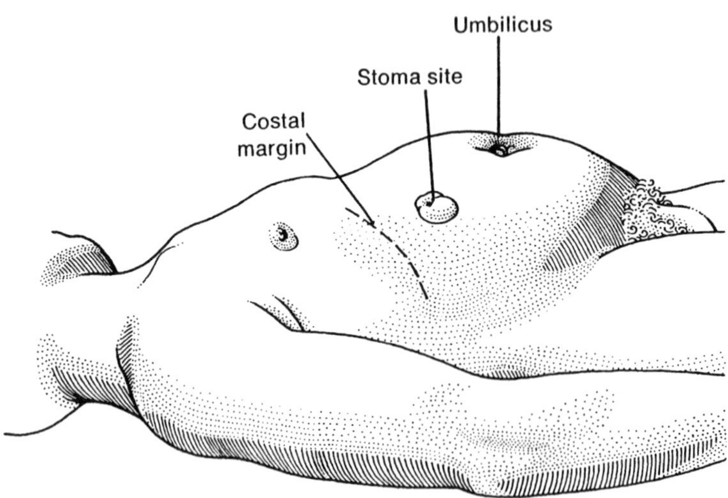

Figure 8 Upper quadrant stoma sites for a supine adult with an obese or enlarged abdomen. (From Ref. 19.)

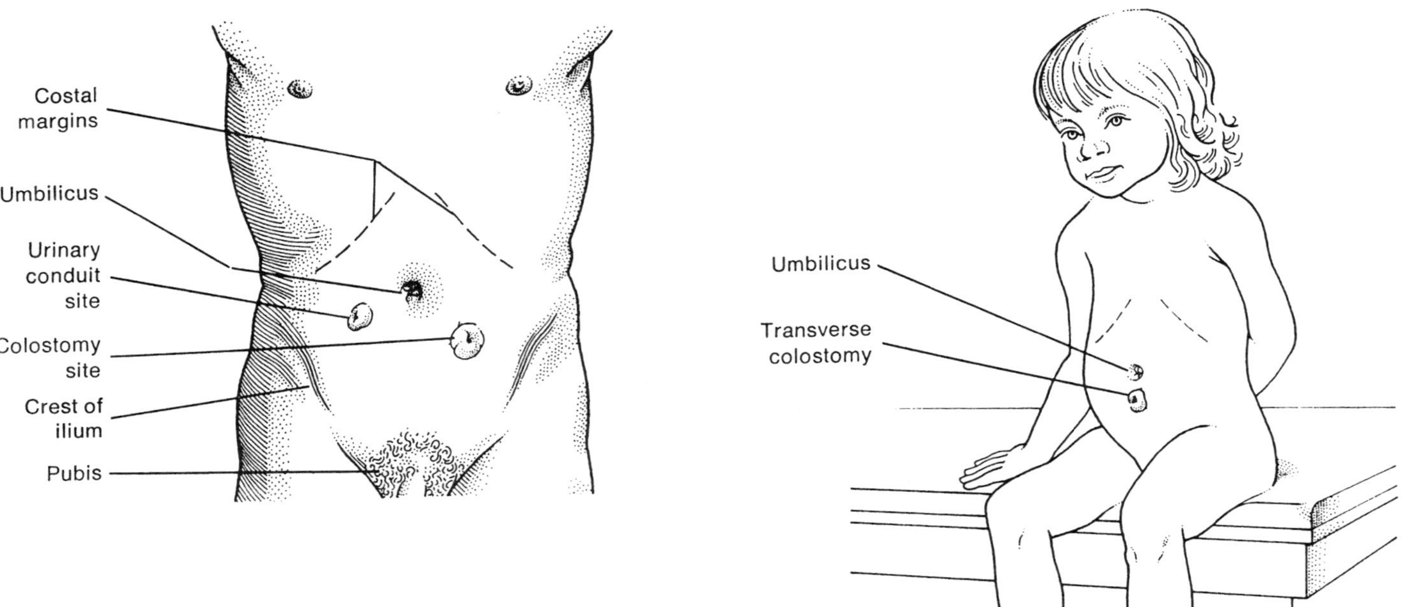

Figure 9 Two abdominal stomas: urinary diversion, right lower quadrant, and fecal diversion, left lower quadrant. (From Ref. 19.)

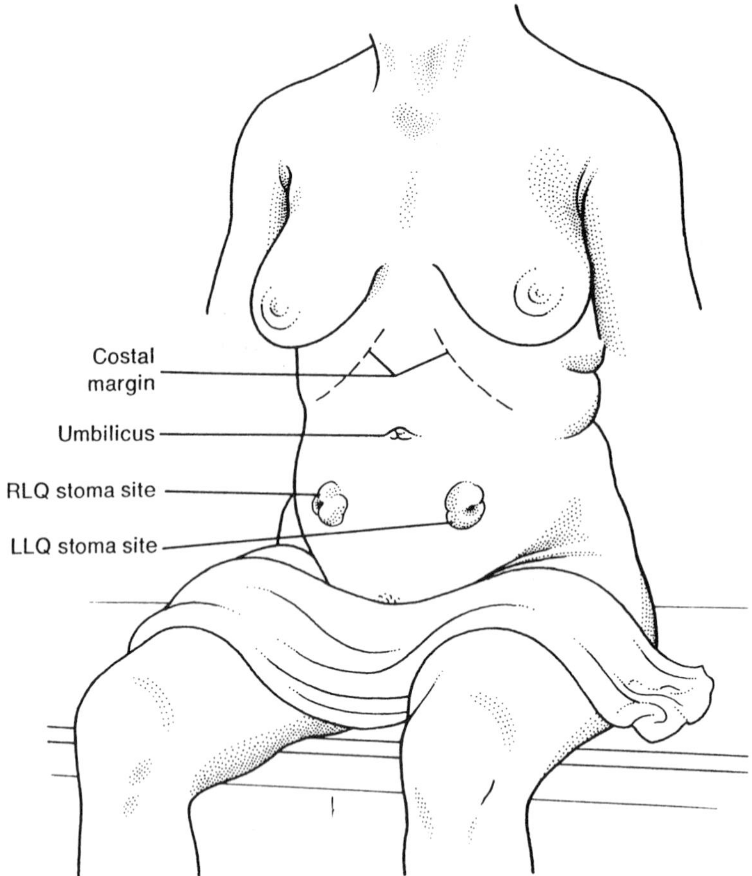

Figure 10 Right and left lower quadrant abdominal stoma sites for a nonambulatory female adult of normal weight. (From Ref. 19.)

If a person is going to have two functioning stomas, the stomas should be on opposite sides of the abdomen. The criteria for locating each stoma should be used in determining location.

3. Nonambulatory Patients (Figs. 10 and 11)

The patient needs to be observed using all prosthetic devices, such as corsets or braces. If the patient uses a wheelchair, the patient is observed in the chair and transferring from bed to chair. In most situations, the stoma is placed above or

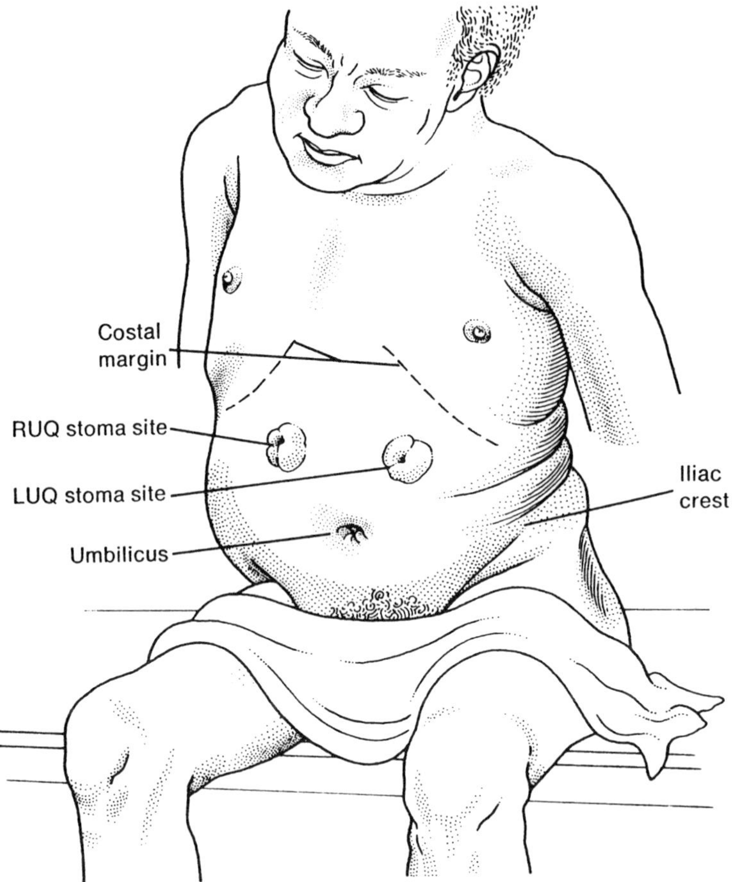

Figure 11 Upper quadrant abdominal stoma sites for a nonambulatory patient with spinal deformity and asymmetrical abdomen. (From Ref. 19.)

level to the umbilicus. Weight gain is common in nonambulatory patients as they age, and often the person gains the weight in the abdomen. Folds are common when the thighs are flexed sitting in a wheelchair. The nonambulatory patient with an extremely difficult abdomen for stoma site selection may benefit from wearing a pouch containing warm water placed at the proposed site for one to two days. Although this technique is not recommended for all patients, the importance of the appropriate stoma location is generally understood and most patients are cooperative and interested.

4. Thinness

Slender men and women may have a different set of considerations. Men tend to have a narrow pelvis, and if they wear their belts below the umbilicus, stoma location may be a problem. Movements and bony prominences may compromise the pouch seal integrity when the stoma placement is in the lower abdominal quadrant. A placement of the stoma higher on the abdomen necessitates clothing changes or else the pouch may be visible. Women tend to have an easier time adapting to a higher beltline than men do. The broader pelvis also makes placement slightly easier.

5. Summary

When a patient has a particularly difficult abdomen for stoma site selection, the surgeon and ET nurse should discuss the situation together. Moving a stoma even a fraction of an inch for these individuals may make a major difference in their ostomy management and in the number of long-term complications encountered following surgery (31). A poor location may even require a second surgery to correct long-term management problems and complications.

V. POSTOPERATIVE TEACHING AND CARE

The care of all diversions begins with the application of a postoperative pouch and skin barrier in the operating room. In most situations, a transparent pouch is used in the hospital to allow for ease of visualization of the stoma, for color and edema, and stomal (mucocutaneous) suture line. In the case of colostomies and ileostomies, normal bowel function may not return for several days, but the pouching system protects the skin from any mucous drainage and unexpected fecal output. With an ileal conduit, the urine drainage from the stoma begins during surgery (32).

A pouching system includes a pouch and some form of skin protection, from solid barrier to paste to liquids. The pouch itself consists of a faceplate, which attaches the pouch to the skin or to the skin barrier. The faceplate may be adhesive or may have a Tupperware-type of connection. The pouch system should be changed on a regular basis in the postoperative period, primarily for teaching the patient and family. Early discharge from the hospital has created a need for family involvement to begin immediately and for the patient to participate in his or her care as soon as feasible. Table 6 provides an outline for changing a pouching system. (Universal precautions must be followed when changing a pouch.) A variety of one- and two-piece drainable pouching systems are available.

Table 6 Principles of Changing a Pouch

1. **Assemble all equipment.**
   a. For cleansing the skin: cotton balls, tissue paper, toilet paper, wash cloths, towels, premoistened towelettes
   b. Pouch
   c. Skin barriers
   d. Pouch closure (rubber band, clip)
   e. Tape or belt.
   f. Equipment for cleansing or disposing of used pouches
2. **Make a pattern.**
   a. During the first pouch change, a pattern will be needed. Use universal precautions during the procedure for developing the pattern. The pouch must be removed to create the pattern.
   b. A paper towel may be used to trace a pattern.
   c. The pattern should hug the stoma, but not ride up on it.
   d. Always label the pattern for "top" or "skin side."
   e. Not only is the stomal opening important in making a pattern, but the outer dimensions of the pattern are also. The pattern should avoid hip bone, pubic area, ribs, and folds at waist or navel.
   f. At subsequent pouch changes, the pattern can be used to prepare the system before the used pouch is removed from the patient's abdomen.
3. **Provide a skin barrier** (always necessary when the stool is not formed and for an ileostomy).
   a. Use one-half, one-fourth, or full wafer (4 × 4 inch wafer) depending on the size of the stoma and abdomen.
   b. Round the corners or conform the wafer to the shape of the adhesive on the pouch.
   c. Trace the stomal pattern on the paper side of the skin barrier.
   d. Cut hole on pattern line; the line will not be visible when it is cut.
   e. Use fingers to smooth sides of the opening.
4. **Preparing the pouch.**
   a. Pouch opening should be *slightly* larger (1/8 to 1/4 inch) than the opening of the skin barrier (paper can cut the stoma).
   b. Trace pattern on the paper side of the pouch (use the opening from the skin barrier that has already been cut).
   c. Cut the hole larger than the line of the pattern (cut outside the line).
   d. The edges around the opening should be smooth.
   e. Remove paper backing from the pouch, center the openings, and apply the shiny side of the skin barrier to the pouch if two are to be applied as one piece. This may help a patient who has difficulty managing the flexible adhesive plate on disposable pouches.
   f. If using a two-piece system, assemble the system before applying to the abdomen in the early postoperative period to prevent discomfort during the application of the system.

Table 6 Continued

5. **Empty the pouch** that the patient is currently wearing. This can prevent spillage of stool or urine during the removal of the pouch. The fewer accidents experienced by the patient the better for his or her overall recovery and attitude about having an ostomy. (Use the universal precautions during the change procedure.)
6. **Remove pouch** (if disposable, place in plastic bag or trash can liner; if reusable, set aside to clean).
7. **Cleanse the skin.**
   a. Use warm water; soaps are not necessary and leave film residue.
   b. It is not necessary to remove the entire skin barrier from the skin; abrasions may be caused by rough cleansing, and other barriers tend to "burn" after applying. This discomfort ceases after a few minutes. Dry the skin gently, but well.
   c. Note any changes in the skin or the stoma, such as color, size, and ulceration.
8. **Apply the clean pouching system.**
   a. Apply skin barrier (if not attached to pouch in step 4).
   b. Center and apply clean pouch.
   c. Close end.
   d. Tape the edges of the pouching system to protect them and improve the seal. A belt may be indicated with some systems.
   e. Check the supplies and reorder as necessary.

Source: Adapted from Ref. 42.

A. Selecting a Pouching System

The steps in selecting the appropriate pouching systems are of utmost importance. Not one single pouch or skin barrier works on everyone. The definition of an effective pouching system is one that contains the effluent and protects the skin in a comfortable, cost-effective manner. This implies a ''good seal'' (19). A good seal is present when the skin protector and pouch are adhered to the skin from the base of the stoma to the outer edge of the faceplate. This is differentiated from a seal that does not allow effluent to escape from the outer edge of the seal and drainage collects between the stoma and outer edge. This is called a ''hidden leak'' (19). The following assessments are needed to select the appropriate equipment for a person with an ostomy:

1. The type of ostomy;
2. The size and contour of the abdomen;
3. The condition of the peristomal skin;
4. The physical and mental status of patient;

5. The physical activities of patient;
6. The financial situation of patient and family; and
7. Personal preference of patient.

The type of ostomy indicates the consistency and content of the drainage from the stoma. This should indicate the need for and type of skin protection, the type of pouch closure, the appropriate pouch material, the need for preventive measures, and potential problems. A urinary diversion pouch should contain an antireflux valve and a spout closure. Colostomy pouches should be odor proof and drainable.

The size and contour of the abdomen and the presence of folds, creases, scars, and bony prominences determine the shape and size of the faceplate of the pouch. In certain situations, the patient may need more convexity in the faceplate selected. When the stoma is flush to the skin or retracted below the skin, and when there are peristomal creases and skin folds and protruding or flabby abdomens, a more firm, convex faceplate may provide the structure needed to hold the pouching system in place. Not every patient can use a convex system. If the patient has pyoderma gangrenosum, caput medusae, or Crohn's ulceration or mucocutaneous separation, convexity is not recommended (33). The pouch length and width are determined by the patient's torso and clothing. The extra long postoperative pouches that are used commonly in hospitals are not appropriate for discharge and are questionable for hospital use.

Peristomal skin condition influences the selection of skin protective products and skin care treatments (34). An effective pouching system should prevent skin breakdown, and once the skin is irritated, the length of time a pouching system is worn is limited. Skin turgor, texture, moisture, and secretions also influence the length of time a pouching system remains intact. Patients who perspire heavily in the summer may need an alternate system during those months.

Physical and mental status assessment of the patient is essential for determining whether the patient is capable of self-care, or whether a family member will help or provide the care at home or a home nurse referral is necessary. The patient and family are the best resource for planning care and teaching programs. The techniques that are required in applying, emptying, and caring for a pouching system should be considered by working closely with the patient (35). One pouch closure may work better for the patient than a second closure.

Physical activities affect the abdomen. Children are more active, in different ways, than adults. Adults who are active sports enthusiasts may experience less success with the length of time a pouch seal remains intact. The hospitalized and recently discharged patient is less active than a person at 3 or 6 months following surgery. The pouching system may need adjusting or changing as the person with an ostomy regains his or her presurgical activity level. This is one major reason that follow-up is so important.

Financial situation is of major concern to the patient and family. The nurse should work with the patient and family to select a cost-effective pouching system. Cost is only one factor to be considered. The other variables to be evaluated include the length of time a pouch can be worn, the prevention of skin problems, the ease of application, and patient comfort and confidence with the system.

Personal preference is a consideration in the selection of a pouch and skin barrier. The choice of color (opaque to clear) precut to starter openings, two versus one-piece, length, and shape varies from person to person (27). The nurse's role in pouch selection is to provide the best possible system to prevent unnecessary leakage, odor escape, and skin breakdown. As the patient gains experience, he or she may experiment with systems, but during the initial postoperative period, the patient may not have the knowledge to make informed choices unless educated to do so. Many patients dislike emptying a fecal pouch into the toilet. Some patients select to use a two-piece closed end pouch that is removed and discarded several times a day. Other patients select a two-piece system that can be removed, emptied, cleansed, and replaced. I do not recommend a closed end system that is removed and discarded because of the cost, but for some people, the cost is not a factor. People explore what is available and ask questions when provided the opportunity. It is important to let a person know what is available and to discuss options with him or her at the appropriate time. Too much information and too many choices early in the postoperative period is not recommended. Help a person find a suitable pouching system that protects the skin and contains the stool or urine. After the person learns to work with and to trust the system, then he or she can try other alternatives more comfortably.

B. Peristomal Skin Integrity

The loss of skin integrity in the peristomal area may be related to several variables: the composition, consistency, and quantity of the effluent; underlying disease process; treatments and medications; surgical construction and location of the stoma; skill of the caregivers; skill and interest of patient in self-care; and availability of proper supplies. In addition, nutrition, age, general health status, personal hygiene, activity, and rest patterns affect the body's ability to maintain skin integrity (36).

The person with an ostomy is at risk for damage to the epidermis around the stoma. Peristomal irritation that may be observed include primary lesions (papules, vesicles, abscesses, and nodules) and secondary lesions (crusts, scales, erosions, ulcerations, and atrophy). Full-thickness wounds involve both the epidermis and the dermis, whereas partial thickness lesions involve the epidermis.

Skin breakdown associated with ostomies may originate from four primary etiologies: allergies, mechanical trauma, chemical reactions, and infections. Although less common, peristomal skin breakdown may be associated with the primary disease of the patient, such as Crohn's disease, or with treatment protocols, such as chemotherapy and radiation therapy.

1. Allergies

Sensitivities have been reported to skin barriers, powders, pouches, clamps, belts, and adhesives. The skin may appear erythematous, edematous, eroded, weeping, or bleeding (37). Patients may report initial symptoms of itching, stinging, or burning. The skin irritation is limited to the area in contact with allergen.

Systemic allergic responses to products in contact with the stoma mucosa have been reported (36). If a person has a history of allergies, the nurse should observe the patient for 30 minutes after applying any new product, pouch, solid barriers, pastes, or powders. Patient teaching can continue during this time. Localized reactions (skin) take longer to appear, but are not life threatening.

Many sensitivities are associated with the misuse of products. Skin barriers applied to wet rather than dry skin, moisture under plastic pouch, and thick applications of bonding agents are frequent causes of skin problems. Many patients report sensitivities to paper or microporous tapes. These sensitivities are often tape burns associated with improper application of tape. When tape is applied to skin and stretched tightly across a dressing, tension is placed on the skin and ''tape burns'' or vesicles appear. A patient may associate this with an allergic reaction. Because many ostomy products are available with a similar tape, the use of these products depends on patient sensitivities rather than with misuse.

2. Mechanical Trauma

Pressure, friction, or stripping of adhesives or skin barriers may result in mechanical trauma to the skin. Repeated, frequent removal of pouching systems is the most common cause (36). The first sign is erythema or redness that does not disappear when the pouching system has been removed for several minutes. Prolonged and continued irritation results in loss of epidermis, with denudation and erosions of the skin being replaced by scales, patches, and crusts.

Prevention of mechanical trauma may be accomplished by regular changes of the pouching system every 4 to 7 days or whenever leakage occurs. If the pouching system is leaking frequently, then the system should be reevaluated and a different system selected.

3. Chemical Irritants

The most common chemical irritants are stool and urine. Any drainage that is left in continual contact with the skin ultimately results in irritation. Skin barriers appropriately sized to fit the stoma and protect the skin prevent problems by eliminating exposure of the skin to stool or urine. The skin barrier can hug the stoma, whereas the pouch opening should be one-eighth inch larger than the stoma.

Although not common in hospitals, accumulation of amorphous ammonium phosphates (urine crystals) may appear on the stoma or skin of a person with an ileal conduit. Urine crystals are more common with alkaline urine. The salts appear as white, gritty particles (38). The prevention of urine crystals includes appropriate cleansing of all equipment, maintenance of an acidic urine, and carefully calibrating stomal openings (38).

Certain chemicals in glues, solvents, soaps, and detergents may irritate the peristomal skin. If burning or stinging sensations are reported by the patient, the system should be removed and the skin cleansed carefully. Soaps are avoided in the peristomal area, because many leave a residue on the skin. This is not to imply that people should never wash the peristomal skin with soap, but it is important to provide a thorough rinsing. When patients return home, they may shower, if possible, during the pouch change; the running water helps remove any soap residue (36).

4. *Infections*

The most common infection is caused by *Candida albicans* (*Monilia*). The skin appears bright with erythema, with papule and vesicle lesions. Satellite vesicles are common. As the infection progresses, scaling and crusting follow serous weeping (36). Candidal infections are more common in urinary diversions and are related to the extensive bowel preparation before surgery and the moist environment of the peristomal area. Diagnosis of *C. albicans* infection can be made by visual inspection and by skin scrapings prepared with potassium hydroxide. Treatment is with nystatin (Mycostatin) powder (36). Steroid sprays are not recommended unless severe inflammation is present and extends beyond the peristomal area.

Bacterial infections are less common. *Staphylococcus aureus* may present as a large patchy, erythematous, crusty area with plaques (37). Organisms should be identified by culture of the affected area. The appropriate topical or systemic antibiotic is then ordered. Initially, skin barriers will not adhere to an ointment. The ointment should be applied and the skin exposed to air, light, and heat. As the ointment begins to be absorbed, the skin barrier can be applied.

5. *Chemotherapy*

The basal cells in the epidermis rapidly divide and, therefore, are more susceptible to the effects of chemotherapy. Skin reactions can be minimized or prevented by adding solid skin barriers to the pouching system if not routinely used, changing pouches when a leak occurs, and early recognition of bacterial or fungal infections. A discoloration, deep red and purple, may be caused by 5-fluorouracil and bleomycin (39). A generalized skin breakdown may occur with methotrexate, bleomycin, and adrenocorticoids that will not subside until the causative agent is discontinued (39).

6. *Radiation Therapy*

Skin reactions with radiation therapy may vary from a mild loss of hair to a deep, purplish erythema with blistering. Prevention includes minimizing trauma and irritation; reducing friction; avoiding solvents, soaps, ointments, and lotions; avoiding direct sunshine and heat; and keeping the area dry (36). The skin should be gently cleansed with warm water and patted dry, not rubbed. If the stoma is in the direct field of radiation, the pouching system should be removed if possible. If the pouch or a segment of faceplate is in the radiation field, the pouch should be moved or removed during treatments. The faceplate or skin barrier can often be adjusted or trimmed to remove it from the field of radiation.

The treatment of peristomal skin is more difficult than prevention. Table 7 provides a summary of common types of peristomal skin problems and steps for treatment.

VI. DIAGNOSTIC PROCEDURES USED FOLLOWING DIVERSIONAL SURGERIES

A. Colostomy

The most common diagnostic procedures following colostomy are diagnostic studies or further intestinal surgery that requires bowel preparation. The first questions to be answered should include the reason for the bowel preparation, the usual consistency and volume of the patient's stool, and the length and function of the proximal bowel (40). If the patient has an end sigmoid colostomy, the bowel preparation is used to cleanse the proximal colon and a combination of liquid diets, oral laxatives, and colostomy irrigations may be used. Suppositories are not used because they are expelled from the stoma before being absorbed. If repeated colostomy irrigations are required, saline, rather than tap water, may be used for the procedure to reduce any fluid and electrolyte imbalance (40). Any colostomy irrigation should be done using a cone rather than an enema tube to reduce the possibility of perforation of the bowel.

If the distal bowel is intact, the nurse should clarify whether both segments of colon are to be cleansed or whether the distal (nonfunctioning) bowel or proximal bowel needs cleansing. When irrigating a distal bowel segment, the returns are expected through the rectum unless a blockage is present in the segment of distal bowel. When a Hartmann's pouch is to be cleansed for surgery, the length

Table 7 Management Strategies for Peristomal Skin Problems

1. Rash

Location: Rash can be located under the tape, under the faceplate, and on any part of the skin where the pouch comes in contact with the skin. Generalized reddish appearance that covers an entire area, similar to a diaper rash, will be seen.

Cause: Leaking appliance
Perspiration
Allergies to tape
Hair follicle irritation

Treatment:

- Use heat lamp or hair dryer to dry the skin.
- Sprinkle a small amount of powder (karaya, stomahesive) on the skin, wipe off the excess, then blot with a skin sealant to seal the powder to the skin.
- Powder the skin on which the pouch lies (not under the faceplate) after the pouch is applied.
- Make or buy a pouch cover.
- Wearing a pouch belt too tight may break the seal.

2. Erythematous skin

Location: Under tape, under the faceplate, or on any part of the skin in contact with the pouch

Cause: Allergic response
Mechanical trauma

Treatment:

- Remove the pouch every 48 to 72 hours or more often if the patient complains of pain.
- Cleanse the skin with warm water, pat dry.
- Expose the skin to light, air, and heat for 20 minutes.
- Use a solid skin barrier covering all erythematous skin.
- Use a different pouching system if erythema is related to an allergic response.

3. Eroded or denuded skin

Location: Under faceplate or tape

Cause: Mechanical trauma
Chemical irritant

Treatment:

- Change system every 24 to 48 hours to treat the skin.
- Cleanse with warm water, pat dry.
- Apply Burow's solution (aluminum acetate) compresses for 20 minutes (optional step).
- Expose skin to air, heat, and light.
- Apply powder or paste (not containing alcohol).
- Apply solid skin barrier.

Table 7 Continued

4. Ulcerated area on stoma

Location: Anywhere on stoma

Cause: Stomal opening of the pouch was too small or activities were causing the faceplate to rub or cut into stoma

Treatment:

- Enlarge the size of the pouch opening. (Opening should be at least one-eighth larger than stoma.)
- Evaluate patient activities; may need a different size or shaped faceplate.
- Loosen the belt; if too tight, the belt may cause the faceplate to ride into stoma.

5. Infected or irritated hair follicles

Location: Under the faceplate, raised red areas (similar to acne) at the shaft of the hair follicle

Cause: Not keeping the area under the faceplate shaved. An electric razor or safety razor can be used to remove the hair under the faceplate.

Treatment:

- Let the irritation improve before removing any more hair by shaving or cutting.
- Use hair dryer or heat lamp to dry the skin, if oozing is present.
- Use a skin barrier between skin and faceplate until irritation improves. Try to leave on 24 to 48 hours.

6. Solvent burns

Location: Burns can be located anywhere under the faceplate, but they usually are found at the outside edges.

Cause: Chemicals in the bonding agents or solvents used to remove adhesives were not allowed to evaporate off the skin surface before applying pouch, or they were too thick and it was unable to dry completely.

Treatment:

- Apply heat lamp or hair dryer to the weeping skin.
- Cover the burn with a solid skin barrier and apply pouch in the usual way. Try to leave the pouch on 24 to 48 hours.
- Avoid the use of the agent in removal of adhesives or barriers.

7. Water-logged skin (urinary diversions)

Location: Between the opening of the faceplate and the stoma

Cause: Urine pools on exposed skin

Treatment:

- Use heat lamp (60-watt bulb) or low heat hair dryer to dry the area.
- Cover with pectin-based skin barrier, hugging the stoma.
- Decrease the size of stomal opening in faceplate.
- Monitor the pouching system for hidden leaks between the inner seal at the stoma and the outer taped seal that can trap urine.

Table 7 Continued

8. *Candida albicans* infections

Location: Skin surrounding the stoma. May extend beyond the faceplate and appears as reddened skin with raised lesions; satellite lesions are common.

Cause: Fungal infection of the skin associated with *Candida albicans.*

Treatment:

- Use low wattage heat lamp or hair dryer on low setting to dry lesions.
- Apply Mycostatin powder to the area, blow off excess powder, and seal with a thin coat of a skin sealant.
- Apply pouch and skin barrier in usual manner.

9. Alkaline urine crystals (urinary diversion)

Location: On the stoma or around the base of the stoma. May be found in some types of pouches.

Cause: Alkaline urine and predisposition for stone formation.

Treatment:

- Swab vinegar solution (one part vinegar to one part water) on the stoma when changing the pouch.
- Insert vinegar solution into the pouch while it is being worn. For a minor formation, insert four times a day.
- Remove the antireflux valve from the pouch to allow the solution to reach the stoma, if using a one-piece system. If possible, a two-piece system can make the treatment easier.
- Empty the pouch and instill 1 to 2 ounces of vinegar solution.
- Encourage the patient to lie down so the solution bathes the stoma. The vinegar solution may discolor the stoma, making it appear blanched or white. The normal color returns in a few minutes.
- Empty the pouch of the solution and rinse with cool water to remove the vinegar odor.
- Use vinyl or plastic pouches until the condition clears, and replace pouches as necessary to keep crystal formation in the pouch reduced.

Source: Adapted from Ref. 43.

of retained distal colon determines the volume of solution. A low volume enema is indicated when the rectosigmoid colon has been left (40).

B. Urinary Diversion: Urine for Culture and Sensitivity Procedures

The most important test done following urinary diversion that is most often performed incorrectly is obtaining a urine specimen for culture and sensitivity from an ileal conduit or other form of urinary diversion. The urine should be obtained from the conduit by introducing a catheter through the stoma using sterile technique. Many times, a specimen is taken from the pouch in the doctor's office, resulting in a positive culture, regardless of whether a urinary infection is present.

After handwashing and donning of sterile gloves, the nurse or physician should establish a sterile field. The stoma is cleansed or ''prepped'' with three swabs soaked in an antiseptic solution. Each swab is washed over the stoma once. A fourth sterile swab is used to remove any remaining solution off the stoma. A lubricated catheter is introduced through the stoma opening into the conduit. The drainage end of the catheter is placed in a sterile container and held below the level of the abdomen to facilitate drainage from the conduit. It is necessary to wait for urine to drain into the container because the conduit is not a reservoir and does not hold urine.

VII. COMPLICATIONS ASSOCIATED WITH DIVERSIONAL PROCEDURES

A. Stomal Complications

In the early postoperative period, the stomal complications that may occur include bleeding, ischemia and necrosis, and skin-mucosal separation. Stomal complications that may occur at any time include melanosis coli, prolapse, hernia, retraction, stenosis, and laceration. Careful observation of the stoma during each pouch change provides for early diagnosis of any complication.

B. Alterations in Sexual Function

Ostomy surgery and adjuvant therapy may directly or indirectly alter the sexual function of the patient. Surgery for low-lying rectal cancers and bladder cancer damages the nerves and structures that are essential for penile-vaginal intercourse. Men experience erectile and ejaculatory problems. The degree of impotence is related to the amount of tissue resected (41). For women, the changes are not as apparent. Women may experience decreased lubrication and coital pain. Gynecological cancers may result in the loss of or shortening of the vagina.

Radiation therapy may result in nerve damage, alteration in vascular flow, and tissue changes that affect sexual function. Chemotherapy may cause impotence, sterility, depressed libido, and the appearance of secondary sex characteristics. Indirectly, both radiation and chemotherapy result in side effects that negatively impact on sexual functions, including depression, nausea, vomiting, and general malaise.

Patients and their partners benefit from open and honest discussions about sexual functioning and alternatives that are available following surgery and recuperation. Referral to a counselor for assistance should be considered for each patient and their partner.

C. Resources for Families

One of the major resources for persons having ostomy surgery is a person who has undergone similar surgery. The International Ostomy Association (IOA), an association of ostomy associations, was formed to provide a forum for people with ostomies to work together to encourage the highest possible standards of surgery and care. Worldwide associations have been organized and formed regional associates to promote the agenda of people living with an ostomy. The IOA contact office is through the British Colostomy Association at 15 Station Road, Reading, Berkshire RG1 1LG, England (telephone 44 1189 391537); the Internet site is http://www.bcas.org.uk. In the United States, the United Ostomy Association (UOA) (19772 MacArthur Boulevard Suite 200, Irvine, CA 92612-2405 or telephone 800-826-0826) is composed of individuals who participate at the national as well as a local level. These self-help groups are designed, developed, and run by people with stomas to help people who have had surgery. The UOA Internet site is http://www.uoa.org.

People with stomas can live successful and productive lives, marry, have children, work, play, and grow. The group meetings allow members to share experiences and solutions. Volunteers are available for hospital or home visits or to make telephone calls to people who have had surgery.

The worldwide web and the use of home personal computers have added a new dimension to self-help groups and to finding personal information. Not only can patients access information in their home country but they also have access to worldwide information, chat rooms, and medical resources.

The American Cancer Society (ACS) (1599 Clifton Road NE, Atlanta, GA 30329) also serves as a major resource for persons undergoing ostomy surgery. The ACS provides education for lay public as well as medical professionals. The American Cancer Society has played an instrumental role in developing screening programs for detecting colorectal cancers. Consumer information is available through their Internet site http://www.acs.org.

The organization Friends of Ostomates Worldwide was founded in 1986 and is a self-supporting association that helps people worldwide through its SHARE program. The SHARE program sends ostomy products and literature to people in need. They accept donations and redirect them to countries that have little resources available for people with ostomies. The Project Share address for correspondence is FOW-UOA, H.R., Bob Hall, 5284 Dawes Street, San Diego, CA 92109. Donations may be made to FOW-UOA, Project Share, c/o ASW Logistics, 1501 Exeter Road, Akron, OH 44306-3889.

VIII. FUTURE PERSPECTIVES

The outlook for people with cancer is brighter than it has been in the past. This trend will continue as long as researchers search for new and better diagnostic methods, genetic markers, preventive causes, and new treatments. Ostomies will continue to be necessary for a small number of people. The focus for surgeons will be in the new techniques developed and refined that will eliminate the need for external devices and stomas. Doctors and nurses need to remember for those individuals for whom ostomy is necessary that they too deserve the best possible care and the most up-to-date and efficient equipment available. The trends and advantages of new surgeries and standards are not available for all. Even in countries with state-of-the-art health care, the major research institutes provide the best and newest procedures first. Years may pass before the standards in the community reflect the standards at research centers. The advantages for future patients include no fears of odor or embarrassing leakages. For some, no pouch will be required, even though other procedures will be needed, such as intermittent catheterization.

REFERENCES

1. American Cancer Society. Cancer Facts and Figures—1997. Atlanta: American Cancer Society, 1997.
2. World Health Organization Report 1997. Fifty Facts for the World Health Report 1997. World Health Organization, Geneva, Switzerland. URL: www.who.int/whr/1997/factse.htm.
3. Hurney C, Holland J. Psychological sequelae of ostomies in cancer patients. CA 1986; 36:26–41.
4. Fry RD, Fleshman JW, Kodner IJ. Cancer of the colon and rectum. Clin Symp 1989; 41(5):2.
5. Perez CA, Knapp RC, DiSaia PJ, et al. Gynecologic tumors. In: DeVita VT, Hellman S, Rosenberg SA, eds. Cancer: Principles and Practice. 2d ed. Philadelphia: JB Lippincott, 1985:1013–1082.
6. Holland J. Psychological aspects of cancer. In: Holland JF, Frei E, eds. Cancer Medicine. 2d ed. Philadelphia: Lea & Febiger, 1982.
7. Sugarbaker PH, Gunderson LL, Wittes RE. Colorectal cancer. In: DeVita VT, Hellman S, Rosenberg SA, eds. Cancer: Principles and Practice. 2d ed. Philadelphia: JB Lippincott, 1985:795–884.
8. Ezzell C. Colon cancer's newly mapped gene puts it all in the family. Journal of NIH Research 1993; 5(6):38–39.
9. Myers RE, Balshem AM, Wolf TA, Ross EA, Millner L. Screening for colorectal neoplasia: physicans' adherence to complete diagnostic evaluation. Am J Public Health 1993; 83(11):1620–1622.

10. Khubchandani IT, Karamchandani M, Kleckner F, et al. Mass screening for colorectal cancer. Dis Colon Rectum 1989; 32:754–758.
11. Simon J. Occult blood screening for colorectal carcinoma: a critical review. Gastroenterology 1985; 88:820.
12. Bryant RA, Buls JG. Pathophysiology and diagnostic studies of gastrointestinal tract disorders. In: Hampton BG, Bryant RA. Ostomies and continent diversions: nursing management. St. Louis: CV Mosby, 1992.
13. Droller MJ. Transitional cell cancer: upper tracks and bladder. In: Walsh PC, et al, eds. Campbell's Urology. 5th ed. Philadelphia: WB Saunders, 1986.
14. Gray M. Genitourinary Disorders. St. Louis: CV Mosby, 1992.
15. Hampton BG. Nursing management of a patient following pelvic exenteration. Semin Oncol Nursing 1986; 2(4):281–286.
16. Fazio VW. Cancer of the colon and rectum. In: Broadwell DC, Jackson BS. Principles of Ostomy Care. St. Louis: CV Mosby, 1982:148–166.
17. Atkinson KG. Abdominoperineal resection of the rectum. In: Broadwell DC, Jackson BS. Principles of Ostomy Care. St. Louis: CV Mosby, 1982:186–205.
18. Dobkin KA, Broadwell DC. Nursing considerations for the patient undergoing colostomy surgery. Semin Oncol Nursing 1986; 2(4):249–255.
19. Broadwell DC, Jackson BS, eds. Principles of Ostomy Care. St. Louis: CV Mosby, 1982.
20. Pernet FPPM, Jonas U. Ileal conduit urinary diversion: early and late results of 132 cases in a 25-year period. World J Urology 1985; 3:140.
21. Rolstad BS, Hoyman K. Continent diversions and reservoirs. In: Hampton BG, Bryant RA. Ostomies and continent diversions. Nursing Management. St. Louis: CV Mosby, 1992:129–162.
22. Dudas S. Rehabilitation concepts of nursing. J Enterostomal Ther 1984; 11:6–15.
23. Broadwell DC. Rehabilitation needs of the patient with cancer. Cancer 1987; 60(suppl):563–568.
24. Mitchel JV. A clinical pathway for ostomy care in the home: process and development. Journal of WOCN 1998; 25(4):200–205.
25. Vella J. Learning to listen, learning to teach. San Francisco: Jossey-Bass Publishers, 1994.
26. Frank-Stromborg M, Wright P. Ambulatory cancer patients' perception of the physical and psychosocial changes in their lives since the diagnosis of surgery. Cancer Nursing 1984; 7:117–130.
27. Jackson DB. Variables affecting ostomy patient outcomes. National Institutes of Health, NIH 1 R15 NRO2929-01, Final Report, 1995.
28. Jackson BS, Broadwell DC. Ostomy surgery: an overview of historical, current, and future perspectives. Semin Oncol Nursing 1986; 2(4):227–234.
29. Druckerman LJ. The management of a permanent colostomy. Am J Dig Dis 1938; 5:382–385.
30. Watt R. Stoma placement. In: Broadwell DC, Jackson BS. Principles of Ostomy Care. St. Louis: CV Mosby, 1982:329–339.
31. Bass EM, Del Pino A, Pearl RK, Orsay CP, Abcarian H. Does preoperative stoma marking and education by an enterostomal therapist affect outcome? Dis Colon Rectum 1997; 40:440–442.

32. Alterescu KB. Colostomy. Nursing Clin North Am 1987; 22(2):281–289.
33. Clinical Fact Sheet. Wound, Ostomy and Continence Nursing Society. Pouching systems: convexity. Laguna Beach, CA: Author, 1998.
34. Wagner VP, Osgood SB. Patient with a recessed, stenosed stoma located in irregular, pendulous abdomen and the presence of pseudoverrucous lesions. J WOCN 1998; 25(5):261–266.
35. Erickson PJ. Ostomies: the art of pouching. Nursing Clin North Am 1987; 22(2): 311–320.
36. Broadwell DC. Peristomal skin integrity. Nursing Clin North Am 1987; 22(2):321–332.
37. Watt RC. Pathophysiology of peristomal skin. In: Broadwell DC, Jackson BS. Principles of Ostomy Care. St. Louis: CV Mosby, 1982:241–256.
38. Watt RC. Nursing management of a patient with a urinary diversion. Semin Oncol Nursing, 1986; 2:265–269.
39. Rodriques DB. Special considerations: care of the ostomy patient receiving cancer therapy. In: Broadwell DC, Jackson BS. Principles of Ostomy Care. St. Louis: CV Mosby, 1982:381–389.
40. Erwin-Toth P, Doughty DB. Principles and procedures of stoma management. In: Hampton BG, Bryant RA. Ostomies and Continent Diversions: Nursing management. St. Louis: CV Mosby, 1992:29–103.
41. Shipes E. Sexual function following ostomy surgery. Nursing Clin North Am 1987; 22(2):303–310.
42. Jackson DB, Sorrells S. Colostomy Care. Plainfield, NJ: Patient Education Press, 1988.
43. Jackson DB, Sorrels S. Urinary Diversion Care. Plainfield, NJ: Patient Education Press, 1988.

27

Fatigue in Patients with Cancer

Agnes Glaus
Center for Tumor Detection and Prevention, St. Gallen, Switzerland

I. INTRODUCTION

Whether fatigue is called a symptom, a sign of disease, a side effect of treatment, or a medical or nursing diagnosis, its manifestation and description is dependent on cultural and linguistic features. In the English and French language, the word ''fatigue'' is being used to express feelings of extreme, unusual tiredness. In some countries, the word fatigue does not even exist and it seems to be replaced by the words ''extreme tiredness'' and by ''general exhaustion.'' Italian speaking individuals usc the word ''stanchezza'' (tiredness) and the German speaking population also simply uses the word ''Müdigkeit'' (tiredness). The Latin word ''fatigatio'' is being translated in German with ''general exhaustion'' (allgemeine Erschöpfung) (1). The linguistic differences, however, reveal the complexity of the word, which not only represents a semantic problem in different languages and cultures but also raises questions of understanding and interpretation of the phenomenon. Surprisingly, the word fatigue is not only used in the context of medicine or psychology, it is also widely used in the technical area of engineering. Material can become fatigued and eventually break down. A similar technical use is seen in medicine, for example, a fatigue-fracture is a breakdown of bone tissue after exertion (2).

In *Stedman's Medical Dictionary*, fatigue in humans is ''that state following a period of mental or bodily activity characterized by a lessened capacity for work'' (3). Even though this definition is of a physiological nature and does not describe how the capacity of work is affected by fatigue, it does point to a multidimensional concept by its origin. Attempts to define fatigue from a psychological viewpoint require the distinction between fatigue as an objective decrease in performance and general feelings of fatigue, which ''are not a simple act, but a psychological state made out of a number of simpler elements which include changes in affect or sentiments corresponding to obscure and sometimes subconscious tactile and muscular sensations'' (4). It seems that the word ''fatigue'' could be used as an umbrella term to describe a variety of sensations or feelings and expressions of decreased capacity at physical, mental, psychological, or social levels.

II. FATIGUE/TIREDNESS—HUMAN RESPONSE TO HEALTH AND DISEASE

A. Fatigue—A Human Adaptation Mechanism to Maintain Health

The biological meaning and aim of tiredness, as described by the fatigue theorist Grandjean (5), lies in the fact that nature conducts the behavior of humans and animals through feelings of fatigue to help the body find its balance between rest and activity, thus being a life-sustaining state, similar to other physiological needs, such as thirst or hunger. It is difficult, however, to capture tiredness, which is in transition from a ''healthy, life-sustaining state'' into a life-distressing sign or symptom of an approaching disaster or breakdown.

In general, fatigue is frequently regarded as something to be avoided. Avoidance of fatigue may not be entirely desirable if it is viewed in relation to the process of adaptation to maintain health. Fatigue sensations may be essential indicators that the physiological equilibrium somewhere in the body is breaking down. Therefore, fatigue could be defined as a defense mechanism, a protective phenomenon, that helps to maintain the physiological equilibrium by stimulating a desire for work decrements or stress avoidance when the response to stress reaches a level of discomfort (6).

Deviations from ''normal'' tiredness are not always easy to recognize. The activity of the human organism is rhythmical and geared toward the maintenance of a dynamic, healthy equilibrium. Well-known processes, such as circadian rhythms, cardiac work-rest cycles, humoral and neural balances, and compensatory mechanisms contribute to maintaining this dynamic equilibrium. Tiredness, which is seen as a regulative, protective mechanism, could be called healthy tiredness. ''Acceptable'' fatigue includes recognition of tiredness and steps taken to overcome it as soon as possible, enabling the person to sustain performance. Persons able to sustain performance perceive themselves as healthily tired; their tiredness does not make them anxious (7).

B. Fatigue-Modulating Factors in the General Population

People generally believe that age plays a role in relation to fatigue, attributing higher levels of fatigue to the older population. Data from a large survey of 2000 American adults between 25 and 74 years of age were used to explore the relationship of self-perceived fatigue and age and gender (8). Chen concluded from his study that there was no association between age and fatigue. A newer study examining fatigue in general practice attendees concluded that there was no correlation between age and the total of fatigue scores for men and women (9). A further study comparing fatigue between 104 breast cancer patients and 93 healthy women did not describe differences in age in the control group (10). Gender has been defined by Chen (8) as a risk factor. He concluded that women had 1.5 times the risk of males of being fatigued. Less fatigue was reported by Pater et al. (11) in the oldest patients and in male patients. David and Pelosi found no difference between men and women in his study (9) and Glaus (12) found higher mean levels of fatigue in women than in men. However, only few fatigue studies include a control group with healthy individuals. Methodological problems in defining and measuring fatigue make it difficult to interpret and compare results.

C. Fatigue—A Sign of Disease

Fatigue has been described as a warning signal of an approaching disaster (13). Excessive tiredness has been observed as preceding 30% to 55% of myocardial infarction or sudden cardiac deaths (14). Fatigue has been identified among the three most significant stressors experienced by hemodialysis and peritoneal dialysis patients, even after initiation of hemodialysis, which improved well-being but did not relieve feelings of fatigue (15). Furthermore, patients suffering from multiple sclerosis (16), rheumatoid arthritis (17), and hyperparathyroidism (18) have been associated with high levels of fatigue. Recently, fatigue associated with acquired immunodeficiency syndrome (AIDS) has become subject of high interest. Much attention has also been devoted to the chronic fatigue syndrome (CFS) in recent years, in which feelings of fatigue are considered to present a disease in itself. A controversy is still going on about the question of whether the CFS is a postviral disease or a psychiatric syndrome (19).

III. FATIGUE—ITS CONCEPT IN PATIENTS WITH CANCER

A. Prevalence

In the past years, fatigue has been recognized as the most common symptom reported by cancer patients (20–23). New therapeutic antineoplastic strategies and advances in the control of treatment-induced nausea and emesis or in treating pain have induced changes in the prevalence of the most common symptoms of cancer. More insight has been gained concerning the incidence of fatigue as a treatment side effect, especially when treatment entered the era of biological response modifiers (24). Methodological problems make it difficult to compare available research in order to assess the exact prevalence of fatigue. A recent study, investigating the incidence and severity of symptoms in 1000 patients with cancer, showed that fatigue, together with pain and anorexia, was consistently among the 10 most prevalent symptoms (25). Data from 2275 patients on 10 clinical trials have been collected to show the relationship between levels of fatigue and patient and disease characteristics, as reported by the patients on the fatigue scale of the EORTC Q 30 quality of life questionnaire. Factors that were associated with greater fatigue levels included female gender, presence of metastatic disease, poorer performance status, and ovarian and lung cancer. Lower fatigue levels were reported by patients with breast cancer and by patients who underwent the antiemetic trials in which emesis was better controlled (11). These recent investigations show the many influencing variables that must be carefully controlled to predict prevalence of fatigue in different cancer populations.

B. Etiology

Although cancer patients might be more vulnerable to fatigability during active disease, they also might experience acute tiredness as a consequence of exertion or daily living activities. This "healthy" type of tiredness might be acute and located in specific parts of the body, and it might be resolved by rest (12). Clinical experience and qualitative research show that cancer patients suffer from a second type of tiredness, better called fatigue, which has recurrent character, is distressing over the whole day, is not relieved by rest, and lasts longer than weeks (26–28). This type can be considered a chronic fatigue state, affecting the whole person in body and mind.

One of the first and most cited models proposed to theoretically explain etiology of fatigue in patients with cancer has been developed by Piper (29). It is the "integrated fatigue model," addressing many potential causes of fatigue in cancer and stresses the multidimensionality of the concept. The many influencing confounding variables represent the complex reality. Biochemical influences, and psychological, social, behavioral, environmental, and treatment factors are included, as are patterns of perception and manifestation. The model gives an overview of related aspects and the researchers need to break down the many elements into observable units and to weight them in order to set priorities for further scientific hypothesis testing. On the basis of the model, the author has developed and validated a fatigue measurement scale (in American English) for cancer patients (30).

C. Primary Causes

A further way of theoretically explaining the causes of fatigue is to use a model including pathophysiological, biochemical, and psychological processes and to distinguish between the primary impact of cancer on specific, affected organs and the secondary effects of cancer on the whole body and mind system (31).

The primary impact of cancer concerning fatigue can be explained by the consequences of the local infiltration of the tumor or its metastasis. For example, tumors of the lung or bone marrow infiltration (severe anemia) can lead to

- Circulatory and metabolic adaptation failure, leading to
- Decreased oxygen carrying capacity, leading to
- Increased fatigue levels

If cancer of the lung inhibits pulmonary function, circulatory capacity for oxygen supply might be impaired. Additional lung infection, severe anemia, or impaired cardiac function might further aggravate the situation.

Infiltration of cancer into other organs, such as kidney, liver, brain, or endocrine glands causes metabolic disorders, endocrine and hormonal disturbances, disruption of central nervous function, and further damage. The aim of supportive care in relation to fatigued cancer patients in this sense includes proper assessment of local tumor infiltration and its consequences or complications and, if possible, to support adaptation failures.

D. Secondary Causes of Fatigue in Cancer

1. *Asthenins*

Apart from the many direct primary causes of fatigue, produced by the local changes through tumor infiltration, other secondary paraneoplastic pathways exist. It has been proposed that the malignant process itself may secrete substances, also called ''asthenins,'' which cause asthenia (32). Asthenia, in this sense, has been defined with pathological fatigability, loss of strength, and generalized weakness (33) and can be seen as a major component of fatigue. Such asthenins cause morphological, biochemical, or physiological changes in tumor-free muscle tissue in cancer patients. These changes in the muscles are thought to be the causes of asthenia (32). In cancer patients with advanced disease, abnormal electrophysiological changes in the muscles can be observed, independent from malnutrition and loss of muscle tissue (34). Whereas it is still unclear whether these asthenins are produced by the tumor or by the immune system, it is also unclear whether the muscle changes are responsible for asthenia or whether they represent an epiphenomenon (35). Muscle wasting occurring in the course of advanced cancer was thought to be responsible for fatigue, because it requires patients to exert an unusually high amount of effort to generate adequate contractile force and changed muscular metabolism may occur (36).

2. Fatigue—An Immunological Response Against the Tumor

A further hypothesis for fatigue has been described as ''the body's inflammatory defense mechanism against the tumor,'' analogous to the situation in infectious disease. The secretion of cytokines, such as interferons, interleukins, and tumor necrosis factors by monocytes and inflammatory cells, activated in response to the neoplastic process, involves a whole cascade of reactions, and fatigue and associated phenomena may be expected to be caused by this underlying process (37). However, not all tumor types activate the immune system and some might even cause immune suppression.

Chronic stimulation by endogenous interferon-gamma can be measured as elevated neopterin levels as an indication of activated macrophages. Decreased levels of tryptophan, associated with increased neopterin levels may impair protein synthesis and may be a defense mechanism against the active proliferation of tumors (38). Tryptophan is a precursor substance of serotonin, which has also been used as sleep medication. A tiring effect could be expected from such a substance. Endogen tumor necrosis factor (TNF) leads, as the word suggests, to tumor necrosis but also to protein degradation, weight and muscle loss, and anorexia (39). Some of the tumor necrosis factors are primarily secreted by macrophages and monocytes but may also be produced by various tumor cells (40). It was hypothesized that different types and stages of cancer are associated with different amounts and types of cytokine production, which goes hand in hand with tumor activity and its devastating consequences, such as cachexia, weakness, and fatigue (31).

3. Fatigue in Paraneoplastic Syndromes

Paraneoplastic syndromes, which might induce fatigue, are known in some types of cancer. Secretions of mediators by the tumor, such as parathormone-related factors, antidiuretic hormone, and similar substances may cause severe metabolic consequences such as hypercalcemia, hyponatremia, and hypoglycemia, all of which may cause fatigue. Hypercalcemia, induced by osteolytic active substances, is frequently seen in patients with skeletal metastasis of breast cancer and in patients with non-small cell lung cancer. This frequently seen secondary disease can lead to muscular weakness, fatigue, dehydration, hyporeflexia, and other symptoms (41).

4. *Fatigue and Energy Transformation Processes*

Patients with advanced cancer and cachexia typically demonstrate modestly increased rates of energy expenditure in the presence of diminished food intake as a result of anorexia and to gastrointestinal disturbances (42). Rates of glucose production by the liver, gluconeogenesis, and glycolysis to lactate (Cory cycle) are increased and fat mobilization and oxidation are accelerated. A redistribution of body proteins away from muscle toward visceral proteins, resulting in marked muscle protein loss, can be observed (42). The resultant loss of muscle tissue might be responsible for muscle weakness, which requires patients to exert an unusually high amount of effort to generate adequate contractile force, as is discussed earlier.

Irvine (10) has developed a theoretical framework of fatigue that pays regard to changes in energy transformation processes. The ''energy analysis model'' focuses on interactions of different energy variables, such as sources (oxygenation of blood), transformation (change in weight), expenditure (activities of daily living), and energy response modifiers (treatment, symptom distress, mood disturbance). It is suggested that this important energy model refers to relevant ''tips of icebergs,'' from where interesting hypotheses need to be further tested.

E. Fatigue—Its Role as a Primary and as Secondary Symptom

The high prevalence of fatigue in patients with cancer might be due to the fact that it can occur as a primary and as a secondary symptom. Clinical experience shows that patients with specific tumor types primarily complain about fatigue as a first symptom of cancer.

Secondary fatigue might be the consequence of other symptoms of cancer. The ''psychobiological entropy model'' developed by Winningham (22) describes a unique relationship between fatigue and other symptoms, based on its effect on activity and functional status. Cancer patients are thought to become less active as a result of symptoms such as primary fatigue, pain, nausea and vomiting, dyspnea, diarrhea, fever, anxiety, depression, fatigue, and others, resulting in a loss of energizing metabolic resources. The outcome of decreased activity is described as secondary fatigue resulting from decreased energetic capacity (decreased oxygen uptake, decreased calories/consumption), leading to reduced functional status. Symptoms that induce more rest and inactivity might lead to secondary fatigue. If anemia is severe and causes inactivity, then secondary fatigue could be the consequence of reduced activity. In light of Winningham's theory, immobilization could be a fatigue-inducing state.

Medications such as antiemetic substances, and pain and sleep medications have potential fatiguing effects. On the other hand, control of side effects, such as nausea and emesis, could be seen as a fatigue relieving factor (11). It remains to be substantiated whether patients experience less fatigue because of good nausea and emesis control or whether good symptom control prevents fatigue-inducing inactivity. The same could be said concerning other symptoms, especially pain.

IV. FATIGUE AS A CANCER TREATMENT SIDE EFFECT

A. When Treatment Relieves Fatigue

If fatigue-associated cancer is being successfully treated, the disappearance of the disease might be associated with disappearance of fatigue. Fatigue levels of patients with lung cancer were observed to be higher before and during radiotherapy than after (43). The decrease of tumor burden can result in lower fatigue levels as a result of better oxygen exchange, less breathing distress, or less production of cytokines. In contrast, patients with localized breast cancer receiving adjuvant radiotherapy experienced higher levels of fatigue after treatment than before (44). In this case, no primary tumor bulk (with cytokine-inducing fatigue) had to be reduced but radiotherapy induced fatigue as a side effect. If functional capacity of an organ can be ameliorated by the treatment, fatigue might be reduced by the treatment. If patients are free of tumor burden and need adjuvant therapy, they are more likely to experience fatigue as a side effect.

B. Radiotherapy-Induced Fatigue

Although it is common to attribute fatigue in patients with radiotherapy to the production of by-products of cell death, little is known to underpin this belief. Destruction of tumor cells by irradiation is an unusual condition for the body, which is left to eliminate the waste products. Cell damage and the reaction of the body to necrotic tissue have been discussed in the context of fatigue in radiotherapy patients.

Type and aim of radiotherapy, for example, adjuvant therapy in breast cancer or palliative treatment in lung cancer, play an important role in the development of fatigue. Side effects of radiotherapy usually are of a localized nature, based on the site of treatment. Fatigue is one of the few systemic side effects and has been found to increase toward the end of radiotherapy (43,45). A decrease of fatigue during the pauses at weekends was observed in a further study (43). Contradictory findings have been reported from a study by Nail and Winningham (46) in which fatigue did not decrease over the weekend in pre- to post-treated women undergoing intracavitary radiation therapy for gynecological cancer. King and Nail (45) interviewed 96 radiotherapy patients and found that they perceived fatigue as intermittent early in treatment but that it became a continuous state by the end of treatment and that it was worse in the afternoon or evening.

C. Chemotherapy-Induced Fatigue

As with radiotherapy, the mechanisms of fatigue development are poorly understood in the context of chemotherapy treatment. Cell damage and reactions to cell necrosis are, again, generally accepted explanations. In contrast to the usually localized effect of radiotherapy, chemotherapeutic cancer treatment, according to its type and intensity, might damage healthy cells as well as cancer cells everywhere in the body. This generalized influence on the whole body system might explain its severe impact. In many studies, fatigue has been demonstrated to be the most prevalent side effect in patients receiving chemotherapy (26,47–50).

Chemotherapy patients often relate fatigue directly to the treatment. Clinical experience shows that their fatigue is most prominent during the first days during and after treatment and that patients exhibit increased energy before the next therapy cycle. Intensity and duration are perceived differently by individuals and might be correlated with regimen and type of drugs. Richardson (51) investigated the onset, pattern, duration, intensity, and distress associated with fatigue in chemotherapy patients. Data indicated that, although fatigue may be essentially similar among groups receiving different chemotherapy regimens, there is a significant individual variation in its severity and the amount of associated distress. An increase of distress has been noted with progression of therapy in patients with ovarian cancer (52). It can be expected that intensity of treatment has an influence on fatigue levels. Hann and Jacobsen (53) investigated fatigue in 43 women with breast cancer undergoing autologous bone marrow transplantation. They concluded that these women experienced considerable fatigue, which interfered with functioning and quality of life. A study investigating fatigue in 715 women with localized breast cancers showed that fatigue scores were highest among those receiving a combination of radiotherapy and chemotherapy (54). However, methodological aspects of measurement, such as timing or the choice of the measurement instrument, are potential biases, especially in chemotherapy patients, making it difficult to compare results between studies.

A variety of other influences need to be analyzed in patients with chemotherapy. Other side effects of treatment, such as nausea, emesis, decrease of nutritional intake, and unusual anemia could be linked with higher fatigue levels.

Antiemetic drugs, especially sedating substances, are expected to increase fatigue.

D. Biotherapy-Induced Fatigue

In addition to the potential mechanisms for treatment-related fatigue as described earlier, biotherapy exposes patients to exogen and endogen cytokines. Interferons, interleukin-2, tumor necrosis factors, and colony-stimulating factors are the most often used substances in cancer treatment. Biotherapy-related fatigue usually presents itself as part of a syndrome, the so-called flu-like syndrome, including fatigue, fever, chills, myalgias, headache, and malaise (55). Fatigue has been seen as a dose-limiting factor of treatment with biotherapy (24). Cognitive deficits, such as the expression of mental fatigue, have been associated with biotherapy side effects. In a study of 10 interferon-treated cancer patients, neuropsychiatric investigations revealed a lack of energy and reduced motivation to initiate activities. The cognitive and affective impairment observed was similar to the symptoms found in patients with pathological processes in the frontal lobe (56) and, therefore, it was concluded that patients with interferon therapy had experienced toxicity of the frontal lobe. The central mechanisms are thought to hold the possible key to explain fatigue in biotherapy patients. The central mechanisms may include impaired spinal cord transmission, or recruitment of motor neurons (24) or ''an exhaustion or malfunctioning of brain cells in the hypothalamic region'' (57).

E. Fatigue After Surgery

The problem of postoperative fatigue is not well understood. Clinical experience shows that it improves with time. It is unclear whether it is a consequence of tissue damage and healing, or whether it results from deconditioning because of immobility. Postoperative pain medication and nutritional demands may play a role. Depending on the type of surgery, the patient is confronted with changes of body image and function and needs energy to adapt to new conditions. If surgery leads to the identification of a diagnosis of cancer, psychological distress, such as anxiety and depression, might lead to a fatigued condition (58).

V. THE INTERRELATIONSHIP BETWEEN FATIGUE AND COPING

Social and psychological adaptation to disease and treatment demands are thought to have a major influence in patients confronted with cancer. Coping with cancer means dealing with a reality that healthy persons usually repress, and fragility of life cannot be denied anymore. The existential outlook of a person affected with a potentially mortal disease may need withdrawal, enabling him or her to cope with the circumstances, and fatigue may be a coping mechanism, expressed as feelings of depression. There is little scientific evidence to support the hypothesis, but it is generally accepted that depressed persons report chronic fatigue. Greenberg (19) noted that 90% of patients with depression report decreased energy and that fatigue remains a criterion of the diagnosis of clinical depression. Weisman (59) described various meanings of ''I feel very tired all the time'' and notes that long, drawn-out fatigue is both a cause and a symptom of emotional distress.

It seems important to distinguish between depression and fatigue, because different treatment approaches might be needed. It is difficult to rely on the results of existing studies because different measurement instruments have been used in different populations, resulting in both positive (20,50,60) and negative correlations (15,61). It can be argued that feeling sad and depressed is a reaction to the whole life-threatening situation of a cancer patient and that tiredness results from the body's attempt to deal with disease, treatment, and its consequences rather than as an expression of fatigue itself. In this sense, tiredness could be seen as a symptom of coping and depression. On the other hand, there is evidence for physical causes of tiredness in cancer patients, as described earlier. It can be hypothesized that these two potential sources of tiredness should be seen as a differential diagnosis, needing careful assessment and different treatment approaches. Consideration of the patient history, such as psychological difficulties in the past, social vulnerability, such as social isolation and lack of a supporting network, as well as disease-specific influences, such as brain tumor lesions or metabolic disorders, seem crucial in diagnosing causes of tiredness. Interesting results have recently been published by Visser and Smets (62) who investigated 250 patients with cancer undergoing radiotherapy (longitudinal). They concluded that fatigue and depression do not follow the same course over time and there was no strong evidence for a cause-and-effect relationship between depression and fatigue. Another study, however, showed a very strong correlation between advanced stages of cancer (correlated with highest fatigue levels) and high levels of depression (31).

Relief of anxiety might result in a depressive state or a failure to resolve causes of the anxious state might lead to exhaustion. Clinical experience shows that cancer disease and its treatment can be sources of intensive anxiety over long periods of time. An interesting observation described by Simms and Rhodes (63) was the finding that inclusion of lorazepam, an anxiolytic medication, into an antiemetic treatment for the prevention of chemotherapy-induced nausea and emesis reduced levels of post-therapy tiredness. It points to anxiety as a possible cause in the development of tiredness and fatigue.

VI. METHODOLOGICAL ASPECTS OF FATIGUE MEASUREMENT

Recent key publications concerning fatigue measurement have made it easier to capture current knowledge (12,31,64). Selection of a measurement instrument heavily depends on the purpose of measurement and on the population concerned. Validity, reliability, and easy and short use are requested for this vulnerable population. If fatigue/tiredness is assessed as one of several quality of life aspects or as a symptom among others, a quality of life questionnaire or symptom distress scale is applicable. In many of these instruments, tiredness/fatigue is mainly addressed as a consequence of fatigue (65–67). If it is the aim to measure the actual experience of fatigue for epidemiological purposes, specific fatigue measurement instruments are needed.

A fatigue subscale was developed for the Functional Assessment of Cancer Therapy Scale (FACT-Fg), which was derived from the FACT Anemia scale (FACT-An) (68). If fatigue is to be measured within the context of quality of life, this tool might be useful. It has to be confirmed, however, whether anemia-associated fatigue is the same experience as fatigue in cancer patients generally. Experience shows that fatigue in cancer patients can but does not necessarily need to be associated with anemia.

The subscale on vigor/fatigue of the Profile of Mood States (69) has been used frequently and proved to be useful in fatigue measurement in cancer patients. Items of this scale, however, are derived from sources other than from cancer patients' experience. Items concerning physical expression of tiredness are scarce and therefore this subscale does not apply in the measurement of multidimensional fatigue.

Many of the symptom distress scales include tiredness as a single item question. This restricted approach measures one dimension of a variety of symptom distress. A defined visual analogue scale with a definition of a reliable, cancer-specific fatigue continuum is needed to quantify the construct and its distress. Most symptom distress scales address fatigue without a cancer-specific continuum. In past research, fatigue was measured with performance indexes, which is difficult because they do not measure tiredness directly but are rather indicators of general well-being and activity status.

General fatigue measurement tools, such as the Pearson-Byars Fatigue Checklist for the measurement of tiredness in airmen (70) or the Yoshitake Fatigue Symptom Checklist for the measurement of tiredness in Japanese industrial populations (71), have been used in many fatigue studies in cancer patients. However, they have been developed for specific purposes and, therefore, their underlying theoretical framework differs. Fatigue research in industrial workers is based on the concept of physiology and needs different phraseology to capture the impact of tiredness on productivity or effectivity. Fatigue in cancer has a different nature, source, and impact: cancer patients might not feel ''refreshed, peppy or full of energy'' in the morning, in contrast to active airmen, who are supposed to feel so after a period of rest (70). Qualitative research has shown that fatigue in cancer patients includes at least partially different themes than those reflected in the items of these general fatigue measurement instruments for healthy populations (27).

Some instruments measure fatigue in cancer patients specifically. The Piper Fatigue Scale, the most often used modern fatigue measurement tool developed for cancer patients specifically, grounded in a multidimensional framework, measures fatigue from different viewpoints with an emphasis on consequences of fatigue (20). It measures subjective fatigue within the temporal, affective, sensory, and severity dimensions. This instrument in American English language might be helpful in assessing consequences of fatigue on activities of daily living and for individual care planning or for developing individual coping strategies. Description of fatigue and potential responses to fatigue, including impact on daily living, are addressed. The instrument has been used in a growing number of studies. It is currently being reduced from 41 items to a 20-item questionnaire and has undergone validity and reliability tests (30).

A recently developed fatigue measurement instrument, developed in Dutch and translated into English, is the Multidimensional Fatigue Inventory (MFI) (72). The 20-item self-report instrument covers five dimensions of fatigue: general fatigue, physical fatigue, mental fatigue, reduced motivation, and reduced activity. These dimensions have been supported by confirmatory factor analyses and its psychometric properties have been tested in cancer patients receiving radiotherapy as well as in noncancer populations. The reduction of scales was recently discussed.

Concurrently with the MFI 20, the Fatigue Assessment Questionnaire (FAQ) has been developed in the German language (31). It is based on qualitative research, in which fatigue in cancer patients was identified as a phenomenon that is expressed at physical, affective, and cognitive levels. A theoretical model of nociception, perception, and manifestation of fatigue in cancer patients was generated, in accordance to a model developed for pain (Table 1) (73). Consecutive research with quantitative methodology confirmed the qualitative foundation. The physical, affective, and cognitive dimensions have been supported through confirmatory factor analyses. The scale can be used to calculate the three subscale scores and a total fatigue score. It has been constructed with the aim of being easy and short for the use in a fatigued population. It is made up of 20 items (11 physical, three cognitive, five affective, and one single item) and, especially for epidemiological research, was first constructed with simple yes and no answers. In the course of its development, a version with four categorical answers was constructed to be able to measure levels of fatigue over time. Measurement concerns the time period of 1 week. Apart from the physical, affective, and cognitive

Table 1 Production, Expression, and Measurement of Fatigue in Cancer Patients

Step	Conditioning factors			
Nociception	Specificity			
	Cancer type and stage-associated cytokine production (e.g., interferon, interleukine, TNF)			
	Immunological defense against the tumor, paraneoplastic syndromes			
	Treatment (toxicity, waste products, cell death, healing)			
	Other symptoms (e.g., nausea, emesis, pain, immobility, primary fatigue)			
↓	Energy transformation changes (e.g., muscle loss, increased expenditure, anorexia, nutritional deficits)			
	Cancer-associated, organ-specific impairment			
	Circulatory adaptation failure (e.g., decreased oxygen-carrying capacity)			
	Metabolic disorders (e.g., hypercalcemia, hyponatremia)			
	Endocrine disorders (e.g., hypoadrenocorticism, hypothyroidism)			
	Coping (depression, anxiety)			
Perception	Decreasing inhibitory pathways, threshold			
↓	Affective state, social and psychological support, beliefs, personality, general well-being			
Expression	Manifestation of fatigue at			
		physical	affective	cognitive level
↓		↓	↓	↓
↑		↑	↑	↑
Measurement	Of fatigue at	physical	affective	cognitive level

dimensions, fatigue quantity and fatigue distress are measured with linear analogue scales to include the quantity and severity dimension. It measures the direct experience of fatigue and thus is suitable to measure fatigue in the context of epidemiological fatigue research or to measure effectiveness of therapeutic strategies. Studies have supported its reliability and validity (31).

VII. SUPPORTIVE CARE STRATEGIES TO ALLEVIATE FATIGUE DISTRESS

A. Fatigue Awareness of Caregivers

Physicians and nurses have only recently become aware of the fact that fatigue in cancer patients has a high prevalence and that it presents one of the most distressing symptoms. Cancer patients might feel that fatigue is an inevitable companion. It can be suggested that a rather nihilistic attitude of caregivers amplifies these feelings. Fatigue awareness of physicians, nurses and relatives can help patients feel better understood and to be allowed to speak about the experienced distress. Fatigue awareness is the first step for the assessment of fatigue. Assessment might mean simply asking "How do you feel?" It means listening to the aspect of fatigue or using a specific fatigue measurement tool for a specific purpose.

B. Support Through Information About Fatigue

Once patients and caregivers speak about the fatigue experience, information about its causes and possible intervention strategies can be exchanged. Patients often feel anxious about their fatigue. Knowledge might prevent feelings of anxiety. Clinical experience shows that patients and relatives feel relieved if they learn that fatigue normally occurs in a given situation and that there is a causal relationship between fatigue and the disease or the treatment. The information can also prevent misinterpretations of the patient's behavior or health state. A special role is given to information when patients receive cancer treatment. Evidence of probable patterns of fatigue is being accumulated and it is crucial to prepare patients for the treatment. Information might help them to anticipate the distress and enable them to use coping strategies, such as decreasing nonessential activities and accepting help to do housework. Adaptation of the working schedule might be considered. Some patients may prefer to interrupt work for certain periods or to reduce it. If therapy is as an extra time-consuming factor, apart from usual work, it could be hypothesized that fatigue will be an outcome of overexertion.

C. Differences of Interventional Strategies Between Patients with Early Disease and Treatment and Patients with Progressing, Advanced Disease

Research has shown that patients with advanced disease experience the highest fatigue levels (11,31). The causes of fatigue in these patients can be expected to be different than in patients with an adjuvant treatment. If fatigue is seen as an inevitable outcome of advanced disease (cytokine-producing tumor bulk), interventional strategies are geared toward "learning to live with the restricted energy account." This can mean learning to accept frequent rest periods. It also means identifying fatigue-promoting activities and learning how to modify or eliminate them. Setting realistic goals not only means adapting to limited energy resources but also learning to cope with progression of disease.

Even though high fatigue levels are often correlated with advanced disease, another vulnerable population has been described recently. Patients with early breast cancer receiving adjuvant chemotherapy (54) or adjuvant radiotherapy (74) indicated having high fatigue levels. As described earlier, the causes of fatigue in these patients might be related to the treatment rather than to the disease (no cytokine-producing tumor bulk). Even though these patients also need fatigue awareness, assessment, and information, and they should be prepared to anticipate a period with possible fatigue distress, the interventional strategies might be different than for patients in palliative situations. Berger (75) documented significantly different activity levels over time in women with breast cancer receiving chemotherapy, with scores being higher at treatments and lower at cycle midpoints. She concluded that patients can be informed that these patterns may be expected to be similar during the first three chemotherapy cycles (75).

D. The Rest–Activity Balance: The Role of Physical Exercise

Activity reduction is commonly recommended in patients to reduce fatigue. However, there is little supporting evidence, and Corcoran (76) even suggested that inactivity may promote fatigue. This idea was supported in a study that identified the correlation between fatigue and stages of cancer: it was hypothesised that fatigue leads to unusual need for rest, which in turn leads to inactivity, weakness, and reduced physical performance, resulting in a lack of energizing metabolic resources (31). This ''vicious circle phenomenon'' needs further testing. Graydon analyzed the strategies used by women receiving chemotherapy or radiotherapy that were perceived as most helpful and concluded that the most effective strategy was ''sleeping;'' however, ''exercise,'' ''doing something different,'' and ''talking to friends'' were also effective strategies (77). In a program using aerobic training in patients undergoing chemotherapy, Mac Vicar and Winningham documented decreased perception of fatigue (78). A further study tested a self-paced, home-based walking exercise program in patients on radiotherapy. The program was significantly effective for physical functioning and symptom intensity, particularly fatigue, anxiety, and difficulty sleeping (74). These interesting strategies need to be considered individually and especially in light of disease stage. Whereas frequent naps might be more beneficial than physical exercise in patients with advanced disease, physical exercise might be recommended in early disease and especially during chemotherapy or radiotherapy. These patients can be encouraged to maintain activity levels balanced with efficient rest periods.

E. Nutrition, Fluid Intake, Vitamins—Suggestions

No evidence has been provided that nutrition influences fatigue levels, apart from the generally accepted fact that fatigue might increase after a meal. Because nutrition plays an important role concerning well-being, it can be suggested to be helpful if meals are frequent, small, and carefully prepared. It has been recommended to encourage patients to increase fluid intake, but there is little knowledge to underpin this suggestion. It at least can be suggested that dehydration impairs well-being and that a higher fluid intake can support the elimination of waste products in the course of a treatment. During cancer therapy and in the course of disease, there might be an increased demand and a reduced intake concerning vitamins; therefore, supplements might improve well-being. Even though there is no substantiating research evidence, clinical experience shows that patients appreciate such supportive care strategies.

F. Medical, Pharmacological, and Psychological Support to Combat Fatigue

The most effective medical intervention against fatigue is the effective treatment of cancer. However, on the way to cure, during the treatment period, and in the palliative phase, some other aspects can be considered helpful. Although it is still difficult to influence cytokine-induced fatigue, treatment of electrolyte imbalance or anemia is possible and seems essential. Good medical care, such as the treatment of cardiac insufficiency, is required. Diagnosis and treatment of hypercalcemia may present a most effective intervention. Treatment of other symptoms, such as nausea and emesis or pain, may be crucial. Accumulation of pharmacological substances, thus intoxication, in patients with hepatic or renal insufficiency must be considered, especially in relation to psychoactive drugs and pain medication.

Some pharmacological treatments have been proposed to treat fatigue in patients with cancer. Corticosteroids are said to have significant effects on overall well-being (79) and therefore are frequently used in low doses to support fatigued, cachectic patients, however, with little research evidence. In a study carried out by Bruera, it was found that patients with cachexia who were receiving megestrol acetate experienced significantly more appetite and less fatigue than the patients without that treatment (80). Substances, described to reduce circulating cytokines, such as thalidomide, melatonin, or clenbuterol (79), could be of interest in future fatigue research. Psychostimulants, such as amphetamines, are proposed, however with little research evidence. The same is the case with the use of antidepressants or anxiolytic substances.

Growing evidence suggests that fatigue is not only a physical but also an emotional and cognitive phenomenon (31,72). Interventional strategies must therefore consider these dimensions. Correlation of fatigue with depression has been documented and it can be suggested that coping with life-threatening disease is associated with fatigue. As a consequence, psychological and social support for cancer patients can be seen as effective intervention, be it through individual psychotherapy, psychological support groups, art therapy, relaxation, recreational activities, distraction, or spiritual support.

REFERENCES

1. Duden. Wörterbuch Medizinischer Fachausdrücke. Stuttgart: Thieme, 1985.
2. Reuter P, Reuter C. Thieme Leximed: Medical Dictionary. Stuttgart: Thieme, 1995.
3. Stedman's Medical Dictionary. 22d ed. Baltimore: Williams & Wilkins, 1973.
4. Berrios G. Feelings of fatigue and psychopathology: a conceptual history. Comprehensive Psychiatry 1990; 31:140–151.
5. Grandjean E. Fatigue: Its physiological and psychological significance. Ergonomics 1968; 11:427–436.
6. Bartley S. The human organism as a person. Philadelphia: Chilton, 1967.
7. Nixon P. The human function curve. Practitioner 1976; 217:765–770.
8. Chen M. The epidemiology of self-perceived fatigue among adults. Prev Med 1986; 15:74–81.
9. David A, Pelosi E. Tired, weak, or in need of rest: fatigue among general practice attenders. BMJ 1990; 301:1199–1202.
10. Irvine D, Vincent L, Graydon J. The prevalence and correlates of fatigue in patients receiving treatment with chemotherapy and radiotherapy. Cancer Nursing 1994; 17: 367–378.
11. Pater J, Zee B, Palmer M, Johnston D, Osoba D. Fatigue in patients with cancer: results with National Cancer Institute of Canada Clinical Trials. Group studies employing the EORTC QLQ-C30. Support Care Cancer 1997; 5:410–413.
12. Glaus A. Assessment of fatigue in cancer- and non-cancer patients and in healthy individuals. Support Care Cancer 1993; 1:305–315.
13. Morris M. Tiredness and fatigue. In: Norris C. Concept Clarification in Nursing. Rockville, MD: Aspen Publishers, 1982:263–275.
14. Appels A, Mulder P. Excess fatigue as a precursor of myocardial infarction. Eur Heart J 1988; 9:758–764.
15. Srivastra R. Fatigue in end stage renal disease patients. In: Funk S, Tornquist E. Key Aspects of Comfort. New York: Springer Publishers, 1989:217–233.
16. Krupp L, Alvarez L. Fatigue in multiple sclerosis. Arch Neurol 1988; 45:435–437.
17. Crosby L. Factors which contribute to fatigue associated with rheumatoid arthritis. J Adv Nursing 1991; 16:974–981.
18. Kristoffersson A, Boströn A. Muscle strength is improved after parathyroidectomy in patients with primary hyperparathyroidism. Br J Surg 1992; 79:1165–1168.
19. Greenberg D. Neurasthenia in the 1980's: chronic mononucleosis, chronic fatigue syndrome, and anxiety and depressive disorders. Psychosomatics 1990; 31(2):129–137.
20. Piper B, Lindsey A. Development of an instrument to measure the subjective dimension of fatigue. In: Funk S, Tornquist E. Key Aspects of Comfort. New York: Springer Publishers, 1989:199–208.

21. World Health Organization. Cancer Pain Relief and Palliative Care. Technical Report Series 804. Geneva: Author, 1990.
22. Winningham M, Nail L, et al. Fatigue and the cancer experience: the state of the knowledge. Oncol Nurs Forum 1994; 21:23–36.
23. Irvine D, Vincent L. A critical appraisal of the research literature investigating fatigue in the individual with cancer. Cancer Nursing 1991; 14:188–199.
24. Piper B, Rieger P. Recent advances in the management of biotherapy-related side effects: fatigue. Oncol Nurs Forum 1989; 16(suppl 6):27–34.
25. Donelli S, Walsh D. The symptoms of advanced cancer. Semin Oncol 1995; 22(suppl 3):67–72.
26. Rhodes V, Watson P. Patients' descriptions of the influence of tiredness and weakness on self-care abilities. Cancer Nursing 1988; 11:186–194.
27. Glaus A. A qualitative study to explore the concept of fatigue/tiredness in cancer patients and in healthy individuals. Support Care Cancer 1996; 4:82–96.
28. Richardson A, Ream E, Wilson-Barnett J. Fatigue in patients receiving chemotherapy: patterns of change. Cancer Nursing 1998; 21:17–30.
29. Piper B, Lindsey A, et al. Fatigue mechanisms in cancer patients: developing nursing theory. Oncol Nurs Forum 1987; 14:17–23.
30. Piper B, Dipple S. The revised Piper Fatigue Scale: confirmation of its multidimensionality and reduction in number of items in women with breast cancer (abstr). Oncol Nurs Forum 1996; 23:352.
31. Glaus A. Fatigue in patients with cancer-analysis and assessment. Recent Results Cancer Res 145. Heidelberg, Springer.
32. Theologides A. Anorexins, asthenins and cachectins in cancer. Am J Med 1986; 81: 296–298.
33. Bruera E. Asthenia in patients with advanced cancer. J Pain Symptom Manage 1988; 4:9–14.
34. Bruera E, Brenneis C. Muscle electrophysiology in patients with advanced breast cancer. J Nat Cancer Inst 1988; 4:282–285.
35. Stiefel F, Morant R. Asthenie bei Tumorkranken. Deutsche Medizinische Wochenschrift 1992; 117:107–111.
36. St. Pierre B, Kaspar C. Fatigue mechanisms in patients with cancer: effects of tumour necrosis factor and exercise on skeletal muscle. Oncol Nurs Forum 1992; 19:419–425.
37. Morant R. Asthenia in cancer patients—a double-edged inflammatory response against the tumor? J Palliat Care 1991; 7(3):22–24.
38. Denz H, Orth B. Weight loss in patients with haematological neoplasias is associated with immune system stimulation. Clin Invest 1993; 71:37–41.
39. Beutler B, Cerami A. Cachectin: more than a tumour necrosis factor. N Engl J Med 1987; 316:379–385.
40. Naylor M, Malik S. In situ detection of tumour necrosis factor in human ovarian cancer specimens. Eur J Cancer 1990; 26:1027–1030.
41. Senn HJ, et al., ed. Checkliste Onkologie. 4. Auflage. Stuttgart: Thieme 1997: 271.
42. Keller U. Pathophysiology of cancer cachexia. Support Care Cancer 1993; 1:290–294.

43. Haylock P, Hart L. Fatigue in patients receiving localized radiation. Cancer Nursing 1979; 2:461–467.
44. Kobashi J, Hanewald G, Van Dam F. Assessment of malaise in cancer patients treated with radiotherapy. Cancer Nursing 1985; 8:306–313.
45. King K, Nail L. Patients' descriptions of the experience of receiving radiation therapy. Oncol Nurs Forum 1985; 12:55–61.
46. Nail L, Winningham M. Fatigue. In: Groenwald S, Frogge M. Cancer Nursing: Principles and Practice. 3d ed. Boston: Jones and Bartlett 1993:608–619.
47. Knoff M. Physical and psychological distress associated with adjuvant chemotherapy in women with breast cancer. J Clin Oncol 1986; 4:678–684.
48. Nerenz DR, Leventhal H. Factors contributing to emotional distress during cancer chemotherapy. Cancer 1982; 50:1020–1027.
49. Meyerowitz B, Watkins I. Quality of life for breast cancer patients receiving adjuvant chemotherapy. Am J Nurs 1983; 83:232–235.
50. Blesch K, Paice J. Correlates of fatigue in people with breast or lung cancer. Oncol Nurs Forum 1991; 18:81–87.
51. Richardson A. The experience of fatigue and other symptoms in patients receiving chemotherapy. Eur J Cancer Care 1996; 5(suppl 2):24–30.
52. Love R, Leventhal H. Side effects and emotional distress during cancer chemotherapy. Cancer 1989; 63:604–612.
53. Hann D, Jacobsen P. Fatigue in women treated with bone marrow transplantation for breast cancer: a comparison with women with no history of cancer. Support Care Cancer 1997; 5:44–52.
54. Woo B, Dipple L. Variations in fatigue scores by treatment methods in women with breast cancer (abstr 182). Annual Meeting Oncology Nursing Society (ONS), Philadelphia, 1996.
55. Haeuber D. Recent advances in the management of biotherapy-related side effects: flu-like syndrome. Oncol Nurs Forum 1989; 16(suppl 6):35–41.
56. Adams F, Queseda J. Neuropsychiatric manifestations of human leucocyte interferon therapy in patients with cancer. JAMA 1984; 252:938–941.
57. Poteliakhoff A. Adrenocortical activity and some clinical findings in acute and chronic fatigue. J Psychosom Res 1981; 25:91–95.
58. Christensen T, Hjortso N. Fatigue and anxiety in surgical patients. Acta Psychiatr Scand 1986; 73:76–79.
59. Weisman A. Coping with cancer. New York: McGraw Hill, 1979.
60. Bruera E, Brenneis C. Association between asthenia and nutritional status, lean body mass, anemia, psychological status and tumor mass in patients with advanced breast cancer. J Pain Symptom Manage 1989; 4:59–63.
61. Pickard-Holley S. Fatigue in cancer patients. Cancer Nursing 1991; 14:13–19.
62. Visser M, Smets E. Fatigue, depression and quality of life in cancer patients: how are they related? Support Care Cancer 1998; 6:101–108.
63. Simms S, Rhodes V. Comparison of prochlorperazine and lorazepam antiemetic regimens in the control of postchemotherapy symptoms. Nursing Res 1993; 42:234–239.
64. Richardson A. Measuring fatigue in patients with cancer. Support Care Cancer 1998; 6:94–100.

65. Padilla G, Presant C. Quality of life index for patients with cancer. Res Nurs Health 1983; 6:117–126.
66. Schipper H, Clinch J. Measuring the quality of life of cancer patients: The Functional Living Index—Cancer: development and validation. J Clin Oncol 1984; 2:123–136.
67. Aaronson K, Ahmedzai S. The European Organization for Research and Treatment of Cancer QLQ-C30: a quality of life instrument for use in international clinical trials in oncology. J Natl Cancer Inst 1993; 85:365–376.
68. Yellen S, Cella D. Measuring fatigue and other anemia-related symptoms with the Functional Assessment of Cancer Therapy (FACT) measuring system. J Pain Symptom Manage. In press.
69. McNair D, Lorr M. EITS Manual for the Profile of Mood States. San Diego, CA: Educational and Industrial Testing Service, 1971.
70. Pearson P, Byars G. The Development and Validation of a Checklist Measuring Subjective Fatigue (Report No. 56-115). Randolph Air Force Base, TX: School of Aviation, 1956.
71. Yoshitake H. Relations between the symptoms and feelings of fatigue. Ergonomics 1971; 14:175–186.
72. Smets E, Garssen B. Application of the multidimensional fatigue inventory (MFI-20) in cancer patients receiving radiotherapy. Br J Cancer, 1996; 73:241–245.
73. Bruera E. New developments in the assessment of pain in cancer patients. J Support Care Cancer 1994; 2:312–318.
74. Mock V, Hassey K, Candance J. Effects of exercise on fatigue, physical functioning, and emotional distress during radiation therapy for breast cancer. Oncol Nurs Forum 1997; 6:991–1000.
75. Berger A. Patterns of fatigue and activity and rest during adjuvant breast cancer chemotherapy. Oncol Nurs Forum 1998; 25(1):51–62.
76. Corcoran P. Use it or lose it—the hazards of bedrest and inactivity. West J Med 1991; 154:536–538.
77. Graydon G, Bubela N. Fatigue-reducing strategies used by patients receiving treatment for cancer. Cancer Nursing 1995; 18:23–28.
78. Mac Vicar MG, Winningham ML. Promoting the functional capacity of cancer patients. Cancer Bull 1986; 38:235–239.
79. Bruera E. Pharmacological treatment of cachexia: any progress? Support Care Cancer 1998; 6:109–113.
80. Bruera E, Ernst S. Symptomatic effects of megestrol acetate: a double-blind, crossover study. Proc Am Soc Clin Oncol 1996; 1716:531.

28

Care of the Patient Close to Death

J. Norelle Lickiss
University of Sydney and Royal Prince Alfred Hospital, Camperdown, New South Wales, Australia

I. INTRODUCTION

Death is a journey to be undertaken (1), eventually by all of us. For most patients with advanced cancer, except those few with curable (as distinct from controllable) disease, death is close.

How close is "close to death?" The situation of the actually dying patient (in the last days of life) may be the focus, or the focus may be on the patient for whom death is clearly on the horizon.

The value and significance of the last phase of life need to be appreciated by all concerned in care. In the Eriksonian (still useful) framework for personal development, the challenge of the last phase of life is the achievement of a sense of wholeness (which he termed "integrity") rather than its contrary, despair (2). Part of the clinical task in relation to a patient in the final phase of life is the facilitation of the emergence of wholeness rather than despair: the implications of this view are considerable and practical.

II. THE PATIENT APPROACHING DEATH

A conceptual frame is essential for sound clinical practice. A human can be viewed (Fig. 1) as being situated within a complex current environment, which

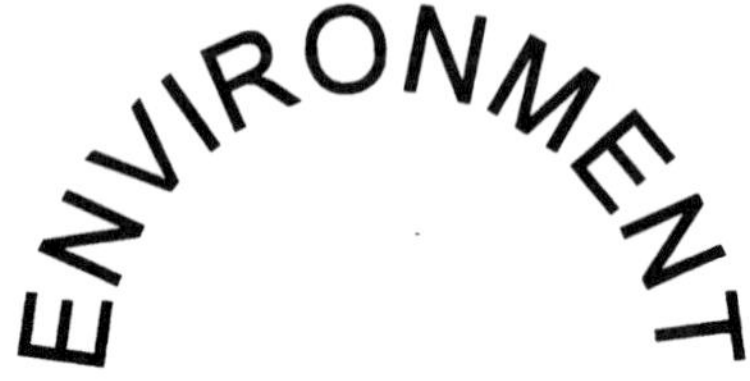

PERSON

H
I
S
T
O
R
Y

INHERITANCE

• BIOLOGICAL • CULTURAL

Figure 1 The human environment.

includes personal (significant others, caregivers) as well as nonpersonal (geographical factors, resources) elements. The person within this complex environment, with mutual interactions, cannot be adequately understood until personal history is also appreciated: for example, place of birth or experience of war, migration, disease, complications of treatment, or family violence. Furthermore, the person ''stands on'' his or her inheritance, both biological (including genetically influenced cancer) and cultural (including attitudes toward decision making, disclosure, disease, suffering, and death). The lineaments of this ecological perspective of the patient can be appreciated only if deliberately and sensitively sought for by appropriate means, usually a simple narrative approach rather than questionnaire, with the portrait becoming more clear over time.

A view of the patient from an ecological perspective is incomplete unless there is recognition of the way out of a possibly closed system, expressed in the dynamic of hope.

For what does this patient (and this patient's family) hope at this time, in this place, in these present circumstances? And, is this hope realistic in the face of the current medical reality and the resources that are realistically available? If so, then planning treatment and care must relate to the central hope of the patient (and not vitiate it, for example, by preventing a patient from attending a longed for family or religious celebration to undergo a marginally useful investigation or treatment modality). If the central hope is not realistic, then the clinician (usually the most senior) must assist the patient in restructuring hope so that it becomes centered on not what could not be achieved or could fail, but rather on what will never fail. It is crucial that a patient hoping for cure or even control of a disease process when, for example, first, second, or even third line therapy has failed (and chance of complete or partial remission for a few months is remote) should not be encouraged to have hope fixed on the outcome of chemotherapy, but rather on matters such as the unfailing love of a spouse (if this is unlikely to fail), the fidelity of the doctor, and ultimately the patient's value as a person. These matters have philosophical significance, requiring deep reflection, especially (although not only) in clinical trials, in which randomization may heighten expectation and focus hope on matters upon which hope should not rest.

The approach of death may be associated, for several reasons, with an increase in suffering. Because the relief of suffering is one of the goals of medicine, it is necessary for the issue of suffering to be respected and understood by any clinician involved in the treatment and care of very ill patients.

In his classic paper, Cassell (3) formulated an operational definition of suffering—a sense of impending personal disintegration. Theoretically, and in informal studies, it is clear that the triggers for such a sense, expressed in common parlance as ''feeling like going to pieces'' may include clinical activities such as having an investigation, experiencing pain, having bad news badly communicated, being in hospital, or being in danger of dying far from home.

Research, formal and informal, demonstrates abundantly that decisions regarding end of life are not taking these matters into account: there is obligation globally to do better with cancer pain relief and end of life decision making.

III. ASSESSMENT OF PATIENTS

Assessment of patients includes the achievement of the understanding of the patient's current personal situation, history, and inheritance in relation to the aforementioned ecological model and the clarification of the thrust of his or her hope. The narrative approach is a useful assessment tool (with therapeutic effects also, if skillfully undertaken). Thereafter, there is need for delineation of specific present needs, both of the patient and of the family and caregivers. These may include a need for symptom relief, emotional support, assistance with care, or more information. The profile of needs and the hierarchy of priorities need to be understood and are not predictable.

IV. SYMPTOM RELIEF

Symptom relief is extensively discussed elsewhere (4). Pain relief remains crucial and is extensively discussed in the literature. At least two-thirds of patients with cancer do experience some cancer-related pain, mostly as a result of the cancer itself, but sometimes pain is a legacy associated particularly with radical radiotherapy. Failures in cancer pain relief, the so-called barriers, are both attitudinal and clinical as well as being due to a lack of availability of essential drugs. The principles of pain relief in cancer have been enunciated in many reports. Assessment involves clarification of site, type, periodicity, and aggravating factors, and a simple scale of severity is useful. Monitoring must be meticulous. The three-step World Health Organization (WHO) ladder, which has transformed pain relief at a global level, wherever it is correctly applied, is familiar to many physicians. A more clinical approach may be useful for some oncologists. Cancer pain relief can be considered to have four steps, best undertaken intellectually in chronological order, even if all are covered in a short period of time.

A. Step 1

Clarify the cause of the pain anatomically and pathologically with careful history taking, careful physical examination, and sometimes precise investigations. Failure to clarify the local cause of the noxious stimulus is a common cause of poor pain relief. Treat the local cause wherever possible and as appropriate. Local measures include some surgical procedures, radiotherapy, antibiotics (if infection is obvious), immobilization (if there is a fracture), and drug therapy with an apparently local action such as nonsteroidal anti-inflammatory drugs (NSAIDs) and paracetamol.

B. Step 2

Raise the patient's pain threshold by all means possible, including diversion, anxiolytic or antidepressant therapy when anxiety or depression is pathological, and general supportive measures. Threshold issues become obvious as the patient's story is told—the narrative approach is therapeutic and assists in diagnosis, not only of the mechanism of the pain but also of the coping style and level of distress.

C. Step 3

Use opioid drugs precisely and appropriately. Codeine in combination with locally acting drugs such as aspirin or paracetamol may well be adequate in the general practice context, but laxatives should always be introduced in patients in whom codeine is to be used, unless the patient has intrinsic bowel disease causing diarrhea. Much misery is caused when patients get severe constipation and even fecal impaction when preparations combining paracetamol and codeine or other opioids are used without concomitant laxatives and adequate hydration. Impaction may be the cause of pelvic pain, diarrhea, ineffectiveness of oral opioids through apparent failure of absorption, or even confusion—preventable disasters.

Morphine is the gold standard of the strong opioids and it is essential that every physician in contact with patients with cancer should understand the principles of modern morphine therapy. There is no place for the attitude that morphine should be "saved up until later." It is the type of pain and the severity of pain which dictates whether morphine is appropriate, not the prognosis of the cancer patient. The use of morphine in patients with pain caused by processes other than cancer is not discussed here and, in general, is to be discouraged because of the problems associated with its use. Furthermore, morphine should be used precisely; the dose calibration is normally by the oral route, using 4-hourly morphine mixture initially to achieve levels of morphine that do not cause sedation.

Calibration should not usually be attempted using controlled released morphine preparations. Many problems are occurring through this practice, however convenient the shortcut appears to be. Controlled release preparations in particular should usually not be used in (1) patients with severe pain (sort out the 24-hour dose of morphine needed by immediate release preparations first, before converting to the controlled release preparation), (2) patients with nausea, vomiting, or constipation, (3) patients with huge intra-abdominal masses, and (4) patients prone to gastrointestinal (GIT) dysmotility or obstruction. Otherwise, and where correctly used, controlled release morphine preparations offer an opportunity for convenient and effective morphine therapy, involving twice daily or even once daily medication.

The dose of oral morphine necessary per day to ensure the optimal effect of morphine in a combined analgesic program (and morphine should rarely indeed ever be used alone) may vary from 20 mg per day to 200 or 500 mg per day. In general, in services with much experience with cancer pain relief, the majority of patients are on less than 200 mg of oral morphine per day as the morphine component of an analgesic program. If more than 200 mg appears to be needed, ideally the patient's case should be discussed with a palliative medicine consultant, in case there are other measures that should be considered. Patients in whom early tolerance to morphine has developed with rapid escalation of doses up to 300 to 400 mg per day do need to be reconsidered fairly urgently; otherwise, problems may be quite unmanageable later in the course of the disease.

Calibration of morphine doses may have to be done under some circumstances using parenteral morphine by the subcutaneous route (using a butterfly needle left in situ for 2 to 3 days). Intravenous (IV) and intramuscular (IM) morphine should rarely, if ever, be used in the management of cancer-related pain. The subcutaneous (SCI) route for morphine when this is needed parenterally is considerably preferable to the IM or IV route in view of simplicity and the advantage of more sustained blood levels. The SCI route offers also the possibility of using a syringe driver combining morphine with drugs other than morphine, normally under supervision of a palliative care service. Good palliative care may be given without syringe drivers, or IV infusions.

The oral to parenteral morphine ratio in patients stabilized on morphine therapy, in brief, is three to one. This implies that 10 mg morphine used parenterally 4 hourly is equivalent to approximately 30 mg of morphine orally 4 hourly in a patient who is already stabilized on morphine therapy. A patient who has been on morphine for some time at 30 mg oral morphine 4 hourly or 90 mg of controlled release morphine (e.g., MS Contin or Kapanol) bd would need to be converted to 10 mg of morphine SCI 4 hourly if for some reason the oral route became unavailable. Such a circumstance could include having to go for an operative procedure or intervention requiring fasting or the onset of severe nausea or vomiting.

It is important to stress that the 3-to-1 ratio (or 2½-to-1) prevails only to patients stabilized on morphine therapy. If morphine therapy is to be initiated, then the oral to parenteral ratio is closer to 6 to 1 because the patient lacks the advantages of steady-state morphine therapy, which may be due to the contribution made by morphine metabolites, to the analgesic effect.

Once morphine therapy is stable, then, in most patients, it is possible to give a double dose late at night, for example, at 10:00 PM, omit the 4 hourly dose due at the small hours in the morning and resume a normal dose at around 6:00 AM. This practice of loading the patient at night does relieve both the patient and carergivers greatly and should be the norm. When controlled release preparations are used in stable situations in suitable patients, there is no problem with regard to middle of the night dosing. However, in some circumstances, it is important to recognize that a breakthrough preparation, or rescue dose, should be available: The 4 hourly dose equivalent is administered in the form of immediate release morphine (i.e., morphine mixture or immediate release morphine tablets). It is not satisfactory to use controlled release morphine tablets as a breakthrough preparation because the effect is not realized for several hours and the cumulative effect of the slow release tablets can cause therapeutic chaos. Once morphine therapy is well established and patients have slowly progressive disease, there should be little variation in dose requirements unless the tumor itself changes fairly rapidly. One of the myths associated with morphine therapy is that tolerance invariably appears (i.e., that the same dose ceases to have effectiveness as time goes on). It has been repeatedly shown that patients may remain on a stable dose of morphine for long periods, with stepwise changes necessary only with stepwise increases in the noxious stimulus associated with the new manifestation of the tumor. Even in such circumstances, there always needs to be review as to whether any other treatment modality could be used to cope with the new complications associated with the tumor, such as a short course of palliative radiotherapy or a nerve-blocking procedure.

It is also not true that precise morphine therapy used along lines previously suggested leads to morphine addiction. The patient becomes physiologically dependent on morphine just as a patient with heart disease is physiologically dependent on cardiac failure drugs, and the withdrawal of essential drugs abruptly leads to serious consequences. A patient on morphine therapy for several months will certainly have withdrawal symptoms if sudden cessation of morphine occurs. There is no place for experimentation to see whether the patient is comfortable without morphine after a great deal of trouble has been undertaken to achieve a satisfactory, steady dose free of side effects. There is place for some maneuvering in experienced hands under some circumstances, and especially after radiotherapy has been introduced, to see whether a lower level of noxious stimulus has been achieved; one of the clues is drowsiness appearing in a patient previously not drowsy on morphine therapy.

Drowsiness in a patient on morphine therapy suggests one of several things:

1. The dose of morphine is too high and a reduction can be undertaken by, for example, 20% in the first instance to see whether this is the case.
2. The patient's renal function has become impaired by either dehydration, a renal tract obstruction, or some other insult to renal function such as renal tract infection.
3. Another cause of drowsiness has come on to the scene such as hypercalcemia or unwitting introduction of a sedative drug such as hypnotic or anxiolytic or other drugs capable of some sedation effect such as anticonvulsants or antidepressants.

In general, there is no benefit to the patient of having morphine levels in the range causing drowsiness. If an anxiolytic is needed, a direct anxiolytic drug is much preferable because the drug is being used for its central action not for toxic side effects. Morphine-induced drowsiness is a manifestation of a toxic effect of morphine, albeit traditionally well recognized. It is not always realized that, if morphine is used in excessive doses, the toxic effects can mitigate against human dignity. Myoclonic jerks can ensue as can encephalopathic features, none of which are welcome, especially when a patient is in the last days or even hours of life. Dehydration in the last days of life may increase the likelihood of morphine toxicity, and occasionally SCI hydration may be justified in a dying patient to improve quality of life (and of dying).

Pethidine or meperidine has virtually no place in cancer pain management, and a patient already on pethidine should be changed, with respect to the opioid component, to morphine (at approximately one-tenth of the dose of pethidine when converting to SCI morphine). Methadone does have a place; the drug is difficult to use well, especially in patients with very severe pain, but should not be forgotten. The problem is the long (and varying) half life—up to days—and the prolonged sedation: calibration of the drug is difficult in the elderly or over a long period of use. Oxycodone (equal to oral morphine in potency) is useful in some patients needing a strong opioid at relatively low dose. Rectal oxycodone (Proladone suppository) is useful as long as it is remembered that one 30-mg oxycodone suppository is equivalent to at least 10 mg oral morphine 4 hourly for two doses. Transdermal opioids, such as TTS Fentanyl, clearly have a place (if cost can be contained). Ketamine has a role also in cancer pain relief in some circumstances (5).

A clinical challenge is presented by the patient on locally acting drugs such as paracetamol or NSAIDs and morphine carefully calibrated up to the level of drowsiness and yet pain is not relieved. One of the causes of this combination is so-called morphine nonresponsive or morphine partially responsive pain. It is necessary to understand that opioid drugs (which alleviate pain by complex methods not wholly understood) do not appear to be very effective in relieving pain caused by certain mechanisms. These include (1) pain of muscle spasm such as may occur with metastases in the spine, associated with palpable paravertebral spasm; (2) pain of existential anguish, in which other means are needed to assist in the distress of a fellow human being, and (3) pain of nerve irritation or nerve injury—neuropathic pain.

D. Step 4

The diagnosis and treatment of neuropathic pain is the fourth step in the schema of pain relief. Physicians are familiar with pain associated with herpes zoster, which may include both local nociceptive elements (associated with blisters, for example) and lancinating neuropathic pain. The latter pain does not respond well to codeine, oxycodone, morphine, and so on, but may be alleviated by the use of anticonvulsants or some antidepressants.

In general, cancer-related neuropathic pain requires close scrutiny. The diagnosis of the problem is not difficult. Careful questioning and examination of the patient with regard to the primary site of the pain, the qualities of the pain, the pattern of radiation of the pain, and the change in the pain over time, usually all indicate clearly that a nerve root or a plexus is involved and often the anatomical pattern is discernible with great precision.

Neuropathic pain is not wholly morphine resistant. Morphine, when used precisely, has far fewer side effects than drugs such as antidepressants, anticonvulsants, and corticosteroids. Morphine therapy should be exploited before these other drugs are instituted in most cases.

The use of steroids in the care of patients with advanced cancer is difficult and controversial. The institution of corticosteroids, such as dexamethasone, when other measures are readily available is not to be encouraged, because corticosteroid therapy, especially when long continued, has side effects that can mitigate against the quality of life for patients. If corticosteroid therapy is used to the level at which cushingoid features appear, then distressing body image changes may reduce quality of life. Furthermore, steroid therapy can aggravate infection, diabetes, and possibly even more importantly can induce emotional changes that are either out of character with the previous personality or somehow dissonant in the face of the whole context. Rarely, serious emotional consequences develop such as extremely discordant and inappropriate euphoria or depression.

Steroid therapy in the palliative care context should be precise, targeted, evaluated, and discontinued if not proving effective. With these provisos, corticosteroid therapy may be valuable in treating neuropathic pain, used at the lowest dose necessary to achieve effect (e.g., dexamethasone 4 mg each morning for a few days, then a decrease in dose 2 mg daily or even every second day). The trusted and tried tricyclic drugs are still useful for alleviating some forms of neuropathic pain. Initially, tricyclic antidepressants such as amitriptyline or imipramine are best used at low dose to check tolerance, but up to 50 to 75 mg a day (at night) or more are used if some benefit is being achieved. Newer antidepressants have a role that is steadily being clarified. Anticonvulsants most commonly used include carbamazepine or a sodium valproate, but both drugs may have unfortunate side effects in the form of skin rashes, GIT intolerance, drowsiness, or even confusion, and normally specialist advice should be sought before such therapy is instituted in cancer-related pain.

Pain therapy, like diabetes therapy, requires continuous vigilance and evaluation. Pain relief is achievable most of the time in most of the patients with cancer by careful use of the aforementioned measures, sometimes with assistance of a palliative medicine or pain consultant, especially when neuropathic pain is problematic or when oral therapy cannot be used. It must be recognized, however, that in a very small minority of patients some problems do arise and, even more rarely, in possibly 1% of patients at some stage in the course of the cancer, the pain may be refractory to the measures outlined earlier. It is necessary to get assistance from doctors experienced in cancer pain management and palliative care under such circumstances.

No patient should die in pain. In the rare situations when pain is proving intractable, there is a case for ensuring that a patient at least sleeps peacefully during the last few days or hours of life, if that is preferred. Morphine, in doses above that used as analgesic therapy, is not the drug to use in such circumstances, because toxic side effects are unfortunate and do not add to the dignity of human life or human dying. If direct sedation is needed, it is more appropriate to use a drug such as midazolam, normally in a syringe driver in doses up to 50 or even 100 mg per day, or clonazepam 1 to 2 mg SCI 12 hourly. Under such circumstances, patients should usually be able to wake to know loved ones or staff and to communicate gently. The care of dying patients is discussed further later.

The fear of dying in pain should be removed from the list of fears that patients with cancer normally and understandably carry in their hearts. Other symptoms also require management, notably nausea, vomiting, constipation, and dyspnea. These are discussed extensively in relevant texts on palliative medicine (4).

1. Gastrointestinal Symptoms

In general, the cause of gastrointestinal symptoms dictates the therapy and the cause is elucidated by careful history taking, careful examination, and sometimes investigation. Nausea in a patient with cancer may have nothing to do with the cancer; it may be related to digoxin toxicity, to renal failure, to infection, to drugs being given for any of several reasons, or to hypercalcemia. Nausea caused by the cancer is liable to be related to mechanical factors associated with pressure on the stomach or small intestine, or to fecal loading (commonly ignored). The most common cause of nausea in patients with cancer or patients on morphine is, in fact, constipation. Morphine therapy otherwise is rarely, in practice, the cause of nausea—it may in theory, however, lead to central nausea (prevented by haloperidol 3 mg nocte) or gastric stasis (relieved by metoclopramide).

Nausea associated with delayed emptying of the stomach in general (e.g., because of pressure from a large liver) may respond to gastrokinetic drugs such as metoclopramide or cisapride, but if there is actual obstruction of the stomach or small intestine, then such gastrokinetic drugs make the situation worse. A judicious trial may be required for a day or two, with the gastrokinetic drug being withdrawn if it is manifestly worsening the situation. Nausea resulting from central causes may also occur in patients with cancer. Hepatic metastases may cause a central type of nausea as well as some squashing of the stomach, with the former being amenable to centrally acting drugs such as oral or SCI haloperidol, 1.5 mg bd, and prochlorperazine, 5 to 25 mg two or three times a day, either orally or rectally. Occasionally, patients with cerebral metastases have a vestibular form of nausea worsened markedly by movements of the head, and such patients may respond dramatically to small doses of antihistamines. When nausea is due to fecal loading, then alleviation of fecal loading, usually with the assistance of a competent palliative care trained nurse, is necessary. The constipation is better prevented than treated and the most common cause of constipation in patients with cancer is opioid therapy unaccompanied by laxative therapy. In such a case, the institution of laxative therapy together with enema may begin to restore normal colonic function, but it will take a week or two. In general, opioid therapy requires a combination of stimulant plus a softener, for example, combinations of coloxyl with senna.

Management of patients with symptoms associated with actual gastrointestinal obstruction requires specialist input, with the surgical option being clarified as soon as possible. In general, many symptoms need to be managed in such patients in addition to nausea or vomiting, and the problem profile is related intimately to the site of obstruction, the rate of progression, the association of other morbidity, and so on. When a decision is made for medical, not surgical, management, most patients with terminal gastrointestinal obstruction do not need nasogastric tubes or intravenous drips, as long as there is superb intensive palliative care available, including expert mouth care and occasionally judicious use of subcutaneous infusions. Dying can be peaceful and dignified as long as all the rules are followed. Occasionally, more expensive drugs such as octreotide, hyoscine hydrobromide infusions, and so on are necessary as adjuncts, normally within a specialized context, but not necessarily in the hospital.

2. *Dyspnea and Other Respiratory Symptoms*

Dyspnea has many causes and, as in the case of pain or gastrointestinal symptoms, the cause of dyspnea needs to be established by careful history taking, clinical examination, and occasionally radiological investigation. The dyspnea may not be directly due to the cancer but may in fact be due to cardiac failure and may be amenable to conventional therapy of cardiac failure. When dyspnea is due to massive pleural effusion, then tapping of the effusion and probably the early use of pleurodesis may be justified, unless the patient is in the last few weeks of life. Dyspnea caused by a blocking of a bronchus may be amenable to radiotherapy. Dyspnea caused by lymphangitis carcinomatosa should respond to a combination of careful morphine therapy plus judicious use of corticosteroid. When infection is aggravating dyspnea, then antibiotics may well be valuable as a symptomatic measure in the patient in the last week or two of life.

Morphine therapy used correctly for cancer pain management does not depress respiration. Morphine therapy used to control dyspnea is also not harmful to the patient, but it is important that the doses of morphine used be very small initially, approximately 2 mg oral morphine 4 hourly, with gradual increase in dosage; not much more benefit is achieved by increasing the dose to more than 20 mg oral morphine 4 hourly. It is commonly found that morphine mixture used intermittently is more effective than controlled release morphine in the relief of dyspnea. Subcutaneous morphine used with the usual oral to parenteral dose ratio is also valuable and sometimes irreplaceable in a patient in the last days of life. Initially, therapy can be guided by the respiratory rate if it is not possible to get clear answers from the patient whether the dyspnea is improving. A patient with labored breathing at a fast rate normally feels better if the respiratory rate is moved down toward more normal rates, and careful use of morphine therapy can achieve this. When patients are already on morphine therapy for pain relief, the dose of morphine needs to be increased by 20–30% to relieve dyspnea.

V. CARE OF THE PATIENT IN THE LAST DAYS OR HOURS OF LIFE

Once it is clear that the patient has only a few days (or even hours) to live, it is essential that all is gently focused on inducing comfort and calm. There are fundamental principles.

General nursing care, especially mouth care (mouth washes, ice to suck, and care of lips) is crucial. There is usually no need for IV fluid, nor for food and drink if the patient either refuses them or is too weak. In dry weather, SCI fluid may be of value, but if mouth care is meticulous, some dehydration will not cause discomfort.

Drugs that have been used for symptom relief in the preceding stages will still be needed in the patient close to death but the routes may need to be changed if the patient ceases to be able to take oral medication without undue effort or if nausea and vomiting have supervened. In such circumstances, the subcutaneous route becomes extremely important using a simple butterfly needle. Syringe drivers are not essential although they may be very helpful.

Drugs not relevant for symptom relief should be stopped. Care should be taken not to stop drugs controlling symptoms not due to cancer (e.g., cardiac failure).

If sedation is wished, needed, and justified to permit death to occur while the patient has been sleeping peacefully, then a direct sedative or hypnotic drug should be used, not morphine (which sedates only through toxic side effects). Midazolam given SCI at a dose of 2.5 to 15 mg usually induces sedation, but the half-life is brief and the drug needs repetition every 2 to 4 hours unless a syringe driver is used. Clonazepam 1 to 2 mg SCI bd induces sedation and can be given sublingually. There is still a place for rectal chlorpramazine in some patients in the last day or two of life, if the patient is not fecally impacted. The use of morphine as a sedative in place of more precise and appropriate drugs has unfortunate pharmacological side effects (including distressing myoclonus in some patients) that impair dignity and it carries a high cost to staff. Nurses (or physicians) involved in the administration of morphine used as sedative (especially if ever used to accelerate death) frequently have difficulty in accepting morphine used precisely for pain relief—for themselves or their families—for many years to come.

Every physician needs to know how to manage a terminal palliation crisis, for example, massive hemoptysis or hematemesis, massive pulmonary embolus (clearly terminal), or other such problems. It is essential to render the patient unaware by the most rapid available route, and doctors need to know the following options:

1. Midazolam: 5–20 mg IV or IM
2. Rectal diazepam: 20 mg PR (via a female catheter). Rapidly causes sedation and can be administered when IV access is difficult. (Do not use diazepam IM or SCI.)
3. Barbiturate: for example sodium phenobarbital SCI 200 mg stat

Once the emergency is over, assistance should be sought regarding further drug therapy.

In the climate created by the current euthanasia controversy, it is important to clarify for patients that carefully used sedation is not euthanasia. To help a patient die in his or her sleep by precise use of sedative drugs at normal doses is not causing death but permitting death from other causes to be peaceful. Distressed doctors also need this reassurance.

VI. SPIRITUAL CARE

Spiritual care is a subject requiring and receiving profound consideration. The following points are noteworthy:

1. Spiritual care is not necessarily or primarily related to religious belief, but it is concerned with issues of meaning of hope, of personal growth, of transcendence—of a move ultimately toward the other (however conceived). These matters are the stuff of profound (not ephemeral) aspects of psychology, philosophy, and religion.

2. Religion is of deep human significance, and physicians at the height of their careers are often surprised at the depth of adherence of patients to religious traditions and practices that appear to have little influence or mention on the surface of their lives. Clinicians need to have respect for and some knowledge of the diversity of religious approaches to the great questions and of practices related to these traditions in the context of serious illness, dying, and death.

VII. THE EVALUATION OF CARE

Outcomes of care of patients close to death are difficult because the key witness and evaluator, after the process is complete, is unavailable. Furthermore, the process of care is complex, and after the event of death, grieving considerably distorts perception.

A simple approach was developed in Central Sydney (6) based on the identification of bad outcomes, defining circumstances of which clinical staff can be aware, and, in the course of busy practice in an acute hospital, hospice, and community, it has proved useful. A weekly inventory of such matters at unit level (hospital, hospice, or community based) can lead to immediate correction of procedures as well as ventilation of concern in a ''no fault atmosphere.'' Matters taken into account include ''deaths without dignity'' referring mainly to external circumstances or observable matters (not intrinsic human dignity) such as uncontrolled distressing symptoms and unplanned (but preventable) admissions to hospital. Each clinical unit needs to be encouraged to develop its own list of ''sentinel'' events to alert the group for possible changes of procedures or need for heightened awareness.

VIII. SPECIAL PROBLEMS IN THE CARE OF PATIENTS WITH DEATH ON THE HORIZON

The issue of personal grieving is complex. It was recognized by Tolstoy a century ago (7) that pretense by others that death is not on the horizon or is very close can aggravate the situation of the patient. The communication of truth in a multicultural world is complex—man cannot bear too much reality but unreality may be even harder to bear. Problems that require mention of specific relevance to oncology services include particularly ambiguity of goals, obstruction of death, and the recognition (and prevention) of the ''battered patient syndrome.''

Ambiguity of goals is commonplace and distressing, and is distinguishable from uncertainty in the face of inadequate information concerning type or extent of tumor, or likelihood of response to anticancer therapy (surgery, radiotherapy, or chemotherapy). There is need for clarity in the mind of the senior and junior clinicians of the goal of current treatment, even if the outcome is uncertain, for the present. When cure is impossible realistically, no patient or family faced with the offer of inclusion in a clinical trial of palliative chemotherapy should be led to think that the questions to be answered in the trial are about cure: the despair when treatment fails may be far greater if there was ambiguity on this matter.

During a period (e.g., a few days) when decision making is proceeding about whether surgery or other intervention would benefit the patient, it may be wiser to use the term ''decision making period'' for patient and family rather than present a situation of unclear goals. This matter comes to a fine focus when it is clear that the patient is actually dying, with the obvious convergence of pathophysiological processes and psychological signs of increasing inwardness and distancing even from significant others. It may be destructive and deforming of the process of dying to continue with efforts to cure or control disease by heroic measures when care requires otherwise. The ''wild death'' described so clearly by Aries (8) is unfortunately still occurring, when a gentle ''tame death'' is possible if current knowledge concerning palliative care is appropriately applied.

Obstruction of death is unethical as well as tragic. The fundamental ethical requirement is to affirm life—but not to obstruct death—two principles possibly best articulated in the Jewish tradition.

Obstruction of death may occur in several ways:

1. Attempts to control (without the slightest chance of cure) and prolong the life of a patient with a tumor already causing local symptoms already very difficult to control by specialist palliative medicine techniques. A temporary reprieve may lead to horrific symptoms later, with much lower chance of good symptom relief.
2. Attempts to prolong the life of such a patient by other means, for example, tube feeding or even total parenteral nutrition, or by correction of electrolytes in a patient very close to death (a relevant matter in medical management of end-stage gastrointestinal obstruction).
3. An attempt at cardiopulmonary resuscitation in a patient with very far advanced cancer but dying peacefully with optimal symptom relief. This should never occur but errors in decision making are not as likely as failure in clear communication to staff concerning treatment policy.

The ''battered patient syndrome,'' a term in use in Central Sydney Palliative Care Service (9) based on unpublished observations, refers to occasional newly encountered patients (usually in acute hospitals) who exhibit some or all of the following characteristics (without neurological disease or history of psychiatric illness): (1) flattened affect or extreme passivity, (2) inability to exercise choice or express wishes—loss of a capacity for autonomy, (3) sense of loss of control over clinical events especially investigations and treatment interventions (even if consent has been formally given), and (4) bewilderment. Depression may be a component of the situation, but it is not an adequate concept.

These patients urgently need personal space, rest, sometimes removal from the current clinical situation, and noninvasive, gentle personal support. They usually recover, sometimes within a few days, and may then be prepared for and be able to face further essential investigations and treatments. The problem may be exacerbated by cross-cultural situations and language gaps.

The final phase of life may, and indeed should, be a time not of failure (no person should die perceiving himself or herself as a ''treatment failure'') but of positive achievement: the last movement of a symphony is worth writing, experiencing—and hearing. The tools are the patients, but clinical staff and activities may influence the possibility of the emergence of the final music, and even its pattern.

It has been said that ''it is the task of medicine to emancipate man's interior splendour'' (10), at least there is need to recognize the existence of the mystery of the splendor within each human person, even and especially at the close of life.

REFERENCES

1. Barbato M. Death is a journey to be undertaken. Med J Aust 1998; 168:296–297.
2. Erikson EH. Identity and the life cycle. Psychological Issues Monograph. New York: International Universities Press, 1968.
3. Cassell E. The nature of suffering and the goals of medicine. N Engl J Med 1982; 306(11):639–645.
4. Doyle D, Hanks GWC, Macdonald N, eds. Oxford Textbook of Palliative Medicine. 2d ed. Oxford: Oxford University Press, 1997.
5. Mercadante S. Ketamine in cancer pain: an update. Palliative Medicine 1996; 10: 225–230.
6. Glare PA, Lickiss JN. Quality assurance in palliative care. Med J Aust 1992; 157: 572.
7. Tolstoy L. The Death of Ivan Illyich. Trans Maud L & A (commentary Arthur C. Carr). New York: Health Sciences Publishing, 1973.
8. Aries P. The Hour of Our Death. Oxford: Oxford University Press, 1981.
9. Lickiss JN, Wiltshire J, Glare PA, Chye RWM. Central Sydney Palliative Care Service: potential and limitations of an integrated palliative care service based in a metropolitan teaching hospital. Ann Acad Med 1994; 23(2):264–270.
10. Mortimer K. The impossible profession: the doctor-priest relationship. Proceedings of Australian Association of Gerontology 1984; 2:81.

29

Delivery of Cancer Care at Home

Vincent Vinciguerra and James T. D'Olimpio
North Shore University Hospital, Manhasset, New York

I. INTRODUCTION

During the past 20 years, the medical community has witnessed an explosion in the delivery of home care services. There are many reasons for this transition from hospital to home care, including the increasing cost of hospital care, the institution of strict guidelines for length of stay for inpatient treatment, the success of the hospice movement for cancer patients, the aging population, and the fact that home care has been shown to be financially feasible and most effective. Many services routinely administered in the hospital have come to be safely and effectively administered in the home care setting. Studies of quality of life have demonstrated patient preferences for home care treatments rather than hospitalization. It is estimated that the annual Medicare budget for home care is more than $19 billion, which has increased 900% in the past 10 years (1). A large percent of home care and the economic burden is directed toward cancer patients because this is a disease of an aging population and is the primary diagnosis in many hospice programs.

Similar to many aspects of health care delivery, home care involves many aspects of treatment, prevention, and support, and requires the expertise of trained specialists. The home care team includes physicians, visiting nurses, physical therapists, occupational therapists, home health aides, laboratory personnel, social workers, dentists, homemakers, speech therapists, dietitians, pharmacists, clergy, and volunteers. The U.S. Medicare budget is currently supporting 160 million home visits per year. The percent of visits by one of the key members of the team, the physician, has recently been found to have dramatically decreased, from 40% in 1930 to 0.6% in 1980 (2). At the present time, however, with the renewed interest in home care, there is currently a reevaluation of the role of house calls by physicians, especially for cancer patients. Also, interest in house calls has been stimulated as a result of developments in the health care environment, including the fact that there is more competition among physicians for patients, and there is perceived a need to train physicians in the special area of home care (3).

Modern cancer care has evolved into a variety of portable choices that can be made by the practitioner in close association with patient and family (4,5). This process is as much driven by recent trends in managed care (6) applications to home care as it is in the ability of refined techniques to deliver that care in the home. This is particularly true when it becomes difficult for a marginally ambulatory, frequently frail, elderly patient to keep scheduled appointments in

Table 1 Important Features of Domiciliary Cancer Care

1. Cancer care at home is unique in medicine given the defined limited prognosis of advanced disease.
2. It can be difficult and burdensome to the patient and family, but has the potential for success with multidisciplinary input.
3. It can seem to be the only alternative offered to patients and their families, especially after a difficult hospitalization.
4. It should be regarded as a family experience and steps need be taken to ensure a family role.
5. Most research has been done on pain management; little has focused on co-associated symptoms.
6. Pain and symptom control can be problematic to certain families because of poor comprehension or lack of education.
7. Quality assurance and overall effectiveness is difficult to analyze when separated from home hospice programs. However, it can be a profoundly meaningful experience that transcends the physical act of dying.
8. Basic management of physical symptoms will reduce the burden of patient and family.
9. House calls by physicians are critical in management of advanced cancer patients.
10. Hospice referral and input should be at the earliest possible time that coincides with a terminal prognosis.

a hospital-based, outpatient department, or office setting. Cancer care delivery at home therefore becomes an important part of the treatment plan, especially as the focus shifts from a curative to a palliative strategy. Indeed, given future trends in cancer treatment and limited financial resources as the insurance reimbursement structures evolve, more and more cancer care will be based at home. This fact is expected to increase burdens on the patient and family, and can only be lessened by a coordinated effort on the part of the health care team to recognize what potentially problematic issues need to be addressed (5,7).

This chapter focuses on domiciliary cancer care. It incorporates some original data based on our experience of the H.O.M.E. Program at North Shore University Hospital. In addition, elements of practical aspects on home cancer care delivery are presented, along with criteria that can be useful to the cancer clinician when trying to organize a program. Current concepts in home cancer care are an amalgam of multiple experiences. Research is being done in different countries, with different sets of resources, so there is no set ''blueprint,'' yet models taken from hospice and palliative care programs have helped enormously in coordinating the kinds of resources that make home cancer care successful. Table 1 summarizes the clinical and psychosocial underpinnings that are important in understanding the complexities of this approach (4,5,7–9).

II. PREVIOUS EXPERIENCE WITH HOME CANCER CARE

In 1978, the Don Monti Division of Medical Oncology, North Shore University Hospital, began a pilot program called the Home Oncology Medical Extension (H.O.M.E.) Program (10–12). This program appeared simultaneously with the introduction of the hospice concept, which was gaining national interest. The Don Monti H.O.M.E. Program was an attempt to deliver home care services for advanced and terminal cancer patients. A medical team consisting of a physician (an oncologist), oncology nurse, dietitian, social worker, and laboratory technologist was transported in a medically equipped van to the patient's home to provide comprehensive, multidisciplinary services.

The most important factor that was required for eligibility for the H.O.M.E. Program included a willingness on the part of the patient and the family to accept home treatment. Also, patients had to have a proven diagnosis of cancer and be under the care of, or be referred to, an attending physician on the hospital staff. A geographical restriction included that patients live within a 10-mile radius of the hospital in order to achieve maximal time efficiency.

A medically equipped van included an appropriate generator, electrical wiring and lighting, and heating and air conditioning systems, along with cabinets and countertops. The medical equipment included a refrigerator for the transport of blood products, a binocular microscope with a phase attachment, a microhematocrit centrifuge, capillary tube reader, and a centrifuge to perform complete blood counts.

In the first 15 years of the program more than 1700 patients have been treated and more than 11,000 home visits have been made. The patient survival on the home van program has been 78 days. (Services provided are listed in Table 1). Chemotherapy administration in the home has been provided for 23% of patients; home blood transfusions have been administered to 8%. Approximately 50% of patients are allowed to remain at home to die. Because the physician was not present at each visit, physical assessments were provided either by the oncologist or the oncology nurse. The coordinator of the program is the oncology nurse who organized the various activities of the medical team and is the main liaison for the staff, patient, and family members. The types of cancers treated at home are listed in Table 2. Chemotherapy was a unique service offered for our home patients, and the types of agents administered are shown in Table 3.

The next step in evaluating the efficacy of the H.O.M.E. Program was to develop a study comparing home versus hospital care for advanced cancer patients (13). Two groups of patients were analyzed, including one group living within a 10-mile radius from the hospital who were assigned to the home care program and another outside the catchment area who received hospital-based care. The services of the H.O.M.E. van medical team were provided for patients on home care. Medical, nutritional, psychosocial, and economic data were obtained from this study, which was supported by a National Cancer Institute grant. The medical information included data on survival, laboratory studies, pain control, and place of death. Nutritional information included weight and anthropometric changes and dietary intake. Social and demographic descriptors and mood profiles and economic information, including comparative cost for home and hospital treatment, were also obtained.

Table 2 Most Frequent Cancer Diagnoses Treated in H.O.M.E. Program

1. Breast
2. Colorectal
3. Lung
4. Leukemia
5. Lymphoma
6. Renal cell
7. Prostate

Table 3 Types of Intravenous Chemotherapy Safely Administered in the Home

1. 5-Fluorouracil
2. Vinblastine
3. Cisplatin, low-dose
4. Adriamycin
5. Mitomycin
6. Plicamycin (mithramycin)
7. Vincristine
8. Cyclophosphamide
9. Methotrexate
10. Cytosine arabinoside

Our study indicated that comprehensive home treatment provided by a multispecialty medical team was an effective alternative to hospitalization for terminal cancer patients. An evaluation of survival indicated that there was no detrimental effect of home treatment on patient survival. Patients with higher Karnofsky performance status had superior survival at home compared to those undergoing hospital treatment. An assessment of pain control was also performed. The average daily morphine equivalent dose of analgesics was significantly less for the home patients compared with those in the hospital group. It was speculated that home treatment may provide a comfortable environment that allows effective pain control requiring smaller amounts of narcotic analgesics. Nutritional evaluation indicated that most terminal cancer patients can be effectively supported with oral intake or food supplements in the home. Selected patients did require enteric tube feedings or total parenteral nutrition. In our study, it was noted that improved body fat stores could be accomplished for female patients undergoing treatment at home as measured by triceps skin fold measurement. Overall, nutritional education and counseling can accomplish a great deal in the home to advance the nutritional status of cancer patients.

A comparative cost analysis of home and hospital treatment was also carried out (14). This was complicated by the fact that economic analyses must take into account direct and indirect costs. Indirect costs include losses in the family income as a result of days or work lost by the patient and the primary caregiver. The per diem cost savings were calculated from the differences between hospital and home costs. The cost of home care during this study was 75% less than hospital care. This study supported the fact that home care can result in significant per diem savings when compared with hospital treatment.

Our experience indicated that a great deal of medical care can be transported to a patient's home and can be done safely and with excellent quality of life results (15). When our home care program began, hospice was being defined and programs were beginning to be developed. While the H.O.M.E. van program provided hospice-type services, the additional services allowed patients to elect continued anticancer treatment, which, for many patients and families, were more acceptable than supportive care only and end of life treatment. This transitional care, which bridged the time from initial diagnosis and aggressive therapy to the terminal phase of cancer, allowed patients the needed time to reflect on which direction for cancer care they would favor and choose. Many patients were eased into the dying process as it became obvious that anticancer treatment was no longer indicated.

III. UNIQUENESS OF HOME CANCER CARE

Domiciliary cancer care is unlike any other in medicine. This patient population is the potentially most problematic, the ''sickest'' in medicine (16). The reality of 50% of cancer patients still living with a limited prognosis and life span is unique to this patient population as is the relative predictability of physical deterioration (7–9,17). Prognostication, especially in the advancing stages of illness, is becoming more precise, and disease trajectory, although still at times biologically indefinite, is becoming easier to gauge (18,19). Therefore, the clinician is more capable of assisting the family and support staff with more accurate information in terms of time-related issues and exhaustion of medical resources and finances. Table 4 lists some important survival considerations (18–20) that are necessary for the proper evaluation of any homebound patient. The clinician must be able to attempt to plan for eventual complications and orchestrate an individualized treatment plan.

It is important that the practitioner be mindful of the tendency to neglect the advantages of home care in a ''high-tech'' world. Cancer is the great disruptor of the rhythm of home life. It can be very difficult for patients to travel back and forth to doctor and pharmacist, laboratory, or radiology suite. Issues of transportation and distance, child or elder care, and the physically taxing act of preparing oneself for the day of the visit can have a negative impact on the quality of life (21). More research dealing with issues of compliance in the setting of physical deterioration is needed, although it must be stressed that the approach is individualized to the patient's particular situation and compromises are always made (7,22,23).

Most cancer patients, especially those with metastatic disease, are polysymptomatic and require polypharmacy-based therapeutics (18). In addition, they fre-

Table 4 Reliable Categories in Predicting Survival in Cancer

1. Karnofsky Performance Status (2)
2. Biological indicators of significance (27):
   - Neutrophil percentage
   - Lymphocyte percentage
   - Total white blood count
   - Serum albumin level
   - Proteinuria
3. Clinical indicators of significance (20):
   - Xerostomia
   - Dyspnea
   - Eating disorder
   - Dysphagia
   - Disorientation
   - Weight loss

quently require durable medical equipment such as respiratory assist devices, nebulizer delivery systems, special hospital beds and mattresses, syringe drivers, and transcutaneous electron nerve stimulation (TENS) units (5,28). Therefore, care at home needs to be symptom focused and coordinated in a multidisciplinary ''team'' format (Table 5). Performance status changes need to be closely monitored. Patients need to stay rested, nourished, and hygienic. The home should be clean and safe. Medication compliance is critical as is education of the patient and family in keeping careful records of medication administration.

Table 5 Interdisciplinary Elements of Domiciliary Cancer Care

1. Physician visit program
2. Nurse visit program/OCN certified HCN certified
3. Social work services program (social workers with experience in cancer care)
4. Pharmaceutical liaison/formulary
5. Nutritional support/liaison
6. Community/church liaison
7. Centralized record keeping
8. Insurance reimbursement liaison
9. Laboratory affiliation for at home phlebotomy

IV. MODERN CONCEPTS IN THE DELIVERY OF CANCER CARE AT HOME AND "BENEFIT VERSUS BURDEN" ISSUES

There are certain basic tenets of care that every patient, regardless of diagnosis, deserve as a basic focus of management. With a diagnosis of cancer and a limited prognosis, the paradigm of care shifts (9,17). Many pitfalls can diminish the home experience, not the least of which is a complicated and debilitating disease course. Table 6 lists characteristic elements to consider along the continuum of care. Not necessarily does cancer treatment allow the luxury of categorization but, in general, the focus shifts from less intensive office-based or hospital-based care to more intensive home-based care as primary treatment options narrow. In theory,

Table 6 Selection Criteria: Home Care Considerations Along the Continuum of Care

Minimal home care requirements	
Potentially curative therapy (combination chemotherapy, surgery, multimodality therapy, RT)	
1. Frequent doctor office visits	(NOT RELEVANT TO HOME CARE IN MOST SITUATIONS)
2. Less frequent hospitalizations	
3. High-tech interventions common/necessary	
4. Patients frequently younger, with KPS ≥ 80	
5. "Burden versus benefit" tolerance at maximum	
6. Prognosis indefinite/long; optimism high	
Moderate home care requirements	
Life-extending therapy (1st or 2nd relapse, onset of metastasis, potential response to hormonal manipulations)	
1. Periodic doctor office visits	
2. More frequent hospitalizations as complications of disease process arise/increase	
3. Older patient population or physically deteriorated with KPS 60–80	
4. "Burden versus benefit" tolerance changing	
5. Prognosis guarded; palliation the focus of care	
High home care requirements	
Comfort care/primary palliative care	
1. Doctor office visits more problematic	
2. Need for hospitalizations increase frequently for dehydration or pain control, general weakness	
3. Physically deteriorated KPS <60	
4. "Burden versus benefit" primarily related to physical or emotional discomfort relief	
5. Prognosis limited	
6. Hospice logical next step	

this should allow time to assist in understanding when a patient should be more home based, but in reality the clinical situation can change more rapidly, blurring the distinctions until it is not practical or desirable to keep a patient home (7,17,24,25). The burden versus benefit equation therefore can change to include home care as not an option to the family (26). Under these circumstances, home cancer care is an ''unacceptable modality'' if the patient cannot tolerate treatment at home or if the family cannot cope with the situation (7,26–28). Under these conditions, hospice/palliative care units have begun to emerge as an alternative, although these programs are frequently home based (29,31,34,37).

There are pitfalls, and in a practical sense, multidisciplinary domiciliary cancer care delivery cannot be done without a cohesive and reliable group of health care resources (26,29,31). Elements of support need to accommodate low-tech and high-tech delivery. This can range from simple oral medication administration and legitimate complementary measures, such as acupuncture and massage therapy, to full intravenous (IV) support at home for administration of blood products, total parenteral nutrition (TPN), anticancer pharmaceuticals, and analgesic drugs (Table 7).

Modern cancer care is expensive and time-consuming. Part of this aspect cannot help but be transferred to potentially vexing problems at home. It also requires committed, competent, and experienced caregivers. Clinical expertise and familiarity with cancer treatment is not a luxury but a requirement. Table 1 lists well-recognized elements of home cancer care that should ensure its success. The problem is that each region, each province, each city, and each country has

Table 7 Components of Therapy at Home

A. Medication administration (flow sheet per agency)
   1. Oral/sublingual delivery, concentrates
   2. Rectal suppository
   3. Transdermal preparations
   4. Subcutaneous infusion pumps/drips
   5. Intravenous infusion drips
   6. Patient-controlled analgesic/computerized
B. Uncomplicated wound care
C. Nutritional support
   1. Total parenteral nutrition (TPN)
   2. Peripheral parenteral nutrition (PPN)
D. Blood products
E. Anticancer pharmaceuticals
   1. Chemotherapy, i.e., infusional 5-fluorouracil
   2. Adjuvant therapies, i.e., monthly pamidronate
F. Portable x-ray diagnostics

strengths and weaknesses in different areas (5,34). In a market-driven, customer satisfaction, total quality management atmosphere that has become the industry in many countries, competition is a mixed blessing and does not lend itself to standards of care that are easy to quantify. Care can be uneven and results uncertain. Hospice programs have helped solve these problems by bringing many of these elements into a focused multidisciplinary model, which has made a major impact in caring for patients once they reach a terminal stage. Certainly earlier referral to home hospice care would facilitate the transition to comfort care, but many patients, families, and physicians are unfamiliar with the practical aspects and advantages of hospice care (31). Any home cancer care program must have either within its organizational structure or in a collaborative community-based setting, a hospice connection. Indeed, part of the model used in home care closely parallels the hospice model, simply applied to an earlier stage in the disease trajectory (31,37).

V. ELEMENTS OF A SUCCESSFUL HOME CANCER CARE PROGRAM

A physician visit program is essential to successful outcomes. Bedside clinical expertise has no equal in efficiency and care coordination. A home visit in the patient's own environment can provide much useful information to the practitioner. For example, how really necessary are high-tech interventions? Could conversions to low-tech measures be equally effective? How has the patient responded to treatments? Is the information given by family and support staff accurate? Has the education component ''sunk in''? Is more repetition necessary to reinforce instructions? Are flow sheets properly done? Is the environment safe? Many questions can be answered firsthand with a home visit. Recent surveys have lamented the disappearance of the house call, although some have indicated a resurgence in some areas. Part of the problem is probably the modern practitioner's reliance on laboratory and pharmacy support. These problems can be solved by assuring the organizational framework listed.

Only a limited quantity of home visits can be made by physicians. A nurse well trained in the clinical aspects of oncology care can provide valuable services for advanced cancer patients. These services include evaluation of patient performance status, state of hydration, pain control, need for antiemetics, laxatives, and nutritional support, safety issues in the home, need for psychosocial support, and family adjustment and coping to continued home care treatment. The nurse is the central coordinator and liaison among patients, physicians, and other members of the home care team. The availability of 24-hour coverage for the nurse is considered an essential feature of any successful home cancer care program.

Well-trained nurses, preferably with oncology/hospice certification, are invaluable in the organization of cancer care at home. Visits can be more flexible, more frequent, and can take more time. Communication with the physician is essential and nursing autonomy is directly related to experience, competence, and ongoing professional relationships.

Completing the core of the home team are social workers. The importance of the social worker interfacing with family dynamics and addressing psychosocial issues is critical to successful home cancer care. As stated previously, cancer care at home is different than with other diseases. The specter of life-limiting or life-threatening conditions makes managing patients and families much more complicated and problematic.

There is a range of psychological ailments that can be encountered in patients with advanced stage cancer. These include varying degrees of depression, anger, hopelessness, acute psychotic reactions to pharmacological therapy, and mood changes. Despite the terminal nature of the patient's condition, suicide is an uncommon event and has been seen only rarely in patients with end stage cancer. Even when cancer pain is severe, few patients have taken their own lives. The ability of a social worker to identify the need for interventions when psychosocial turmoil exists is critical. Consultation with a psychologist or psychiatrist may also be required in certain clinical situations.

The remainder of the resources that should be made available for adequate home cancer care reflects community-based resources, agencies, and vendors (34). These can be complicated and difficult to administer, but when in place, they are very useful for quality of care assurance at the bedside. Pharmaceutical support with an acceptable and efficacious formulary should be available to compound and formulate drugs tailored to patient needs. When this is not available, at a minimum, a designated pharmacist needs to be available 24 hours a day, 7 days a week, with home delivery capability. Orders can be telephoned or faxed, if necessary, to temporize the situation for documentation. Novel drug delivery systems can simplify the ordering process and frequency, especially if the oral route becomes a problem and parenteral delivery is unacceptable. Table 8 lists common drugs especially useful in domiciliary care.

When physical symptoms are well controlled, and the patient and family feel that care is attentive and competent, this being accomplished with the personal intervention of practitioners and team members, then the care runs smoothly. Additional components such as nutritional liaison and community-based volunteers and church liaison would be much more effective when the care services are performing well. When the physical condition of the patient deteriorates, the system needs to respond to it in a timely and efficient manner. Using bedside diagnostic x-ray machines is becoming popular in some regions and a chest or skeletal x-ray study is possible to be done in the home. Laboratory

Table 8 Oral Concentrate, Transdermal, Rectal, Sublingual Preparations Available for Homebound Patients

Pharmacological agent	Route of delivery	Indications
Concentrated morphine solution 20 mg/mL	PO/SL	Pain, breathlessness, agitation
Lorazepam "Intensol" 0.5 mg/cc	PO/SL	Anxiety, nausea, breathlessness, depression, myoclon
Duragesic fentanyl 25 mg	TD (other?)	Pain
Hydromorphone suppositories 3 mg	PR	Pain
Choline magnesium salicylate 500 mg/5 mL	PO	Pain, inflammation
Indomethicin rectal suppositories 50 mg	PR	Pain, inflammation
Haloperidol 2 mg/mL	PO/SL	Agitation, nausea, pain
Thioridizine 30–100 mg/mL	PO	Agitation, sleep disturbance (nocturnal, wakefulness), depression, anxiety
Chlorpromazine suppositories 25 mg	PR	Nausea, agitation, psychosis
Chloral hydrate 500 mg/5 mL	PO	Sleep disturbances
Pentobarbital suppositories	PR	Severe sleep disturbances
Hyoscyamine 0.125 mg	SL/PO chewable	Antispasmodic, nausea, diarrhea, T secretions
Megestrol acetate 400 mg/10 mL	PO	Appetite stimulant
Sandostatin	SC	Early bowel obstruction
Scopolamine	TD	Nausea, secretions

Abbreviations: PO, orally; SL, sublingually; PR, per rectum; TD, transdermal; SC, subcutaneous.

support of phlebotomy and a designated STAT lab is required if physical deterioration or change takes place, and interventions are being contemplated to provide palliative care.

Centralized record keeping and the ability to properly bill for services rendered have become major accreditation, antifraud, and quality assurance issues for government sponsored programs and cannot be underestimated in their importance. The reality is that, as home cancer care programs mature and evolve into

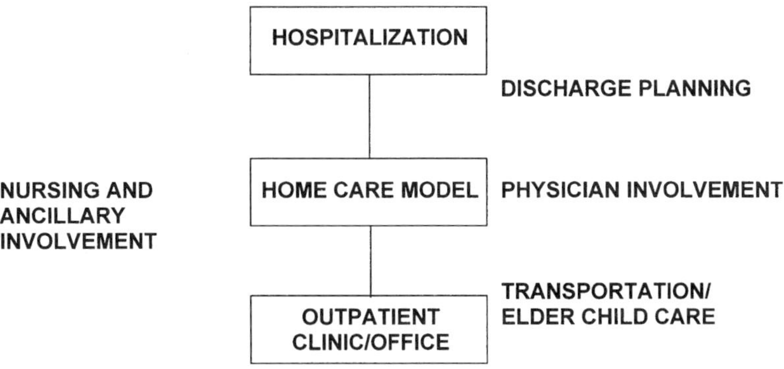

Figure 1 Factors influencing care continuum success.

cohesive, continuous models of care, programs will not survive unless practical logistic solutions keep up with the changing pace of care delivery at home.

Figure 1 summarizes the interaction of factors that influence these issues. Each element, from discharge planning in the hospital to the details of transportation, factor into the decisions about committing resources for home cancer care. To summarize, the word interdisciplinary, not multidisciplinary, describes the care of success in this type of program. It seems simplistic, but the model for home cancer care will not succeed unless the practical aspects of care are fully integrated, with the physician taking responsibility for a major role.

VI. FUTURE TRENDS IN HOME CANCER CARE

The world's population is aging and the diagnosis of cancer as a leading cause of death is increasing. These are incontrovertible facts. The cost of health care will continue to increase and patient choice of care is logically moving toward models of delivering what will best accommodate these inevitable changes. The deficiencies of a complete clinical data base that reflect current and future trends in cancer therapy need to be corrected for the future anticipated increase in the numbers of patients with advanced cancer needing home care services. The development of quality of life evaluation, and tools that are easy to manage and catalog is essential in developing future care refinements. In addition, the development of palliative care teams that have been organized and enabled by hospitals as part of their continuum of care will become more frequently used in this setting. The development of a core curriculum and the proliferation of new monographs and texts in this field has grown in less than a generation. The efficacy of these teams, coupled with an integrative community-based hospice program, should allow for the expected growth in this area of supportive oncology.

REFERENCES

1. Pear R. Home health care. The New York Times, July 27, 1997.
2. Meyer GS, Gibbons RV. House calls to the elderly—a vanishing practice among physicians. N Engl J Med 1997; 337:1815–1820.
3. Cammpion EW. Can house calls survive? N Engl J Med 1997, 337:1840–1841.
4. Ferrel BR. In: Principles and Practice of Supportive Oncology. New York: Lippincott-Raven 1998:709.
5. Doyle D. In: Oxford Textbook of Palliative Medicine. Oxford: Oxford University Press, 1998:958.
6. Dodd K, Coleman J. Homecare and managed care—prospective partners. Caring 1994; March: 68.
7. Bruere E. In: Oxford Textbook of Medicine. Oxford: Oxford University Press. 1998: 179.
8. Jones RVH, et al. Death from cancer at home—the carers perspective. BMJ 1993; 306:249–251.
9. Tuscani F, Mancini C. Adequacies of care in far advanced cancer patients. Palliative Medicine 1989, 4:31–36.
10. Vinciguerra V, Degnan T, Drena J, et al. Home oncology medical expenses: a new home treatment program. CA A Cancer Journal for Clinicians 1980; 30:182–185.
11. Vinciguerra V, Degnan T, O'Connell M, et al. Bringing terminal care home. Your Patient and Cancer 1983; October.
12. Vinciguerra V. Home Oncology Medical Extension (H.O.M.E.)—an effective alternative to hospital care. Adv Cancer Control 1983; 319–326.
13. Vinciguerra V, Degnan T, Sciortino A, et al. A comparative assessment of home versus hospital comprehensive treatment for advanced cancer patients. J Clin Oncol 1986; 4:1521–1528.
14. Vinciguerra V, Degnan T, Budman D, et al. Comparative cost analysis of home and hospital treatment. Adv Cancer Control 1986; 155–164.
15. Vinciguerra V. How it can be done: a pilot project in comprehensive home cancer treatment. J Palliat Care 1988; 4:53–55.
16. Brivio E, Gamba A. Home care for advanced cancer patients: the efficacy of domiciliary assistance. Eur J Cancer Care 1992; 1(2):24–28.
17. Cartwright A. Balance of care for the dying between hospital and the community. B J Gen Pract 1991; 41:271–274.
18. Reuben DB, et al. Clinical symptoms and length of survival in patients with terminal cancer. Arch Intern Med 1988; 148:1586–1591.
19. Donnelly S, Walsh D. The symptoms of advanced cancer. Semin Oncol 1995; 22(2 suppl 3):67–72.
20. Coyle N, Layman-Goldstein M, et al. Development and validation of patient needs assessment tool (PNAT) for oncology clinicians. Cancer Nursing 1996; 19:81–92.

21. Bryan JL, et al. An evaluation of the transportation needs of disadvantaged cancer patients. J Psychosocial Oncol 1991; 9:23.
22. Hinton J. Can home care maintain an acceptable quality of life for patients with terminal cancer and their relatives. Palliat Med 1994; 8:183–196.
23. Maltoni M, et al. Biological indices predictive of survival in 519 terminally ill cancer patients. J Pain Symptom Manage January 1997; 13(1):1–9.
24. Ferrell BR, Schneider C. The experience and management of cancer pain at home. Cancer News 1988; 11(2):84.
25. Taylor EJ, et al. Managing of cancer pain at home; the decisions and ethical conflicts of patients, family caregivers and home care nurses. Oncol Nurs Forum 1993; 20(6): 919–927.
26. MacAdam DB. A review of 715 terminal patients cared for at home by a hospice palliative care service. Cancer Forum 1985; 9:101–104.
27. Indeck BA, Bunney MA. In: Section 6 community resources. Cancer Principles and Practice of Oncology. New York: Lippincott-Raven, 1997.
28. Caro FG, Blank, AE. Quality impact of home care for the elderly; post hospital care arrangements. Home Health Care Services Q 1988; 9:59.
29. Wortman GB. Social support and the cancer patient. Cancer 1984; (10 suppl): 2339–2362.
30. Griffiths M, Leek C. Patient education needs opinions of oncology nurses and their patients. Oncol Nurs Forum 1995; 22:139.
31. Parkes CM. Terminal care: home, hospital or hospice? Lancet 1985, 1:155.
32. Davies B. Family functioning and its implications for palliative care. J Palliat Care 1994; 10:29.
33. Yost LS. Cancer patients and home care: extent to which required services are not received. Cancer Pract 1995; 3:83.
34. Hays JC. High-technology and hospice home care: strange bedfellows. Home Health Care 1988; 23:329–340.
35. Longman AJ, et al. Care needs of home based cancer patients and their caregivers. Cancer Nurs 1992; 15(3):182–190.
36. Kennedy BJ. Aging and cancer. J Clin Oncol 1988; 6:1903–1911.
37. Ventafridda V, DeConno F, et al. Comparison of home and hospital care of advanced cancer patients. Tumori 1989; 75:619.

30

Complementary Medicine*

Stephen C. Schimpff
University of Maryland Medical System and University of Maryland School of Medicine, Baltimore, Maryland

I. INTRODUCTION

Complementary medicine has a clear role in palliative care of cancer and acquired immunodeficiency syndrome (AIDS). If one is to follow a holistic approach to medical care, one in which the focus is on healing and not just an attempt at cure of the underlying disease, then complementary medicine techniques are clearly appropriate. True, they have not received the type of scientific validation that might be desirable, but to the extent that the patient finds relief and has an improved quality of life as a result of these techniques, thcn the use of complementary techniques is clearly valid and appropriate. Furthermore, it is clear that patients use complementary approaches with or without their doctor's knowledge or recommendation, and it therefore behooves physicians to recognize that their patients may well be visiting complementary medical practitioners. That being the case, it is better that physician and complementary medicine practitioner work together as a team, understanding what each team member can add to the overall care and healing of the patient.

---

* Adapted with permission from Schimpff SC. In: Eguchi K, et al, eds. Complementary Medicine in Palliative Care of Cancer and AIDS. New York: Springer Verlag, 1998.

II. TOWARD A HOLISTIC MODEL OF MEDICINE

The fundamental goals of medicine are cure, promoting health, preventing illness and injury, restoring functional capacity, avoiding premature death, relieving suffering, and caring for those who cannot be cured. American medicine and indeed that of most countries that have a predominance of ''science-based medicine,'' or ''conventional medicine,'' focuses primarily on only the first of these goals, namely, cure. Ellen Fox, in a recent editorial of the *Journal of the American Medical Association* (1), spoke of the predominance of the curative model of medical care and defines this as a model focused on eradication of the cause of illness or disease but which tends not to focus on the other aforementioned goals of medicine. The curative model by its very nature carries with it certain attitudes, assumptions, and values. Among them is an analytical and rationalistic approach to medicine in which the object of the practitioner's attention is not the patient but the disease. The symptoms are clues to diagnosis but, in and of themselves, are not the object of treatment. Because cure is contingent upon diagnosis and then therapy, the practitioner of conventional medicine is highly invested in the scientific approach. Thus, the physician values scientifically based data over all others. For example, there is a high focus on and attention to the results of laboratory tests and radiological studies and a lesser appreciation for the subjective elements of the history. Another attitude is that psychological factors that arise through the history are regarded as rather trivial despite the fact that these psychological factors may play a large role in determining the patient's quality of life. As a result, facts become differentiated from feelings and the body becomes differentiated from the mind. We frequently hear on morning rounds ''the gallbladder in room 706'' rather than ''the lady in room 706 who has symptoms which suggest gallbladder disease.'' In like manner, practitioners tend to perceive a patient in terms of component parts rather than as a total person. Finally, and perhaps most importantly, the curative model conflicts with the notion of a ''good death.'' To the physician, death is the ultimate failure and the patient or the patient's disease ends up being labeled as ''untreatable.'' The result, Dr. Fox suggests, is a neglect of palliative care (1).

Because death is seen as a medical failure, it sends a message to medical students and residents in a sense of a ''hidden curriculum.'' This undermines the attitudes that form the basis for compassion and effective care of the dying (2). This focus on cure as the critical goal of medicine and with it the neglect of palliative care drives the resident in training, who feels the need to be as efficient as possible, to ''turf'' psychosocial tasks, to avoid intimacy with patients and family, to embrace hierarchical structures, and to float above commitment (3). The physician in training tends to believe that psychosocial activities with patients are less important or, to the extent that they are important at all, can be taken care of by other members of the health care team. The avoidance of intimacy comes with the resident's (and later the practicing physician's) inability to be intimate with the patient because of his or her own sense of inadequacy if not failure at the inability to cure the disease. This also leads to the creation of hierarchical structures of the medical team with the physician as superior and the one who deals with the "truly important" issues related to cure, whereas "lower" individuals within the hierarchy, such as nurses, and social workers, can deal with the compassionate aspect of care. The result is that the team is not made up of individuals all respected equally for their expertise, actions, and commitment but rather as those who are more or less important. All of these attitudes, assumptions, and values are carried over into the physician's lifelong practice patterns.

How then does palliative care fit into conventional medicine? The World Health Organization defines palliative care as the active total care of the individual when disease is not curable. The goals are the relief of suffering, the control of symptoms, and the restoration of functional capacity. These goals are addressed not only through conventional medical approaches but also through psychological, social, cultural, and spiritual approaches. The practitioner involved in palliative care is sympathetic to subjective phenomenon such as pain, anxiety, and depression and focuses on treating these symptoms directly as important phenomena to address. Similarly, the practitioner is tolerant of incomplete medical knowledge. For example, if the patient has pain, the approach is to treat the pain without necessarily obtaining a computed tomography (CT) scan to prove that the metastasis has developed in a particular bony location. Finally and importantly, death is considered as not a defeat but rather the natural conclusion of life. As such, the physician and the entire health care team is devoted to dealing with the patient and the patient's family in a way to ensure comfort.

But, it is not only in the setting of an incurable disease in which the patient's demise is expected in some fairly definitive time period where this approach to medicine is important. I propose that science-based medicine, or conventional medicine, needs to shift from the curative model of medical care to a holistic model of medical care. This model is not unlike the model practiced a few generations ago, albeit without the benefits of modern, scientifically delivered technologies. Such care would take current science-based medicine and add to it symptom-based therapy, and give attention to preventive medicine, attention to psychosocial needs, and attention to spiritual needs. Thus, the relief of pain, a focus on diet and exercise, attention to stress reduction, and the use of techniques such as massage would all help relieve symptoms and prevent future illness. Arranging for financial counseling and developing effective measures of home health care would assist the psychological and family needs of the patient. Teaching the patient meditation would help reduce stress, and being comfortable discussing prayer would help attend to the spiritual needs of the patient. Thus, the purpose of the physician begins to shift from one in which cure is the major focus of attention to one in which healing becomes the primary focus. The term ''healing'' implies much more than just cure or care, but rather suggests an attention to all of the needs of the patient regardless of whether an underlying disease can ultimately be cured. It is within this context that complementary medicine is addressed herein; I believe complementary medicine can be of assistance in a holistic approach to medicine, one in which the model is that of healing.

A. Alternative and Complementary Medicine—Definitions, Prevalence, and Techniques

There is no generally accepted definition of alternative, complementary, or unconventional medicine (Table 1). Until recently, the terms tended to connote ''unproved,'' ''untested,'' ''quackery,'' and ''charlatanism,'' and organized medicine made strong efforts to not only discourage their use but also to actively ban many approaches, to prevent licensing by nonallopathic practitioners, and to bring suit against those who claimed effectiveness for their therapies. Alternative medicine tends to focus on elements of nature, vitalism, observational rather than experimental science, and spirituality. The term ''alternative medicine'' is in more common usage than the term ''complementary medicine.'' Alternative medicine is a somewhat unfortunate term, in that it suggests approaches to be used instead of conventional or science-based medicine as opposed to the term ''complementary,'' which tends to suggest approaches that are to be used in conjunction with conventional medicine. I prefer the term ''complementary medicine.''

Complementary medicine might include diet, exercise, stress reduction methodologies, or techniques commonly used in the Orient, such as acupuncture, acupressure, meditation, herbal medicine, and the like. Many, if not most, of these approaches are unproved by the standard scientific method, are not taught in

Table 1 Terminology—Alternative Versus Complementary

Alternative medicine
Implies avoidance of conventional medicine and practitioners
Complementary medicine
Implies working in conjunction with conventional medicine and practitioners
Both alternative medicine and complementary medicine
Science-observational rather than experimental
Generally not taught in medical schools
Practitioners not accepted by dominant practitioners

medical school or residency programs, and, in general, have been on the fringes of orthodox medicine. Complementary approaches, however, have become more and more common, and a number of medical schools (University of Maryland, Stanford) and hospital systems (Sharp in San Diego, Beth Israel in Boston) are developing formal programs. The National Institutes of Health, in part as a result of congressional pressure, has created the Office of Alternative Medicine (OAM), which has been established to scientifically evaluate some of these processes and procedures (4).

In January, 1993, Eisenberg et al. (5) published an article in the *New England Journal of Medicine* on the prevalence, costs, and patterns of use of unconventional medicine in the United States of America. They noted that the extent and costs of unconventional therapeutic practices were unknown and conducted a national telephone survey during 1990 of 1,539 adults. With a response rate of 67%, they determined that fully one-third (34%) of respondents had used at least 1 of 16 predefined interventions in the past 12 months (Table 2). Furthermore, one-third of these individuals visited a provider an average 19 times at an average cost per visit of $27.50 during the past year. Interestingly, the highest use was reported by middle-aged adults who had relatively more education and higher incomes. There were more visits to alternative medicine practitioners than to primary care physicians (Fig. 1), with a ratio of about 4:3 (5).

The 16 unconventional therapies included relaxation techniques (13% usage reported in prior 12 months), chiropractic (10%), massage (7%), imagery (4%), spiritual healing (4%), commercial weight loss program (4%), life style diets (e.g., macrobiotics) (4%), herbal medicine (3%), megavitamin therapy (2%), self-help groups (2%), energy healing (1%), biofeedback (1%), hypnosis (1%), homeopathy (1%), acupuncture (<1%), and folk remedies (<1%). Those who saw a provider were especially likely to do so if using acupuncture, chiropractic therapy, hypnosis, and massage therapy.

Table 2 Prevalence of Alternative Medicine Usage in the United States

1990 Survey—*New England Journal of Medicine*
33% used one or more complementary medicine therapies in past year
70% did not tell their physician
Mostly used for chronic conditions
If generalized to entire U.S. population
More visits to complementary medicine practitioners (425 million) than to primary care physicians (388 million)
Total costs = $13.7 billion
Insurance: $3.4 billion
Out of pocket: $10.3 billion

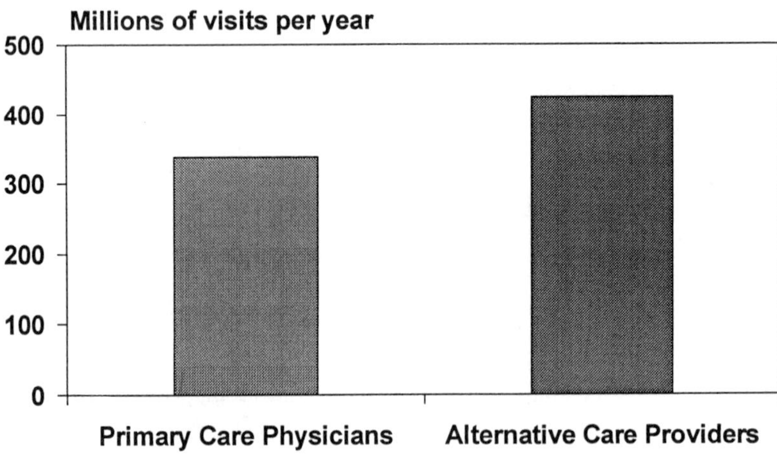

Figure 1 Medical visits: alternative versus primary care practitioners.

Some of the most common medical problems for which these therapies were used included back pain, headache, anxiety, and other musculoskeletal dysfunction. Among those who used one or more of these approaches for serious medical conditions, 83% also sought care from a physician. Nearly one-fourth (24%) of those interviewed who reported having cancer had used one or more unconventional approaches. Most commonly used were relaxation techniques, chiropractic therapy, and massage.

Most of those who reported using an unconventional therapy did not report such to their medical doctor. Other than reimbursement for chiropractic, biofeedback, and herbal therapists by some insurance carriers, most unconventional medicine was paid entirely out of pocket. The authors extrapolated the survey to the entire United States population to estimate a total annual outlay of $13.7 billion, of which $10.3 billion was out of pocket. The authors concluded that use of unconventional therapy was much greater than generally appreciated and, again, noted that most usage went unreported to the individual physician.

The use of alternative, or complementary, approaches in other countries is likewise common and probably higher than most physicians would anticipate. In the United Kingdom, Finland, The Netherlands, Germany, and France, the use of alternative medical therapies ranges from 25% to 75% of the population seeking medical care. In Japan, it is estimated that $1.3 billion is spent annually for Kampo (herbal) remedies. In China, traditional Chinese medicine (e.g., herbal therapy, acupuncture) is more common in many areas of the country than is conventional medicine. Ayurvedic approach to medical care is the dominant medical methodology in India. A *Wall Street Journal* article on April 14, 1997, re-

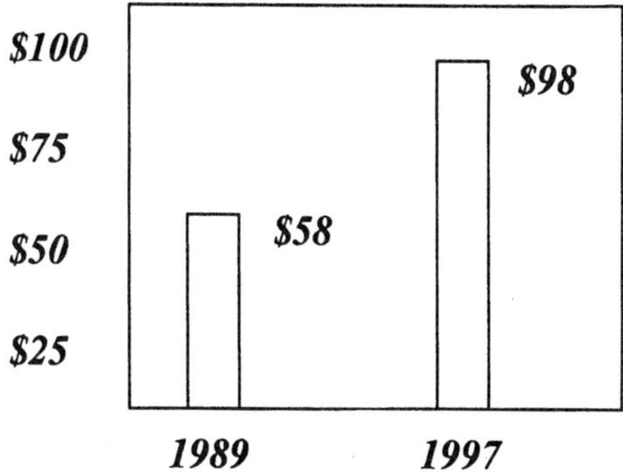

Figure 2 Spending on alternative medicine ("other professional services," i.e., chiropractic, reflexology, acupuncture) in the United States rose 69% between 1989 and 1997. (From *The Wall Street Journal*, Monday, April 14, 1997.)

ported (Fig. 2) that spending for alternative medicine, such as chiropractic, acupuncture, and reflexology amounts to $98 billion per year in the United States, an increase of about 69% since 1989, according to the article (6).

One of the most notable evaluations of complementary medicine is that conducted by Dean Ornish and colleagues (7,8) into the reversal of coronary artery disease by a combination of stress management, exercise, and diet modification combined with group support sessions. Patients were middle-aged men and women who had coronary artery disease documented by arteriography and who were then randomly allocated to a program that included a low-cholesterol (<5 mg/d), low-fat (<10% of total energy intake) vegetarian diet with 15% protein and 75% complex carbohydrate augmented with vitamin B_{12}. All patients had to stop smoking and practice stress management techniques for 1 hour daily, which included a meditation technique. They participated in mild to moderate aerobic exercise 3 hours per week and participated in group support mechanisms. Experimental and control patients had initial and follow-up coronary arteriograms and had positron emission tomography (PET) before and 5 years after initiation of risk factor modification. Although one cannot determine from this study whether all or only certain of the modifications were critical to the outcome, the patients showed modest but definitive regression of coronary artery stenosis and decreased size and severity of perfusion abnormalities on rest-dipyridimole PET images. Although this work has been published in the *Journal of the American Medical Association* by Gould et al. (7), it is also recorded in greater detail in a book by Dr. Ornish entitled "Program for Reversing Heart Disease" (9).

Complementary, alternative, and unorthodox medical practices have become common topics for lay publications. Anyone standing in line at the local supermarket is bombarded with articles in magazines such as *Natural Health, Prevention*, and *Ladies Home Journal. Life* Magazine had a major article on alternative medicine during the summer of 1996, and *Consumer Reports* had a three-part series entitled ''Alternative Medicine: The Facts'' in the January 1994 issue (10).

Why do individuals seek out complementary medicine? A number of studies give some indications. Different attitudes on health and illness appear important. In a study of 202 adult working Germans (11), those seeking complementary medicine were more critical and skeptical as to the effectiveness of orthodox medicine but were not necessarily personally disappointed with the lack of effectiveness in a first-hand manner from their physician. Rather, they simply carried a deep-seated belief that complementary medicine should or would work for them. In a British study of 250 individuals who used acupuncture, homeopathy, or osteopathy, the key reasons for using complementary medicine were the following: ''I value the emphasis on treating the whole person,'' ''I believe complementary medicine will be more effective than orthodox medicine,'' and ''I believe complementary medicine will allow me to take a more active part in maintaining my health'' (12).

Much of complementary medicine is paid for out of pocket, either in cash or with credit cards. Insurance companies in the United States frequently cover chiropractic therapy, occasionally cover acupuncture (more often if administered by a physician), rarely cover massage, support groups, herbal remedies, or other mind–body techniques (unless administered by a psychiatrist), and almost never cover herbal prescriptions. There are some innovative programs developed by insurance carriers, usually managed care organizations. Aetna has accepted the Ornish program for specific subgroups of patients. Oxford Health Plan advertises that it covers many complementary approaches but patients complain that access is difficult, at best. Nevertheless, the tide does seem to be turning.

In other countries, not only are complementary approaches more common, they are often practiced in tandem by physicians. For example, German physicans prescribe about as many herbal products as they do pharmaceuticals, often using them together.

When the National Institutes of Health created the OAM in the early 1990s, largely in response to congressional pressure, the concept was to ensure that alternative approaches would be given appropriate research support and, perhaps, ''fairer hearing.'' A number of research centers have received support for specific studies, often in concert with sponsorship by one of the institutes. Furthermore, center grants have been awarded to a few institutions to look critically at specific areas. The University of Maryland, for example, has a center grant to study musculoskeletal pain, and the University of Texas has a center grant for cancer. The office still receives relatively little funding but it is growing as valid work becomes published. The office also has sponsored some consensus conferences such as one on acupuncture in November 1997, which accepted acupuncture as efficacious for certain pain conditions. Also, a conference was held jointly with the National Cancer Institute in August 1997 to address approaches for defining endpoints in cancer studies.

B. Framework for Use of Complementary Medicine

In focusing on complementary medicine for the palliative care of patients with cancer, I suggest that the concepts enunciated by Lerner (13) form a sound framework. He begins by noting the distinction between healing and curing akin to the concept of the medical model of holistic, or healing, care. Lerner notes that healing may be physical, mental, spiritual, or any combination of the three. Healing enhances the quality of life and it may or may not lengthen the span of life. Importantly, healing is in the domain of the patient not the physician. The patient is the one in charge and the physician and other health care providers are in the service of the patient.

Using these concepts, it follows that conventional medicine should be the primary approach to the treatment of cancer. In all likelihood, there are no complementary approaches that are curative. On the other hand, complementary approaches may well assist in the supportive care of the patient and equally, if not more importantly, complementary approaches may help in healing.

The uses of complementary medicine in cancer should be considered from the following perspective. First, complementary medicine techniques are not curative, and there is little scientific evidence for their effect on symptomatic relief. On the other hand, there is strong anecdotal evidence for improved quality of life. It is notable that the average user is above average in education, income, and motivation, and the average practitioner is both licensed and charges fees (13).

In searching for choices in healing, Lerner focuses on several approaches. Spiritual approaches, including prayer and hands-on approaches; psychological approaches, including support groups and guided imagery or creative visualization; nutritional approaches, including diet and other supplements; and physical approaches, including massage, yoga, and perhaps chiropractic therapy. Lerner believes that these four approaches represent a ''vital quartet'' that may enhance the quality of life and improve functional status for patients with cancer. He adds a fifth approach, which is the use of traditional medical systems such as Chinese acupuncture and herbal therapy, Ayurvedic medicine, which uses mental and emotional approaches plus a variety of herbal compounds; traditional European herbal medicines; and traditional Native American approaches. The Chinese, India Ayurvedic, and Native American approaches have long empirical traditions, and European herbal remedies were well known and followed by Americans from colonial times until just a generation or two ago.

III. SPECIFIC COMPLEMENTARY MEDICINE APPROACHES

Table 3 lists specific complementary medicine approaches to supportive care of cancer and AIDS.

A. Acupuncture

Acupuncture has been used in China for more than 2,000 years and has been developed on an empirical basis. The Western medical mind cannot relate easily to the concept of acupuncture adjusting the body's ''energy,'' but there should be little difficulty relating to the results of relieving symptoms. Acupuncture probably works by stimulating nerve endings just under the skin and thereby affecting the central nervous system. Various studies have demonstrated the release of endorphins from the brain following acupuncture.

Acupuncture is clearly effective in reducing or eliminating some types of pain including musculoskeletal, postoperative, and migraine. There are few data on its use for deep-seated pain of cancer related to organ or nerve root involvement. Acupuncture can reduce chemotherapy and radiation-induced nausea and emesis and likewise the nausea and vomiting associated with some postoperative states.

Acupuncture has been shown to be an effective adjunct to reduce emesis after chemotherapy. Vickers (14) reviewed 33 controlled trials in the literature from which he selected 12 as being of particularly high quality as both randomized and placebo controlled. In each of these investigations, the P6 acupuncture site was used. In 11 of the 12 trials with more than 2,000 patients studied, acupuncture proved to be statistically superior to placebo.

Table 3 Complementary Medicine—Some Practices to Consider

Acupuncture
Herbal medicine
Support groups
Mind–body approaches
Meditation
Relaxation response
Creative visualization
Prayer
Massage

Acupuncture needles can be inserted and left alone, can be twirled, or can be attached through minor electric current. A related approach is transcutaneous electrical nerve stimulation (TENS), which has been found useful for pain control. Acupuncture, electroacupuncture, and TENS have all been found to be useful in reducing chemotherapy-induced nausea and vomiting. In an Irish study involving 130 patients with repeated episodes of chemotherapy-induced emesis, electroacupuncture was either completely or considerably effective in 97% of patients. Sham acupuncture sites, even though electrically stimulated, do not have the beneficial effects. The effect, however, is relatively short-lived. TENS was then studied by the same investigators (15), and they found that, in more than 100 patients with chemotherapy-induced emesis, 75% had considerable benefit. Although less than electroacupuncture, the benefit of TENS was that it could be self-administered by patients every 2 hours for a longer lasting relief (15).

There are substantial data on the use of acupuncture for pain relief (16). Some studies at the University of Maryland School of Medicine are illustrative of the use of acupuncture for musculoskeletal pain. Brian M. Berman, MD, was recruited to establish a complementary medicine program in 1991. Starting with a $1 million grant from the Maurice Laing Foundation and the Thera Trust in London, Berman has set out to establish a scientific basis for a number of complementary medical procedures, such as acupuncture. In this regard, he and his colleagues have shown in pilot controlled trials that patients with severe osteoarthritis of the knee receiving best medical therapy will have decreased need for pain medication and increased mobility through the added use of acupuncture. This was a double-blinded trial in which Berman gave real or sham acupuncture to patients who then recorded their use of pain medication while their rheumatologist recorded range of motion (17). In another study, individuals having their wisdom teeth removed were or were not given acupuncture (18). Those who received acupuncture treatments reported less pain following the procedure, used less pain medications, and used them for a shorter period of time. In an animal model, Berman and colleagues have demonstrated that acupuncture releases endorphins into the cerebrospinal fluid, suggesting at least one aspect of the potential physiological effect of acupuncture.

B. Herbal Remedies

Herbal approaches to medicine are as old as civilization. Four different traditions (Table 4) developed over time, with input from each other in many cases. Chinese herbal approaches are a definitive part of traditional Chinese medicine as still taught and practiced extensively in China, in parallel with Western medicine. Indeed, schools of both traditions are highly regarded. The practice has a defini-

Table 4 Herbal Medicine: Four Traditions

Chinese
As part of traditional Chinese medicine
Japanese Kampo as derivative
Indian
As part of traditional Indian medicine (Ayurveda)
Egyptian/European
Native American

tive approach to diagnosis using, as noted previously, a thought process hard for a Western-trained physician to relate to. Nonetheless, the system has stood the test of millennia and leads to a therapeutic approach that incorporates diet, herbal prescriptions, and acupuncture plus other elements. An outgrowth of the Chinese approach is Japanese Kampo medicine, brought to Japan from China more than 1,000 years ago and usually incorporating combinations of 10 or more herbs in a single prescription. Some Japanese physicians incorporate Kampo into their daily practice but most largely ignore, reject, or are simply uninformed about the practice.

The fundamental medical practice of India is known as Ayurveda and incorporates herbal remedies as an integral aspect of this practice.

Native Americans also made extensive use of herbal preparations in their medical approach.

Finally, there is the Egyptian/European tradition of herbal remedies, which was extensively used until the 20th century arrival of science-based medicine. Compounds that our grandparents and great grandparents used on a daily basis have largely been ''lost'' but are rapidly returning in many areas as individuals seemingly take more responsibility for their health and wellness with exercise, diet, and dietary supplements.

Common ''folk remedies'' of the past became standard prescriptions of today. For example, in England, foxglove contained the digitalis compound, which has since been synthesized. Chinchona bark was used in South America for fever and was later found to have quinine as the active ingredient. The cocoa leaf in South America was the origin of cocaine for pain relief and the Peyote plant of Mexico contains a hallucinogen.

Some commonly used herbal compounds (Table 5), that is, the current ''best sellers'' are St. John's wort, which has been used extensively in Germany for depression and in just the past year has become popular in the United States where it received major attention by National Public Radio in 1997. It is said to work by affecting a group of neurotransmitters in the brain. Echinacea is used extensively to prevent and treat upper respiratory viral infections. Presumably it

Table 5 Commonly Used Herbal Remedies

Remedy	Application
St. John's Wort	Depression
Echinacea	Common colds
Licorice	Cough
Chamomile	Indigestion
Garlic	Cholesterol Hypertension
Ginseng	General tonic
Dong quai	Menopausal symptoms

works by augmenting immune function and by reducing the spread of the virus from cell to cell. Chamomile is well known as a tea for an upset stomach. Apparently its effect is mediated by relaxing stomach muscle contractions. Garlic is an age-old remedy for multiple ailments, but, recently, there has been some evidence that it reduces cholesterol, limits the formation of blood clots, and reduces blood pressure. Licorice makes a good candy but also has a salutary effect on coughing by thinning secretions and soothing mucous membranes. Ginseng is a staple in China and other oriental countries where it is used as a general tonic. Also from China is use of dong quai for its plant estrogen compound to reduce the symptoms of menopause.

C. Mind–Body Techniques

1. *Meditation/Relaxation Response*

Mind–body techniques have been described in a network television series moderated by Bill Moyers and subsequently published as a best seller (19). A commonly used mind–body technique is meditation that has been shown to reduce blood pressure, induce a sense of well-being, and reduce both anxiety and depression (20,21). One of the earliest persons to scientifically study mind–body approaches was Herbert Benson, M.D., a cardiologist originally of Harvard and later of Tufts Medical School, who popularized what he calls the ''relaxation response'' (22). He had been studying approaches to hypertension when he met some individuals from India who said that they could teach him meditation techniques that would lower blood pressure. Initially skeptical, he began to study meditation and determined that, indeed, it did reduce blood pressure and change pulse rate in addition to creating a general calming effect and inducing a sense of increased energy. In developing his methodology with patients, he chose to avoid the term ''meditation'' because of its sometimes ''exotic'' connotations and instead coined the term "relaxation response." This is a fairly simplified form of meditation in which the patient is asked to focus on a single word or short phrase. The word can have some religious connotation to the individual, such as "Lord," or it can be a word with little or no other meaning, such as "one." The purpose, however, is to quiet the mind and focus it on this one word to prevent the wandering or "chattering" that occurs within the conscious brain all of the time. Individuals who practice this technique have been regularly shown to reduce their blood pressure, reduce or eliminate their need for antihypertensive medications, especially when done in concert with diet and exercise (22).

2. Hatha Yoga

Hatha yoga, a technique of simple, quiet stretching exercises with a quiet peaceful attitude, tones the musculature, creates a serene, quiet mind, and is often used as an adjunct or as a precursor to meditation (9,23).

3. Visualization/Guided Imagery

Visualization and guided imagery are related mind–body techniques. With creative visualization, individuals seek a quiet resting state in a semimeditative mode in which they imagine themselves as healthy, free of disease, free of certain habits such as smoking or overeating, or enthused about positive attributes such as exercise. The concept is that if one repetitively embeds a desired state into the subconscious mind, the mind–body connections will work toward that state in an ongoing fashion. Guided imagery is a similar technique in which the patient imagines elements of the body actively affecting a disease; e.g., macrophages and natural killer cells are imagined as moving toward the tumor and destroying it.

4. Support Groups

There are more than 45 studies demonstrating that support groups, or psychosocial interventions, enhance the quality of life (24). It is important to recall that the cancer patient's major concerns are the fear of dying alone (literally or figuratively) and of unmanaged pain. These are not necessarily the physician's primary concerns in dealing with the patient. In support groups, the concept is to help patients learn how to cope better so they can have improved interaction with physicians and other medical team members and so that they can manage pain on their own to a greater degree through relaxation techniques and self-hypnosis, through teaching various relaxation skills such as meditation or deep breathing, and through teaching problem-solving skills (Table 6). The group setting is generally conducive to these approaches, in part, because patients can gain from one another and recognize that they are not alone in their concerns, anxieties, and frustrations. As a generalization, the studies of support groups have demonstrated that overall quality of life is much improved, that the patients have better pain

Table 6 Support Groups—General Observations

Patients' major concerns
Dying alone (literally or figuratively)
Unmanaged pain
45 studies of support groups on quality of life
Overall quality of life much improved
Better pain coping
Less psychological distress
Reduced anxiety
Reduced depression
Increased physical activity

management and coping skills, that there is less psychological distress, including reduced anxiety and reduced depression, and that there is increased physical activity. Complementary medicine practitioners typically spend more time with their patients, more time addressing symptoms as opposed to the underlying disease, and more time focusing on the patient's concerns. Thus, complementary medicine practitioners are much more likely to be involved with support group type activities in a direct or indirect way than are physicians.

Three studies totaling 250 patients demonstrated longer survival or reduced mortality rates as a result of psychosocial interventions (24). One of these studies, conducted by David Spiegel and associates at Stanford, has been commonly referred to since its publication in *The Lancet* in 1989. Eighty-six women with metastatic breast cancer were randomly allocated to psychosocial interventions (50) or not (36). All patients had standard oncologic care, whereas those randomized to intervention had weekly supportive group therapy that lasted for 90 minutes and were trained in self-hypnosis for pain. The study was prospective; it was not designed to study survival but rather to address psychological distress and pain management. Thus, the authors did not control for potential survival factors so that there was no attempt to balance, for example, the disease stages other than that all women had metastases. At the end of the first year, the results demonstrated that there was decreased anxiety and decreased pain among the patients (Fig. 3). At follow-up 10 years later at which time only three of the patients were still alive, there was a clear difference in survival. The control patients had lived an average of 19 months, whereas the support group patients had lived an average of 37 months, a statistically significant difference. When analyzed with a Kaplan-Meier survival plot, it was demonstrated that a divergence of survival began at 20 months after randomization (or 8 months after intervention ended), again statistically significant (25).

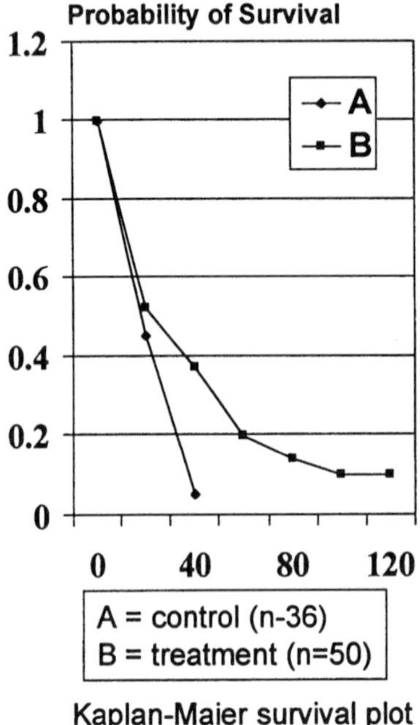

Figure 3 Kaplan-Maier survival plot. Results: decreased anxiety, decreased pain, and improved survival (control group—19 months, support group—37 months).

In another study, Fawzy et al. at UCLA School of Medicine evaluated the recurrence or survival of 68 patients with malignant melanoma who participated in a 6-week structured psychiatric group intervention that took place shortly after their diagnosis and initial surgical treatment. The groups were then observed for about 6 years. Patients were randomly allocated to either no intervention or intervention, which consisted of teaching psychosocial intervention, which, among other things, taught coping skills, relaxation, pain management skills, and problem-solving skills. The researchers found that these interventions enhanced effective coping and reduced affective distress. Furthermore, they found that there were more deaths (10 of 34) among the control patients than among intervention patients (3 of 34), a statistically significant difference (26). A study by Richardson et al. shows a survival advantage as a result of a supportive educational program among patients with leukemias and lymphomas. In this latter study, the supportive program was relatively brief and was designed to enhance medical compliance, unlike the other studies in which there was a more defined approach to psychosocial intervention. The researchers found an increase in social support, self-care, and sense of control by the patients in addition to a survival advantage (27). These are relatively small studies and generally were not designed to address survival; nonetheless, they are intriguing. In any event, they each demonstrate improved quality of life.

5. Prayer

Finally, prayer is a form of complementary medicine that needs to be considered as part of mind–body techniques. Larry Dossey, M.D., editor of *Alternative Therapies, A Journal of Alternative Medicine*, has written a ''best seller,'' which focuses, in part, on prayer as an adjunct to medical care (28). E. Targ recently reviewed some of the research in this field (29). One scientific evaluation of prayer therapy was done at San Francisco General Hospital. Cardiologist Randolph Byrd of UCSF conducted a 10-month study in which 393 patients admitted to the coronary care unit were randomly allocated to either be in a group that was prayed for by home prayer groups or to a group that was not remembered in prayer. It was a randomized, prospective, double-blind trial. The prayer givers were individuals recruited for this purpose with no personal knowledge of the patients and with no specific instructions as to how they should pray other than to do so at least once each day. Prayer groups were given the names of patients; each patient had five to seven people praying for him or her. The prayed-for patients were five times less likely than the unremembered patients to require antibiotics (3 versus 16 patients); pulmonary edema was less likely to develop (6 versus 18); they were less likely to require endotracheal intubation (0 versus 12 patients); and fewer prayed-for patients died, although the difference was not statistically significant (30).

Tying mind–body medicine together as a scientific discipline is the concept of psychoneuroimmunology, or the study of central nervous system function on physiological processes. This area has grown rapidly in the past 10 to 15 years as evidenced by a symposium entitled ''Psychoneuroimmunology and Cancer: Fifteenth Sapporo Cancer Seminar'' (31). The report of the symposium in *Cancer Research* gives a good overview of the inteaction, as currently understood, between the brain and the endocrine/immune systems.

D. Massage

The word ''massage'' comes from Arabic meaning ''to stroke.'' There are records of massage having been used in China at least 3,000 years ago and in Egypt 4,200 years ago. Hippocrates was a very strong advocate of the use of massage, and it was a common form of medical therapy in Europe until the Middle Ages when the Catholic Church denounced it as ''the work of the Devil.'' More recently, the association of massage with prostitution has given it a bad reputation, but the increasing emphasis on healthy lifestyles has brought massage back in the United States to a position of relatively common acceptance. For example, some companies employ massage therapists as an employee benefit to reduce stress and increase relaxation for their employees.

In some medical studies of massage, it has been well demonstrated that premature infants who receive massage compared to those who are not massaged are more alert, active, and responsive; they gain weight nearly 50% faster; they sleep more deeply; their hospital stay is about 6 days shorter; and the total cost is about $10,000 less. Even so, the use of massage for premature infants has not become an insurance covered expense and is rarely a standard therapeutic practice (32).

Massage has been shown to lead to improvement for some patients with asthma; it has been demonstrated to cause some increase in immune function in human immunodeficiency virus (HIV) infected patients; it increases concentration in autistic children; it substantially lessens anxiety in burn victims about to undergo debridement; it lessens depression; and it reduces frequency of migraine headaches (32). Massage is well known to reduce stress and to alleviate some of the symptoms of stress in everyday life such as neck and back pain. Many companies provide on-site massage for their employees; it can be a simple clothes-on seated massage done during a break or lunch period for 10 to 20 minutes once a week with positive results.

There is some controversy as to whether some patients with cancer should undergo massage. Those who are opposed suggest that it might increase circulation to areas of cancer and, hence, increase tumor growth or that it might promote metastases. On the other side are those who give and those who receive massage who report profound relaxation, reduction of chronic pain, and reduction of tension. In addition, the psychological benefit of the hands-on effect of massage can be very positive. Kay Warren in *Nursing Times* (33) recommends slow stroke back massage along with distraction, guided imagery, and progressive muscle relaxation to enhance relaxation and the general feeling of well-being among patients with cancer. Also in *Nursing Times* (34), S. Sims, in a pilot study, reported that breast cancer patients had fewer symptoms and had more tranquility and more vitality with less tension and tiredness as a result of massage therapy.

Massage by a massage therapist is well known to have stress-reducing benefits that can be of value to a cancer patient without having any direct effect on the cancer per se. Other approaches are modern offshoots of the ancient concept of ''laying on of hands.'' The concept is that there is an energy field that exists around each person and that this energy field can be altered through the efforts of a practitioner. These types of approaches have become fairly popular in the United States in recent years.

E. Other Touch Therapies

The concept of ''laying on of hands'' goes back into the far reaches of history. One technique used is known as ''therapeutic touch,'' which was developed from this background largely by Dora Kunz, a healer, and Delores Krieger, a professor of nursing at New York University (35). Krieger teaches the concept and believes that essentially anyone can learn the technique of therapeutic touch. The approach includes three phases. In the first phase, centering, the healer enters a meditative state to become acutely open to any input from the client. In the second phase, assessing, the therapist scans a patient's body with hands held a few inches above the skin to detect disturbances in the energy field around the body. The third phase, rebalancing, uses the therapist's hands to smooth out the energy field. The procedure takes about 15 to 20 minutes. Therapeutic touch has been taught to nurses across the country and is used at multiple institutions, hospices, and offices. In research studies, therapeutic touch seems to be effective in reducing acute pain in postoperative patients, in relieving pain in general, decreasing anxiety in hospitalized patients, improving behavior in premature infants, and decreasing headache pain in adults.

IV. COMMENTS

Ornish's studies of cardiac disease used multiple interventions at once: diet, smoking cessation, exercise, relaxation techniques, meditation, hatha yoga, and group support. Even though it is impossible to dissect out which elements were or were not critical to the improved outcome, the results were clear: a demonstrable reduction in coronary artery narrowing and improved cardiac muscle perfusion. Perhaps with cancer patients, the same approach can be considered. General recommendations are listed in Table 7 and an approach to a holistic model of medical care is outlined in Table 8. Physicians should consider use of those techniques that seem to add benefit to the patient's symptoms and improve quality of life. Concurrently, the outcome of scientific studies of each modality are awaited.

Complementary medicine has a clear role in palliative care of cancer. If one is to follow a holistic approach to medical care, one in which the focus is on healing and not just an attempt at cure of the underlying disease, then complementary medicine techniques are clearly appropriate. True, they have not received the type of scientific validation that might be desirable, but to the extent that the patient finds relief and has an improved quality of life as a result of these tech-

Table 7 General Recommendations

Complementary medicine is used commonly by patients, but physicians largely ignore its use and are uneducated.
Most techniques are not subjected to scientific evaluations.
Anecdotal evidence and thousand-year traditions suggest efficacy.
Palliative care physicians should consider:
Acupuncture for relaxation and pain
Herbal therapies for relaxation
Meditation for stress reduction
Support groups to improve quality of life and coping skills
Massage for muscle relaxation and general sense of well-being
Prayer for spiritual needs
Use holistic model for medical care.

niques, then the use of complementary techniques is clearly valid and appropriate. Furthermore, it is clear that patients use complementary approaches with or without their doctor's knowledge or recommendation, and it therefore behooves physicians to recognize that their patients may well be visiting complementary medical practitioners. That being the case, it is better that physician and complementary medicine practitioner work together as a team, understanding what each team member can add to the overall care and healing of the patient (36). Acupuncture, electroacupuncture, and transcutaneous nerve stimulation can all be used to reduce chemotherapy-induced nausea and emesis, reduce pain, and be useful for other syndromes such as migraines. Herbal remedies have been used for thousands of years and some seem to be useful in reducing stress, giving a calming influence, perhaps reducing the side effects of chemotherapy, acting as a "tonic," and just providing the general pleasant effects of a good cup of tea. The mind–body approaches of meditation can reduce stress or create a positive mental atti-

Table 8 Holistic (Healing) Model of Medical Care

Standard (science-based) medicine
Symptom-based therapy
Example: Relief of pain
Attention to preventive medicine
Example: Diet, exercise, stess reduction, massage
Attention to psychological needs
Example: Financial counseling, home health care
Attention to spiritual needs
Example: Meditation, prayer

Table 9 Goals of Medicine

Cure
Promoting health
Preventing illness and injury
Restoring functional capacity
Avoiding premature death
Relief of suffering
Caring for those who cannot be cured

tude. Massage can reduce stress, reduce pain, and, in general, energize the recipient. These practices need to be incorporated into the curricula of academic medical centers so that the physicians know and understand these techniques; more importantly, there is a need for a fundamental shift from the curative model to the holistic model of medical care, which focuses on the patient and not the disease. The holistic medical model recognizes that the cure of disease is not the only goal of medicine (Table 9), recognizes that disease symptoms are worthy of direct treatment, accepts death as the natural conclusion of life when the underlying disease cannot be cured, and accepts that true holistic medicine includes attention to psychological, social, cultural and spiritual concerns, and needs of the patient and the patient's family. Once the holistic model of medical care is accepted, complementary approaches will become part of the mainstream.

REFERENCES

1. Fox E. Predominance of the curative model of medical care. A residual problem. JAMA 1997; 278:761–763.
2. Billings JA, Block S. Palliative care in undergraduate medical education. Status report and future directions. JAMA 1997; 278:733–738.
3. Christakis DA, Feudtner C. Temporary matters: the ethical consequences of transient social relationships in medical training. JAMA 1997; 278:739–743.
4. Gordon JS. Alternative medicine and the family physician. Am Fam Phys 1996; 54: 2205–2210.
5. Eisenberg DM, Kessler RC, Foster C, et al. Unconventional medicine in the United States. N Engl J Med 1993; 328:246–252.
6. *Wall Street Journal*, April 14, 1997, p B1.
7. Gould KL, Ornish D, Scherwitz L, et al. Changes in myocardial perfusion abnormalities by positron emission tomography after long-term, intense risk factor modification. JAMA 1995; 274:894–901.
8. Ornish D, Brown SB, Scherwitz LW, et al. Can life style changes reverse coronary heart disease? The Lifestyle Heart Trial. Lancet 1990; 336:129–133.

9. Ornish D. Program for Reversing Heart Disease. New York: Ballantine Books, 1990.
10. Alternative medicine: the facts. *Consumer Reports*, January, 1994.
11. Furnham A, Kirkcaldy B. The health beliefs and behaviors of orthodox and complementary medicine clients. Br J Clin Psychol 1996; 35:49–61.
12. Vincent C, Furnham A. Why do patients turn to complementary medicine? An empirical study. Br J Clin Psychol 1996; 35:37–48.
13. Lerner M. Choices in Healing: Integrating the Best of Conventional and Complementary Approaches to Cancer. Cambridge, MA: MIT Press, 1994.
14. Vickers AJ. Can acupuncture have specific effects on health? A systematic review of acupuncture antiemesis trials. J R Soc Med 1996; 89:303–311.
15. Dundee JW. Belfast experience with P6 acupuncture antiemesis. Ulster Med J 1990; 59:63–70.
16. Thomas M. Acupuncture studies on patient. Acupunc Med 1997; 15:23–31.
17. Berman BM, Lao L, Greene M, et al. Efficacy of traditional Chinese acupuncture in the treatment of symptomatic knee osteoarthritis: a pilot study. Osteoarth Cartil 1995; 3:139–142.
18. Lao L, Wong RL, Berman BM. Efficacy of Chinese acupuncture on postoperative oral surgery pain. Oral Surg Oral Med Oral Pathol 1995; 79:423–428.
19. Moyers B. Healing and the Mind. New York: Doubleday, 1993.
20. Cooper M, Aygen M. Effect of meditation on blood cholesterol and blood pressure. Harefuah 1978; 95:1–2.
21. Chopra D. Quantum healing: exploring the frontiers of mind-body medicine. New York: Bantam Books, 1989.
22. Benson H. The Relaxation Response. New York: William Morrow, 1975.
23. Gore MM. Effect of yogic treatment on some pulmonary functions in asthmatics. Yoga Mimamsa 1982; 20:51–58.
24. Dreher H. The scientific and moral imperative for broad-based psychosocial interventions for cancer. Advances: J Mind-Body Health 1997; 13:38–49.
25. Spiegel D, Bloom J, Kraemer HC, et al. Effect of psychosocial treatment on survival of patients with metastatic breast cancer. *Lancet* 1989; 2:888–891.
26. Fawzy FI, Fawzy NW, Hyun CS, et al. Malignant melanoma: effects of an early structured psychiatric intervention, coping, and affective state on recurrence and survival 6 years later. Arch Gen Psychiatry 1993; 50:681–689.
27. Richardson JL, Shelton DR, Krailo M, et al. The effect of compliance with treatment on survival among patients with hematologic malignancies. J Clin Oncol 1990; 8: 356–364.
28. Dossey L. Recovering the Soul: A Scientific and Spiritual Search. New York: Bantam Books, 1989.
29. Targ E. Evaluating distant healing: a research review. *Alternative Therapies* 1997; 3:74–78.
30. Byrd RC. Positive therapeutic effects of intercessory prayer in a coronary care unit population. South Med J 1988; 81:826–829.
31. Besedovsky HO, Herberman RB, Temoshok LR, et al. Psychoneuroimmunology and Cancer: Fifteenth Sapporo Cancer Seminar meeting report. Cancer Res 1996; 56: 4278–4281.

32. Field T. Massage therapy for infants and children. J Develop Behav Pediatr 1995; 16:105–111.
33. Warren K. "Will I be sick, nurse?" Nurs Times 1988; 84:53–54.
34. Sims S. Slow stroke back massage for cancer patients. Nurs Times 1986; 82:47–50.
35. Krieger D. Therapeutic touch: the imprimatur of nursing. Am J Nurs 1975; 75:784–787.
36. Eisenberg DM. Advising patients who seek alternative medical therapies. Ann Intern Med 1997; 127:61–69.

31

Hospice and Palliative Care

Elizabeth LeTourneau-Lee
Hospice of the Valley, Phoenix, Arizona

Michael E. Frederich
San Diego Hospice, San Diego, California

I. INTRODUCTION

Improving care of persons as they near the end of life is receiving more attention than ever from the medical profession. The debate on assisted suicide and euthanasia has focused both medical and public attention on dying. Whereas death has often been viewed as an enemy to be fought and abhorred at all costs, a more realistic acceptance of its inevitability has led many health care providers and professionals to acknowledge a need for more information to improve care for patients who are terminally ill.

Death is difficult to talk about, even difficult to think about. Death is neither a concept nor a medical rarity, yet dying is not to be viewed as a simple event. Death is a family disease. Nobody dies in isolation, despite the current trends to keep the dying patient remote. Death occurs in a context, and the most immediate context is that of the family. The family ''dies'' along with the patient and no longer continues in its previous form. The family context must be renegotiated and redefined, and it must reemerge, using a new set of givens that do not include, except for memories, the deceased (1). The relatively quick dying trajectories of a few days or weeks as a result of infectious diseases has been replaced by the often years of dying with cancer. With the small nuclear family scattered across a mobile society replacing the larger extended families of the past, the burdens that the dying places on the family are greater than ever. In response, society attempts to remove death from being a personal experience to being an institutional experience. Despite the existence of effective in-home palliative care in hospice, most individuals still die outside their home environment, in hospitals and nursing homes.

Part of the problem in integrating hospice and palliative care into mainstream medicine is the continued lack of acceptance by health care professionals and patients that, regardless of the quality or quantity of sophisticated medical treatment available, cure is not always possible for all cancer patients. Acceptance of this fact is understandably difficult for many health care professionals, particularly if associated with individual patients with whom providers have built a very close relationship of trust. If the goal of acute medical care is to restore patients to their once healthy normal lives, then the failure to reach this goal with terminally ill patients is ultimately frustrating (2). The only rational approach is to change the goal of cure to one of providing comfort and quality time for the patient nearing the end of life.

In a sense, the ever increasing integration of hospice and palliative care with traditional health care delivery systems is a symbol of the maturation and evolution of health care in the United States, United Kingdom, and other countries. This is a symbol that medicine has begun to accept its limitations and has matured sufficiently as it continues to grow in different, viable directions. When cure may no longer be possible, the need for patient and family comfort becomes more compelling (2). Eric Cassell, M.D., stated the following (3):

> It is a sad fact that serious illness is attended by sorrow and pain. Bad when medical care fails to relieve them, it is even worse when medical care adds to the suffering.

If the attempt to reverse the course of malignant disease is futile and only leads to prolonged pain and suffering for the patient and family, then the decision to change the pattern and goal of care to provide more satisfying results become a logical one. In an age when medical science and technology have affected overwhelming advances in health care, embracing the hospice philosophy of palliation and patient and family comfort requires both a willingness to accept limitations and the ability to anticipate opportunities for growth (2).

Providing patient and family comfort through hospice requires, by definition, a holistic approach that encompasses medical, nursing, psychosocial, spiritual, and ultimately bereavement care. The patient and the family are the unit of care. This approach makes hospice unique in the health care field (2). But hospice is more than just support and hand-holding. Interventions for comforts are just as intense and innovative as those invasive techniques required to save lives. In fact, palliative care requires more attention to detail to be effective than acute care does, in that it deals with the whole person, not just a disease.

Through exposure to medical information in the media, patients are better informed and have greater expectations of medicine. Patients and their families are becoming more responsible for their own health care and are asking intelligent, direct questions and expecting honest answers. Reviewing some of these questions highlights issues to be addressed during end of life care:

Will the pain be worse as I get closer to death?
What if I cannot talk and I am in pain. How will anyone know?
If I take medication now, what will I use toward the end?
I am afraid I will not be safe and will be abandoned.
Will medical care be available any time of day or night?
Will my doctor be open and honest with me?
Can I express my feelings about my illness and personal matters?
Will I be able to maintain normal relationships with my family?
Will I be a burden on my family?
Will the doctor and nurses respect my wishes when I am unable to speak?
Will I be able to finish all my business?
What will my illness and my death be like?
Will visitors understand how tired I am?
Will my family be comfortable touching and holding me?
Is this disease contagious?
Will I be able to cry without upsetting everyone?
Will I be treated as a living person, not someone who is already dead?

Hospice has meant a place of rest or shelter on the journey from birth to death. Particularly as death approaches and symptoms may be making the journey more difficult, hospice programs offer care and comfort combined with expert professional services. Many people think that hospice means a place to die. It is not. It is a program and philosophy of health care to provide comfort for individuals approaching the end of life. Many of those who enter a hospice program are near the close of their lives, yet all hospice programs are able to discharge a small proportion of their patients. Indeed, it sometimes happens that the care and refreshment offered enables the patient to take a new lease on life, leave the hospice for a period of time, and continue further active living (4).

II. HISTORY OF HOSPICE

During the Middle Ages, the words hospice, hospital, and hostel were used almost interchangeably. These entities, known generally as "traveler's rest," provided food and shelter, as well as care for those sick or dying. Two of these original hospices founded in the 10th century AD still exist: The Hospices of the Great St. Bernard and the Little St. Bernard in Switzerland.

Hospices continued to evolve for care of the sick and incurable. The word hospice became synonymous with care of the terminally ill in the late 19th century with the founding of Our Lady's Hospice in Dublin, Ireland, by Sister May Aikenhead of the Sisters of Charity, who was a contemporary of Florence Nightingale. St. Joseph's Hospice was established in 1900 in London and later became a training ground for Dame Cicely Saunders.

In the 1960s, Dame Cicely Saunders began refining the treatments and protocols that formed the cornerstone of modern hospice care. Starting her health care career as a nurse, she became a social worker and later a physician who developed her own postgraduate training in palliative care. In 1967, she founded St. Christopher's Hospice in London, which has served as the model for modern hospice care. Dame Saunders believed that, whereas modern medicine was primarily motivated toward cure or prolonged survival of cancer patients, such aggressive care was often inappropriate and even counterproductive for dying patients. She has continued to teach this philosophy, influencing the worldwide hospice movement, and St. Christopher's Hospice has pioneered techniques and palliative interventions that have come to be considered standards of care for the terminally ill.

Development of hospice in North America followed that in the United Kingdom. The Palliative Care Service at the Royal Victoria Hospital in Montreal, Canada, was started by Balfour Mount, M.D., in 1975. Following a lecture by Dame Cicely Saunders at Yale University, Florence Wald, Dean of the Yale School of Nursing, founded The Connecticut Hospice in 1974. This hospice opened a 44-bed inpatient unit in 1979, the first such inpatient facility in the United States.

In 1983, The Tax Equity Fiscal Responsibility Act created the Hospice Medicare Benefit in the United States. This act provided financial reimbursement for the first time for hospice care in the United States, which prior to this time had been provided on a completely voluntary basis. In the intervening 15 years, more than 2500 hospice programs have been created in the United States so that, currently, most communities have hospice care available. The Hospice Medicare Benefit defined hospice in a way that has influenced other countries to explore a more comprehensive hospice program.

III. PHILOSOPHY OF CARE

Hospice is not a place or facility. It is a philosophy of care that can be applied to care for terminally ill patients in any setting (2). Perhaps the largest reason for the rapid growth in popularity of hospice care has been the comfort and support provided to the patients and families. While hospice care is often considered ''high-touch,'' not ''high-tech,'' palliative care and hospice have been on the forefront of new interventions, complex pain management, and techniques that make symptom management more effective. Dying patients and their families are concerned that pain and symptoms remain controlled and thus seek out available hospice care. A significant measure of comfort is also provided by allowing the patients to be in the familiar surroundings of their homes, surrounded by loving family and friends. Peace of mind is assured for the patient, because hospice inpatient care is readily available in case needs arise that cannot be met in the home.

The following are key concepts of the hospice philosophy of care:

1. The patient and family (as defined by the patient) are the single unit of care.
2. The hospice uses a core interdisciplinary team (physician, nurse, social worker, and chaplain) to address the physical, social, emotional, and spiritual needs of the patient and family.
3. The hospice provides for the medical treatment and control of pain and other distressing symptoms associated with the terminal illness, but does not provide interventions to cure the disease or prolong life.
4. The interdisciplinary team develops the overall plan of care, in collaboration with the patient and family, to provide coordinated care that emphasizes supportive services such as home care, respite care, pain management, and inpatient services.
5. The hospice actively engages the community by using volunteer support in coordination with paid professional staff in delivering its services.
6. The patient's home, or place of primary residence (such as a nursing home), is the primary site of care.
7. The philosophy of hospice emphasizes comfort, dignity, and quality of life, with the focus on the patient's spiritual and existential issues.
8. The hospice empowers the patients and families to achieve as much control over their lives as possible.

The National Hospice Organization Arlington, Virginia, describes hospice as a specialized form of interdisciplinary health care designed to provide palliative care (relief of pain and uncomfortable symptoms as opposed to curative care); alleviate the physical, emotional, social, and spiritual discomforts of an individual who is experiencing the last phase of life as a result of the existence of a terminal disease; and provide supportive care to the primary care giver and the family of the hospice patient.

The hospice philosophy of care allows the physician, nurse, social worker, counselors, and clergy to create a supportive environment where a terminally ill patient may die with dignity and without pain. Dignity, of course, is defined by the patient as dying in ''their character.'' The hospice philosophy commands that both the patient and family be viewed as the unit of care, allowing the patient as much control as possible while attending to physical, spiritual, emotional, and psychological issues. This is not to imply that the hospice philosophy of care is not part of the traditional health care system, hospice was started, at least in part, in response to patients' dissatisfaction and often frustrations to failures of traditional health care to provide adequately for the needs of the terminally ill, especially in the area of pain relief.

As the hospice philosophy of care continues to become an acceptable option for terminally ill patients, it is clear that traditional curative health care and hospice palliation are neither mutually exclusive nor in competition, but rather they complement each other.

IV. INTERDISCIPLINARY CARE

Palliative care requires an interdisciplinary team (IDT) to provide holistic care to the dying patient and his or her family. An IDT differs from the more familiar health care model multidisciplinary team (MDT) in several important ways, the most distinguishing characteristic being the relationship between team members. In an IDT, the identity of the team supercedes individual professional identities and leadership is shared among team members depending on the task at hand. The IDT members share information directly and work together to develop goals, whereas MDT members share information using the medical record. Most importantly, in an IDT, the team is the vehicle of action and the interactional process is vital to success, whereas in an MDT, the interactional process is somewhat irrelevant. In an IDT, all members are aware of the overall plan of care and often provide care that is not strictly within the limits of their professional roles. They often experience a blurring of roles.

This is the beauty of the hospice interdisciplinary team—the distinct disciplines of medicine, nursing, social work, clergy, counselor, volunteer, and others—working together without barriers with the patient and family so that the patient's needs may be met. Managing the pain and the symptoms associated with terminal illness, the IDT members emphasize inpatient medical interventions that are appropriate and adequate for each hospice patient. Providers also concentrate on providing appropriate psychosocial interventions to ease the stress that patients and families experience (5). The top three goals must be patient/family, patient/family, patient/family. It is crucial that the team focuses on the patient's quality of life. Open communication, critical thinking, and a supportive environment are paramount to ensure these needs are met (6).

Although the role of the physician is crucial to the success of the interdisciplinary team, it may be somewhat complicated and is discussed in a separate section of this chapter.

The nurse plays a significant role on the team. The nurse bears most of the responsibility for carefully assessing the patient's condition and for organizing and integrating the care. The nurse must communicate frequently with the attending physician or the hospice physician and the other interdisciplinary team members. Hospice nurses usually serve as primary care providers and, with time and experience, become the experts in palliative interventions. For this reason, it is crucial that physicians respect hospice nurses and their suggestions for care, even beyond the traditional level. If a hospice inpatient unit has a defined set of protocols and standing orders, signed by the physician, the nurses may initiate interventions and referrals both within and outside traditional hospice and palliative care.

The hospice social worker often serves as counselor in addition to providing traditional medical social work interventions. Helping with advance directives, living wills, funeral arrangements, and initiating bereavement support are common hospice social work tasks not often provided by social workers in other medical fields.

Hospice clergy and chaplains communicate and relate with the patient and family's own spiritual leader to coordinate care to assure that spiritual needs are being met. After developing close relationships with patients, it is the hospice chaplain who often is asked to participate in, if not officiate at, the funeral service. Both the social worker and chaplain offer special support to the IDT and other staff members and volunteers, especially in an inpatient unit.

Volunteers provide many services to patients and their families. These include providing support and visits to lonely individuals, as well as performing tasks and errands that the patient and family are unable to perform themselves. The most needed service they provide is staying with the patient while the family relaxes, relieving them of the continuous pressures of caring for their loved one. Volunteers are expected to complete a structured training program and commit to several hours a week. They are an integral part of the IDT, bringing life experiences, personal talents, and the community to the patient.

Therapists are available in the care of the patient and include but are not limited to the following: physical therapists, occupational therapists, respiratory therapists, music therapists, art therapists, speech therapists, pharmacists, and dietitians. Both music and art therapy can be quite helpful, especially when the patient has trouble with self-expression. If a therapist is involved with a patient, then the therapist becomes a member of the IDT.

V. PAIN MANAGEMENT AND PALLIATIVE CARE

Palliative medicine (the term came from the Latin word pallium, meaning "cloak," and connotes a sense of protection) emerged from the hospice movement begun by Dame Cicely Saunders. Hospice does not mean to imply custodial care. Palliative care (symptom control) requires the clinician to be able to carefully evaluate and assess pain or an uncontrolled symptom and then to apply interventions and techniques to relieve the pain or symptom.

Palliative care is defined by the World Health Organization as follows (7):

> The active total care of patients whose disease is not responsive to curative treatment. Control of pain, of other symptoms, and of psychological, social, and spiritual problems, is paramount. The goal of palliative care is achievement of the best quality of life for patients and their families. Many aspects of palliative care are also applicable earlier in the course of the illness in conjunction with anticancer treatment.
>
> Palliative care: . . . affirms life and regards dying as a normal process, . . . neither hastens nor postpones death, . . . provides relief from pain and other distressing symptoms, . . . integrates the psychological and the spiritual aspects of care, . . . offers a support system to help patients live as actively as possible until death, . . . offers a support system to help family cope during the patient's illness and in their own bereavement.

A simpler definition of palliative medicine proposed by Sir William Osler is as follows:

To cure sometimes
To relieve often
To comfort always

Whereas palliative care is dependent on a defined body of knowledge, specific interventions are tailored to meet individual patient goals. There are, however, three goals, which, if met will ensure excellent palliative care for most individuals. These were first written by Eric Cassell, M.D., in his book *The Nature of Suffering and the Goals of Medicine* (3):

> All diagnostic or therapeutic plans be made in terms of the sick person, not the disease.
> To maximize the patient's function, not necessarily the length of life.
> To minimize the suffering of the patient and family.

An example of palliative care is to provide corticosteroids that will improve function but may in fact shorten life in an immunocompromised individual. Routine testing, for instance weekly hemoglobin measurement or radiological assessment, is usually not done in palliative care, unless therapeutic intervention depends on the result of the test. Testing is not done merely to follow the course of the disease progression.

Pain management was revolutionized through the work of Dame Cicely Saunders at St. Christopher's Hospice in London. Development of the prescription of oral opioids on a routine scheduled basis became a significant part of palliative care. This system of opioids scheduled "around-the-clock" rather than on an ''as-needed'' basis has greatly influenced and changed the way physicians order medications for the management of chronic pain.

Patients experiencing an agonal phase of chronic pain may require initially higher doses of an opioid to break the pain-anxiety cycle; therefore, a high initial dose of opioid is often indicated. The clinician should realize that severe pain is exhausting and usually precludes restful sleep. Thus, it is common for a patient to sleep for many hours after an adequate dose of analgesic. Such sleep alone does not indicate overdosage or sedation (8). Many well-done studies have confirmed that addiction and tolerance are not issues for individuals receiving strong opioids for chronic cancer pain. There should be less paranoia on the part of physicians that may inhibit prescription of adequate doses of opioid for pain management.

The optimal dose of an opioid is determined through titration and assessment for effectiveness. Allowing a smaller, immediate-release opioid dose for breakthrough or incidental pain in addition to a routine scheduled dose completes opioid management. Continuous pain requires regular preventive therapy. The aim is to balance the dose of the analgesic against the patient's pain, gradually increasing the dose until the patient is pain free. The next dose is given before the effect of the previous one has worn off. In this way, it is possible to erase the memory and fear of pain (8). Using adjunctive medications such as anti-inflammatories, antidepressants, anticonvulsants, and anxiolytics in addition to the opioids ensure control of opiate-resistant pain (Tables 1, 2, and 3).

Dr. Robert Twycross has drawn up a list of ten commandments for physicians dealing with the pain of cancer (9):

1. Thou shalt not assume that the patient's pain is due to the malignant process.
2. Thou shalt try simple analgesics in the first instance.
3. Thou shalt not be afraid of narcotic drugs.
4. Thou shalt not prescribe inadequate amounts of any analgesic.
5. Thou shalt not use the abbreviation PRN.
6. Thou shalt take into consideration the patient's feelings.
7. Thou shalt provide support for the whole family.
8. Thou shalt not limit thy approach simply to the use of drugs.
9. Thou shalt not be afraid to ask colleague's advice.
10. Thou shalt have an air of quiet confidence and cautious optimism.

Complications of dying come before death and it is the responsibility of the health care team to use keen and intelligent assessment skills, including listening carefully to the patient and family members. The response and treatment decision require excellent clinical skills and often, imagination. The entire interdisciplinary team is involved. Reviewing current medications and making necessary changes for the patient's comfort, sitting with the patient and listening, and occa-

Table 1 Hospice Inpatient Facility Protocols

Pain management	
1. Mild	a. Enteric coated ASA 5–10 gr PO/PR q4–6 h. b. Acetaminophen 500–1000 mg PO q4–6 h or 650 mg PR q4–6 h (limit 4000 mg/24 h). c. Ibuprofen 200–400 mg PO/PR q4–6 h (limit 3200 mg/24 h).
2. Moderate	a. Acetaminophen with Codeine #3 1–2 tabs PO q4–6 h. b. Roxicet tabs or liquid 5–10 mg PO q4–6 h.
3. Severe	Initiating and Titrating Morphine and/or Dilaudid: a. Morphine sulfate immediate release (MSIR) dose: MSIR 10–80 mg PO/PR/SL q1–4 h PRN. May give additional dose q30 min × 2 for severe pain; or, 3–30 mg SQ q1–4 h or, 2–5 mg IVP q10–15 min. May titrate by increasing dose 25%–50% of last dose as stated in AHCPR guidelines. b. Morphine long-acting dose (MS Contin): May convert to long-acting form of morphine after titration of immediate release morphine over past 24–48 h. Conversion does not include doses for incident pain. To calculate: add total mg of MSIR in past 24 h and divide by 2 to get correct MS Contin 12-h dose. After conversion, MSIR dose for breakthrough pain is 1/4–1/2 of long-acting 12-h dose or 1/6 of 24-h dose q1–4 h PRN. After 3–4 doses of breakthrough MSIR, convert to higher dose of MS Contin and increase breakthrough dose accordingly. c. Dilaudid 2–8 mg PO/PR q3–4 h; or 0.25–1 mg SQ q3–4 h.
Adjunctive pain management	
1. Skeletal/bone	a. Ibuprofen 200–800 mg PO/PR q4–6 h (limit 3200 mg/24 h.) Give with food.. b. Trilisate 750–1000 mg PO/PR BID (will not upset GI tract or deplete platelets; available in liquid). c. Decadron 2–4 mg PO/PR q6 h. Give with food.

2. Neuropathic	a. Pamelor 10–50 mg PO qhs. b. Depakene 250 mg qhs × 2 nights; if pain continues, 500 mg qhs × 2 nights; if pain continues, 750 mg qhs × 2 nights; if pain continues, 1000 mg qhs (valproic acid level needed). Note: May combine Pamelor and Depakene for severe neuropathic pain. c. Neurontin 300 mg qhs × 2 nights; if pain continues, 300 mg BID × 2 days; if pain continues, 300 mg TID. Note: May combine with Pamelor and/or Depakene for severe uncontrolled neuropathic pain. If pain continues, call physician for further orders.
3. Mass effect	a. Decadron 12–24 mg PO/PR Q/d in divided doses. Give with food.
Anxiety/agitation	a. Ativan 0.5–2 mg PO/SL/PR/SQ/IV q2–3 h PRN or ATC. b. Haldol 1–5 mg PO/PR/IM q6–8 h PRN or ATC. c. Valium 5–10 mg PO/PR q4–6 h PRN or ATC. Note: To avoid Ativan and Valium withdrawal symptoms, do not abruptly discontinue either unless exchanging Ativan for Valium. May combine Ativan and Haldol or Valium and Haldol.
Nausea/vomiting	a. Compazine 5–10 mg PO/IM/SQ/IV or 25 mg PR q4–6 h; may add Benadryl 25 mg PO/PR q4 h and/or Reglan 10 mg SQ/IM/IV/PO q6–8 h PRN/ATC. b. May use Haldol 0.5–1.5 mg PO/SL or 1–2 mg IM q1–2 h with above, or alone for nausea due to opioids. c. Phenergan 12.5–25 mg PO/PR q4–6 h PRN. d. For continuous, uncontrollable nausea/vomiting, start Metoclophen PO/PR (compound by pharmacist to include: Reglan 20 mg, Cogentin 1 mg, Decadron 10 mg, Haldol 1 mg, Dramamine 50 mg). Give 1 PO/PR q6–8 h ATC. This is not a PRN medication. If/when desired response is noted, gradually decrease dosage to q12 h, then to q24 h, then DC. Note: DC all prior medications for nausea/vomiting when starting Metoclophen. For phenothiazine-induced EPS side effects, give Cogentin 1 mg IM, may repeat × 1 in 10 min, or Benadryl 50 mg IM/IV × 1.
Dyspnea	a. Morphine Sulfate (MSIR) 5–20 mg PO/SL/PR q1–4 h PRN or 2–8 mg SQ q1–4 h. Titrate until desired response keeping respiratory rate >10–12/min. b. Ativan 0.5–2 mg PO/SL q2–4 h PRN. c. SVN unit dose albuterol sulfate q2 h PRN for respiratory distress. d. SVN 5 mg MSIR in 3 cc N/S q2–4 h PRN for respiratory distress.

Table 1 Continued

Chest pain	a. Nitroglycerin (NTG) tabs 0.4 mg (1/150gr). Give 1 tab SL q5min × 3 doses. If no relief, refer to pain management protocol and follow.
Terminal restlessness/severe agitation	a. Ativan 0.5–2 mg PO/SL/PR/SQ/IV q1–2 h PRN or ATC. Call physician for increased dosages, no limit on Ativan. b. Haldol 10 mg PO/SL/PR/IM q30min × 1 or 2 loading dose; then Haldol 2–5 mg PO/SL/PR/IM q6–8 h PRN or ATC. May use with Ativan. c. For severe agitation/combativeness/psychosis or if above medications ineffective, add Thorazine 50–100 mg PO/SL/PR/SQ/IM q1–2 h until sedation achieved, up to 400 mg/24 h. d. For unrelieved severe agitation/combativeness/psychosis, phenobarbital 65–200 mg IM/IVP × 1 loading dose. Notify physician. Note: To avoid Ativan withdrawal symptoms, do not abruptly discontinue Ativan.
Pulmonary congestion	a. Atropine sulfate 1% drops, 1–2 gtt SL q4–6 h PRN. b. Scopolamine (250 mcg/0.1 cc) gel, 0.1 cc topically q6 h ATC. c. Scopolamine enemas (0.5 mg/cc in 5 cc water, solution made by pharmacist) PR q4–12 h PRN or ATC. Note: May combine any of the above for severe pulmonary congestion.
Insomnia	a. Benadryl 25–50 mg PO/PR qhs. May repeat × 1 PRN. b. Ambien 5–10 mg PO qhs. May repeat × 1 PRN. c. Restoril 15–30 mg PO qhs PRN. May repeat 15 mg × 1 in 1 h PRN. d. Ativan 0.5–2 mg PO/SL/PR qhs. e. Desyrel 50–400 mg PO qhs (preferable for insomnia with depression).

Candidiasis	a. Nystatin swish and swallow liquid (100,000 U/mL) 4–6 mL PO QID × 5 d. May repeat. b. Diflucan 200 mg PO × 1 d; then 100 mg QID × 5 d. c. Sporanox 10–20 mL QID × 7 d.
Bowel regimen	a. Senna 1 tab PO for every 30 mg of long-acting morphine sulfate and Colace 100 mg PO for every 30 mg of long-acting morphine sulfate up to 8 tabs Q/d. b. Dulcolax tabs 2–8 PO or Dulcolax suppository PR Q/day. c. Magnesium citrate, 1–2 doses PO daily. d. If no results in 3 days, use sorbital/lactulose up to 30–60 mL PO BID.
Bladder spasms	a. Ditropam 5–10 mg q6–8 h until symptoms resolve. b. Urispas 100–200 mg PO q6 h PRN. c. B & O suppository PR q6 h PRN.
Itching	a. Benadryl 25–50 mg PO q4–6 h PRN. b. If not responding within 4 h, may use Vistaril 25 mg PO q3–4 h PRN.
Seizures	a. Ativan 2 mg SL q2 h or 2 mg/min slow IVP up to 20 mg b. If no IV access, then give Valium enema PR (10 mg in 5 mL water, solution made by pharmacist) up to 4 times in 30 min. c. If no response, give 1 dose of phenobarbital 200 mg IM and notify physician. d. If status epilepticus, start Dilantin 20 mg/kg IV at 50 mg/min. Notify physician.
Intractable hiccups	a. Thorazine 25–50 mg PO/SL/PR/IM q4 h PRN or ATC. b. Baclofen 5–10 mg PO/PR q8 h ATC. May use with Thorazine.
Anaphylactic reaction	a. Epinephrine (1:1000) 0.5–1 mg SQ/IM or 0.25–0.5 mg IV. May repeat at 10–15 min intervals until desired response.

Table 2 Hospice and Palliative Care Drugs Used in Table 1

Ambien	zolpidem tartrate
ASA	acetylsalicylic acid (aspirin)
Ativan	lorazepam
Atropine sulfate	1% opthalmic solution
Benadryl	diphenhydramine HCL
Cogentin	benztropine mesylate
Colace	docusate sodium
Compazine	prochlorperazine
Decadron	dexamethasone
Depakene	valproic acid (therapeutic blood level 50–100 μg/mL)
Desyrel	trazodone HCL
Diflucan	fluconazole
Dilantin	phenytoin
Dilaudid	hydromorphone
Ditropan	oxybutynin chloride
Dramamine	dimenhydrinate
Dulcolax	bisacodyl
Haldol	haloperidol
MSIR	morphine sulfate, liquid concentrate 20 mg/mL, 100 mg/mL; suppositories 10 mg, 20 mg, 30 mg
MS Contin	morphine sulfate, controlled release 15 mg, 30 mg, 60 mg, 100 mg, 200 mg (may be given PR)
Neurontin	gabapentin
Pamelor	nortriptyline
Phenergan	promethazine HCL
Reglan	metoclopramide
Restoril	temazepam
Roxicet (Percocet)	tablets: 500 mg acetaminophen and 5 mg oxycodone liquid: 325 mg acetaminophen and 5 mg/5 mL oxycodone
Scopolamine	hyoscine
Sporanox	itraconazole
Trilisate	choline magnesium trisalicylate (<1500 mg/d—pain relief only; >1500 mg/d—pain relief and anti-inflammatory)
Thorazine	chlorpromazine HCL
Urispas	flavoxate HCL
Valium	diazepam
Vistaril	hydroxyzine HCL
Other Drugs Commonly Used in Hospices	
Elavil	amitriptyline HCL
Klonopin	clonazepam
Mellaril	thioridazine HCL
Oxycontin	oxycodone HCL controlled-release tablets 10 mg, 20 mg, 40 mg (may be given PR)
Versed	midazolam (used SQ in combination with other drugs for aggressive palliation)

Table 3 Hospice Inpatient Facility Standing Orders

1. Admit to hospice inpatient facility.
   Patient has a diagnosis of ______ and is in the later stages of a terminal illness.
2. Do not resuscitate.
3. Activity and diet as tolerated.
4. Continue current opioid. Titrate to maintain patient comfort according to pain management protocols.
5. May continue current medications at time of admission.
6. May insert indwelling urinary catheter PRN; may use lidocaine gel on catheter tip PRN for comfort.
7. Bowel care of choice.
8. Skin care/wound care as appropriate.
9. Patient may have over the counter medications PRN for comfort.
10. Oxygen at 2–4 L/min per nasal cannula, PRN for comfort only.
11. May use normal saline solution or sterile water for routine irrigation including catheters, G-tubes and NG tubes.
12. May use protective device or bed siderails only as needed for patient safety.
13. May give medications PRN and/or ATC (around the clock) as appropriate for the patient's comfort/needs.
14. May discontinue medications or change route of administration as related to patient tolerance.
15. Patient may go out on pass if not on GIP (acute) status.
16. IV or SQ access device may be initiated PRN to establish route for implementation of parenteral medication. Care of IV or SQ site and tubing per hospice protocol.
17. May insert NG tube to gravity or low intermittent suction PRN for nausea/vomiting.
18. Oral/pharyngeal suction PRN for airway congestion.
19. Pharmacy may substitute generic equivalent.
20. Hospice medical director may consult when indicated.
21. If unable to reach attending physician within 4 h, may contact hospice medical director for orders.
22. May institute hospice standing orders and protocols.
23. Attending physician may delete or add to this list as needed.

Abbreviations: PRN, as needed; IV, intravenous; SQ, subcutaneous; G, gastric; NG, nasogastric; ATC, around the clock; GIP, general inpatient.

sionally intervening with a medical procedure are equally important parts of palliative care. This total concept of care must be available 24 hours per day, regardless of the location of the patient.

A patient's pain, physical and/or emotional, could serve as a roadblock from the important work of closure or "putting my house in order," before dying. For patients who choose hospice, the clinician can offer a variety of services, medication, and support to begin to eliminate these roadblocks.

It is the responsibility of every health care provider to provide adequate pain and symptom relief for patients nearing the end of life. If an individual is unable or unwilling to provide such relief, consultation or referral should be completed.

VI. APPROACHING DEATH, HELPFUL CLARIFICATIONS FOR FAMILIES

When a person enters the final stage of the dying process, two different dynamics are at work that are closely interrelated and interdependent. On the physical plane, the body begins the final process of shutting down, which will end when all the physical systems cease to function. Usually this is an orderly and undramatic progressive series of physical changes that are not medical emergencies requiring invasive interventions. These physical changes are a normal, natural way in which the body prepares itself to stop, and the most appropriate kinds of responses are comfort-enhancing measures.

The other dynamic of the dying process at work is on the emotional-spiritual-mental plane and is a different kind of process. The spirit of the dying person begins the final process of release from the body, its immediate environment, and all attachments. This release also tends to follow its own priorities, which may include the resolution of whatever is unfinished of a practical nature and reception of permission to "let go" from family members. These events are the normal, natural way in which the spirit prepares to move from this existence into the next dimension of life. The most appropriate kinds of responses to the emotional-spiritual-mental changes are those that support and encourage this release and transition.

When a person's body is ready and wanting to stop but the person is still unresolved or unreconciled over some important issue or with some significant relationship, he or she may tend to linger to finish whatever needs finishing, even though he or she may be uncomfortable or debilitated. On the other hand, when a person is emotionally, spiritually, and mentally resolved and ready for this release but the body has not completed its final physical shutdown, the person continues to live until that shutdown process ceases.

The experience called death occurs when the body completes its natural process of shutting down and when the spirit completes its natural process of reconciling and finishing. These two processes need to happen in a way appropriate and unique to the values, beliefs, and lifestyle of the dying person (10).

The following are a few signs and symptoms that impending death is close. Not all of these signs and symptoms occur in every patient, nor do they always occur in this particular sequence. Refer to Table 1 for medication suggestions to ease some of the symptoms.

Coolness and color of skin changes
Sleeping
Disorientation
Incontinence
Pulmonary congestion
Terminal restlessness
Decreased urine and/or bowel output
Decreased fluid and food intake
Breathing pattern changes
Withdrawal from family and/or friends
Decreased socialization
Unusual communication and nearing death awareness
Visual sightings that others cannot see

Patients have communicated their time of death in many ways to family members and staff. When dressing a patient in a ''fancy'' dress for the day, one woman stated, ''Are you dressing me for the casket?'' Another patient stated, ''I am going to join my deceased husband today.'' A patient, who was very restless, finally said, ''I have seen all the people I know who have died, but one. I think it is Gayle who will come to take me. I will wait for her.'' A young woman whose mother was ill stated, ''My mother told me she is hosting 'this party' and that when she decides 'the party' is over, she will leave.'' All four patients died within 2 days.

The professional staff must begin to prepare the loved ones of the possible signs and symptoms of the approaching death and near death communications. During this time, emotional support and active listening are paramount.

VII. THE ROLE OF THE PHYSICIAN

In hospice, the physician often behaves in ways that may be called countercultural to that of his or her professional peers. The hospice physician is most competent when he or she stops seeking cure of the disease as a goal and substitutes skills in easing the approach of death, meets basic needs of daily comfort and support, assists in training of staff, and works cooperatively with the hospice team. The hospice physician learns to internalize a reward system, recognizing that quality care for a dying person is a form of high competence (1). Unwillingness to acknowledge the terminal state, that is, pursuing new tests and treatments, prevents the patient from exercising the option of hospice care as an alternative. The physician often justifies this behavior as an attempt to maintain hope in the patient. Yet, experience shows that, although the things hoped for change as the patient faces his or her condition, hope is alive and refocused on more immediate desires: seeing a loved one, staying pain free, dying peacefully, and being brave. These latter hopes are not destroyed by speaking honestly with the patient; rather, the patient is given an opportunity to entertain these hopes, to enjoy them, and to take strength and comfort from them (1). As an authority figure in the hospice environment, the hospice physician, must be comfortable giving the patient, through actions and words, permission to deal openly with the social, emotional, and spiritual issues surrounding death. This physician must focus on more than the details of the physical care or else the very essence of hospice care is undermined (1). The hospice physician has four main roles: (1) he or she advises and constantly reviews the control of distressing symptoms—chronic pain being the most common; (2) he or she helps the patient and the family by listening, responding appropriately, and being freely available; (3) he or she has a teaching role; and (4) the physician has a research role to constantly assess and improve methods of care (11). By working alongside the patient's own medical attendants in the hospital or hospice and with other general practitioners, broad-based multidisciplinary teaching is achieved not only through the advice given, but also by example through their attitude toward death and dying. Teaching is considered to be one of the most important aspects of the physician's role. In the past, most formal teaching sessions were with nurses.

The role of the physician in hospice and palliative care is different depending on the relationship between the hospice and the physician. For the private attending physician who wishes to continue managing his or her own patient, the role is simple. This includes continuing to see the patient in the office or hospital while ordering medications and interventions. The intent of hospice is not to disrupt the previously beneficial doctor–patient relationship.

As the illness progresses and the patient becomes more debilitated, it is often beneficial for the attending physician or the hospice physician to visit the patient at home or the inpatient unit. Medical management is often facilitated through the expertise of the hospice nurse who evaluates the patient and then suggests or requests interventions through telephone contact with the physician.

If there is a hospice or palliative care physician available for consultation, the attending physician may request a home visit from this physician to evaluate his or her patient. Using a recognized specialist in this way allows additional input and suggestions for care and interventions. Often, the best alternative is for the attending physician to remain primarily responsible for the patient's care with the assistance of the palliative care or hospice expert as a consultant in difficult areas such as pain management. The hospice or palliative care physician has more contact with the hospice nursing staff on an ongoing basis; therefore, there is an understanding of the strengths and abilities of the nurse in assessing the patient, pain, and symptoms. This can be invaluable in patient management. With time, some attending physicians will also enhance this expertise, but it is an advantage the hospice physician readily possesses and may put to good use in managing patients.

Even when the palliative care or hospice physician is not requested to become involved directly in patient care as a consultant, this physician continues to remain responsible in the role of hospice medical director to oversee the total medical care provided by the hospice program. This happens most frequently in the form of attendance at interdisciplinary team meetings when patient cases are reviewed. Even though, the private attending physician is welcome to attend these meetings, as a practical matter of time management, few do so. Therefore, the hospice physician is in a position to make medical recommendations to team members and the attending physicians.

Usually, the sharing of patient responsibility in a congenial professional relationship among several physicians is the best system for the patient and family. It is to be hoped that friction and disagreement will be kept to a minimum to avoid adding physician conflict to the problem list of an already stressed dying patient and family. As trust is developed, attending physicians often request the palliative care or hospice physician to manage the patient's pain and symptoms and they remain involved by receiving weekly updates. This has worked well when a patient enters an inpatient unit. The attending physician reviews the hospice inpatient protocols and standing orders (see Tables 1,2, and 3) and if he or she agrees, signs them as orders. When and if a patient returns to a home setting, the attending physician becomes responsible for the overall care again. Most hospices are creative in maintaining a relationship with both the attending and hospice physician for total care for the patient.

Recently, some innovative oncologists have added a palliative care specialist to their practice. In this situation, the oncologists continue to practice curative and palliative interventions while the palliative care specialist manages pain and symptoms. These innovative partnerships offer a unique opportunity to combine acute and palliative care. Their existence and success underline the ability of acute and palliative care to coexist and complement one another.

VIII. LEVELS OF CARE

Hospice, as defined and regulated by the Health Care Finance Administration in the United States, requires that a Medicare-certified hospice provide four levels of care. Although this regulatory system is only required in the United States, it is a useful model for the division of levels of care.

Routine home care is the most common and is provided in a patient's place of residence, being offered on an intermittent basis, based on physical, emotional, and family needs. This same level of care refers to those whose principal place of residence is the nursing home. Under this level of care, the family and one designated primary caregiver are responsible for the ongoing continuous needs of the patient.

Respite care is provided on a short-term basis (5 days or less) to offer relief for the family and caregivers. This emphasizes the family as the unit of care by recognizing the need for families to have a break from day to day responsibilities. This respite may be provided by moving a patient to a hospice inpatient unit or nursing home, or by providing in-home hired or volunteer caregivers for the duration of the respite.

Continuous nursing care is provided, usually in the patient's residence, during a medical crisis. This 24-hour care is available only for short periods of time and, because of staffing difficulties or medical complexities, are often replaced by transfer of the patient to a hospice inpatient unit.

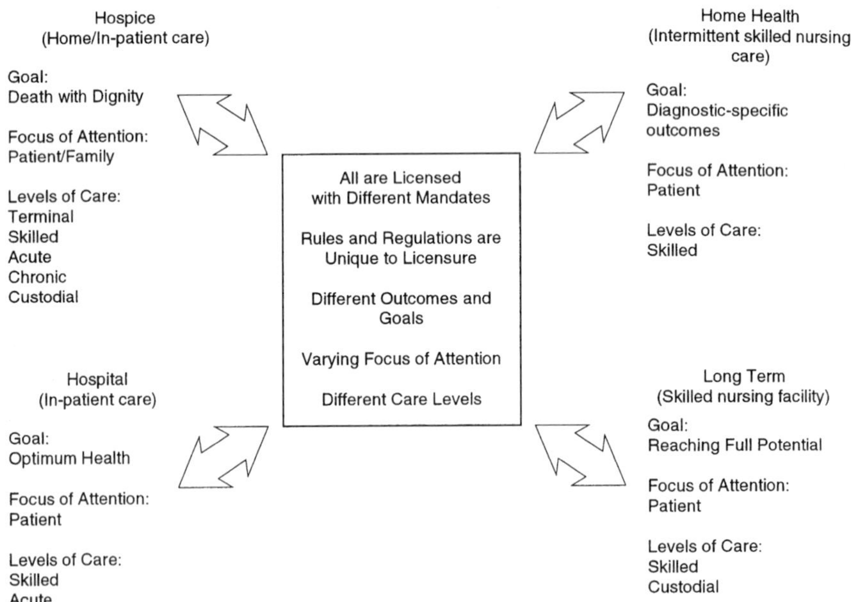

Figure 1 Four cornerstones of the health care system. (Copyright 1993 Elizabeth LeTourneau-Lee, B.A., R.N., C.R.N.H.)

Table 4 Focus of Care

Hospice	Home Health Care
1. TERMINALLY ILL: A disease process which, regardless of known medical treatment, will be the cause of death or a major contributing factor to a person's death. The patient does not need to be home bound.	1. ACUTELY ILL: The patient must be home bound. Signs of improvement or decline must be present.
2. PALLIATIVE CARE: The focus of care is on pain and symptom control and comfort measures.	2. SKILLED NEEDS: The patient must have skilled needs requiring the services of a nurse. Comfort measures are not the focus. The focus is on "getting better."
3. UNIT OF CARE: The unit of care is the patient and the family or significant caregivers. Physical, emotional, psychosocial, and spiritual needs are addressed.	3. UNIT OF CARE: The unit of care is the patient and the skilled needs.
4. ON-CALL: The hospice team is on-call 24 hours a day, 7 days a week for all needs.	4. ON-CALL: The home health team is on-call 24 hours a day, 7 days a week for skilled nursing needs only.
5. VOLUNTEERS: Trained volunteers are offered to each family, through the bereavement period.	5. VOLUNTEERS: Usually no volunteers are provided for the patient or family.
6. SERVICE: Hospice service continues across all settings, nursing home, private home, inpatient units and hospitals.	6. SERVICE: Home health services do not continue across all settings, only in the private home of the patient.
7. BEREAVEMENT: Bereavement follow-up from the hospice team is routinely available for 12 months after a death.	7. BEREAVEMENT: Home health does not offer bereavement follow-up for the family after the death.
8. GOAL: The goal is pain relief (physical and emotional) and death with dignity. This means allowing the patient to die in his/her own character, surrounded by loved ones.	8. GOAL: The goal and focus of care is on curative or rehabilitative measures. Hopefully the patient will return to optimum health.

General inpatient or acute hospice care is usually provided in either a free-standing hospice unit or in a designated area in a contracted nursing home or hospital facility. The management of the free-standing unit and case management of the patient remain the responsibility of the hospice interdisciplinary team.

Hospice is thus one of the few forms of health care that is allowed to provide continuity of care for patients regardless of their environmental needs. Hospice has become one of the four cornerstones of health care (Fig. 1). There are also several pertinent differences between hospice care in the home and traditional home health care (Table 4).

IX. HOSPICE INPATIENT UNIT CARE

The majority of hospice care is provided in the patient's private home. However, if a patient's pain or symptoms become out of control or if there is a breakdown in the patient's caregiver system, an admission to an inpatient hospice unit may be necessary, particularly if the patient requires close medical monitoring. The patient's quality of life and personal wishes continue to be the primary goal of the hospice team. In this way, a hospice inpatient setting is very different from an acute care or long-term care or nursing home facility setting.

The hospice inpatient unit offers an environment that is homelike and relaxed without the traditional rules and regulations of an acute care hospital. Vital signs and other disease-monitoring interventions are usually not done on a routine basis. There is a uniqueness within the unit that provides a special tranquility and a feeling of safety for the patients. Holistic care is provided by a well-trained and competent staff with a sense of blended community through the trained volunteers. A variety of services are available that are directed solely toward the patient's quality of life. Provisions for privacy for patients and families are essential, as is private space for staff members. Gardens, special visiting areas, and places to share a meal are also provided. Family members, friends, children, even pets are welcome on a 24-hour basis.

> I remember Alice, a 92-year-old woman with carcinoma of the breast metastatic to bone. She was sitting quietly in her room with her face toward the window. When invited to join the music therapy group, she declined, stating "I'm too sad." Apparently, she was very active and it was her habit to spend time with Toby, her horse, on a daily basis, until her admission to the unit. "I have been separated from my only friend." With some maneuvering, Toby was brought to the garden area of the hospice unit and Alice was wheeled outside. The joining of these two friends brought great joy to everyone. After Toby left, Alice said, "Now I can let go and die peacefully. I talked with Toby and he will be all right without me."

Ben, a large dog with a wonderful face who belonged to one of the night nurses on the hospice inpatient unit, often accompanied her to work. A few weeks ago, Ben laid in front of a doorway, making it difficult for a mother of a young patient from leaving his room. Ben refused to move. The mother, laughing at Ben, decided Ben was giving her a message to spend the night with her son. In the early morning, she put her arms around her son and said, "I brought you into this world and I will hold you until you leave this

Table 5 Patient/Family Bill of Rights

We believe that patients and families enrolled in the Hospice program have the following rights:

1. The right to privacy and confidentiality of information and the right to refuse to be photographed.
2. The right to be treated with respect and dignity regardless of age, sex, disability, ethnicity, religion or ability to pay.
3. The right to expect that services will be provided by skilled, licensed, certified and humane professionals. The right to a nurse's consultation 24 hours a day, 7 days a week.
4. The right to be informed and involved in the physician-approved, individualized plan of care provided by the Hospice.
5. The right to be informed of the sevices, based on need, provided by Hospice and the frequency of visits by each discipline that is involved, and the right to be informed of charges for service provided by the Hospice.

6a. The right of self-determination, i.e., to make your own health care decisions. This includes the right to accept or refuse treatment, the right to refuse to participate in experimental research and the right to be informed about advance directives.

Advance Directive(s) executed ☐ Y ☐ N

6b. The right to withdraw from Hospice services if desired.

7. The right to express dissatisfaction with any hospice service according to the written guidelines.

PATIENT SIGNATURE ______________________ DATE __________

AUTHORIZED REPRESENTATIVE & RELATIONSHIP ______________

____

HOSPICE REPRESENTATIVE SIGNATURE & TITLE ______________

____

PATIENT NAME ______________________________________

> world.'' The young man died in her arms. After the death, Ben got up and walked into the room and looked at the mother and young man, then moved away from the doorway, allowing space for the mother to leave the room.

The climate on the inpatient unit is one of warmth, love, respect, and caring. Caring, a gothic word meaning ''getting into someone's pain,'' is an invitation to share a most intimate time of one's life. This holds tremendous power and responsibility for the staff. The unit staff offer a sense of peace and expert knowledge in palliative care under the direction of a hospice medical director. Physicians affect the success or failure of a hospice inpatient unit by their attitude and ability to integrate palliative medicine with traditional medicine. They are an integral part of the interdisciplinary team.

Although the ultimate outcome is death, the patients are in an environment where they are encouraged to live as fully and comfortably as possible until they die. These units are not death houses, but homes for the living, a place to receive physical, emotional, and spiritual care and to complete unfinished business. Patients living in the unit observe the care and dignity provided for others and this helps them overcome their own fear of death (Table 5).

X. HOSPICE CARE IN THE NURSING HOMES

There is little question that hospice principles can contribute to long-term care environments in many ways (13). However, providing hospice care in the nursing home is complicated by the need to work with and relate to the nursing home staff. Initially, this may be problematic if nursing home personnel are not comfortable with death and caring for dying patients. They may also be unaware of palliative principles of care, particularly providing regular scheduled dosing of opioid pain medication. In many nursing homes and long-term care facilities, a true relationship eventually develops between hospice providers and the nursing home staff to improve care to nonhospice residents nearing the end of their lives. When nursing home staff begin to see hospice personnel, primarily nurses and social workers, as resources to help them, real cooperation may develop. Often, hospice nurses are invited to attend care plan conferences where their expertise and suggestions for good palliative management may be applied by the nursing home staff. When the other hospice interdisciplinary team members provide educational inservices for the nursing home staff, the working relationship continues to improve. The nursing home has the potential to provide a focus for individual efforts, promote team interaction, encourage family involvement, improve community relations, and offer residents and families a more complete continuum of care (12).

The nuances of care, including interventions and medications, do not vary from setting to setting in hospice, and therefore principles used in the home and inpatient units are easily applied to the nursing home environment. The coordination and continuity of care (professional management) for hospice patients among all levels and settings are the responsibility of the hospice team. This includes being an advocate for the patient and family. If educational inservices can be provided along with a formal letter of agreement between the nursing home and hospice, the care of the patient will remain palliative care.

XI. BEREAVEMENT CARE

Bereavement is an event: the loss, the death of a loved one. Grief is the emotional feeling to the perception of the loss. Mourning is the process of resolving the grief. Mourning has a beginning, the loss, and it can have an ending, the resolution. Anticipatory grief is the emotional feeling to the perception of the impending loss (13).

Hospice bereavement care begins with helping the family through anticipatory grief while the patient is alive. Helping the family accept the impending death of their loved one makes the nearing bereavement and grieving process easier. Support at the time of death of the patient is important, with attendance by hospice professional staff easing the burden on the family. Attendance at memorial services and funerals also is important to let the family know the hospice team cares and will continue to be involved during the mourning process.

Support is offered for at least 1 year, with frequent contacts being made with surviving family members to ensure the grieving and mourning process is proceeding normally. If there is ever any indication that abnormal grief is present, an additional referral for specific counseling can be made to a community service. This support is especially crucial at anniversary dates and holidays, which are well-known and documented times of increased risk for grieving family members.

Bereavement support groups for specific types of grieving individuals are also provided by most hospice programs. These usually consist of groups for adults, teenagers, children, and elderly persons. Support groups for hospice professional staff and volunteers also exist for assistance in dealing with the many losses. Some hospice programs even provide special grief camps for children. These have been especially effective in reaching this young population.

XII. CONCLUSION

Hospice care emphasizes supporting a patient to live fully during a time of decline. This care may provide a quality of life that includes opportunity for extraordinary personal spiritual growth. Focusing on the needs of the dying is like watching the ripples from a pebble cast into a lake; their effect touches caregivers, family members, friends, and professionals, and can reach the furthest limits of our culture. It has been said that a civilization can be measured by how it regards and takes care of the dying. Confronting our own death or being confronted by the dying challenges the basic belief systems and values of society (14).

The challenge comes from within ourselves, as health care professionals, to provide the dying patient and his or her family personal concern, dignity, excellent pain control, and thorough symptom management in a loving, nonjudgmental environment. It may require a simple change in our attitudes, rethinking of old traditions, being open to learning new ways to administer medications, or even studying palliative care and learning from those more advanced than ourselves, to care for these special patients. When the disease has won and traditional treatment has lost, we need to listen carefully to the goals of the patient and family and, if appropriate, offer palliative care as the next formal treatment available to them. Hospice is an option. If it is presented in a positive manner offering new goals and hopes, not for survival, but for physical and emotional comfort and dignity, most patients and their families would choose hospice care, either in their homes or in an impatient setting. Hospice is the best form of health care available to the dying.

HOSPICE AND PALLIATIVE CARE SPECIAL ORGANIZATIONS

1. American Academy of Hospice and Palliative Physicians, web site: http://www.aahpm.org, e-mail: aahpm@aahpm.org
2. Association for Death Education and Counseling, 638 Prospect Avenue, Hartford, CT 06105, phone: 860-586-7503, web site: http://www.adec.org
   ADEC is dedicated to improving the quality of death education and death related counseling and caregiving.
3. Bereavement and Hospice Support Netline, web site: http://www.ubalt.edu/www/bereavement
   This is a web page listing bereavement support groups and services, state by state.
4. Children's Hospice International, 2202 Mt. Vernon Avenue, Suite 3C, Alexandria, VA 22301, phone: 702-684-0330, e-mail: chiorg@aol.com, web site: http://www.chionline.org
   Provides medical and technical assistance, research and education for children with life threatening conditions and their families.
5. European Journal of Palliative Care, edited by Dr. Andrew Hoy, web site: http://www.ejpc.co.uk/ejpc.online

Published in English and French 6 times a year.

6. The Growth House, web site: http://growthhouse.org
   A comprehensive international gateway to resources on the web related to life-threatening illnesses and end-of-life issues.
7. Hospice Foundation of America, 2001 S. Street NW, Suite 300, Washington, DC 20009
   Sponsors an annual Living with Grief teleconference series, a monthly bereavement newsletter, and other publications.
8. National Hospice Organization, 1901 N. Moore Street, Suite 901, Arlington, VA 22209, phone: 703-243-5900, web site: http://www.nho.org
   NHO provides referral services to link individuals with hospices in their local communities, and various educational programs.
9. Pediatrics Home Care Guide, web site: http://hmc.psu.edu/depts/pedsonco/Homeguide.html
   Hosted by the Pediatric Oncology Group, this site is dedicated to providing information useful to those caring for children with cancer at home.

REFERENCES

1. Werner PT. Providing hospice care: the changing role and status of physicians. In: Paradis LF, ed. Hospice Handbook and Guide for Managers and Planners. Rockville, MD: Aspen Publication, 1985:345–362.
2. Gardner K, ed. Quality of Care for the Terminally Ill. Chicago: A Special Publication of the QRB, 1985.
3. Cassell E. The Nature of Suffering and the Goals of Medicine. New York: Oxford Press, 1992.
4. Cockburn M. Nursing care of dying persons and their families. In: Corr CA, Corr DM, eds. Hospice Care Principles and Practice. New York: Springer, 1983:120.
5. McCann BA, Hill KL. The hospice project. In: Gardner K, ed. Quality of Care for the Terminally Ill. Chicago: A Special Publication of the QRB, 1985:11.
6. Berry P, Zeri K, Egan K. The Hospice Nurses Study Guide: For Certification. 2d ed. Pittsburgh, PA: Hospice Nurses Association, 1997.
7. Cancer Pain Relief and Palliative Care. Report from the World Health Organization, Geneva, 1994.
8. Twycross RC. Principles and practice of pain relief in terminal cancer. In: Corr CA, Corr DM, eds. Hospice Care Principles and Practice. New York: Springer, 1983: 81.
9. Stoddard S. The Hospice Movement. Briarcliff Manor, NY: Stein and Day Publishers, 1978.
10. Adapted from North Central Florida Hospice, Inc., 1996.
11. Bates TD. At home and in the ward: the establishment of a support team in an acute general hospital. In: Wilkes E, ed. The Dying Patient. Ridgewood, NJ: George A. Bogden and Son, 1982:275–276.

12. Owen G. The application of hospice principles in long-term care. In: Paradis LF, ed. Hospice Handbook and Guide for Managers and Planners. Rockville, MD: Aspen Publication, 1985:124.
13. Berry P, Zeri K, Egan K. The Hospice Nurses Study Guide: For Certification. 2d ed. Pittsburgh, PA: Hospice Nurses Association, 1997:177–178.
14. Hoy T. Hospice chaplaincy in the caregiving team. In: Corr A, Corr M, eds. Hospice Care Principles and Practice. New York: Springer, 1983:179.

BIBLIOGRAPHY

1. Armstrong-Daley AG. Hospice Care for Children. New York: Oxford Press, 1993.
2. Barley N. Grave Matters: A Lively History of Death Around the World. New York: Henry Holt, 1997.
3. Byock I. Dying Well: The Prospect for Growth at the End of Life. New York: Riverhead Books, 1997.
4. Doka KJ, Davidson J, eds. Living with Grief: When Illness Is Prolonged. The Hospice Foundation of American. Washington, DC: Taylor & Francis, 1997.
5. Godkin MA, Krant JJ, Doster JJ. The impact of hospice care on families. Int J Psychiatry Med 1983:153–165.
6. Grey A. The spiritual component of palliative care. Palliat Med 1994:215–221.
7. Irish D, ed. Ethnic Variations in Dying, Death, and Grief: Diversity in Universality. Washington, DC: Taylor & Francis, 1993.
8. Johanson G. Symptom Relief in Terminal Care. Sonoma County Academic Foundation for Excellence in Medicine, Santa Rosa, CA, 1994.
9. Kaye P. Symptom Control in Hospice and Palliative Care. 9th ed. Essex, CT: Hospice Education Institute, 1994.
10. McCaffery M, Beebe A. Pain: Clinical Manual for Nursing Practice, St. Louis: CV Mosby, 1989.
11. National Hospice Organization. Medical Guideline for Determining Prognosis in Selected Non-Cancer Diseases. 2d ed., NHO Publisher, Arlington, VA, 1996.
12. Purtillo R. Ethical Dimensions in the Health Professions. Philadelphia: WB Saunders, 1993.
13. Salerno E, Willens JS. Pain Management Handbook. St. Louis: CV Mosby, 1996.

32

Information, Education, and Counseling: Essentials of Supportive Cancer Care

Agnes Glaus
Center for Tumor Detection and Prevention, St. Gallen, Switzerland

Gertrude Grahn
Lund University, Lund, Sweden

I. INTRODUCTION

Supportive care in cancer patients is a concept that has evolved in the past 2 decades. The struggle against cancer as a life-threatening disease was primarily understood in terms of the destruction of cancer cells, the stopping of tumor growth, and the increase in survival time. The progress of medical science in the 20th century allowed many patients to understand that even cancer could be cured, or at least controlled, over years. Thus, success has inspired hope and improved quantity and quality of life for many patients. Once it became possible to increase survival time, the quality of life debate became more relevant. Death was no longer seen as the greatest and sole enemy of quality of life.

Quality of life is of concern for cancer patients in all stages of the disease. Supportive care therefore deals with patients from the time of diagnosis to the time of cure, relapse, or death. Palliative care can be seen as part of supportive care, which deals especially with the suffering of patients with incurable disease during the terminal phase of their lives. Supportive care bridges so-called curative care with palliative care, because its activities, feelings, and attitudes pay regard to physical, psychological, and social coping with progressive illness and survival (1).

Supportive care also bridges the efforts of different health care professionals; it is an interdisciplinary endeavor. To be supportive means to care for patients from different viewpoints, accepting other professionals as specialists and patients as competent claimants (2). Information, education, and counseling are one part of supportive care, which needs a strong link between professions and patient to be effective and complementary. It has been said that the ability to care for oneself and to exercise control over daily activities may improve psychological as well as moral well-being, which again is considered the most significant dimension of quality of life (3). This implies that information, education, and counseling are major concerns for patients and, from their viewpoint, probably the most relevant aspects of supportive care.

II. THE CONCEPT OF SUPPORTIVE CARE AND ITS RELATION TO INFORMATIONAL NEEDS

Providing support for others is considered a key aspect of nursing. However, definitions about the nature and behaviors of support are vague. A supportive care model was developed by O'Berle to articulate a specific palliative nursing role. This model includes six interwoven dimensions: valuing, connecting, empowering, doing for, finding meaning, and preserving one's own integrity (4). This model raises the question of whether being supportive is different from caring and whether it is representative of a specific role. Support is cited as an integral component of care, which is defined by Leininger as "those assistive, supportive or facilitative acts towards or for an individual or group, intended to ameliorate or improve a human condition or life way" (5). Similarly, Paternoster defines caring as "warmth, compassion, support and concern" (6). The supportive care model by O'Berle seems to be highly compatible with the holistic view of caring as described by the experts Benner and Wrubel (7).

In this sense, support for cancer patients seems to be an integral component of nursing, medical, and psychosocial care. This support could be explained as helping methods to deal with specific physical and psychological problems, but also as attitudes and feelings that mediate the supporter to act. In cancer care, this refers, apart from any tumor therapy, to assisting in adjustment to new circumstances (physical and psychological), to understanding treatments, to combating the side effects of therapy, to relieving symptoms, and to helping the patient cope. Orem describes support as encouragement, assurance, communication, and physical help with the aim of enabling the patient to control and direct action in the situation, once support has been received (8). However, some cancer patients cannot, or can no longer, control and direct actions. For those who are able to do so, information, education, and counseling become crucial prerequisites to gaining control and directing action.

III. INFORMATION

A. Definition and Aim

Information giving is described as an important element of teaching. It may not be the same as teaching, the latter inferring an interactive process whereby learning takes place, which may subsequently be used to influence behavior. From research conducted in patients who were due for tests or surgery, clues emerge to explain the mechansim of how information giving or patient teaching helps individuals (9):

1. Anxiety is alleviated by reducing the area of ''unknown'' experiences, fears and fantasies being corrected by providing a realistic account of what will happen.
2. The role of instruction helps patients to know what is expected of them and how to do things, which will improve their experiences and recovery. Through this confidence they can behave in a useful way and feel less dependent and helpless.

Information giving is described as a process in which there is only one-way exchange. Topics may be limited and unquestioned, data factual only, and the relationship neutral but authoritative (10). Information giving in itself provides only a small amount of interaction or assessment of individual needs. The level of negotiation on content is usually low. Goals may not be discussed, and continuing sessions may be lacking. This kind of information can easily be obtained but not easily retained. A bad example of one-way information is the misuse of written, informed consent, in which patients sign a paper with information on procedures and possible outcome. In practice, patients badly understand the text and unfortunately often cannot discuss it with anyone.

It becomes evident that the underlying ethical attitudes of the health care professionals may play a major role in how information is given. On one side, these professionals, especially doctors and nurses, mostly lack education concerning communication skills. Nursing and medical education in Europe usually does not include teaching principles. On the other side, the relationship between patient and caregiver plays a crucial role. Whenever a paternalistic attitude prevails, patients are not involved in the information process. What can they be told about, if they are not allowed even to know the diagnosis? Patients are coming to understand that knowledge about illness and medical care is not the exclusive property of health professionals (11). Information is essential if respect for the autonomy of the patient is to be considered.

Sound knowledge, communication, and teaching skills, as well as a partnershiplike relation between caregiver and patient, allow mere information to become a process with a two-way exchange. They build the framework for the actual impartation of information (Fig. 1).

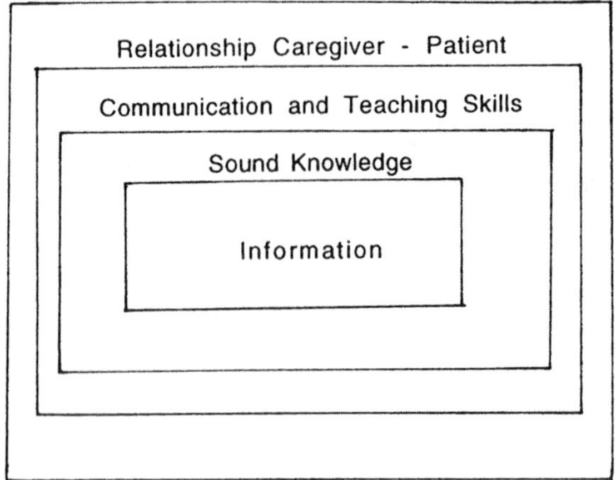

Figure 1 Framework for imparting the cancer diagnosis.

B. Imparting Information

Clear guidelines have become commonly accepted for the actual imparting of information (12). New oral information must have the following characteristics:

Carefully planned, sequential, and logical
Covers the most important points first
Related to the next event
Limited amount of information
Includes questions to elicit patient's understanding
Complemented by written or audiovisual material if possible

Informal patient information may represent the most common type of information and refers to all unplanned patient-staff communication. Even though this may be effective, it can scarcely be pursued or measured by outcome. Essential information must be given in a methodological and timely planned intervention.

Formal, planned information giving has a specific content, for example, information about the diagnosis. Questions related to the person of the informer, to the receiver of the information, and to the how and where of information giving, are described later in the specific context of cancer care.

IV. INFORMATION ABOUT CANCER: STILL A QUESTION?

Paterson found in 1954 that cancer was regarded as the most alarming disease a person could contract, and 50% of the sample believed that it was incurable

(13). There is still something about cancer that causes more fear and anxiety in individuals than any other disease, even though one-third to one-half of these patients are treated successfully and can be cured (14). There is still no worldwide agreement about whether to inform the patient about cancer. In 1979, however, Novack and Plumer suggested that 95% of patients in the United States were told the diagnosis when cancer was discovered (15). In some other countries, a consensus has emerged that it is best to tell the "truth." This does not seem to be the case in Latin countries, where cancer is still treated as a taboo and the sociocultural background stipulates withholding the diagnosis cancer. A study from Spain shows that establishing a "conspiracy of silence" around the patient is the usual manner of "communicating." A survey of 167 cancer patients reveals that only 15% of them were aware of their diagnosis (16). In view of the trends toward unification of Europe and inevitable intermigration of populations, disclosure of a cancer diagnosis to patients of different cultural origins becomes an important issue.

A. Aim of Communicating the Diagnosis of Cancer

In countries where patients are told about the disease, health care professionals and patients believe in the right to know. From the ethical point of view, this refers to the principle of respect for autonomy. Who, if not the patient, can decide which course of action maximizes his or her welfare? The information allows the patient to gain knowledge about illness and treatment and helps to decide further steps. It gives the opportunity to set priorities in life, to set realistic goals, to understand treatments, and to comply with or refuse them. If the patient is kept in ignorance, he or she cannot know how to cope with the situation.

B. Who Communicates the Diagnosis?

There is no question about the fact that the truth is communicated by more than merely words. Professionals and relatives or friends may express their knowledge in nonverbal signs. The expression on the physician's face, silence, increased attention, and avoidance strategies, as well as signals from body language, may promptly inform the patient. Everyone around the patient is communicating in some way.

1. *Role of the Physician*

If the information about cancer is a formal, planned intervention, the responsibility is likely to be the physician's. Because many physicians are involved in the diagnostic procedure, the questions evolves as to which is meant to be the informer. Many primary care physicians initially convey warnings or suspicions to patients and schedule them for consultation with surgeons or oncologists. Lind documented that the majority of patients first learned the diagnosis of cancer from a surgeon who performed a biopsy and only a minority were told by their primary care physicians (17). Advances in radiological imaging complicate the question of who should do the telling. Experience suggests that the physicians who are involved only at the diagnostic stage should pass the results to the primary physician or to the oncologist, who will also discuss treatment options. Further research is needed to identify whether the person telling the diagnosis is of importance to patients or if this concern is overridden by the diagnosis itself.

2. Role of Nurses and Other Health Care Professionals

It has been said that hospital staff can be divided into announcers and nonannouncers. Physicians are the primary announcers. When it comes to information about the patient's condition, nurses are nonannouncers (18). There seems to be a gap between the primary announcers and the nonannouncers. The primary announcement, in everyday practice, soon becomes a message that must be repeated. This repetition can be classified as an announcement, and at that time, the telling person is often likely to be the experienced nurse. Translation into the patient's own vocabulary, in which hiding behind medical terms is no longer possible, can be very painful. At this stage, information is transformed into counseling.

There are few official instructions about the type of information nurses are allowed to release. There is anecdotal evidence that nurses sometimes cannot or do not want to escape from breaking the rule of withholding information. Their closeness to patients makes it difficult to hide anything. Experience shows that nurses push withholding doctors to tell the truth because they, like the patient, suffer from the "silent conspiracy." It has been suggested that the greater the power of a nurse and the lesser the social distance between the doctor and nurse, the less the nurse feels bound to hospital rules (18). Here, power is not defined; it can be interpreted as knowledge, experience, position, and communication skills. It becomes evident that the degree of collaboration between doctor and nurse and the expert role of nurses, as well as their ideological perspective, have immediate influence on truth telling.

Tilley found that patients acknowledged nurses as sources of certain information. They preferred to receive information from the nurse concerning the event of illness and about what to expect in the future. However, patients preferred to receive medically oriented information from doctors (19). These findings suggest that nurses and doctors can and must have different emphases in information giving.

Little research has been done on the role of auxiliary staff, physiotherapists, social workers, cleaners, or the clergy in the informal communication. It is not known how much information, if any, these individuals pass on to patients and relatives.

C. When and Where Should the Diagnosis Be Told?

Patients relate that the time of uncertainty is difficult. The period between suspicion and the results of a biopsy or radiological procedure seems endless to patients. They may push doctors to rapid conveyance of information, immediately after biopsy or radiography. Because the revision of an initially benign diagnosis is an unlikely but potentially traumatic consequence, many institutions respect the following rule:

> Never inform a patient about the cancer diagnosis before the final proving report is available (biopsy or cytology).

This rule prevents unnecessarily burdening patients with a cancer diagnosis that might turn out to be only a suspicion or later, false.

However, delaying until the biopsy report is available lengthens the time of uncertainty. To overcome this problem, physicians may relate the diagnosis over the telephone. Lind and Delvecchio found that 42% of a studied patient population in the United States was told either in the recovery room or over the telephone. A significantly greater percentage of the patients told over the telephone expressed negative feelings about the timing of information, compared with those told in a hospital room or doctor's office (17). Negative feelings were related to being upset when caught off-guard or in a nonprivate setting. To overcome this problem, the following rule might be helpful:

> Making an office appointment to tell the patient the diagnosis is preferable to telling the patient the diagnosis over the telephone. If an office appointment is not possible, the telephone call should be scheduled to give the patient the opportunity to prepare psychologically and choose an adequate locality.

In the same study, patients indicated that learning the diagnosis of cancer sooner is not necessarily better. The circumstances and mode of telling bad news seem to be crucial. If the diagnostic results are negative, telling the good news over the telephone has not been received negatively (17). As outpatient diagnosis of cancer becomes more common, the question of how to tell patients who are not hospitalized will be increasingly relevant, not only in American but also in European countries, from where there is little knowledge concerning information via telephone calls.

Another important point is the readiness of the patient to be informed. Patients distressed about being told in the recovery room believed that they had not fully recovered from anesthesia and did not have sufficient mental clarity to cope effectively with learning the diagnosis at that time (17).

> Psychoactive medication, inability to concentrate, discomfort (e.g., pain), or anxiety interferes with the patient's readiness to receive information.

It is not evident from research whether the presence of a spouse, relative, or close friend is important to patients when receiving bad news. Experience shows that many patients come to the office together with a significant person. If the principle of respect for autonomy is to be regarded and if it is not allowed by law to inform someone other than the patient, then the patient must agree to the involvement of another person.

> It remains the patient's choice to share the truth with someone else.

Experience shows that patients find it helpful if they are offered to learn the diagnosis together with a significant other person.

> If the information is given in a patient's room, care should be given that no other patients are in the room. Never inform patients "en passant" in a corridor. Ensure that everyone is seated comfortably. As an informer, never remain standing in front of patients who are seated or in bed.

D. How to Inform Patients About Cancer

Many questions concerning the "how" of truth telling are still unexplored. What do patients understand by the terms used by doctors and nurses? What does "tumor" or "malignancy" mean to them? If doctors use terms other than cancer, do they want to leave the patient with more hope? Or, perhaps it is a reflection of the fears and anxiety of the doctor (18). Bearing in mind how difficult it is to disclose such a diagnosis, this reason is understandable. Caregivers are vulnerable people, too.

To care for someone means to respond to a person who matters. It means to feel an interest in, to feel concern for. Caring in this sense is the essence of a helping relationship (20). If this concept of care underlies medical, nursing, or social care, how a life-threatening diagnosis is told cannot be cold, neutral, or without sympathy. This is the opposite of paternalistic withholding of the truth. Physicians who comfortably and confidently convey clear information and who can ask sensitively about the patient's reaction are usually perceived as more empathic, concerned, and trustworthy (21).

The Swiss Working Group for Clinical Cancer Research (SAKK) developed a method for assessment of the efficacy of the first interview between an oncologist and a cancer patient (22). Videotaped interviews were analyzed. Three dimensions formed the basis for assessment of the first information concerning cancer diagnosis.

1. Dimension: Content of Information (Cognitive Aspects)

This dimension deals with the cognitive aspects of the information. It refers to diagnostic, therapeutic, and prognostic information. Ideally, the language of the informer is clear and well understood by the patient.

Information is understandable to the patient (words and content): there are no unexplained medical terms and the diagnosis is clear and unequivocal.
Style and structure of talk are not rigid, allowing the patient to interrupt.
Informer realizes that questions may already contain information.
Informer listens to already available knowledge and builds on it or corrects misunderstanding.
Informer does not talk down to the patient.
Informer uses the word *I*, not *we* or *one*.
Informer pays attention to the equal contribution of speaking time between informer and patient.
Content of information is not too dense; informer does not speak too fast and asks questions to elicit understanding.
Informer listens and responds to the patient's comments.
Information is topic centered: there is no mention of minor things or unlikely events.
Relationship to patient is more important than completeness of information.
Informer avoids cross-examination style or induction of guilt.

2. Dimension: Emotional Warmth (Affective Aspects)

In oncology, there remains this unresolvable conflict between the emotional involvement and the distance needed to be able to help. This closeness-distance problem is determined by the personality of the informer and by the patient. Emotional warmth manifests itself by the degree of attachment, positively but also negatively. An informer who takes over the depressed feelings of the patient and thus also becomes depressed is a negative example.

Informer shows respect and esteem for the individual's reaction and experience.
Informer remains friendly and considerate.
Informer encourages patient.
Informer shows interest and remains natural.
Verbal and nonverbal expressions remain congruent (e.g., friendly words are not accompanied by hostility).
Informer must realize that the information is more constructive and supportive with some patients and more defensive and distant with others, depending on the relationship with the patient.

3. Dimension: Patient Centeredness (Interactive Aspect)

This dimension allows the patient to feel personally understood. It refers to taking up all direct (verbal) and indirect patient information (affect, facial expression, and gestures). Critiques or doubts can be verbalized. It also refers to the need to explain the personal meaning or cause of the disease or to the expression of anxiety concerning death.

Anxiety concerning death and suffering can be verbalized.
Informer does not trivialize or console without objective facts.
Informer is reassuring and calming on the basis of objective facts.
Patient can express his or her reactions.
Informer does not blame anyone involved in treatment and care.
Informer listens and responds to individual interpretations of causes and meaning of disease; is ready to keep the talk flexible.

High patient centeredness may lead to ''overidentifiction'' by the informer. This overidentification can go along with fear and anxiety and can make it difficult for physicians and nurses to carry on with aggressive treatments, for example, in research protocols.

Ideal information giving involves all three dimensions equally (Fig. 2). The information is clear and understandable; the informer shows emotional warmth and pays attention to the patient's personal way of reacting. Practice shows that this balance is often difficult to achieve because individual factors of both parties

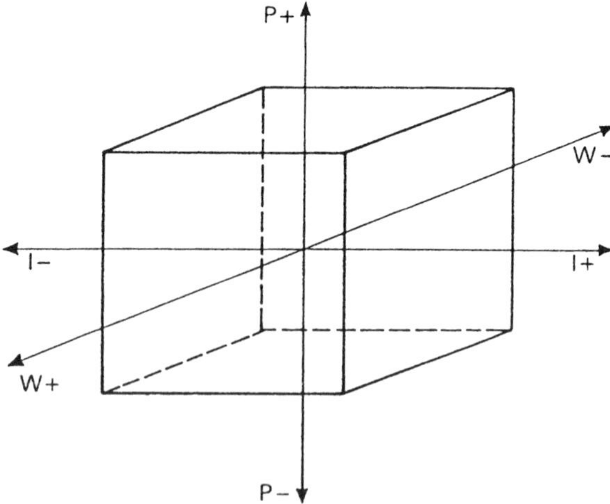

Figure 2 The balance of the three dimensions in truth telling: I, information; P, patient centeredness; and W, emotional warmth.

are involved; circumstances also play a crucial role. Videotaping of such important talks and subsequent analysis with regard to the three dimensions together with peers and psycho-oncologists could be a good learning method for nurses and doctors to prevent routinized and poor information giving. Routinized health care professionals are in danger of forgetting that their information might change everything in the life of the person concerned.

V. INFORMATION: AN ONGOING PROCESS IN CANCER CARE

Information is much more than disclosure of the diagnosis of cancer; it remains essential throughout the course of the illness. It is a continuing need when patients must cope with the disease and also with treatments or symptom control and when they have to live with a limited life expectancy.

Helpful information enables the patient to have control over side effects or symptoms, such as pain, and it enables them to live with obstacles. It helps them to understand why specific reactions happen and why specific measures are being taken. Some patients say that they do not want to know about every detail because it would scare them. Others want to know and document all analyses, including leukocyte counts and drug doses. ''Good news,'' such as indications of tumor regression or of recovery from such side effects as leukopenia, are helpful to inspire hope and to encourage the patient.

During the course of illness and treatment, complications unrelated to tumor progression may arise. Such events must be explained to patients carefully because they observe changes very precisely and interpret them as tumor progression and are unnecessarily scared. This refers, for example, to prolonged therapy-induced leukopenia, to thrombosis or pulmonary embolism, or to unrelated infection.

Some other information seems to be harmful to patients. This especially relates to blunt information concerning the prognosis. Even though it may be realistic from statistical evidence that some patients have a short and determined life expectancy, it remains questionable when doctors speak of a ''specific'' survival time, because this is never known for an individual patient. Experience shows that patients being told a specific survival time (in weeks or months), but who then live longer, additionally suffer because they feel they are ''over their time,'' which makes living difficult. Modern diagnostic procedures, such as relevant tumor markers, may enable patients and caregivers to follow the course of illness much more precisely. However, relating such fluctuations may be absolutely irrelevant for advanced cancer patients, because they in turn may induce additional anxiety. The following German proverb might be a helpful guide in many situations:

> Everything you say should be true, but not everything that is true needs to be told.

VI. EDUCATION: A BASIS FOR COPING WITH CANCER

Interest in the psychosocial aspects of being a cancer-diagnosed patient has grown considerably during the past decade. Supporting patients by means of education to achieve an *understanding* of occurrences in their efforts to cope with the cancer experience has become acknowledged within cancer care but more seldom is it given the attention it deserves.

A. Understanding the Cancer Experience

Research studies have shown that many cancer patients and their significant others want to understand better the events to which they are exposed and experience throughout the course of cancer. They seek information regarding the disease and treatment. They want support in passing through and making sense of the situational demands, which they perceive to exceed their personal resources. They want to be actively involved during the period of treatment as well as during the rehabilitation phase or the terminal phase (23–26).

For health care professionals, supportive care in this respect means to describe and explain for the patient what can be expected or to provide the patient with a means of coming to grips with what has been experienced. It entails outlining and organizing core features in the unfamiliar situation in a meaningful way, and to do so in light of recognizing and respecting the patient as a person with a unique history, with unique expectations, and with unique meaning attached to the experience of illness. Patients seeking an understanding, an ability to infer from the information they have received, might have their coping efforts facilitated by *learning* more about the disease and their own reactions to it, as expressed by Marie Curie: ‘‘Nothing in life is to be feared; it is to be understood.’’ Thus, providing a means to understand the cancer experience merges into the field of education (27).

B. Theoretical Frame for Learning and Coping

Health care professionals must describe and explain many things for the patient who wants to learn about and understand the current situation. Informing patients is generally oriented, for example, toward explaining the diagnosis and describing the treatment modalities and their side effects in a one-way communication. Skill acquisition demonstrations commonly are used.

Education, because it is an interactive process, moves beyond imparting information to increase the knowledge base and beyond demonstrations for skill acquisition. Education aims at growth and changes in the way a person thinks, feels, and acts in a holistic sense. For an *understanding* of events to occur, the cognitive and affective domains concurrently are influenced to increase, modify, or bring about changes in knowledge, attitudes, values, and skills to direct actions. In the teaching-learning process, information, demonstration, and emotional support are interwoven strands.

Growth and *change* are two dynamic words to describe learning and advancement in an educational endeavor. Varying learning theories have made attempts to capture the phenomena of growth and change related to core features in the current context, social structures, and individual differences. The perception of education and its pedagogical consequences has varied from ancient to modern time (28). Fundamental conditions for learning and understanding to take place have been investigated and described in classic pedagogical learning models (e.g. refs. 29–31). To apply knowledge of human learning processes is judicious in supporting patients and their significant others to achieve understanding.

The process of teaching and learning consists of educational experiences planned to meet individual learning needs, readiness, interests, and capabilities. Providing concrete experiences within the learner's world and allowing the learner to take on an active role give rise to increased ability and readiness for actions. Patient education is a valuable tool in empowering patients to make the informed choices that will have an impact on their maintenance or improvement of well-being and quality of life. It is a powerful device in building up confidence for living with cancer when approaching death (32).

People use different strategies to give the events of daily life a decent order and to achieve understanding of unfamiliar events. When an event is perceived as a threat to well-being or touches the very core of life, as does a cancer diagnosis, the situational demands could, according to Lazarus and Folkman, be appraised as exceeding personal resources. Common strategies of daily life become insufficient or inappropriate. In attempts to manage a situation, which thus is changed beyond control, the person constantly tries to modify cognitive, emotional, and behavioral efforts to solve the problem or reappraise the current situation in a process of coping (33–35). Changes in thoughts, feelings, and actions are intertwined and interdependent strands in the process of coping. This parallels the process of learning in which cognitive and affective domains are influenced to bring about changes in knowledge, attitudes, values, and skills to direct actions. That is why education is a valuable tool in developing and supporting coping strategies.

Education, as a base for coping with events throughout the course of cancer, is very much a question of finding congruence between what the patient expects, what the patient is exposed to, and the patient's experiences. When patients and their significant others struggle with demands they consider to exceed their personal resources, support in learning and becoming familiar with facts and feelings releated to the cancer experience will influence their coping ability (32).

The essence and aim of patient education within the frame of psychosocial interventions in cancer care are to provide for intellectual and emotional growth and change. This aim is accomplished by giving patients opportunities and tools that are supportive of coping with the cancer experience, and supportive also of living with cancer when life expectancy is limited.

C. Assessing Learning Needs

The first step in the interactive process of education is to identify the need for knowing something or for gaining an ability to do something. Before staff members enter an educative process, it is important to establish the patient's own needs in terms of information and support. Assessing learning needs comprises an assessment of the content to be taught as well as the method to be used in accordance with assessed learning capacity and motivation. An accurate assessment results in mutually agreed goals for the teaching-learning endeavor. Learning occurs over time, and assessment of learning needs is an ongoing activity.

Because the need for information about the disease and treatment, and the request for support in efforts to cope with the cancer experience are well documented within cancer care, the assessment area is mostly easy to review. However, even if items are well known, it is important in needs assessment to notice obstacles, if any, and to notice patients who are unable to identify or express their learning needs.

Learning requires emotional readiness or motivation. Needs identified by the learner promote learning efforts and stimulate the learning process. Most important in assessing learning needs is thus to help patients and their significant others in identifying *their* learning needs. Not seldom are a patient's learning needs defined from the staff members' viewpoint.

In a paternalistic way, staff members tend to "know best" the learning needs of their patients; they decide what their patients ought to know about procedures before and after surgery, about chemotherapy-induced side effects, and so on. The patients' perceptions of what is essential for them to know about in their coping efforts, their expectations, their experiences, and the meaning they attach to the situation, as well as their learning capacity, may not be congruent with what the caregivers perceive.

The predominantly identified learning needs of cancer patients are cognitive and connected to the disease, treatment and side effects, and procedures. Assessments tend to ignore emotional dimensions, which are profound determinants of the coping capacity. The emotional detachment of health care professionals is mainly a result of lack of training in communication and counseling (36).

A complete and accurate assessment provides a base, which, in a holistic sense, has the potential to meet individual learning needs and to provide comprehensive information and sufficient support. For the beginner, a checklist with itemized learning needs complemented by items suggested by the patient can sometimes be useful when teaching individuals as well as groups (37).

1. *Adult Learners*

Within the theory of adult learning, it is emphazised that the adult learner has a desire to articulate his or her own needs and to make choices in moving from dependence toward self-direction when the climate communicates acceptance and support. Much of adult learning entails relearning. Adult learners are highly motivated to learn when their past experiences are considered and later used as a resource for further learning. Successful adult learning is also based on recognizing and respecting the learner's efforts, competence, and progress when reassessing learning needs. A ''learning by doing'' style is a challenge for adult learners, and their desire for active participation should be noticed when needs are assessed (38).

Because adult learners may be of advanced age, impairment of vision or hearing may interfere with proper understanding. Assessment of such age-related factors is crucial.

2. *Learners with Low Literacy Skills*

To assess the learning needs of patients with low literacy skills is not easy. It takes specialized knowledge to estimate their literacy and comprehension. To reach them in patient education sessions and to find the level at which communication is possible is a challenge for staff members. Efforts to simplify language in verbal communication and written materials, for example, are not always successful, because persons with low literacy skills process information differently from other persons. It is important to work with special sensitivity in assessing the needs of these patients; despite the intellectual handicap, their need for information and emotional support is equal to that of other patients (38).

3. *Learners with Different Cultural Backgrounds*

A diversity of cultural beliefs and values may complicate educational ventures if not assessed properly. Some issues are of special importance to consider, and staff members involved in patient education must learn about salient cultural features. Religious beliefs or cultural traditions may determine what could be communicated and disclosed. Such concepts as the human body, health, disease, and illness are perceived in different ways and have different meanings in different cultures, and nonverbal signals can be interpreted in many ways.

D. Planning and Implementing

Patient education is a psychosocial intervention aimed at supporting the patient in coping with the cancer experience. As such, patient education should become an integral part of cancer care: planned for, accomplished, and evaluated, as is the rule for other interventions. Although there are many similarities between providing supportive education to reduce confusion regarding the cancer experience and, for example, giving antiemetics to reduce nausea and vomiting, one is mandatory whereas the other is incidental. Based on the needs assessment and the mutually agreed goals for teaching and learning, a structured plan must be outlined. In planning for patient education, the guiding principles should be as follows (when the patients' significant others participate, the same principles are applicable):

Confirm and respect the patient as a person with individual expectations, experiences, and reactions.
Consider the contextual influence on distress and coping.
Adopt the patient's perspective, and structure the content to allow reflections.
Focus information vividly and consistently on core features in a comprehensive and applicable way.
Use pedagogical principles for adult learning, modified to accommodate assessed learning needs, capability, readiness, motivation, and attentional fatigue.
Take correct timing into consideration.

It is crucial to adjust the amount of information to assessed learning capacity; otherwise, the educational intervention is overwhelming and confusing. As a consequence of predominantly assessed cognitive learning needs, the main learning activities used in patient education are lectures, group discussions, and demonstrations. Cognitive learning is thus emphasized. The emotional dimension is more seldom addressed. Thus the patient's experiences and reflections are not used to develop values compatible with his or her quality of life and supportiveness of self-esteem and confidence, for example.

For each topic, staff members must select the activities that are most conducive to the intended change. It is important that topics be presented in sequence, interspersed with pauses to give opportunities for repetition, feedback, and questions. Videotapes, slides, and printed material, for example, are useful complements. If produced locally, the written material should reflect the guiding principles earlier mentioned. When elderly patients participate, it is especially important that the letters in printed material be large. For participants to be comfortable, it is a good rule to start with simple concepts presented slowly. Consistency as to content and method should be considered when planning as well as when accomplishing educational sessions. When patient education is a team effort, the members of the team should reach a consensus in answering the questions: What content? For what purpose? With what method? Before staff members take on responsibility for patient education, a training course for patient educators is necessary.

Learning requires directed attention. Concentration difficutly is occasionally a problem even for healthy adult learners. When illness and treatment are added, the difficulties may be more manifest and reduce the patient's attentional capacity. Attentional fatigue must be considered in the education of patients (39). Readability-tested printed material (40) used in combination with pictures facilitates attention.

Patient education should start as soon as patients want. For some patients, the optimal time is directly after the diagnosis; for others, it is weeks or months later. The plan developed for education at these different stages of the cancer experience have very different structures based on the needs assessment.

Careful planning considers timing as a very important factor, but it could sometimes be difficult to squeeze in educational interventions at the time most appropriate from the patient's point of view. However, poor timing causes much unnecessary anxiety and confusion. When patient education is placed within the frame of cancer rehabilitation, there is a risk that education is considered first when discharge from the hospital is discussed.

What best serves the aim of an educational venture determines the choice of teaching format. Group teaching has been reported to be just as effective as individual teaching (41). Both strategies have their advantages and disadvantages. The main advantages to group education are similar to the disadvantages in individual teaching: opportunities of sharing with and gaining support from other patients with similar experiences, amount of time available, and cost of staff time. Increased consistency and congruence between assessed needs and planned interventions, together with flexibility and opportunities to facilitate patients to play an active role, despite depression, anxiety, or impairment are some of the advantages of individual teaching.

E. Evaluation

Evaluation aims to investigate whether the participants have attained the mutually agreed on goal. When patient education is evaluated, it is with almost no exception a question of measuring to what extent behavioral objectives used to define expected outcome have been achieved. Evaluation is straightforward; what is expected can be measured. Several methods are used to evaluate goal achievement. Self-care activities, such as the performance of breast self-examination, can be evaluated by direct observation. Tests are used before and after a teaching session to measure progress in learning. Sometimes patients and family members are asked to answer questions in structured interviews and questionnaires. All these forms of evaluations focus explicitly on learning outcomes, which are defined in detail (38).

When facilitating coping efforts, the desired outcome to be evaluated is the process, not the product. The process of coping, with its intertwined and interdependent strands of changes in thoughts, feelings, and actions, can hardly be fragmented into measurable variables, however. Unstructured interviews in terms of narrative is one approach in which information about increased ability to cope with the cancer experience can be systematically collected.

F. Patient Education—an Evidence-Based Practice

A great number of research-based studies in which the effect of patient education has been investigated give evidence of beneficial alterations. In a meta-analysis of 116 studies, significant outcomes such as increased physical and psychological well-being, increased cancer-related knowledge was found (42). Other studies have given evidence of increased compliance (43), reduced unscheduled readmission (44), and increased pain control (45). Some studies have focused the patient's coping ability related to educational interventions. Evaluation of the U.S. program *I can cope* showed an increased ability to adapt to living with cancer (46). The Swedish program entitled *Learning to live with cancer* has, in evaluations, given evidence that familiarity with facts and feelings throughout the course of cancer influenced the coping capacity by increasing self-esteem and confidence in living with cancer. To make the program an opportunity for the patient's significant others was much appreciated. The program is unique in the education of patients, in that patients and their significant others have been actively involved in developing and evaluating not only the program but also the learning material (32). Recently, the program has also been implemented for clinical practice in many European countries. *Learning to live with cancer* provides a framework for individual needs to be met and individual resources to be cultivated. The educational intervention to support coping efforts is characterized by

Paying due respect to the patient's expectations and experiences
Being based on assessed learning needs
Being anchored in pedagogical principles regarding the learning process

Patient education perceived as one of the patient's rights has been shown to be a powerful intervention, but in many health care settings, it is still a new concept and a new way of thinking, slowly recognized. Patient education is, however, an appealing concept, and interest in using education as an intervention to support patients and their significant others to cope with the cancer experience is growing.

VII. COUNSELING: PART OF INFORMATION AND EDUCATION

In this chapter, counseling refers only to information and education of patients with cancer. The following definition is used by the British Association for Counselling: "The task of counselling is to give the client an opportunity to explore, discover and clarify ways of living more satisfyingly and resourcefully" (47). This definition indeed shows that counseling is part of the information and education process. It goes a step further than informing and educating: it supports people in finding individual ways of living and coping with their disease or in mobilizing for recovery. Counseling in this sense can be seen as coaching. The coaching function in nursing has been described as follows: nurses who have come to grips with the culturally avoided or uncharted and can open ways of being and coping for the patient and the family (48).

Nurses and physicians usually are not counselors but health care professionals who can have counseling skills. To "do" counseling has also been described as "giving personalised care" (49). It usually does not have to do with sessions on a formal basis but rather with situations within everyday care. The effectiveness of counseling might be related to the relationship between patient and caregiver. Those caring for patients understand as a result of their own experience, awareness, and vulnerability (50).

Counseling in cancer patients can therefore be seen as an individual two-way exchange, loosely structured, with the aim to learn and to cope. Topics are agreed on but not limited, and there is an emphasis on feelings with reference to facts and action (10).

Counseling can allow people to interpret the illness and work from their own perspective. This includes the meaning of the disease, the cause, or the treatment. It gives those concerned an opportunity to inform nurses and doctors about their beliefs. This does not exclude the possibility of offering a different interpretation or eliciting harmful fantasies. Realistic facts may help the patient to reduce guilt feelings or anxiety or prevent them from harmful alternative therapeutic strategies.

Counseling also comprises the interpretation of the patient's condition. Experience shows that talking about deterioration of the disease is very difficult if the destruction of realistic hope is to be prevented. Realistic hope here refers to living without physical, spiritual, and psychological distress and to the support offered to achieve this aim. Here, discussing goals and negotiation, as well as finding new perspectives, becomes crucial. What can the perspectives be, when death is impending or when physical or psychological limitations cannot be overcome? A deep connection between patient and physician, based on thorough information, described as "connexional dimension," has the attribute of a relationship and may be much more supportive and helpful than mere information giving (51).

Interpretation of the side effects of therapy or complications not related to tumor progression is another part of counseling. In curative situations, it also can mean convincing patients overwhelmed by the cancer diagnosis that there is hope of successful treatment and cure. Many patients still believe that there is no chance to survive such a disease. Many also need to be reassured that cancer is a noncontagious illness. Questions on family planning or sexual problems are important points of counseling when helping to cope with disease and treatment.

Apart from information giving and education through physicians and nurses, specific counseling may be the professional counselor's task. The role of the psychologist, psychiatrist, clergy, or art therapist in cancer care is not described in this chapter.

VIII. CONCLUSIONS AND PERSPECTIVES

Although in some parts of the world it is the right of patients to be informed about cancer, in others it is still tradition to withhold the truth. Whether the ''silent conspiracy'' is part of culture and whether this needs to be changed need further, thorough research. This becomes especially true when facing the inevitable intermigration of populations in Europe. Apart from the ''whether or not'' question, there are many details to be explored when telling the truth. Changing medical technology and methods creates new situations, and research will also have to focus on very old topics concerning communication, relationship, and given circumstances that are essential to caring information giving, education, and counseling.

Professional information giving and education through nursing and medical personnel are part of effective counseling. To communicate effectively, nurses and physicians need to develop their communication skills. Unfortunately, medical and nursing education, at least in Europe, usually does not include sufficient time in teaching and communication principles, which explains the often experienced lack of such skills. Health care professionals obviously need different teaching strategies, which again need to be underpinned by future research.

REFERENCES

1. Senn HJ, Glaus A. Supportive Care in Cancer, Vol. II. Recent Results in Cancer, Vol. 121. Heidelberg: Springer, 1991.
2. Gaut D. Development of theoretically adequate description of caring. West J Nurs Res 1983; 5(4):313–324.
3. Padilla G, Grant M. Quality of life as a cancer nursing outcome variable. Adv Nurs Sci 1985; 8:45–60.

4. O'Berle K, Davies B. Support and caring: exploring the concepts. Oncol Nurs Forum 1992; 19(5):763–767.
5. Leininger M. The phenomenon of caring. In: Leininger M, ed. Caring: An Essential Human Need. Proceeding of the Three National Caring Conferences. Thorofare, NJ: Slack, 1981:3–15.
6. Paternoster J. How patients know that nurses care about them. J N Y S Nurs Assoc 1988; 19(4):17–21.
7. Benner P, Wrubel J. The primacy of caring. Stress and coping in health and illness. Menlo Park, CA: Addison-Wesley, 1988.
8. Orem D. Nursing concepts of practice. New York: McGraw-Hill, 1985.
9. Wilson-Barnett J, Osborne J. Studies evaluating patient teaching: implications for practice. Int J Nurs Stud 1983; 20(1):33–44.
10. Wheeler D. Counselling colleagues—the role of the staff counseller. Counselling 1984; 47:17–19.
11. Parker M. A nursing inservice curriculum for patient education. Nursing and Health Care 1983; 4(3):142–146.
12. Wepp P. Teaching patients and relatives. In: Tiffany R. Oncology for Nurses and Health Care Professionals. London: Harper and Row, 1988.
13. Paterson R, Aitken J. Public opinion on cancer. Lancet 1954; 857.
14. Pitot H. Fundamentals of Oncology. New York: Marcel Dekker, 1986.
15. Novack D, Plumer R. Changes in physicians' attitudes toward telling the cancer patient. JAMA 1979; 241:897–900.
16. Estapo J, Palombo E. Cancer diagnosis disclosure in a Spanish hospital. Ann Oncol 1992; 3:451–454.
17. Lind S, DelVecchio M. Telling the diagnosis of cancer. J Clin Oncol 1989; 7(5): 583–589.
18. McIntosh J. Processes of communication, information seeking and control associated with cancer. Soc Sci Med 1974; 8:167–187.
19. Tilley J. The nurse's role in patient education: incongruent perceptions among nurses and patients. J Adv Nurs 1987; 12:291–301.
20. Travelbee J. Interpersonal aspects of nursing. Philadelphia: FA Davis, 1966.
21. Holland J. Now we tell—but how well? Editorial. J Clin Oncol 1989; 7(5):557–559.
22. Meerwein F. Das Erstgespräch auf der Abteilung für Medizinische Onkologie. Bern: SAKK Publication, 1985.
23. Grahn G, Johnson J. Learning to cope and living with cancer. Learning needs assessment in cancer patient education. Scand J Caring Sci 1990; 4:173–181.
24. Houts, et al. Information needs of families of cancer patients: a literature review and recommendations. J Cancer Educ 1991; 6(4):255–261.
25. Derdiarian A. Informational needs of recently diagnosed cancer patients. Cancer Nurs 1987; 10(2):107–115.
26. Hinds C. Suffering: a relatively unexplored phenomenon among family caregivers of non-institutionalized patients with cancer. J Adv Nurs 1992; 17:918–925.
27. Grahn G. Coping with the cancer experience. Part I. Developing and implementing an education and support program. Eur J Cancer Care 1996; 5:182–187.
28. Grahn G. Educational situations in clinical settings. A process analysis. Acta Univ

Upsaliensis. Ph.D. dissertation. Uppsala Studies in Education. Vol. 27. Stockholm: A & W International, 1987.
29. Piaget J. Psychologie et pédagogie. Paris: Editions Denoël, 1969.
30. Dewey J. Experience and education. New York: Collier Books, 1980.
31. Montessori M. From childhood to adolescence. New York: Schocken Books 1973.
32. Grahn G, Danielsson M. Coping with the cancer experience. Part II. Evaluating an education and support program. Eur J Cancer Care 1996; 5:176–181.
33. Lazarus R, Folkman S. Stress, appraisal and coping. New York: Springer, 1984.
34. McHaffie HE. Coping: an essential element of nursing. J Adv Nurs 1992; 17:933–940.
35. White N, Richter J, Fry C. Coping, social support and adaptation to chronic illness. West J Nurs Res 1992; 14:211–224.
36. Fallowfield L. Problems in communication to cancer patients. In: Glaxo Symposium: Progress in Supportive Care, Wien, 1992.
37. Wilson E, Desruisseux B. Stoma care in patient teaching. In: Wilson-Barnett J, ed. Patient teaching. London: Livingstone, 1983:95–118.
38. Rankin S, Stallings K. Patient education. New York: JB Lippincott, 1990.
39. Cimprich B. A theoretical perspective on attention and patient education. Adv Nurs Sci 1992; 14 (3):39–51.
40. Folz A, Sullivan J. Reading level, learning presentation preference, and desire for information among cancer patients. J Cancer Nurs Educ 1996; 11:32–38.
41. Lindeman C. Patient education. Ann Rev Nurs Res 1988; 6:29–60.
42. Devine E, Westlake. The effects of psycho-educational care provided to adults with cancer: meta-analysis of 116 studies. Oncol Nurs Forum 1995; 22 (9):1369–1381.
43. Rimer B, Levy M, Keintz M, et al. Enhancing cancer pain control regimens through patient education. Patient Educ Councelling 1987; 10:267–277.
44. Grant M, Ferrell B, Rivera, et al. Unscheduled readmission for uncontrolled symptoms. Nurs Clin North Am 1995; 30(4):67–82.
45. Rimer B, Kedziera P, Levy M. The role of patient education in cancer pain control. Hosp J 1992; 8:1–2, 171–191.
46. Johnson J. The effects of a patient-centered educational program on persons' adaptability to live with a chronic disease. Ph.D. dissertation, University of Minnesota, 1979.
47. Godden M, Charles D. What is counselling? BAC Newsletter 1984; 27:14.
48. Benner P. From novice to expert. Menlo Park, CA: Addison-Wesley, 1984.
49. Jourard SM. The transparent self. New York: Van Nostrand Reinhold, 1971.
50. Tschudin V. Counselling skills for nurses. London: Bailliére Tindall, 1987.
51. Surbone A. The information to the cancer patient: psychosocial and spiritual implications. Support Care Cancer 1993; 1:89–91.

Index

About the Editors

JEAN KLASTERSKY is Chief of the Department of Medicine and Professor of Medicine, Medical Oncology, and Physical Diagnosis at the Institut Jules Bordet, Université Libre de Bruxelles, Belgium. The editor or coeditor of more than 10 books and the author or coauthor of more than 340 professional papers, Dr. Klastersky is a member of the European Society of Medical Oncology, the European Society for Clinical Investigation, the American Society of Clinical Oncology, the American Association for Cancer Research, the American Society for Microbiology, and the Infectious Diseases Society of America, among others. He received the M.D. degree (1965) and the Ph.D. degree (1972) in medical sciences from the Université Libre de Bruxelles, Belgium.

STEPHEN C. SCHMIPFF is Chief Executive Officer of the University of Maryland Medical Center, a component of the University of Maryland Medical System where he is also Executive Vice President, and Professor of Medicine, Oncology, and Pharmacology at the University of Maryland School of Medicine, Baltimore. Formerly Director of the University of Maryland Cancer Center, Baltimore, Dr. Schimpff is the author or coauthor of more than 170 professional papers in the fields of oncology and infectious diseases, and the coeditor of several books. He serves on the editorial board of the *Journal of Supportive Care in Cancer* and is a reviewer for numerous other scientific journals. He is coeditor of the major oncology reference work *Comprehensive Textbook of Oncology*. Trained and certified in both medical oncology and infectious diseases, he is a Fellow of the American College of Physicians and the Infectious Diseases Society of America, as well as a member of the American Association for Cancer Research and the American Society of Clinical Oncology, among others. Dr. Schimpf received the B.A. degree (1963) in biological science from Rutgers University, New Brunswick, New Jersey, and the M.D. degree (1967) from Yale University Medical School, New Haven, Connecticut.

HANS-JÖRG SENN is Medical and Scientific Director, Center for Tumor Detection and Prevention, St. Gallen, Switzerland, as well as Associate Professor of Internal Medicine and Oncology at Basel University Medical School, Switzerland. Dr. Senn is a former chairman of the Scientific Audit Committee of the European Organization for Research and Treatment of Cancer in Brussels, Belgium, and past president of the International Breast Cancer Study Group. He also serves as Editor-in-Chief of the *European Journal of Cancer*, the *Journal of Supportive Care in Cancer*, and of the series *Recent Results in Cancer Research*. A member of the American Society of Clinical Oncology as well as a board member of the European Society of Medical Oncology, he is author or editor of 14 oncology books and the author or coauthor of more than 270 professional publications. Dr. Senn received the M.D. degree (1961) from Zurich University, Switzerland.